TOPICS IN THORACIC SURGERY

Edited by **Paulo F. Guerreiro Cardoso**

Topics in Thoracic Surgery
Edited by Paulo F. Guerreiro Cardoso

Published by InTech

Janeza Trdine 9, 51000 Rijeka, Croatia

Publishing Process Manager Vedran Greblo

Technical Editor Teodora Smiljanic

Cover Designer InTech Design Team

Additional hard copies can be obtained from orders@intechopen.com

Topics in Thoracic Surgery, Edited by Paulo F. Guerreiro Cardoso
p. cm.
ISBN 978-953-51-0010-2

For EU product safety concerns:
IN TECH d.o.o., Prolaz Marije Krucifikse Kozulić 3, 51000 Rijeka, Croatia,
info@intechopen.com or visit our website at intechopen.com.

Meet the editor

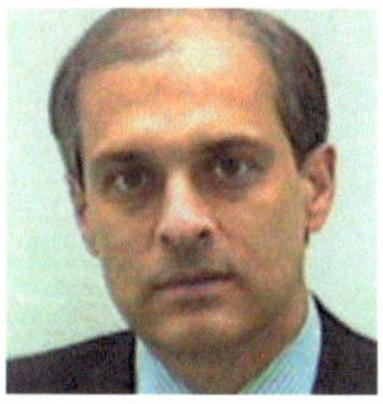

Graduated in Medicine at the Medical School of Rio de Janeiro of the Gama Filho University, Brazil (1979). Trained in General Surgery and Thoracic Surgery and had a MaSc in Thoracic Surgery at the Federal University of Rio de Janeiro, Brazil (1980-87). Research and Clinical fellowship in Thoracic Surgery at the University of Toronto, Canada (1987-1992) and a Ph.D. in Pneumology at the Federal University of Rio Grande do Sul, Brazil (2000). Dr. Cardoso is currently an Associate Professor of Thoracic Surgery at the Department of Cardiopneumology, Division of Thoracic Surgery of the Faculty of Medicine of the University of Sao Paulo, Brazil. He is also an attending thoracic surgeon at the Division of Thoracic Surgery of the Heart Institute (InCor) of the Hospital das Clinicas, Faculty of Medicine of the University of Sao Paulo, Brazil.

Contents

Preface

Open Access publishing has finally become available to Thoracic Surgery. This is a rather simple publishing concept that removes the charges and the need for compulsory subscription. This therefore enables readers worldwide to broaden their access to scientific publications online and, best of all, for free. The numbers are staggering. As I was writing this Preface, I went to the publisher's web site and found the following: 3,8 million downloads for all books published, championed by Electrical Engineering (29,2%) whereas Medicine is making its way up (13,9%). This is the reason why I believe that Open Access Publishing has become a powerful educational and research tool on a global level. Thoracic Surgery can now extend this benefit to both their specialists and trainees. Furthermore, it offers a new gateway for authors around the world to convey their information in a less formal frame, in a faster way and with a more international flavor. The end result is an excellent opportunity for authors to share their experiences and for readers to have access to more information.

The current Thoracic Surgery book has format that differs radically from the usual surgical textbooks. Instead of organizing the book into a pre-formatted table of contents with chapters, sections and then ask authors to submit their respective chapters based on this frame, the authors were encouraged by the publisher to submit their chapters based on their area of expertise. The editor is then commissioned to examine the reading material and put it together as a book. In Thoracic Surgery, the material was rich and encompassed so many interesting chapters that I elected to put it into a single volume with some sense but with no divisions, thus enabling a wider range of topics to be featured. It starts with a comprehensive and objective "Pre-operative Assessment of patients for Thoracic Surgery" by Drs. Rasheed and Raghuraman and moves on to challenging topics such as "Pulmonary Resection for Lung Cancer in Patients with Liver Cirrhosis" by Dr. Iwata from Japan. It then moves into the more specific articles such as "Post-thoracotomy pain management", chest wall malformations and a provocative new technique for pectus repair along with a historical overview provided by Dr. Masaoka and as well as a historical overview on chest wall malformations by Dr. Torre. On the lung cancer topics, the reader will enjoy the review and technical aspects of VATS major pulmonary resections along with more traditional topics such as Pancoast tumors and recurrence patterns of stage I lung disease. The book also includes articles on hyperhidrosis, surgery for bronchiectasis, lung transplantation, surgical and endoscopic management of emphysema among many others.

For the reader who seeks information on research applicable to clinical situations, we chose a few interesting topics such as Dr. Laubach's research on compensatory lung growth and Drs. Miserocchi's and Beretta's studies on extravascular water in lung and pleural cavity following lung surgery.

This inaugurates a novel method of sharing thoracic surgical information and, above all, accessible to everyone with very good publishing quality. I do hope this will succeed as an alternative surgical information output and encourage authors to embark on Open Access.

Paulo F. Guerreiro Cardoso MD, Ph.D.
Associate Professor of Thoracic Surgery
Faculty of Medicine of the University of Sao Paulo
Brazil

1

Preoperative Evaluation of Patients for Thoracic Surgery

Shanawaz Abdul Rasheed and Raghuraman Govindan
Birmingham Heartlands Hospital NHS Trust,
United Kingdom

1. Introduction

Lung cancer is the most common cancer in the world with 1.61 million new cases diagnosed every year (1). The vast majority of lung cancers are caused by cigarette smoking. It has been estimated that the lifetime risk of developing lung cancer in 2008 is 1 in 14 for men and 1 in 19 for women in the UK.

Approximately 2400 Lobectomies and 500 Pneumonectomies are undertaken in the UK annually, the majority for malignancy. For this group of patients, in-hospital mortality rates are 2-4% and 6-8% respectively in the UK, although world mortality rates as high as 11% have been cited for Pneumonectomy(2)

To guide decisions, one must not only consider the extremely poor prognosis for inoperable patients but also be familiar with the operative risks, and understand how surgery impacts on pulmonary function both in short term and long term.

The aim of the preoperative pulmonary assessment is to identify patients who are at increased risk of having peri-operative complications and long term disability from surgical resection using the least tests available. The purpose of this preoperative physiologic assessment is to enable adequate counselling of the patient on treatment options and risks so that they can make a truly informed decision (3)

Preoperative evaluation of a patient with lung cancer involves answering three questions: 1) is the neoplasm resectable? (Anatomic resectability), 2) Does the patient have adequate pulmonary reserve to tolerate pulmonary resection? (Operability or physiologic resectability); 3) is there any major medical contraindication to the proposed surgery?

2. Anatomical resectability

After a tissue diagnosis of lung cancer has been made, the neoplasm should first be assessed for anatomic resectability. A neoplasm is considered resectable if the entire tumour can be removed by surgery. Knowing the extent of tumour both within and outside the thorax is the key in determining resectability. Surgical resection is considered the treatment of choice in physiologically operable patients with up to stage IIIA tumour. (4)

2.1 Operability (physiologic resectability)

2.1.1 Physiologic alterations after thoracotomy and lung resection

If, after adequate staging, the tumour is found to be anatomically resectable, the next step is determination of operability or physiological resectability. To understand operability the physiologic changes due to surgery and the pulmonary reserve require discussion. When thoracic surgery is performed, several physiological effects occur which can be discussed under changes in Lung volume, compliance and pulmonary blood flow.

2.1.1.1 Changes in lung volume

Even if no lung is resected, vital capacity declines by approximately 25% in the early postoperative period and slowly returns to baseline in a few weeks. In patients with underlying lung disease, the reduction in vital capacity by lung surgery may result in acute and chronic respiratory failure, or even death. However, it should be noted that while in most circumstances lung resection leads to reduction in lung function; this is not always the case. Patients who undergo resection of large bullae may actually have improvement in lung function postoperatively because of better lung mechanics. On occasion, lung resection only involves removal of non-functioning lung parenchyma and there is little or no change in resultant lung function after recovery. Moreover, in some highly selected cases, in particular upper lobe tumours in patients with centrilobular emphysema, there may be a lung volume reduction surgery (LVRS)-like effect. In these selected circumstances, the resultant lung function after recovery from resection is actually better than the preoperative measurements. This effect is difficult to anticipate given the obvious important differences between lobectomy and LVRS protocols, but it has been noticed in anecdotal cases (8).

2.1.1.2 Changes in lung compliance

Chest wall compliance also decreases to less than 50% and work of breathing increases to more than 140% of the preoperative level. The cough pressure is reduced to 30% of the preoperative value and increases to 50% by 1 week (5–7).

2.1.1.3 Changes in pulmonary blood flow

Removal of lung parenchyma results in reduction of the pulmonary capillary bed. The decrease in pulmonary capillary bed is well tolerated by patients with otherwise normal lungs but in patients with pulmonary dysfunction this may result in postoperative pulmonary hypertension.

Unlike most general surgical procedures where cardiovascular complications are the major cause of perioperative morbidity and mortality, in thoracic surgical population respiratory complications are the predominant cause of perioperative morbidity and mortality (9,10).

The principles described will apply to all other types of non-malignant pulmonary resections and to other chest surgery. The major difference is that in patients with malignancy the risk/benefit ratio of cancelling or delaying surgery pending other investigation/therapy is always complicated by the risk of further spread of cancer during any extended interval prior to resection. This is never completely "elective" surgery (10).

3. Assessment of patients for lung resection

Each patient's management requires planning by a multi-disciplinary team (MDT), which includes a respiratory physician, a thoracic surgeon, an oncologist and other staff such as physiotherapists and respiratory nurses. If the MDT feels that surgery is appropriate, then the surgeon will decide if the tumour is technically resectable based on chest X-ray and CT scan images (Figure 1).

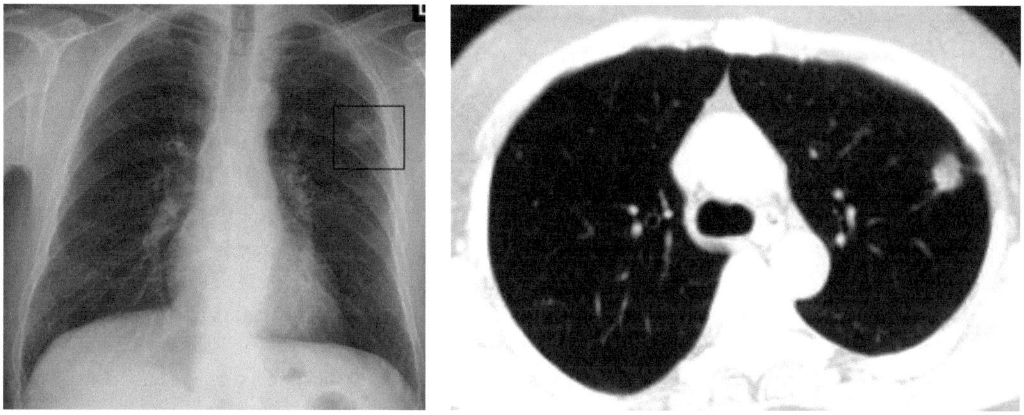

Fig. 1. Chest X ray and CT scan showing Lung Cancer in Left Lung.

4. General assessment

Prevention of postoperative complications requires a detailed medical history and examination. History should address the presence of dyspnoea, exercise tolerance, cough, and expectoration, wheezing, and smoking status. Examination should also focus on respiratory rate, pattern of breathing, wheezing, and body habitus.

4.1 Assessment of risks of the surgery

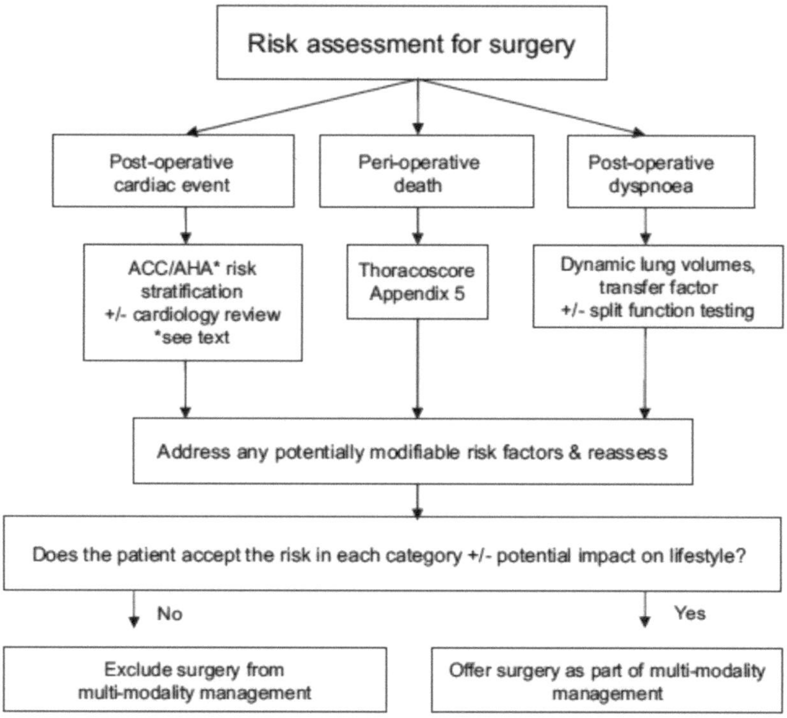

Fig. 2. Tripartite Risk Assessment.

Recent British Thoracic Society guidelines 2010 (BTS) presents a Tripartite risk assessment model that considers risk of operative mortality, risks of perioperative myocardial events and risk of postoperative dyspnoea.
This model facilitate the calculation and assessment of individual outcomes that may be discussed by the MDT and enables the patient to make truly informed decision.

4.2 Assessment of risks of the surgery

Estimating the risk of in-hospital death is one of the most important considerations for surgeons and patients when they evaluate the option of surgery for lung cancer.The 30 day mortality for lobectomy and pneumonectomy in England from National Lung Cancer Audit is 2.3% and 5.8% respectively.
Thoracoscore is currently the largest and most validated global risk score . It is a logistic regression derived model which is based on nine variables like Age, sex, ASA score, performance status, dyspnoea score, priority of suregry, extent of surgery, malignant diagnosis and a composite comorbidity score(11).

Thoracoscore

Variable	Value	Code	β-coefficient
Age	<55 years	0	
	55–65 years	1	0.7679
	>65 years	2	1.0073
Sex	Female	0	
	Male	1	0.4505
ASA score	≤2	0	
	≥ 3	1	0.6057
Performance status	≤2	0	
	≥3	1	0.689
Dyspnoea score	≤2	0	
	≥3	1	0.9075
Priority of surgery	Elective	0	
	Urgent or emergency	1	0.8443
Procedure class	Other	0	
	Pneumonectomy	1	1.2176
Diagnosis group	Benign	0	
	Malignant	1	1.2423
Comorbidity score	0	0	
	≤2	1	0.7447
	≥3	2	0.9065
Constant			−7.3737

Table 1.

Methods for using the logistic regression model to predict the risk of in-hospital death:

1. Odds are calculated with the patient values and the coefficients are determined from the regression equation:

$$\text{Odds} = \exp\,[e7.3737 + (0.7679 \text{ if code of age is 1 or } 1.0073 \text{ if code of age is 2})$$
$$+ (0.4505\ 3 \text{ sex score}) + (0.6057\ 3 \text{ ASA score}) + (0.6890\ 3 \text{ performance status Classification})$$
$$+ (0.9075\ 3 \text{ dyspnoea score}) + (0.8443\ 3 \text{ code for priority ofsurgery})$$
$$+ (1.2176\ 3 \text{ procedure class}) + (1.2423\ 3 \text{ diagnosis group})$$
$$+ (0.7447 \text{ ifcode of comorbidity is 1 or } 0.9065 \text{ if code of comorbidity is 2})].$$

2. The odds for the predicted probability of in-hospital death are calculated: probablity + odds/(1 + odds).

ASA, American Society of Anesthesiologists.

4.3 Age

All patients should have equal access to lung cancer services regardless of age(12). British Thoracic Society (BTS) guideline recommendations with regards to age are:

1. Perioperative morbidity increases with advancing age. The rate of respiratory complications (40%) is double that expected in a younger population and the rate of cardiac complications (40%), particularly arrhythmias, triples that which should be seen in younger patients(10)
2. Elderly patients undergoing lung resection are more likely to require intensive perioperative support. Preoperatively, a careful assessment of co-morbidity needs to be made. (13)
3. Surgery for clinically stage I and II disease can be as effective in patients over 70 years as in younger patients. Such patients should be considered for surgical treatment regardless of age. (13,14)
4. Age over 80 alone is not a contraindication to lobectomy or wedge resection for clinically stage I disease.
5. Pneumonectomy is associated with a higher mortality risk in the elderly. Age should be a factor in deciding suitability for pneumonectomy

4.4 Weight loss, performance status and nutrition

Weight loss>10%, a low BMI or serum albumin may indicate more advanced disease or an increased risk of postoperative complications.(16) The National VA Surgical Risk Study reported that a low serum albumin level was also the most important predictor of 30-day perioperative morbidity and mortality. Mortality increased steadily from less than 1.0% to 29% as albumin declined from values greater than 4.6 g/dl to values less than 2.1 g/dl.(17)

4.5 Cardiovascular assessment

Cardiac complications are the second most common cause of perioperative morbidity and mortality in the thoracic surgical population. As with any planned major operation, especially in a population that is predisposed to atherosclerotic cardiovascular disease due to cigarette smoking, a preoperative cardiovascular risk assessment should be performed.

The European Respiratory Society/European Society of Thoracic Surgery (ERS/ESTS) provides an algorithm based on a well validated score system, the revised cardiac risk index (RCRI), to estimate the patient's risk (18). The calculation of this index is simple, since it is based on the medical history, physical examination baseline ECG and plasma creatinine measurement.

Calculating the revised cardiac risk index (RCRI) based on history, physical examination, baseline ECG and serum Creatinine:

Each item is assigned 1 point.
• High Risk Surgery (including Pneumonectomy or Lobectomy) • History of Ischemic Heart disease (Prior MI or Angina pectoris) • History of Heart failure • Insulin dependent Diabetes • Previous Stroke or Transient ischemic attacks • Pre-operative Serum Creatinine 2 mg/dl.
If
• RCRI is ≥ 2 • The patient has any cardiac conditions requiring medications • The patient has a newly suspected cardiac condition • The patient is unable to climb 2 flight of stairs
A cardiological consultation is needed.

Table 2.

Algorithm for cardiac assessment before lung resection for lung cancer patients:

RCRI: Revised cardiac Risk Index; ECG: electrocardiogram;
AHA: American Heart Association; ACC: American College of Cardiology;
CABG: coronary artery bypass graft; PCI: primary coronary intervention;
TIA: transient ischaemic attack

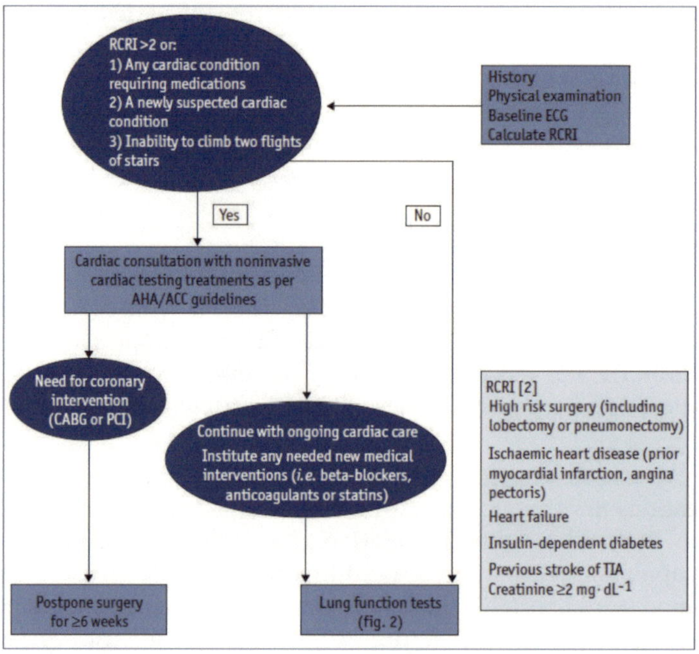

Fig. 3.

Adapted from ERS/ESTS clinical guidelines on fitness for radical therapy in lung cancer patients (14)

4.6 Arrhythmias

Dysrhythmias, particularly atrial fibrillation, are a frequent complication of pulmonary resection surgery (8,15). Factors known to correlate with an increased incidence of arrhythmia are the amount of lung tissue resected, age, intraoperative blood loss, and intra-pericardial dissection (16). Prophylactic therapy with Digoxin has not been shown to prevent these arrhythmias. Diltiazem has been shown to be effective (22).

4.7 Smoking

Smoking cessation should be advised to all patients. Abstinence from smoking will decrease carboxyhemoglobin acutely but improvement in mucociliary function and small airway obstruction may take up to 10 weeks (21). Stein and Cassara established that 3 weeks of smoking cessation combined with perioperative incentive spirometry in a group of patients undergoing nonthoracic general surgery improved outcomes (23,24). Three weeks of smoking cessation should be considered standard for all non-emergent major surgical procedures.

4.8 COPD

COPD patients have 6 fold increased risk of post-operative pulmonary complications like atelectasis, pneumonia, exacerbation of COPD and Respiratory failure. Inhaled anesthetic depresses the respiratory drive in response to both hypoxia and hypercapnia even at sub-anaesthetic doses. Many COPD patients have an elevated Paco2 at rest. To identify these patients preoperatively, all moderate-to-severe COPD patients need arterial blood gas analysis. COPD patients desaturate more frequently and severely than normal patients during sleep (9).

As many as 50% of COPD patients will have RV dysfunction mostly due to chronic hypoxemia. The dysfunctional RV is poorly tolerant of sudden increases in afterload such as the change from spontaneous to controlled ventilation (9,15). Pneumonectomy candidates with a ppoFEV1 ≤40% should have transthoracic echocardiography to assess right heart function (23).

Overall medical condition of patients with COPD who are scheduled for surgery should be optimized. Patients with evidence of suboptimal reduction in symptoms, physical examination demonstrating airflow obstruction, or submaximal exercise tolerance warrant aggressive therapy.

Use of bronchodilators and glucocorticoid agents, and cessation of smoking, aggressive chest physiotherapy are paramount. Antibiotic therapy should be administered if there is evidence of pulmonary infection.

4.9 Renal dysfunction

Renal dysfunction after pulmonary resection surgery is associated with a very high incidence of mortality (19%) (25). History of previous renal dysfunction, concurrent diuretic therapy, Pneumonectomy surgery, postoperative infection, and blood transfusion are all associated with high risk for perioperative renal dysfunction. Fair evidence supports serum blood urea nitrogen levels of 7.5 mmol/L as a risk factor. However, the magnitude of the risk seems to be lower than that for low levels of serum albumin.

5. Specific assessment

5.1 Pulmonary function tests & lung resection

The best assessment of respiratory function comes from a history of the patient's quality of life (9). A unique consideration in patients considered for thoracotomy is the effect of pulmonary parenchymal resection on postoperative pulmonary function and exercise capacity. There is no single test that can reliably predict the patients' likelihood of tolerating thoracotomy and lung resection without excessive postoperative morbidity and mortality.

5.2 Current guidelines

Guidelines from the American College of Chest Physicians and the British Thoracic Society suggest that patients with a preoperative Forced Expiratory volume in 1 second (FEV1) in excess of 2 L (or >80 percent predicted) generally tolerate pneumonectomy, whereas those with a preoperative FEV1 greater than 1.5 L tolerate lobectomy (4,15) However, if there is either undue exertional dyspnea or coexistent interstitial lung disease, then measurement of Diffusing capacity(DLCO) should also be performed (2). Patients with preoperative results for FEV1 and DLCO that are both >80 percent predicted do not need further physiological testing. Although pulmonary function that is better than the aforementioned threshold levels predicts a good surgical outcome, it has been difficult to identify a single absolute value of preoperative FEV1 below which the risk of surgical intervention should be considered prohibitive for all patients. Responsible factors for this lack of a single value include the following:

- Differences in the amount of lung tissue to be resected, as the extent of the planned resection will affect the choice of an acceptable preoperative FEV1.
- Differences in the severity of underlying lung disease and the contribution to total lung function of the portion of lung to be resected.
- Differences in size, age, gender, and race of patients undergoing lung resection.

Below these values further interpretation of the spirometry readings is needed and a value for the predicted postoperative (ppo-) FEV1 should be calculated. As the FEV1 decreases, the risk of respiratory and cardiac complications increases, mortality increases and patients are more likely to require postoperative ventilation.

5.3 Calculating the predicted postoperative FEV1(ppo FEV1) & TLCO (ppo TLCO)

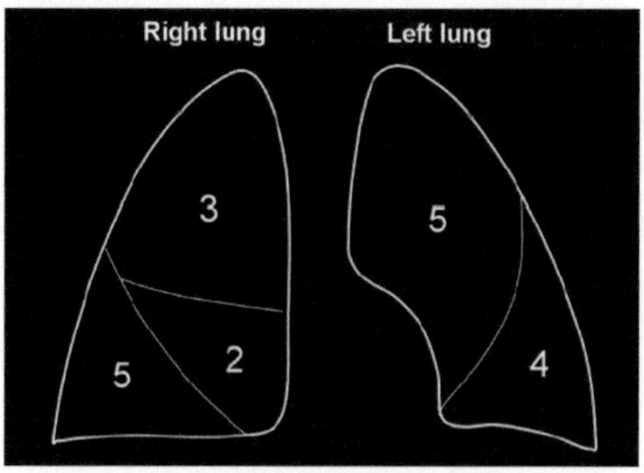

Courtesy from Portch & McCormick.

Fig. 4.

Radiological imaging (usually a CT scan) identifies the area of the lung that requires resection. There are five lung lobes containing nineteen segments in total with the division of each lobe (shown in figure 2).
Knowledge of the number of segments of lung that will be lost by resection allows the surgeon and anaesthetist to estimate the post resection spirometry and TLCO values. These can then be used to estimate the risk to the patient of undergoing the procedure (22). Predicted postoperative function is calculated using preoperative values of FEV1 or DLCO and measurement of lobar or whole lung fractional contribution to function as determined by quantitative perfusion lung scanning, ventilation, or CT lung scanning.

$$\mathbf{ppo\ FEV1 = Preoperative\ FEV1 \times \frac{no.\ of\ segments\ left\ after\ resection}{18}}$$

The value obtained is then compared to the predicted value for FEV1 for that individual's height, age, and gender to obtain the percent predicted postoperative FEV1.

$$\mathbf{ppoDLCO = preoperative\ DLCO \times \left(1 - \%functional\ lung\ tissue\ removed / 100\right)}$$

Predicted post-operative DLCO is the single strongest predictor of complications and mortality after lung resection, although it is important to note that DLCO is NOT predictive of long term survival,only perioperative mortality (28). Interestingly, ppoDLCO and ppoFEV1 are poorly correlated, and thus should be assessed independently (29)
A patient is considered to be at increased risk for lung resection with predicted postoperative values for either FEV1 or DLCO <40 percent predicted. Nakahara et al. (10) found that patients with a ppoFEV1 $\geq 40\%$ had no or minor post-resection respiratory complications. Major respiratory complications were only seen in the subgroup with ppoFEV1 $\leq 40\%$ and patients with ppoFEV1 $\leq 30\%$ required postoperative mechanical ventilatory support. The use of epidural analgesia has decreased the incidence of complications in the high-risk group
The European Respiratory Society and the European Society of Thoracic Surgery (ERS/ESTS) advise that the cutoff value for predicted postoperative FEV1 or DLCO may be lowered to 30 percent rather than 40 percent, due to improvements in surgical technique and the belief that removal of hyperinflated, poorly functioning lung tissue during surgery ameliorates the calculated loss in lung function through a "lung volume reduction effect" (15,16). However, evaluation with cardiopulmonary exercise testing (CPET) is needed prior to making a final decision on operability.

5.4 Exercise tests

5.4.1 Formal cardiopulmonary exercise tests

Exercise tests are thought to mimic the postoperative increase in oxygen consumption and have been used to select patients at high risk of cardiopulmonary complications after thoracic, but also abdominal surgery. The aim of exercise tests is to stress the whole cardiopulmonary system and estimate the physiological reserve that may be available after lung resection. The most used and best validated exercise parameter is V'O2, max. In the literature, V'O2, max appears to be a very strong predictor of postoperative complications, as well as a good predictor of long-term post-operative exercise capacity.
Patients with a preoperative V'O2, max of 15 to 20 mL/kg/min can undergo curative-intent lung cancer surgery with an acceptably low mortality rate. In several case series, patients with a V'O2, max of ≤ 10 mL/kg/min had a very high risk for postoperative death (3,16).

Interpreting the VO_2 Max	
20 ml/kg/min or > 15ml/kg/min and FEV1 >40% predicted	- No increased risk of complications or death.
<15ml/kg/min	- High Risk
<10ml/kg/min	- 40-50% mortality consider non surgical treatment

Table 3.

5.5 Low technology exercise tests

Formal CPET with VO2'max measurements may not be readily available in all centres. Therefore, low-technology tests have been used to evaluate fitness before lung resection, including the 6-min walk test (6MWT), the shuttle test and the stair climbing test.

5.5.1 6MWT

The 6MWT is the most used low-technology test, but the distance walked does not correlate with the VO_2, max in all (especially in fit) patients. Moreover, post-operative complications have been found to be associated with the distance walked in some but not all studies. As a result, the 6MWT is not recommended to select patients for lung resection (3,19).

5.5.2 Shuttle walk test

The shuttle walk test is the distance measured by walking a 10 m distance usually between two cones at a pace that is progressively increased. This test has good reproducibility and correlates well with formal cardiopulmonary exercising testing (VO2max) (44,45) Previous BTS recommendations that the inability to walk 25 shuttles classifies patients as high risk has not been reproduced by prospective study(46) Some authors report that shuttle walk distance may be useful to stratify low-risk groups (ability to walk >400 m) who would not need further formal cardiopulmonary exercise testing.(47)

5.5.3 Stair climbing test

Because calculation of VO2 max is expensive, stair climbing has been proposed as an alternative. It is commonly cited that the ability to climb five flights of stairs without stopping (20 x 6″ steps) is equivalent to a VO2 max of 15 mL/kg/min, and two flights correspond to 12 mL/kg/min.] However, the data are difficult to interpret as there is a lack of standardisation of the height of the stairs, the ceiling heights, different parameters used in the assessment (eg, oxygen saturations, extent of lung resection) and different outcomes.

5.6 Blood gas tension and oxygen saturation at rest

Recent studies have shown that hypercapnia in itself is not predictive of complications after resection, particularly if patients are able to exercise adequate(28) However, such patients are often precluded because of other adverse factors—for example, postoperative FEV1 and TLCO <40% predicted.
Ninan *et al* found that there was a higher risk of postoperative complications among patients who either had oxygen saturation (SaO2) on air at rest of <90% or desaturated by >4% from baseline during exercise (34).

6. Effects of lung cancer

Lung cancer patients should be assessed for "4Ms".

- Mass effects (SVC, Pancoast, obstructive pneumonia, laryngeal nerve paralysis, phrenic paresis)
- Metabolic effects (hypercalcemia, hyponatremia, Cushing's, Lambert-Eaton)
- Metastases to brain, bone, liver& adrenal
- Medications (bleomycin [avoid high FiO2], cisplatin [avoid NSAIDs])

7. Effects of incisions

FEV1 and FVC are decreased by up to 65% on the first postoperative day after thoracotomy. Resolution of these changes takes up to 2 months. The effects can be mitigated somewhat through use of appropriate incisions.

8. Combination of tests

No single test of respiratory function has shown adequate validity as a sole preoperative assessment. Before surgery an estimate of respiratory function in all three areas: lung mechanics, parenchymal function, and cardiopulmonary interaction should be made for each patient (9).
Slinger et al has described "The 3-Legged Stool" of Pre-thoracotomy Respiratory assessment.

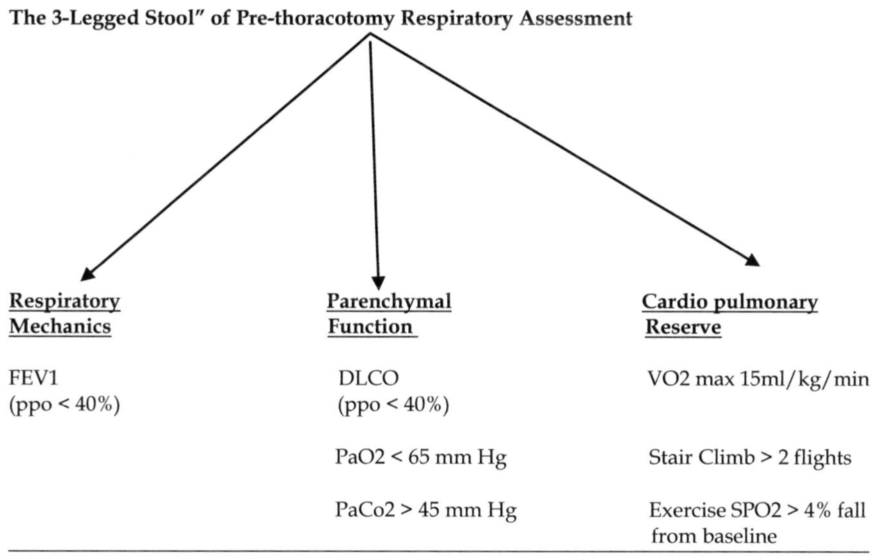

Courtesy of Slinger and Johnson

Fig. 5.

9. Methods of altering the perioperative risks

The following are the risk-reduction strategies which can be considered to reduce the risks in patients undergoing lung resection

- Cardiopulmonary rehabilitation
- Permit recovery from induction therapy
- Nutritional repletion
- Smoking cessation
- DVT and arrhythmia prophylaxis
- Perioperative pulmonary physiotherapy
- Changing extent of or approach to operation

Postoperatively, use of deep-breathing exercises or incentive spirometry, use of continuous positive airway pressure, use of epidural analgesia ,use of intercostals nerve blocks where applicable helps to reduce the postoperative pulmonary complications.

10. Post thoracotomy anaesthetic management based on predicted postop FEV1

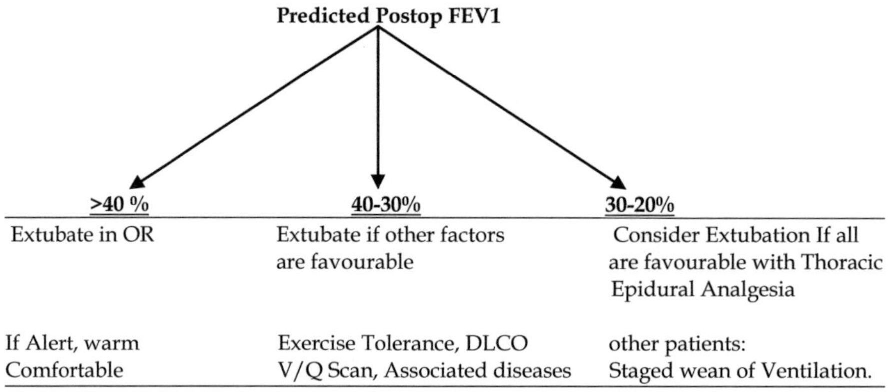

Courtesy of Slinger and Johnson

Fig. 6.

11. Imaging studies

Assessment of patient anatomy is important in order to anticipate a difficult endotracheal, or endobronchial intubation. Any deviation of the trachea from the midline should alert the anaesthetists to a potentially difficult intubation or to the possibility of airway obstruction during induction of anaesthesia. In addition to the physical exam, Chest X-rays, CT scans, and bronchoscopy reports can all be of use. Important factors include tumour that impinges on the chest wall, traverses the fissures between lobes or is in close proximity to major vessels. In some cases, and where available, a PET scan (positron emission tomography) may be performed to further identify the anatomy of the tumour and to clarify whether nodal spread or metastasis has occurred (Figure2). As an anaesthetist it is important to view these scans in order to understand the planned surgery(27). For example:

- chest wall resection may be necessary,
- close proximity to the pleura with pleural resection may make paravertebral analgesia impossible,
- proximity to the pulmonary vessels or aorta makes major blood loss more likely.

12. Algorithm for preoperative evaluation of patients for lung resection

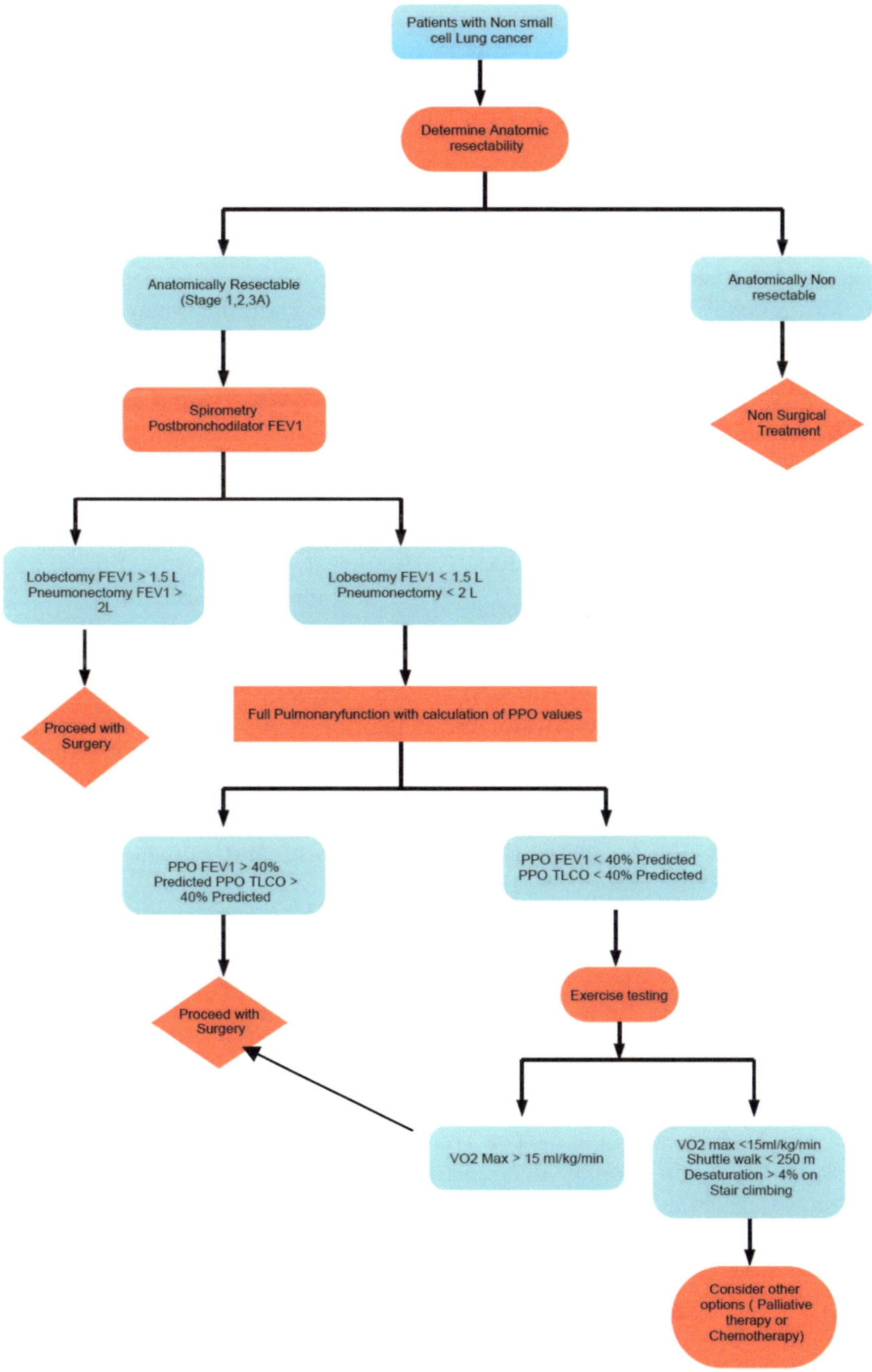

Fig. 7.

13. Summary

Surgical pulmonary resection and chemo radiotherapy both induce significant mortality and morbidity in lung cancer patients. A targeted preoperative assessment combined with multidisciplinary approach can help individualize the morbidity and mortality risk of surgery for each patient and provide the surgeon and patient with the information needed for operative decision making.

14. References

Amar D, Roistacher N, Burt ME, et al. Effects of diltiazem versus digoxin on dysrhythmias and cardiac function after Pneumonectomy. Ann Thorac Surg 1997; 63:1374–81.

Ambrogi MC, Luchhi M, Dini P, et al. Percutaneous radiofrequency ablation of lung tumour: results in midterm. Eur J Cardiothorac Surg 2006;30:177-183.

Batra et al. Preoperative Evaluation in Lung Cancer. *Clin Pulm Med 2002; 9(1):46–52*

Benzo RP, Sciurba FC. Oxygen consumption, shuttle walking test and the evaluation of lung resection. Respiration 2010; 80: 19–23.

Benzo RP, Sciurba FC. Oxygen consumption, shuttle walking test and the evaluation of lung resection. Respiration 2010; 80: 19–23.

Bolton J, Weiman D. Physiology of lung resection. *Clin Chest Med.* 1993; 14:293–303.

Brunelli A, Charloux A, Bolliger CT. ERS/ESTS clinical guidelines on fitness for radical therapy in lung cancer patients (surgery and chemo-radiotherapy). Eur Respir J 2009; 34: 17-41.

BTS guidelines: guidelines on the selection of patients with lung cancer for surgery. Thorax 2001; 56: 89–108

Colice GL, Shafazand S et al. The physiologic evaluation of patients with lung cancer being considered for resectional surgery. ACCP evidenced-based clinical practice guidelines (2nd edition). Chest 2007; 132; 161S-177S.

DeMeester SR, Patterson GA, Sundaresan RS, Cooper JD. Lobectomy combined with volume reduction for patients with lung cancer and advanced emphysema. J Thorac Cardiovasc Surg 1998; 115:681.

DeRose JJ Jr, Argenziano M, El-Amir N, et al. Lung reduction operation and resection of pulmonary nodules in patients with severe emphysema. Ann Thorac Surg 1998; 65:314.

Didolkar MS, Moore RH, Taiku J. Evaluation of the risk in pulmonary resection for bronchogenic carcinoma. Am J Surg 1974; 127:700 –5.

Expert Advisory Group to the Chief Medical Officers of England and Wales. *A policy framework for commissioning cancer services.* London: Department of Health, 1995.

Falcoz PE, Conti M, Brouchet L, et al. The Thoracic Surgery Scoring System (Thoracoscore): risk model for in-hospital death in 15,183 patients requiring thoracic surgery. J Thorac Cardiovasc Surg 2007; 133:325e32.

Ferguson MK et al. J Thor Cardiovas Surg 109: 275, 1995

Ferlay J, Parkin DM, Steliarova-Foucher E. Estimates of cancer incidence and mortality in Europe in 2008 Eur J Cancer. 2010 Mar; 46(4):765-81. Epub 2010 Jan 29

Fernando HC, De Hoyos A, Landreneau RJ et al.Radiofrequency ablation for the treatment of Non small cell lung cancer in marginal surgical candidates. J Thorac Cardiovasc Surgery 2005;129:639-644.

Gibbs J, Cull W, Henderson W, Daley J, Hur K, Khuri SF. Preoperative serum albumin level as a predictor of operative mortality and morbidity: results from the National VA Surgical Risk Study. Arch Surg. 1999; 134:36-42. [PMID: 9927128]

Golledge J, Goldstraw P. Renal impairment after thoracotomy: incidence, risk factors and significance. Ann Thorac Surg 1994; 58:524–8.

Gould G, Pearce A. Assessment of suitability for lung resection. Contin Educ Anaesth Crit Care Pain 2006: 97-100.

Korst RJ, Ginsberg RJ, Ailawadi M, et al. Lobectomy improves ventilatory function in selected patients with severe COPD. *Ann Thorac Surg.* 1998; 66:898–902.

Lagana D, Carrafiello G,Mangini M, et al. Radiofrequency Ablation of primary and metastatic lung tumours: preliminary experience with single centre device. Surg Endosc 2006;20:1262-1267.

Lee TH, Marcantonio ER, Mangione CM, et al. Derivation and prospective validation of a simple index for prediction of cardiac risk of major noncardiac surgery. Circulation 1999; 100: 1043–1049

Linden PA, Bueno R, Colson YL, et al. Lung resection in patients with preoperative FEV1 < 35% predicted. Chest 2005; 127:1984.

Lyrd RB, Burns JR. Cough dynamics in the post-thoracotomy state. *Chest.* 1975; 67:654 -657.

MacNee W. Pathophysiology of cor pulmonale in chronic obstructive pulmonary disease. Am J Respir Crit Care Med 1994; 150:833–52.

Massard G, Moog R, Wihlm JM, *et al.* Bronchogenic cancer in the elderly: operative risk and long term prognosis. *Thorac Cardiovasc Surg* 1996;44:40–5.

McKenna RJ Jr, Fischel RJ, Brenner M, Gelb AF. Combined operations for lung volume reduction surgery and lung cancer. Chest 1996; 110:885.

Morgan AD. Simple exercise testing. Respir Med 1989; 83:383e7.

Nakahara K, Ohno K, Hashimoto J, et al. Prediction of postoperative respiratory failure in patients undergoing lung resection for cancer. Ann Thorac Surg 1988; 46:549 -52.

Ninan M, Summers KE, Landreneau RJ, et al. Standardised exercise oximetry predicts postpneumonectomy outcome. Ann Thorac Surg 1997; 64:328–333

Olsen GN, Bolton JWR, Weiman DS, et al. Stair climbing as an exercise test to predict postoperative complications of lung resection. Chest.1991;99:587-590

Peters R, Wallons H, Htwe T. Total compliance and work of breathing after thoracotomy. J Thorac Cardiovasc Surg. 1969; 57:348–355.

Poonyagariyagorn H,Mazonne P J: Preoperative Evaluation of Lung resction Semin Respir Crit Care Med 2008;29:271-284.

Portch D,McCormick B Update in Anaesthesia: Pulmonary Function Tests and Assessment for Lung Resection.

Ritchie AJ, Danton M, Gibbons JRP. Prophylactic digitalisation in pulmonary surgery. Thorax 1992; 47:41–3.

Schulman DS, Mathony RA. The right ventricle in pulmonary disease. Cardiol Clin 1992; 10:111–35.

Singh SJ, Morgan MD, Hardman AE, et al. Comparison of oxygen uptake duringa conventional treadmill test and the shuttle walking test in chronic airflow limitation. Eur Respir J 1994; 7:2016e20.

Slinger PD Preoperative assessment for pulmonary resection AUTORES EXTRANJEROS Vol. 27. Supl. 1 2004 pp 19-26.

Slinger PD, Johnston MR. Preoperative assessment: an anesthesiologist's perspective. Thorac Surg Clin 2005; 15:11–25.

Stein M, Koota G, Simon M. Pulmonary evaluation of surgical patients. JAMA 1962; 181:765–770

Wang J et al. J Thoracic Cardiovasc Surg 17: 5811, 1999.

Weinberger S E, King T E Jr, Hollingsworth H Preoperative evaluation for lung resection Edwards JG, Duthie DJ, Waller DA. Lobar volume reduction surgery: a method of increasing the lung cancer resection rate in patients with emphysema. Thorax 2001; 56:791.

Win T, Jackson A, Groves AM, et al. Comparison of shuttle walk with measured peak oxygen consumption in patients with operable lung cancer. Thorax 2006; 61:57e60.

Win T, Jackson A, Groves AM, et al. Relationship of shuttle walk test and lung cancer surgical outcome. Eur J Cardiothoracic Surg 2004; 26:1216e19.

Xia T, Li H, Sun Q, et al. Promising clinical Outcome of Stereotactic body radiotherapy for patients with inoperable stage1/2 Non small cell lung cancer. Int J Radiat Oncol Biol Phys 2006; 66: 117 - 125.

Yellin A, Hill LR, Lieberman Y. Pulmonary resections in patients over 70 years of age. *Israel J Med Sci* 1985;21:833–40.

2

Pulmonary Resection for Lung Cancer in Patients with Liver Cirrhosis

Takashi Iwata
Department of Thoracic and Cardiovascular Surgery, Kansai Rosai Hospital,
Department of Thoracic Surgery,
Osaka City University Graduate School of Medicine,
Japan

1. Introduction

Liver cirrhosis is characterized by an advanced irreversible fibrotic change in hepatic tissue as a terminal stage of the chronic progressive injury of the liver.(1) The cause of the liver injury is various, and most common causes are chronic viral infection and alcoholism. In non-endemic area of hepatitis B and C virus such as the United States and European countries, the most frequent cause is long-term alcohol consumption. In the endemic area, especially among Asian and African countries including Japan, chronic infection of hepatitis B or C virus is the most common cause of liver cirrhosis.(2-5) Prognosis is not significantly different according to the cause of cirrhosis, such as alcoholic or viral due to hepatitis B or C virus, however, development of hepatocellular carcinoma is more likely to complicate in hepatitis C virus (HCV) infected-patients than in alcoholic patients.(6, 7) Today, HCV infection is spreading worldwide, even in non-endemic area such as the United States or Europe.(8-12) In these non-endemic areas, the main cause of viral infection has been blood transfusion and healthcare-related transmission. But the prevalence of blood test before transfusion and improvement of healthcare environment are decreasing the risk of HCV infection in daily medical practice. However, continuous increase of intravenous drug user and immigration from endemic countries are now bigger risks for HCV infection in these countries. Because HCV is strongly associated with the development of hepatocellular carcinoma, incidence of hepatocellular carcinoma is also increasing all over the world along with the increasing incidence of HCV-related cirrhosis.

On the other hand, incidence of lung cancer is still epidemic worldwide.(13-18) In some area of industrialized countries such as the United States, the various effort to educate the public about harmfulness of tobacco and importance of quitting smoking, and another effort to decrease air pollution and exposure of workplace carcinogenetic agents are successfully decreasing the incidence of lung cancer declining in the last decade. However, in the rest majority of the countries, incidence of lung cancer is still increasing especially in the developing countries. Thus, opportunity to encounter patients with lung cancer comorbid with liver cirrhosis will be increasing. These two diseases are both lethal. We will face the difficult question how to treat these patients with the both critical conditions.

In this chapter, I describe about pathophysiology of liver cirrhosis, its effect upon pulmonary function, and safety, risk and feasibility of pulmonary resection for lung cancer in cirrhotic patients, introducing my recent three cases with a review of the literature.

2. Pathophysiology of liver cirrhosis

The patients with mild to moderate liver cirrhosis are usually asymptomatic and look very well for years. But the fibrotic change in the liver is irreversible and progressing gradually. Common symptoms of such early-staged disease are non-specific, as general fatigue, loss of appetite, and body weight loss. Degrade of estrogen is performed in the liver and this estrogen metabolism is impaired in patients with liver cirrhosis. As a result of emphasized effect of estrogen, gynecomastia and testicular atrophy could be demonstrated in male patients. Severe fibrosis in the liver causes congestion of blood flow in the portal vein, so-called "portal hypertension." Portal hypertension complicates gastroesophageal varices. The rupture of gastroesophageal varices is an important cause of death in patients with liver cirrhosis. Portal congestion also evokes splenomegaly. Splenomegaly leads chronic anemia by destroying the blood cells. Platelet cell count is also decreased in the advanced cases. Congestion of the small intestine may cause malabsorption of various nutrient and moreover, increased susceptibility of infection due to decay of mucosal barrier, so-called "bacterial translocation" which allowed intraluminal microorganism in the intestine to move into the portal blood flow. Dilatation of the skin vessels is also seen; "vascular spider" is a small capillary dilatation mainly seen in the anterior chest, caput medusa is a sign of venous congestion in the abdominal wall. The flow of biliary juice is also interrupted. Chronic stasis of bile can lead to jaundice, itching, and xanthoma in bilateral eyelids. Decrease of biosynthesis of bile acid results malabsorption of fat and fat-soluble vitamins. Lowered production of coagulating factor increases a risk of bleeding. Palmer erythema, Dupuytren's contracture, muscular atrophy, swelling of salivary glands, axillary alopecia, peripheral nerve disorder are another sign of liver cirrhosis. When the liver congestion gets so severe, ascites and/or pleural effusion are also seen. Impaired synthesis of albumin in the liver also accelerates the production of ascites and/or pleural effusion. Finally, interruption of nitrous metabolism are occurred and leads encephalopathy.

3. Severity of the disease and its evaluation methods

Severity of the disease is evaluated and graded according to various physical and clinical parameters. Modified Child-Pugh classification is widely used all over the world, and the detail of its grading is shown in Table 1.(19-22) Patients with 8 – 9 points of Child-Pugh score are likely to die within a year. Patients with more than 10 points are likely to die within 6 months. Table 2 shows the details of Liver damage class that is another more useful method than Child-Pugh class to evaluate the severity of liver injury. This was made by the Liver Cancer Study Group of Japan, and is also widely used in Japan.(23) Liver damage class was developed for the diagnosis and treatment for hepatocellular carcinoma, and it is very useful to expect the patient's life expectancy because the result is more correlated with clinical outcome than Child-Pugh class.(23, 24)

Model for End-Stage Liver Disease (MELD) score is a new system that exclude the uncertainty and subjectivity from the evaluation process because it is based on mathematical calculation by the results of three blood tests, such as serum value of total bilirubin (mg/dL), prothrombin test and international normalized ratio; PT-INR, and serum value of creatinine (mg/dL).(25-27) The MELD score is calculated using the following equation:

$$3.8\times\log(e)(\text{bilirubin mg}/\text{dL})+11.2\times\log(e)$$
$$(\text{PT}-\text{INR})+9.6\log(e)(\text{creatinine mg}/\text{dL})+6.43\,*$$

*This 6.43 points should not be added if the cause of liver damage is alcoholic or biliary stasis. If not, i.e. the liver damage is due to hepatitis virus infection, 6.43 points should be added.

MELD score is useful to predict short-term prognosis and for its fairness and accuracy it is used for the waiting list of the patients who wishes liver transplantation for end-stage cirrhosis.

Clinical and laboratory findings	Scores		
	1 point	2 points	3 points
Encepalopathy	None	Mild	Coma, occasionally
Ascites	Absent	Slight	Moderate
Serum bilirubin (mg/dL)	<2.0	2.0-3.0	>3.0
Serum albumin (g/dL)	>3.5	2.8-3.5	<2.8
Prothrombin time (sec. prolonged)	1-4	4-6	>6
or Prothrombin time INR*	<1.7	1.7 - 2.3	>2.3

Child-Pugh class is determined due to total score for all findings according to the chart below.

	Total scores	Grade
Child-Pugh	5-6	A
	7-9	B
	10-15	C

INR; international normalized ratio.
from Pugh RNH, et. al. Brit. J. Surg. 60: 646-654, 1973.
*Lucey MR, et al. Liver Transpl Surg, 3: 628-637, 1997.
This table is modified with permission from #23 and #32

Table 1. Child-Pugh classification

	Grade		
Clinical and laboratory findings	A	B	C
Ascites	None	Controllable	Uncontrollable
Serum bilirubin (mg/dL)	<2.0	2.0-3.0	>3.0
Serum albumin (g/dL)	>3.5	3.0-3.5	<3.5
$ICGR_{15}$ (%)	<15	15-40	>40
Prothrombin activity (%)	>80	50-80	<50

Degree of liver damage is recorded as A, B, or C, based on the highest grade containing at least 2 clinical or laboratory findings liseted above in the chart. ICGR15; indocyanine green retention rate at 15 min.
This table is modified with permission from #23 and #32

Table 2. Liver damage classification by Liver Cancer Study Group of Japan

4. Effect of liver cirrhosis upon pulmonary function

Dysfunction of the liver could lead abnormality in pulmonary function and gas exchange. Aller and coworkers reported that mean partial pressure of O_2 in arterial blood in patients with cirrhosis was not significantly different from those in healthy control.(28) However, more than 70% of cirrhotic patients showed hypocapnea in arterial blood gas analysis. Mean partial pressure of CO_2 in arterial blood was 32.2 torr. Abnormality in the result of pulmonary function test was observed in 38%, and hypoxia and decreased diffusing capacity of carbon monoxide were significant in these patients. Pulmonary vasodilatation was also observed in approximately 30% of the patients, and was associated with hypocapnea and higher grade of Child-Pugh class. Yigit and coworkers also reported that hypoxia was not significantly affected by severity of liver dysfunction but diffusing capacity was.(29) These abnormalities of pulmonary function are called as Hepatopulmonary syndrome.(30) In patients with severely impaired liver function, the clearance of vasodilator substances is interrupted in the liver. As the result, excess vasodilator substances stay longer in pulmonary circulation, resulting pulmonary capillary vasodilatation in alveoli or formation of pulmonary arteriovenous shunting in the lung parencyma, or both. These changes could occur and get worse along with the progression of liver dysfunction. Increased amount of pulmonary arteriovenous shunting leads hypocapnea. Because the blood flow is too fast in the dilated pulmonary capillary or simply due to increased shunting flow, without getting enough oxygenation, hyperventilation is occurred to compensate hypoxemia, and resulted hypocapnea. Oxygenation is maintained in the most of the cases, because alveolar membrane itself is not damaged by liver dysfunction. Dilated capillary in the alveoli and/or increased flow of pulmonary shunt also lead decrease in diffusing capacity.

5. Feasibility of pulmonary resection in patients with liver cirrhosis

Feasibility of thoracic surgery in patients with liver cirrhosis is little known. There are only a few reports about this issue in the literature.(31-33) Iwasaki and coworkers reported a series of 17 patients with liver cirrhosis underwent pulmonary resection for primary lung cancer in 2006.(33) Pulmonary resection showed no mortality and morbidity in 4 patients with cirrhosis graded Child-Pugh class A. In 13 patients with cirrhosis graded Child-Pugh class B, morbidity was 4 out of 13 and mortality was 1. This one patient with Child-Pugh class B was died on the day 11 due to pneumonia and multiple organ failure secondary to acute liver failure. We also reported that one patient with Child-Pugh class A and one with class B died of sepsis on the day 6 and 46, respectively, in the series of 37 patients that included 28 patients with class A and 9 with class B.(31)

In 2006, 26,351 patients with lung cancer were surgically treated in Japan and 230 of them died in hospital.(34) The overall in-hospital mortality rate of surgically treated patients with primary lung cancer was 0.9%. Overall postoperative in-hospital death after pulmonary resection in patients with liver cirrhosis was reported as 5.8% and 5.4%, by Iwasaki and us, respectively. The mortality rate is approximately 5 or 6 times higher than the entire result of lung cancer surgery in Japan.

6. Early complications of pulmonary resection associated with liver cirrhosis

We also reported the details of early postoperative complications and their affecting factors from the results of these 37 patients with lung cancer comorbid with liver cirrhosis in

2007.(31) Cirrhosis-related early postoperative complication had occurred in 7 patients of 37 (18.9%). Intrathoracic bleeding was complicated in 4 patients (10.8%) that needed perioperative blood transfusion, and one of them had another bleeding from gastroduodenal ulcer simultaneously (2.7%). All could be saved by blood transfusion only in 3 cases and one needed successive thoracotomy. Liver failure was complicated in 2 patients (5.4%) and both of them had been recovered by liver supporting therapy. In another 2 patients (5.4%), sepsis was occurred and they all died. Preoperative serum value of total bilirubin was the only independent factor predicting postoperative liver failure. The complication of postoperative sepsis was associated with preoperative nutrition status. We could not find any useful factors predicting postoperative bleeding in this study. To prevent postoperative complications, it seems essential to improve preoperative systemic status, especially liver function and nutrition status.

Iwasaki and coworkers also reported perioperative complications, as well. They reported 9 patients (52.9%) out of 17 complicated intra- or postoperative bleeding so that they needed perioperative blood transfusion. Liver failure was complicated in 1 patient (5.9%) who was simultaneously complicated with pneumonia and die on the day 11. Infectious disease, such as pneumonia, was complicated in 2 patients (11.8%) including 1 already mentioned. Prolonged air leak from pulmonary fistula was complicated in 1 patient (5.9%).

7. Postoperative intrathoracic bleeding

According to the depletion of platelets counts and decreased synthesis of coagulation factor in the liver, a risk of postoperative bleeding is increased in cirrhotic patients.(35, 36) Rate of complication with postoperative intrathoracic bleeding that needed blood transfusion were from 10.8% to 52.9%, as described.(31, 33) In our previous report, of 4 patients with intrathoracic bleeding, 1 patient needed re-thoracotomy to control persisted bleeding on the day 1. These four patients showed remarkable decrease in platelet count, preoperatively. However, statistical analysis did not demonstrate that the preoperative platelet count was not a significant risk factor for postoperative bleeding. On the other hand, the size of the tumor was significantly associated with postoperative bleeding. Bigger tumors might have required wider dissections. Performance of wedge resection was correlated with the bleeding, also. This would be because we had selected the less risk operative method, such as wedge resection, than standard lobectomy for patients with comparatively higher risk among advanced cirrhotic patients. Perioperative blood transfusion, including platelet and fresh frozen plasma, should be considered when the patient seemed to complicate severe coagulopathy.(31, 33)

8. Upper gastrointestinal bleeding

We have also reported a case (0.3%) of acute gastrointestinal bleeding complicated after pulmonary resection in the same series of patients.(31) This patient also complicated with intrathoracic bleeding simultaneously. This patient was successfully saved by blood transfusion and endoscopic intervention. However, cirrhotic patients that complicated variceal bleeding have high risk of rebleeding or death and poor prognosis.(37, 38) Preoperative gastrointestinal endoscopy is recommended and sclerotherapy should be performed if needed. Administration of perioperative histamine H_2 blocker or proton pump inhibitor is also essential to prevent bleeding from acute gastrointestinal ulceration.(39)

9. Liver failure

Liver failure is another concern for patients with liver cirrhosis after surgery. This usually occurred in comparatively late period, such as several days or weeks after the surgical intervention. Hepatic encephalopathy could be developed by accumulation of intrinsic neurotoxic substances.(40) Ammonia is the most common cause of hepatic encephalopathy. Administration of oral branched chain amino acid, improvement of intestinal bacterial flora to decrease toxic substance production and absorption, and shunt obliteration are treatment options. However, the cirrhotic patient with encephalopathy has poor prognosis.

Ascites is another critical concern in patients with liver failure. Especially after abdominal surgery, control of postoperative increase of ascites or lymphorrhea is sometimes difficult.(41, 42) Interestingly, we did not experienced uncontrollable lymphorrhea or overproduction of pleural effusion after pulmonary surgery, even with mediastinal dissection. Probably lymphangitic stasis would be less in thoracic cavity than in abdominal cavity in cirrhotic patients. Perioperative maintenance with decreased transfusion and proper usage of diuretics would be important.

Jaundice is another important symptom of liver failure, and is clinically manifested with serum value of total bilirubin 3 mg/dL or more. When the value is between 1 to 3 mg/dL, it is called latent jaundice. Serum value of total bilirubin reflects the severity of liver dysfunction very well. Our studies revealed that preoperative serum value of total bilirubin was useful to predict both postoperative liver failure and long-term survival of the cirrhotic patients who underwent pulmonary surgery.(31, 32)

10. Complications associated with malnutrition and infectious diease

Cirrhotic patients sometimes complicated with malnutrition. Malnutrition is mainly evaluated with hypoalbuminemia, lower serum value of total cholesterol. Damaged tissue by surgical intervention would not be quickly repaired in such poor nutrition status. Delay of the healing of surgical site may lead prolonged air leakage or complication of bronchopleural fistula; those would finally invite intractable infection. Malnutrition also affects immunological insufficiency. Thus, a risk of infectious disease would be increased in such patients. This is more problematic when the patient undergoes surgical intervention.(35, 43, 44) In our study, 2 of 37 patients died of sepsis, postoperatively. Iwasaki and coworkers lost 1 of all 17 patients due to liver failure complicated with pneumonia. Severe infectious disease would be critical in cirrhotic patients after pulmonary resection. Not only perioperative antibiotics administration, preoperative improvement of nutrition status is essential.

11. Long-term outcome of lung cancer surgery in cirrhotic patients

We also reported the long-term outcome after pulmonary surgery in cirrhotic patients with lung cancer in 2007, analyzing 33 cases.(32) Mean survival time was 44.8 months. Overall 5-year survival rate after pulmonary surgery in patients with lung cancer comorbid liver cirrhosis was 37.6% (Fig. 1). During the observation period, lung cancer death had occurred in 9 patients. Mean survival time until lung cancer death was 33.5 months and 5-year survival rate from lung cancer death was 59.7%. Hepatic death had been occurred in 6 patients. Mean survival time until hepatic death was 60.1 months and its 5-year survival was 62.9%. Within 3 years after surgery, main cause of death was secondary to lung caner.

After 3 years, the main reason of death was hepatic cause, as shown in Fig. 1. Factors influencing lung cancer death were nodal extension and limited surgery, and factors influencing hepatic death were preoperative serum values of total bilirubin, choline esterase and alpha-fetoprotein, platelet count, and the result of prothrombin test. Local extensiveness of the tumor, limited surgery, mediastinal dissection, and pathological stage of the disease also affected the occurrence of hepatic death in the long-term period. However pulmonary resection itself might affect liver function in long-term, pulmonary resection for lung cancer is still beneficial also in patients with comorbid liver cirrhosis.

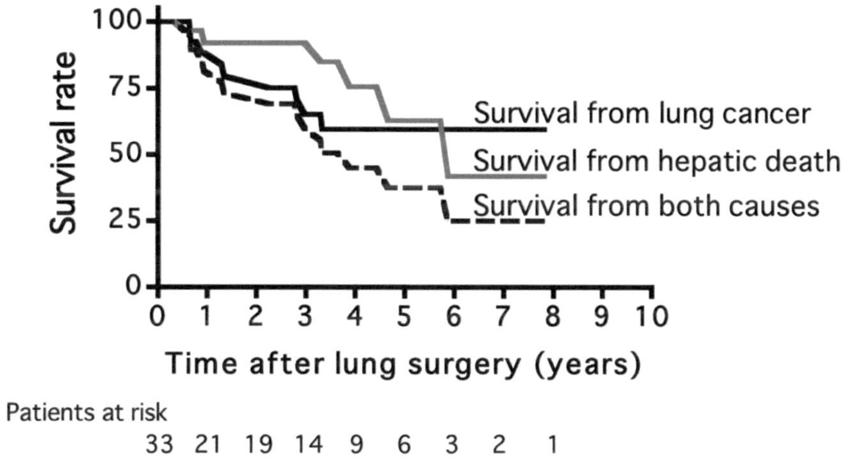

Fig. 1. Survival curves after lung cancer surgery in 33 patients with comorbid liver cirrhosis for lung cancer death (black solid line), hepatic death (gray solid line), and deaths from both causes (broken line). (This figure is taken from the article #32 with permission of Elsevier)

Iwasaki and coworkers also described long-term outcome, shortly. Of all 17 patients, 4 patients died of liver failure, 3 patients died of lung cancer recurrence, 1 died of cardiac event, and 1 died of unknown cause. The rest 8 patients were reported alive.

12. Complication with hepatocellular carcinoma and lung cancer surgery

Hepatocellular carcinoma (HCC) is another critical condition that is commonly found in patients with liver cirrhosis.(7) We also investigated the result of pulmonary surgery performed in 11 patients with both lethal malignancies, lung cancer and hepatocellular carcinoma, all comorbid with liver cirrhosis.(45) As early postoperative complication, liver failure occurred in 2 patients, intrathoracic bleeding did in 2 patients. One of them complicated gastrointestinal bleeding simultaneously. There was no postoperative in-hospital death. Five-year survival rate from lung cancer death was 74.1%, whereas 5-year survival from hepatic death was 39.8% (Fig. 2). Five-year survival from overall death was 29.5%. Complication of hepatocellular carcinoma showed worse long-term outcome than comorbidity of simple liver cirrhosis compared with the previous study.(32) Factors influencing survival in patients with both lung cancer and HCC were preoperative serum values of total bilirubin here again, choline esterase, platelet count, and the result of prothrombin test.

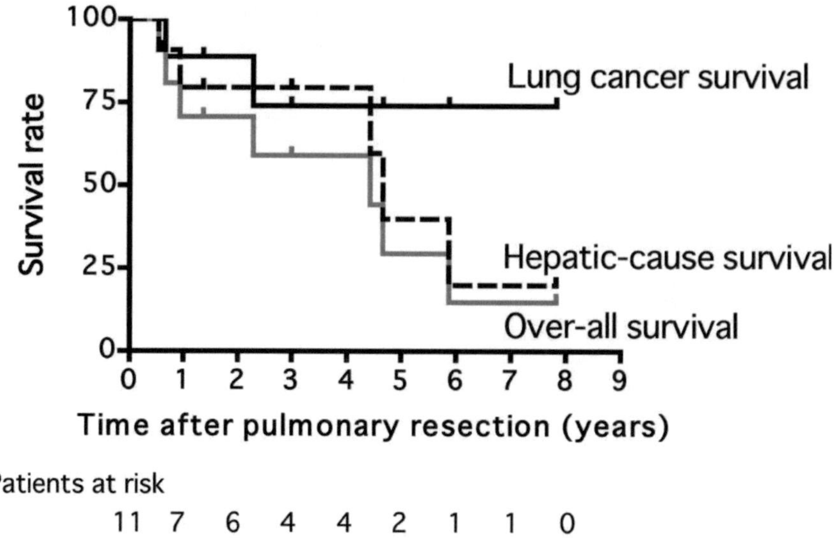

Fig. 2. Survival curves after pulmonary resection for non-small cell lung cancer in patients with hepatocellular carcinoma. Survival from lung cancer (black line), survival from hepatic causes, including both hepatocellular carcinoma and liver cirrhosis (broken line), and overall survival (gray line). (This figure is taken from the article #45 with permission of Springer-Verlag)

13. Decision making; Which patient would tolerate pulmonary resection?

From our previous data, regardless of comorbidity of HCC, if the life expectancy is predicted as more than 3 years according to the liver function, lung cancer surgery should be considered.(32, 45) Modified Child-Pugh grading system is reported to be useful to predict postoperative outcome by multiple investigators, including our results.(22, 41, 42) We have also investigated MELD score to predict postoperative complications and outcome, however, from our unpublished data, we could not find that the usefulness of MELD score for such purpose. The operative method is another problem in patients with cirrhosis; which is better, limited surgery or lobectomy with mediastinal dissection? Our previous data showed that mediastinal dissection, tumor size, and pathological stage have some impact on hepatic death in long-term.(32) Therefore minimal invasive method is favorable to preserve liver function. However, death from lung cancer mainly occurred within 3 years after surgery, and hepatic death after that. Thus, when the extensiveness of the lung cancer is advanced, usual standard operation with lobectomy and/or mediastinal dissection is recommended, while the patient's general status is tolerated for the surgical invasiveness. Basically we would take standard surgical strategy for patients with lung cancer comorbid with Child-Pugh class A cirrhosis. Operative method will be determined upon the extensiveness of the disease and pulmonary function. For patients with Child-Pugh class B cirrhosis, operative method will be determined upon symptoms and the result of blood chemical study, but limited surgery is recommended basically. And for patients with Child-Pugh class C cirrhosis, we recommend another substitution methods, such as stereotactic radiation therapy or radiofrequency abrasion.

14. Case reports and discussions

We are introducing our recent cases that underwent pulmonary resection for primary lung cancer comorbid with liver cirrhosis.

Case 1.

A 79-year-old woman who had diagnosed with chronic type C hepatitis at the age of 72 and was also diagnosed with Child-Pugh class B liver cirrhosis last year, was referred to our department for incidentally-discovered abnormal shadow on a chest radiograph (Fig. 3).

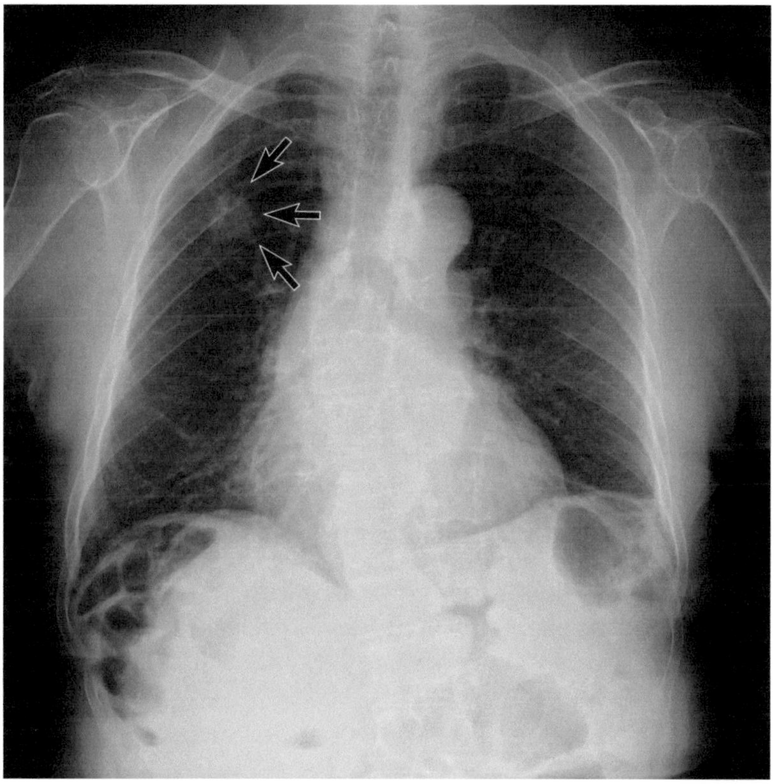

Fig. 3. A chest radiography demonstrates a spiculated mass of approximately 2cm in diameter, in the right upper field of the lung.

Chest computed tomography (CT) demonstrated a spiculated mass with cavity formation, of 23mm in diameter in the posterior segment in the right upper lobe of the lung. Maximum standardized uptake value (SUVmax) of the lesion was 19.19 by 18-fluoro-2-deoxy-D-glucose positron emission computed tomography (PET/CT). Nodal extension was not demonstrated both in chest CT and PET/CT scans. Brain magnetic resonance imaging did not show any metastatic lesions. Dynamic multi-detector-row CT demonstrated high-stained low-density area of 20 mm in diameter, suspecting hepatocellular carcinoma in posterosuperior segment and a typical hemangioma stain in posterosuperior segment of the right hepatic lobe. Ultrasonic scan showed irregular surface and nodular pattern of the liver and very small amount of ascites, a low echoic mass lesion that had partial hyper echoic lesion inside in posterosuperior segment of the right lobe. The lesion that was suspected as hemangioma could not be detected by CT. Esophageal varices were observed without red color signs by Fiberoptic gastroscopy. She had currently smoked 50 cigarettes a day since 23 years old of age. Branched chain amino acid, spironolactone, folic acid, and menatetrenone (vitamin K2) had been orally administrated for a year. Result of blood chemical study showed in Table 3. Result of pulmonary function test revealed vital capacity as 2.39L, forced expiratory volume in 1 sec as 1.78L/sec, forced expiratory volume in 1 sec % as 75.74%, and diffusing capacity of carbon monoxide was 59.4%. She showed a good performance status so that she could climb up the stairs to the third floor all by herself. Right lung cancer of clinical T1aN0M0 stage 1A disease was suspected. Child B cirrhosis was confirmed and needle biopsy of the liver mass was planned after pulmonary surgery by a hepatologist. Thus, wedge resection of the right upper lobe was carried out via video-assisted thoracoscopic approach. Operative time was 1 hr 27 min. Blood loss was 20 g. The histopathology was squamous cell carcinoma without nodal extension, and she was diagnosed with p-T1bN0M0 p-stage 1B disease. The result of postoperative blood chemical study on the day 2 was also shown in Table 3. The patient was uneventfully discharged on the day 5. However, approximately 50 days after surgery, the patient noticed abdominal fullness and visited the out-patient. The hepatologist diagnosed her with liver failure by Child-Pugh class C cirrhosis, according to the result of blood chemical study (Table 3) and increased amount of ascites shown by ultrasonography. The patient was treated with liver supporting therapy, and the ascites was subsequently disappeared and the laboratory data got improved also (Table 3). Needle biopsy of the liver was performed 4 months from pulmonary surgery, and revealed only necrotic tissue, nor metastatic or primary malignancy. The patient is well without recurrent disease or exacerbation of cirrhosis 13 months after the surgery.

Discussion

Case 1 demonstrated a late onset of liver failure after pulmonary surgery, mainly developed as acute increase of ascites. The patient had been graded as Child-Pugh class B cirrhosis due to hepatitis C virus infection, preoperatively. She needed treatment for liver failure 60 days after pulmonary surgery, and she was then diagnosed as liver failure with Child-Pugh class C cirrhosis at that time. There was no other possible cause of acute exacerbation of the liver function for her. We have learned that late onset of liver failure could develop even 60 days after pulmonary resection.

Case 2.

A 61-year-old man presented with leukocytosis and elevation of c-reactive protein level in the serum by regular check up for alcoholic cirrhosis of Child-Pugh class A and chronic pancreatitis. His father and mother died of hepatocellular carcinoma and liver cirrhosis, respectively. A chest radiograph demonstrated a mass lesion of 7cm in diameter in the right upper lung field (Fig. 4). Bronchoscopic biopsy was not diagnostic. He lost 5kg of weight during the past 2 months. Systemic check up did not reveal metastatic disease. Result of blood chemical study showed in Table 3. Pulmonary function tests revealed vital capacity as 4.09L, forced expiratory volume in 1 sec as 2.49L/sec, forced expiratory volume in 1 sec % as 62.18%, and diffusing capacity of carbon monoxide was 56.9%. Preoperatively, delirium, offensive behavior, and hallucination that was related to small insects or dwarfs crawling on the ceiling, were developed suddenly 3 days after the hospitalization. We diagnosed him with alcohol withdrawal syndrome from the typical symptoms including weird hallucinations associated with insects and dwarfs, lack of flapping tremor, and low serum level of ammonia. Thus, surgical treatment was carried out as scheduled by maintaining the

					Case 1				Case 2		Case 3	
					Preop	2POD	60POD	79POD	Preop	6POD	Preop	2POD
Child-Pugh class					B	B	C	B	A	A	A	A
Ascietes					Trivial	None	Yes	None	None	None	None	None
WBC	9	-	4	10^3/μL	3.2	6.3	3.6	4.0	15.3	5.7	5.4	4.4
RBC	5.4		3.8	10^6/μL	2.56	2.10	2.61	2.57	3.89	2.91	4.29	3.79
Hb	15	-	11.5	g/dl	9.7	8.2	10.1	9.9	13.6	10.2	14.3	12.6
Ht	45	-	35	%	28.6	23.6	29.7	28.9	39.9	29.3	42.2	37.6
Plt	350	-	150	10^3/μL	59	32	75	87	311	362	109	103
PT-INR					1.21		1.30	1.18	1.30		1.06	
PTsec				sec	13.2		14.4	13.1	14.4		11.8	
PT%	70	-	140	%	71.0		62.0	78.0	63.0		91.0	
APTT	40	-	25	sec	43.6		41.3	37.7	41.1		37.9	
HCV	-				+				-		+	
HBVag	-				-				-		-	
CEA	5	-	0	ng/mL	11.6				4.3		5.7	
AFP	10	-	0	ng/mL				7			144	
CA19-9	37	-	0	U/mL	45.0				<10.0		130.0	
T-Bil	1.2	-	0.2	mg/dL	1.1	1.8	1.8	1.2	0.7	0.3	0.7	0.4
D-Bil	0.4	-	0	mg/dL	0.8				0.5		0.2	
AST	35	-	12	U/L	56	32	40	39	40	51	45	26
ALT	30	-	5	U/L	35	21	18	31	12	18	37	24
ALP	344	-	109	U/L	372	184	285	581	636	343	220	144
ChE	249	-	97	U/L	49		73	68	58		306	
LDH	240	-	110	U/L	225	199	225	217	150		276	169
γ-GTP	35	-	7	U/L	31		18	21	357		46	
T-Cho	219	-	120	mg/dL	92		90	83	107		190	
Na	147	-	136	mmol/L	140	131	138	132	137	132	142	
Cl	110	-	98	mmol/L	110	101	110	101	97	98	102	
K	5	-	3.5	mmol/L	5	4.2	4.3	4.2	4.0	4.0	4.1	
BUN	20	-	8	mg/dL	12.1	25.8	8.8	19.2	6.4	11.1	13.4	13.3
Cre	0.8	-	0.4	mg/dL	0.85	0.99	0.76	0.71	0.72	0.58	0.61	0.55
AMY	120	-	30	U/L	107		100	157	41		160	
Alb	5	-	3.2	g/dL	2.7	1.9	2.3	2.5	2.5	2.0	4.6	3.0
T-P	8.1	-	6.1	g/dL	6.1	4.5	6.0	6.0	7.4	5.8	8.6	6.2
NH3	60	-	15	μg/dL	18		39	59				
CRP	0.3	-	0	mg/dL	0.1	4.1	0.2	0.1	13.6	3.6	<0.1	1.1
type4 collagen 7s	6	-	0	ng/mL	7.3		12	12				

WBC; white blood cell counts, RBC; red blood cell counts, Hb; hemoglobin, Ht; hematcrit, Plt; platelet counts,

Table 3. Results of preoperative blood chemical studies

symptoms with risperidone. Because the tumor was growing rapidly, we thought that the patient had no time to overcome alcoholism before pulmonary resection. Limited resection was planned at first, but we thought that adjuvant chemotherapy would be difficult due to his mental disorder and liver dysfunction. Therefore, right upper lobectomy of the lung, combined resection of the chest wall, and hilar dissection were carried out. Total fibrous adhesion was observed in the right pleural cavity. Operative time was 4 hrs 6 min. Blood loss was 205 g. He was singing loudly just after extubation. Histopathology revealed pleomorphic carcinoma with chest wall invasion of p-T3N0M0 p-stage 2B disease. Malnutrition status was persisted and serum level of albumin was around 2.0 mg/dL for a week (Table 3). Bronchopleural fistula was also persisted and surgical direct closure of the fistula was performed two weeks after the first surgery. The clinical course after the second surgery was uneventful and he was transferred to a psychiatric hospital for treatment of alcoholism. After 5 months, his nutrition was dramatically improved then postoperative adjuvant chemotherapy with carboplatin and paclitaxel was introduced. After the adjuvant chemotherapy, by too much nutrition and improved liver function, he got 14kg of weight and subsequently developed diabetes mellitus. However, he is well without recurrent disease 13 months after lung cancer surgery.

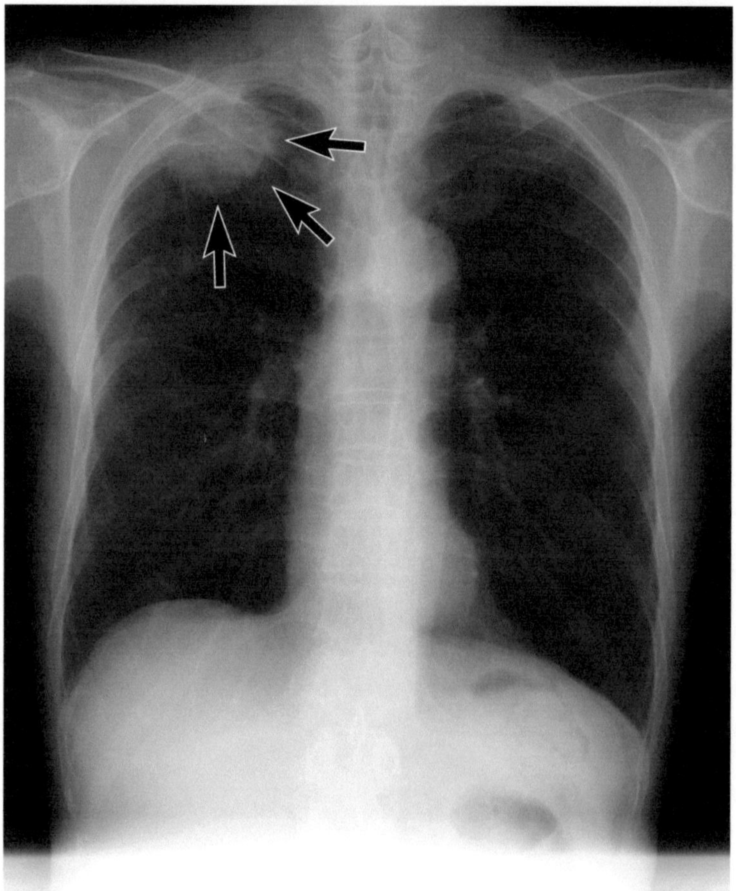

Fig. 4. A chest radiography demonstrates a large mass adjacent to the chest wall in the right apical area.

Discussion

Case 2 developed alcohol withdrawal syndrome preoperatively and persistent bronchopleural fistula that was also occurred due to malnutrition complicated with liver dysfunction. In such cases, differential diagnosis with hepatic encephalopathy is important. Typical symptoms including wired hallucinations associated with insects and dwarfs, lack of flapping tremor, and low serum level of ammonia were useful to exclude hepatic encephalopathy from alcohol withdrawal syndrome. Liver cirrhosis sometimes complicated with malnutrition, especially if it was due to alcoholism. Malnutrition would prolong the healing process at the operated site.

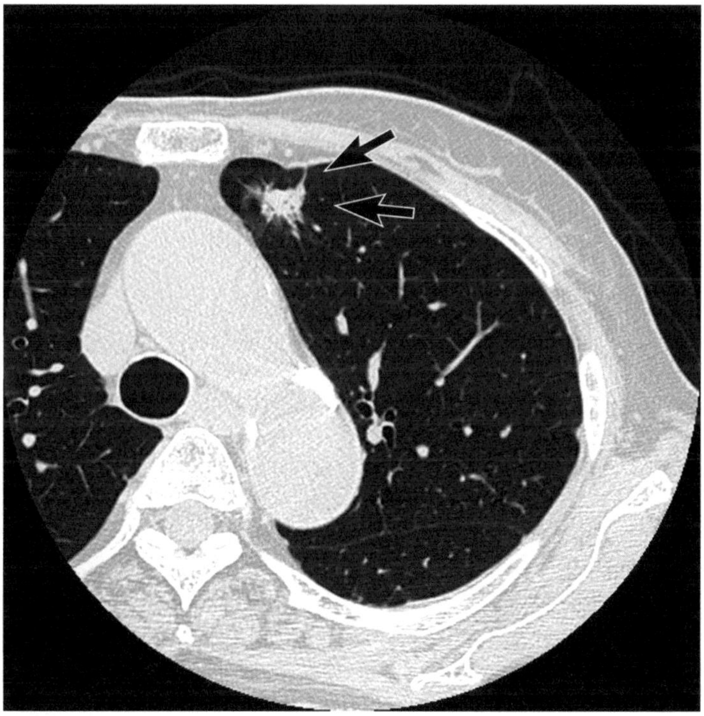

Fig. 5. Computed tomography demonstrates a small spiculated lung mass periphery in the left upper lobe of the lung.

Case 3.

A 77-year-old woman presented with high serum level of carcinoembryonic antigen during observation for Child-Pugh class A cirrhosis with type C hepatitis virus infection. A chest radiograph and chest CT demonstrated a spiculated mass of 1cm in diameter in the anterior segment of left upper lobe (Fig. 5). SUVmax of the lesion was 2.08 by PET/CT. The result of preoperative laboratory test was shown in Table 3. Abdominal ultrasonography revealed irregular-surfaced atrophic liver and multiple high echoic lesions were drawn within. Two of them were suspected as hepatocellular carcinoma and others were diagnosed as hemangiomas. Ascites was not visualized. Result of other systemic check-up did not demonstrate metastatic disease. The patient was never-smoker and the results of pulmonary function test were within normal ranges. Thus, excisional biopsy via video-assisted thoracoscopic approach and subsequent left upper lobectomy with mediastinal dissection were carried out after confirmation of malignancy by frozen sectioning. The operative time was 1 hr 57 min and the blood loss was 5 g. Histopathology revealed adenocarcinoma with mixed subtype of p-T1bN0M0 p-stage 1A disease. She was uneventfully discharged on the day 5. Exacerbation of the liver function was not shown with regular check-up by a hepatologist. She is well without recurrent disease 7 months after the surgery and surgical treatment for hepatocellular carcinoma is now scheduled.

Disucssion

Case 3 was complicated with HCC. Prognosis from liver function and that from lung cancer should be compared to determine the therapeutic strategy, but sometimes it is not easy. Even after successful pulmonary resection, prediction of the patient's life expectancy is very difficult, and we will face another difficult problem if metastatic disease is developed in future.

15. References

[1] Sherman IA, Pappas SC, Fisher MM. Hepatic microvascular changes associated with development of liver fibrosis and cirrhosis. Am J Physiol. 1990 Feb;258(2 Pt 2):H460-5.

[2] Kuniholm MH, Lesi OA, Mendy M, Akano AO, Sam O, Hall AJ, et al. Aflatoxin exposure and viral hepatitis in the etiology of liver cirrhosis in the Gambia, West Africa. Environ Health Perspect. 2008 Nov;116(11):1553-7.

[3] McCaughan GW. Asian perspectives on viral hepatitis: hepatitis C virus infection. J Gastroenterol Hepatol. 2000 Oct;15 Suppl:G90-3.

[4] Zeniya M, Nakajima H. [Liver cirrhosis: statistics in Japan]. Nippon Rinsho. 2002 Jan;60 Suppl 1:233-41.

[5] Michitaka K, Nishiguchi S, Aoyagi Y, Hiasa Y, Tokumoto Y, Onji M. Etiology of liver cirrhosis in Japan: a nationwide survey. J Gastroenterol. 2009;45(1):86-94.

[6] Toshikuni N, Izumi A, Nishino K, Inada N, Sakanoue R, Yamato R, et al. Comparison of outcomes between patients with alcoholic cirrhosis and those with hepatitis C virus-related cirrhosis. J Gastroenterol Hepatol. 2009 Jul;24(7):1276-83.

[7] Trevisani F, Magini G, Santi V, Morselli-Labate AM, Cantarini MC, Di Nolfo MA, et al. Impact of etiology of cirrhosis on the survival of patients diagnosed with hepatocellular carcinoma during surveillance. Am J Gastroenterol. 2007 May;102(5):1022-31.

[8] Alter MJ. Hepatitis C virus infection in the United States. J Hepatol. 1999;31 Suppl 1:88-91.

[9] Hassan MM, Frome A, Patt YZ, El-Serag HB. Rising prevalence of hepatitis C virus infection among patients recently diagnosed with hepatocellular carcinoma in the United States. J Clin Gastroenterol. 2002 Sep;35(3):266-9.

[10] Esteban JI, Sauleda S, Quer J. The changing epidemiology of hepatitis C virus infection in Europe. J Hepatol. 2008 Jan;48(1):148-62.

[11] Naoumov NV. Hepatitis C virus infection in Eastern Europe. J Hepatol. 1999;31 Suppl 1:84-7.

[12] Trepo C, Pradat P. Hepatitis C virus infection in Western Europe. J Hepatol. 1999;31 Suppl 1:80-3.

[13] Youlden DR, Cramb SM, Baade PD. The International Epidemiology of Lung Cancer: geographical distribution and secular trends. J Thorac Oncol. 2008 Aug;3(8):819-31.

[14] Little AG, Gay EG, Gaspar LE, Stewart AK. National survey of non-small cell lung cancer in the United States: epidemiology, pathology and patterns of care. Lung Cancer. 2007 Sep;57(3):253-60.

[15] Alberg AJ, Ford JG, Samet JM. Epidemiology of lung cancer: ACCP evidence-based clinical practice guidelines (2nd edition). Chest. 2007 Sep;132(3 Suppl):29S-55S.

[16] Yoder LH. Lung cancer epidemiology. Medsurg Nurs. 2006 Jun;15(3):171-4; quiz 5.

[17] Alberg AJ, Brock MV, Samet JM. Epidemiology of lung cancer: looking to the future. J Clin Oncol. 2005 May 10;23(14):3175-85.

[18] Lam WK, White NW, Chan-Yeung MM. Lung cancer epidemiology and risk factors in Asia and Africa. Int J Tuberc Lung Dis. 2004 Sep;8(9):1045-57.

[19] Lucey MR, Brown KA, Everson GT, Fung JJ, Gish R, Keeffe EB, et al. Minimal criteria for placement of adults on the liver transplant waiting list: a report of a national conference organized by the American Society of Transplant Physicians and the American Association for the Study of Liver Diseases. Liver Transpl Surg. 1997 Nov;3(6):628-37.

[20] Pugh RN, Murray-Lyon IM, Dawson JL, Pietroni MC, Williams R. Transection of the oesophagus for bleeding oesophageal varices. Br J Surg. 1973 Aug;60(8):646-9.

[21] Bell CL, Jeyarajah DR. Management of the cirrhotic patient that needs surgery. Curr Treat Options Gastroenterol. 2005 Dec;8(6):473-80.

[22] del Olmo JA, Flor-Lorente B, Flor-Civera B, Rodriguez F, Serra MA, Escudero A, et al. Risk factors for nonhepatic surgery in patients with cirrhosis. World J Surg. 2003 Jun;27(6):647-52.

[23] Japan Liver Cancer Study Group. General rules for the clinical and pathological study of primary liver cancer. 2nd English ed. Tokyo: Kanehara & Co., Ltd.; 2003.

[24] Nanashima A, Sumida Y, Morino S, Yamaguchi H, Tanaka K, Shibasaki S, et al. The Japanese integrated staging score using liver damage grade for hepatocellular carcinoma in patients after hepatectomy. Eur J Surg Oncol. 2004 Sep;30(7):765-70.

[25] Farnsworth N, Fagan SP, Berger DH, Awad SS. Child-Turcotte-Pugh versus MELD score as a predictor of outcome after elective and emergent surgery in cirrhotic patients. Am J Surg. 2004 Nov;188(5):580-3.

[26] Said A, Williams J, Holden J, Remington P, Gangnon R, Musat A, et al. Model for end stage liver disease score predicts mortality across a broad spectrum of liver disease. J Hepatol. 2004 Jun;40(6):897-903.

[27] Brown RS, Jr., Kumar KS, Russo MW, Kinkhabwala M, Rudow DL, Harren P, et al. Model for end-stage liver disease and Child-Turcotte-Pugh score as predictors of pretransplantation disease severity, posttransplantation outcome, and resource utilization in United Network for Organ Sharing status 2A patients. Liver Transpl. 2002 Mar;8(3):278-84.

[28] Aller R, Moya J, Moreira V, Boixeda D, Picher J, Garcia-Rull S, et al. Etiology and frequency of gas exchange abnormalities in cirrhosis. Rev Esp Enferm Dig. 1999 Aug;91(8):559-68.

[29] Yigit IP, Hacievliyagil SS, Seckin Y, Oner RI, Karincaoglu M. The relationship between severity of liver cirrhosis and pulmonary function tests. Dig Dis Sci. 2008 Jul;53(7):1951-6.

[30] Huffmyer JL, Nemergut EC. Respiratory dysfunction and pulmonary disease in cirrhosis and other hepatic disorders. Respir Care. 2007 Aug;52(8):1030-6.

[31] Iwata T, Inoue K, Nishiyama N, Nagano K, Izumi N, Tsukioka T, et al. Factors predicting early postoperative liver cirrhosis-related complications after lung cancer surgery in patients with liver cirrhosis. Interact Cardiovasc Thorac Surg. 2007 Dec;6(6):720-30.

[32] Iwata T, Inoue K, Nishiyama N, Nagano K, Izumi N, Mizuguchi S, et al. Long-term outcome of surgical treatment for non-small cell lung cancer with comorbid liver cirrhosis. Ann Thorac Surg. 2007 Dec;84(6):1810-7.

[33] Iwasaki A, Shirakusa T, Okabayashi K, Inutsuka K, Yoneda S, Yamamoto S, et al. Lung cancer surgery in patients with liver cirrhosis. Ann Thorac Surg. 2006 Sep;82(3):1027-32.

[34] Ueda Y, Fujii Y, Udagawa H. Thoracic and cardiovascular surgery in Japan during 2006: annual report by the Japanese Association for Thoracic Surgery. Gen Thorac Cardiovasc Surg. 2008 Jul;56(7):365-88.

[35] Thalheimer U, Triantos CK, Samonakis DN, Patch D, Burroughs AK. Infection, coagulation, and variceal bleeding in cirrhosis. Gut. 2005 Apr;54(4):556-63.

[36] Amitrano L, Guardascione MA, Brancaccio V, Balzano A. Coagulation disorders in liver disease. Semin Liver Dis. 2002 Feb;22(1):83-96.

[37] Bosch J, Abraldes JG. Management of gastrointestinal bleeding in patients with cirrhosis of the liver. Semin Hematol. 2004 Jan;41(1 Suppl 1):8-12.

[38] Odelowo OO, Smoot DT, Kim K. Upper gastrointestinal bleeding in patients with liver cirrhosis. J Natl Med Assoc. 2002 Aug;94(8):712-5.

[39] Rabinovitz M, Schade RR, Dindzans V, Van Thiel DH, Gavaler JS. Prevalence of duodenal ulcer in cirrhotic males referred for liver transplantation. Does the etiology of cirrhosis make a difference? Dig Dis Sci. 1990 Mar;35(3):321-6.

[40] Moriwaki H, Shiraki M, Iwasa J, Terakura Y. Hepatic encephalopathy as a complication of liver cirrhosis: an Asian perspective. J Gastroenterol Hepatol. May;25(5):858-63.

[41] Lee JH, Kim J, Cheong JH, Hyung WJ, Choi SH, Noh SH. Gastric cancer surgery in cirrhotic patients: result of gastrectomy with D2 lymph node dissection. World J Gastroenterol. 2005 Aug 14;11(30):4623-7.

[42] Franzetta M, Raimondo D, Giammanco M, Di Trapani B, Passariello P, Sammartano A, et al. Prognostic factors of cirrhotic patients in extra-hepatic surgery. Minerva Chir. 2003 Aug;58(4):541-4.

[43] Merli M, Nicolini G, Angeloni S, Riggio O. Malnutrition is a risk factor in cirrhotic patients undergoing surgery. Nutrition. 2002 Nov-Dec;18(11-12):978-86.

[44] Vilstrup H. Cirrhosis and bacterial infections. Rom J Gastroenterol. 2003 Dec;12(4):297-302.

[45] Iwata T, Nishiyama N, Nagano K, Izumi N, Mizuguchi S, Morita R, et al. Pulmonary resection for non-small cell lung cancer in patients with hepatocellular carcinoma. World J Surg. 2008 Oct;32(10):2204-12.

3

The Effect of One Lung Ventilation on Intrapulmonary Shunt During Different Anesthetic Techniques

Gordana Taleska and Trajanka Trajkovska
University Clinic of Anesthesiology, Reanimation and Intensive Care, Medical Faculty, University "Sv.Kiril I Metodij", Skopje, Macedonia

1. Introduction

To facilitate the work of the thoracic surgeon it has become accepted procedure in certain circumstances to collapse the diseased lung being operated upon. To accomplish this, the technique most frequently used by the anaesthetist calls for the insertion of a double lumen endobronchial tube. This makes it possible to isolate the intact dependent lung from the diseased upper one and thus to prevent contamination of the sound lung. On the other hand, collapse of the uppermost lung causes serious functional respiratory modifications which call for special compensatory measures to avoid hypoxaemia. The purpose of this study is to stress again that optimum maintenance of oxygenation is crucial for the prevention of sustained cellular hypoxia and to show how this may be achieved (1-3).
During one-lung ventilation (OLV) with patients in the lateral decubitus position, there is a potential risk of considerable intrapulmonary shunting of deoxygenated pulmonary arterial blood, which may result in hypoxemia. The consequences of an increase in pulmonary vascular resistance (PVR) in the nondependent (nonventilated) lung is to redistribute blood flow to the ventilated dependent lung, thereby preventing PaO2 from excessive decrease. This increase in nondependent lung pulmonary vascular resistance is predominantly due to hypoxic pulmonary vasoconstriction (HPV) (4-8).

2. Physiological consequences of the lateral decubitus position

Sometimes, even in normal situations, and especially when there is a disease, a number of zones in the lungs are well ventilated, but the blood doesn't run through their vessels, while there are other areas with extraordinary blood flow, but with poor or no ventilation at all. It is clear that in each of the mentioned conditions the gas exchange through the respiratory membrane is seriously damaged, leading to severe respiratory difficulties, although the total ventilation and the total blood flow through the lungs are regular. A new concept is formulated on this basis, helping understand the respiratory gas exchange even when there is a disturbance of the relation between alveolar ventilation and alveolar blood flow. This term is so called ventilation/perfusion ratio, expressed in quantitative sense as Va/Qt.
In the awake subject, there is little or no additional ventilation/perfusion mismatch in the lateral position. The situation changes during anaesthesia. In the spontaneously breathing subject, there is a reduction in inspiratory muscle tone (particularly the diaphragm) and a

decrease in the volume of both lungs with a reduction in functional residual capacity. The compliance of the non-dependent upper lung increases and it receives more ventilation. Paralysis and intermittent positive pressure ventilation are used during thoracotomy and the compliance of the non-dependent lung is increased even further. In practice, it is usual to selectively ventilate the lower lung (OLV) at this point and allow the upper lung to collapse. This eliminates the preferential ventilation and facilitates surgical access, but creates the more serious problem of ventilation/perfusion mismatch (9).

3. Venous admixture

Pulmonary blood flow continues to the upper lung during one-lung anaesthesia, creating a true shunt in a lung where there is blood flow to the alveoli but no ventilation. This shunt is the major cause of hypoxaemia during OLV, although the alveoli with low ventilation/perfusion ratios in the dependent lung also contribute. In addition, the blood to the upper lung cannot take up oxygen and therefore retains its poorly oxygenated mixed venous composition. This mixes with oxygenated blood in the left atrium causing venous admixture and lowering arterial oxygen tension (PaO2). Total venous admixture can be calculated from the shunt equation which estimates what proportion of the pulmonary blood flow would have bypassed ventilated alveoli to produce the arterial blood gas values for a particular patient. Venous admixture and shunt (Qs/Qt) are often used synonymously. Venous admixture increases from a value of approximately 10% - 15% during two-lung ventilation to 30% - 40% during OLV. The PaO2 can be maintained in the range of 9–16 kPa with an inspired oxygen concentration between 50% and 100% in the majority of patients.

4. Hypoxic pulmonary vasoconstriction and one-lung ventilation

Hypoxic pulmonary vasocontriction (HPV) is a mechanism whereby pulmonary blood flow is diverted away from hypoxic/collapsed areas of lung. This should improve oxygenation during OLV. Volatile anaesthetic agents depress HPV directly, but also enhance HPV by reducing cardiac output. There is therefore no change in the HPV response with volatile agents during thoracotomy and OLV.

Intravenous agents, such as propofol, do not inhibit HPV and should improve arterial oxygenation during OLV. There is some evidence to support this contention (10-17).

5. Cardiac output

Changes in cardiac output affect arterial oxygenation during thoracotomy. A decrease in cardiac output results in a reduced mixed venous oxygen content. Some of this desaturated blood is shunted during OLV and further exacerbates arterial hypoxaemia. Cardiac output can decrease for a number of reasons during thoracotomy. These include blood loss/fluid depletion, the use of high inflation pressures and the application of positive end-expiratory pressure (PEEP) to the dependent lung. Surgical manipulation and retraction around the mediastinum, causing a reduction in venous return, are probably the commonest causes of a sudden drop in cardiac output during lung resection (18-20).

6. Principles of ventilation

OLV should be established to adequately inflate the lung but also minimize intra-alveolar pressure and so prevent diversion of pulmonary blood flow to the upper lung. In practice, this is not easy to achieve. It is reasonable to use an inspired oxygen concentration of 50% initially, which can be increased to 100%, if required. This cannot affect the true shunt in the upper lung but improves oxygenation through the alveoll with low V/Q ratios in the lower lung. Overinflating the single lung ('volutrauma') can be detrimental and lead to acute lung injury. Deflation and inflation of the operative lung with the potential for ischaemia/reperfusion injury has also been implicated in lung damage. The use of low tidal volumes improves outcome in ventilated patients with adult respiratory distress syndrome (ARDS) and this may also apply to OLV. Limiting ventilation can lead to carbon dioxide retention, but a degree of permissive hypercapnia is preferable to lung trauma (21-25).

7. Hypoxia during one-lung ventilation

It is difficult to predict which patients are likely to be hypoxic (SpO_2 < 90%) during OLV. Patients with poor lung function are sometimes accepted for lung resection on the basis that their diseased lung is contributing little to gas exchange and this can be confirmed by V/Q scanning. Conversely, patients with normal lung function are more likely to be hypoxic during OLV because an essentially normal lung is collapsed to provide surgical access. The most significant predictors of a low arterial oxygen saturation during OLV are (1) a right-sided operation, (2) a low oxygen saturation during two-lung ventilation prior to OLV and (3) a high (or more normal) forced expiratory volume in 1 sec. preoperatively. Once hypoxia occurs, it is important to check the position of the endobronchial tube and readjust this if necessary. A high inflation pressure (> 30–35 cmH_2O) may indicate that the tube is displaced. It may be helpful to analyse a flow/volume loop or at least manually reinflate the lung to feel the compliance. If a tube is obstructing a lobar orifice, only one or two lobes are being ventilated at most and hypoxia is likely to occur. Suction and manual reinflation of the dependent lung may be useful.Other measures which can be used to improve oxygenation include increasing the inspired oxygen concentration, introducing PEEP to the dependent lung, or supplying oxygen to the upper lung via a continuous positive airway system, thereby reducing the shunt. In the face of persistent arterial hypoxaemia during OLV, it is pertinent to ask 'What is a low PaO_2 for this patient?'. An oxygen saturation below 90% is commonly tolerated. This arbitrary figure is affected by a variety of factors, including acidosis and temperature. Many patients will have a low PaO_2 when measured while breathing air preoperatively; hence, the usefulness of this preoperative measurement. Arterial hypoxaemia is obviously undesirable but it may be preferable to accept a PaO_2 slightly lower than the preoperative value, rather than undertake measures such as upper lung inflation which may hinder and prolong surgery (26-31).

8. Thoracic epidural anesthesia

Thoracic epidural anesthesia (TEA) with local anesthetics during OLV is increasingly being combined with general anesthesia (GA) in our clinical practice for thoracic surgery. A combination of TEA with GA might maximize the benefits of each form of anesthesia. Furthermore, epidural anesthesia and postoperative epidural analgesia with their effects that exceed pain release, may improve outcome in high-risk patients (32,33).

Thoracic epidural anesthesia reduces the incidence of respiratory complications as well as thoracic morbidity. Besides the excellent postoperative analgesia, it improves the strength and coordination of respiratory muscles; blocking the inhibitory phrenic reflex recovers the function of the diaphragm and the lungs, decreasing the occurrence of athelectasis as well as lung infections. On account of all these effects, the thoracic epidural anesthesia permits early extubation along with decreased length of ICU treatment.

This type of anesthetic technique provides particular advantage in COPD patients as well as cardiac patients: controls tachyarrhythmia, lessens thrombotic complications, liberates from the angina pectoris, reduces myocardial straining, improves left-ventricular function, and makes the balance of myocardial oxygen supply better. By blocking sympathetic nervous system, the high thoracic epidural technique leads to vasodilatation and hypotension, reducing cardiac output. Furthermore, the consequence mentioned above enhances skin perfusion and improves the oxygen supply of peripheral tissues (34).

The blockade of the afferent nervous impulses made by the thoracic epidural anesthesia prevents and modifies neuro-endocrine, metabolic, immune, as well as autonomic response of the human body to surgical stress.

Potential disadvantages include the time required to establish epidural anesthesia, intravascular fluid administration needed to avoid hypotension, and the potential for technical complications, such as epidural hematoma.

The effect of intraoperative TEA with local anesthetics on HPV during thoracic surgery and OLV is unclear. Up till now, there isn't sufficient number of studies in the literature, capable to offer a definite answer to this dilemma. The pulmonary vasculature is innervated by the autonomic nervous system, and the sympathetic tone is dominant in the pulmonary circulation relative to parasympathetic activity. Theoretically, a TEA-induced sympathectomy might attenuate HPV (35). However, in one recent experimental study, TEA did not affect the primary pulmonary vascular tone, but it improved $PaO2$ because of enhanced blood flow diversion from the hypoxic lobe (36-38).

Our aim in this study was:

- To determine the quantity of intrapulmonary shunt during general anesthesia and OLV.
- To determine the quantity of intrapulmonary shunt during combination of thoracic epidural anesthesia and general anesthesia with OLV.
- To compare the values of intrapulmonary shunt in both mentioned techniques.

9. Material and methods

This prospective, longitudinal, randomized, interventional clinical study was performed at the Clinic of Anesthesiology, Reanimation and Intensive care and the Clinic of Thoracic-vascular surgery in Skopje, after getting an approvalal by our ethics committee, and signed, informed consent from each patient.

We studied 60 patients who underwent elective lung surgery (by thoracotomy / thoracoscopy), or other surgical procedure which required OLV in lateral decubitus position (LDP). Patients were randomized to one of two study groups by lottery: general iv anesthesia (GA group = Group A) or general iv anesthesia combined with TEA (TEA group = Group B).

Inclusion criteria:

- Patients undergoing lung resection (by thoracotomy: pneumonectomy, bilobectomy, lobectomy,segmentectomy) or thoracoscopic procedures;
- Procedures other than lung resection, requiring OLV in LDP;
- Age between 15 and 75 years;

- ASA 1, 2;
- Preoperative values of $SaO_2 \geq 90\%$.

Exclusion criteria:

- Renal insufficiency (creatinine>114 umol/L);
- Liver dysfunction (aspartate amino transferase-AST >40 U/L, alanine amino transferase-ALT >40 U/L);
- Documented coronary or vascular disease (EF<50%);
- Previously existing chronic respiratory disease of non-operated lung;
- FVC, FEV1 < 50%,
- Patients who intraoperatively needed $FiO_2>0.5$.

Exclusion criteria from TEA group:

- Patients with serious haemostatic disorders and/or those under anticoagulant therapy (<12 hours since the last dose of LMWH);
- Patients with serious deformities of the vertebral column, neurological diseases, and/or
- Infection in the thoracic or lumbosacral region of the spine.

The methods used in this study included as follows:

Clinical evaluation: For all patients, preoperative assessment included: clinical examination, chest X-ray, echocardiography, measurements of forced vital capacity (FVC), forced expiratory volume in 1 sec. (FEV1), these values as a percentage of predicted values (FVC%, FEV1%), coagulation tests, standard biochemical analysis, and arterial blood gas analysis on the evening before surgery.

Anesthesia: In the GA group (group A), general anesthesia was induced using fentanyl iv (3 μg/kg), midazolam (2–3 mg), and propofol (2 mg/kg); rocuronium (0.6 mg/kg) or succinyl cholin (1 mg/kg) was given to facilitate intubation of the trachea with a double-lumen endobronchial tube. Anesthesia was maintained with propofol at continuous perfusion (6–7 mg/kg/h), with increments of fentanyl (2 μg/kg) to maintain the systolic blood pressure within 15 mm Hg of post induction values and rocuronium at continuous perfusion (0.3 mg/kg/h), or pancuronium (0,01 mg/kg).

In the TEA group - group B (combined anesthesia), an epidural catheter was placed at the Th5-6, Th6-7 or Th7-8 interspaces and advanced 3 cm in the epidural space before anaesthesia induction. TEA was then induced using an initial 6 to 8-ml dose of plain bupivacaine 0.5%; if necessary, additional increment doses up to 14 ml were administered until a thoracic-sensitive blockade was induced. The level of anesthesia was determined by the loss of pinprick sensation. During the onset of epidural anesthesia, colloids were infused (7 ml/kg); crystalloids (8 ml/kg/h) were subsequently infused throughout the study (the same rate as in group A), and when systolic arterial blood pressure decreased to 100 mm Hg, ephedrine was planned to be injected in increments of 5 mg (yet, no patient received ephedrine). GA was induced using the same method as in group A. After tracheal intubation, with a double-lumen endobronchial tube, anesthesia was maintained by continuous epidural infusion (6–8 ml/h) of bupivacaine 0.25%, plus propofol in continuous perfusion (6–7 mg/kg/h) and rocuronium (0.3 mg/kg/h) in continuous perfusion, or pancuronium (0.01 mg/kg), as well as fentanyl.

In both groups, fluid replacement and transfusion management were based on hemodynamic monitoring and were under the direction of the attending anesthesiologist.

After the induction of anesthesia, an arterial catheter was placed in the radial artery, contra lateral from the operated side, with the intention of extraction of arterial blood samples and consequent blood gases and intrapulmonary shunt analysis.

After clinical confirmation of correct double-lumen tube placement (by inspection and auscultation) with the patient in both supine and lateral decubitus position, ventilation was controlled (volume-controlled mechanical ventilation – VC) by using 50% oxygen in air (for all patients) and tidal volume of 6-8 ml/kg at a respiratory rate to maintain PaCO2 between 35 and 40 mm Hg (4, 5 – 6 kPa). Effective lung isolation was determined by the absence of leak from the nonventilated lumen of the endobronchial tube. When the pleura was opened, the isolation was confirmed by direct observation of the collapsed nonventilated lung and the absence of leak from this lung. During OLV, the same tidal volume, respiratory rate, and fraction of inspired oxygen were used; the bronchus of the lung not being ventilated upon was excluded and open to atmospheric pressure.
Monitoring during anesthesia:

- heart rate (HR)
- ECG
- mean arterial pressure (MAP)
- respiratory rate (RR)
- oxygen saturation from pulsoxymetry – SAT%
- inspired oxygen fraction – FiO2
- partial pressure of carbon dioxide in arterial blood – PaCO2

Measurments – in 4 stages (always in lateral position):

- **T0** - during TLV
- **T1** - immediately after beginning of OLV
- **T2** - 10 min. after beginning of OLV
- **T3** - 30 min after beginning of OLV

Blood samples were drawn simultaneously from the arterial catheter and analyzed within 10 min., using the blood gases analyzator AVL **Compact 3 BLOOD GAS** (which is used in our Intensive Care Unit).
Parameters evaluated in these 4 stages:

- partial pressure of oxygen in arterial blood **(PaO2)**
- oxygen saturation of arterial blood **(SaO2)**
- intrapulmonary shunt value **(Qs/Qt).**

The Qs/Qt% is usually calculated using the venous admixture equation:

$$\mathbf{Qs / Qt\,\% = (Cc'O2 - CaO2) / (Cc'O2 - CvO2) \times 100}$$

$$\mathbf{Cc'O2 = (Hb \times 1.39) \times SaO2 + (PaO2 \times 0.0031)}$$

$$\mathbf{C(a\ or\ v)O2 = (1.39 \times Hb \times SaO2) + (0.0031 \times PO2)},$$
$$(PO2 = PaO2 \text{ or } PvO2)$$

But for the purpose of this study, the quantitative value of **Qs/Qt %** was mathematically calculated by the blood gases analyzator **AVL Compact 3 BLOOD GAS**.
Statistical analysis was performed using specific computer programs. Collected data were processed with standard descriptive and analitical bivariant and multivariant methods. Statistical significance of discrepancies between atributive series was tested using Student t – test and Mann-Whitney U test. The probability for association between distributions of frequencies of two atributive variables was evaluated with x^2 - test.

Statistical relevance of dissimilarities inside groups was analysed with ANOVA test, which was additionaly confirmed with post hoc test - Tukey honest significant difference (HSD) test.
For CI (confindence interval) was considered $p<0,05$.
Results were displayed with table and graph illustrations.

10. Results

10.1 Demographic data

60 patients were enrolled in the study, 47 of which were men, and 13 were women (p=0,020). The examinated patients were divided in two groups, each with 30 pts: group A, whose patients underwent thoracic surgery with OLV in general anesthesia, and Group B, subjected to the same operative procedure, performed in combined general and thoracic epidural anesthesia.
Graph 1 demonstrates patients' gender in groups, showing that no statistically significant difference exists between two examinated groups of patients.

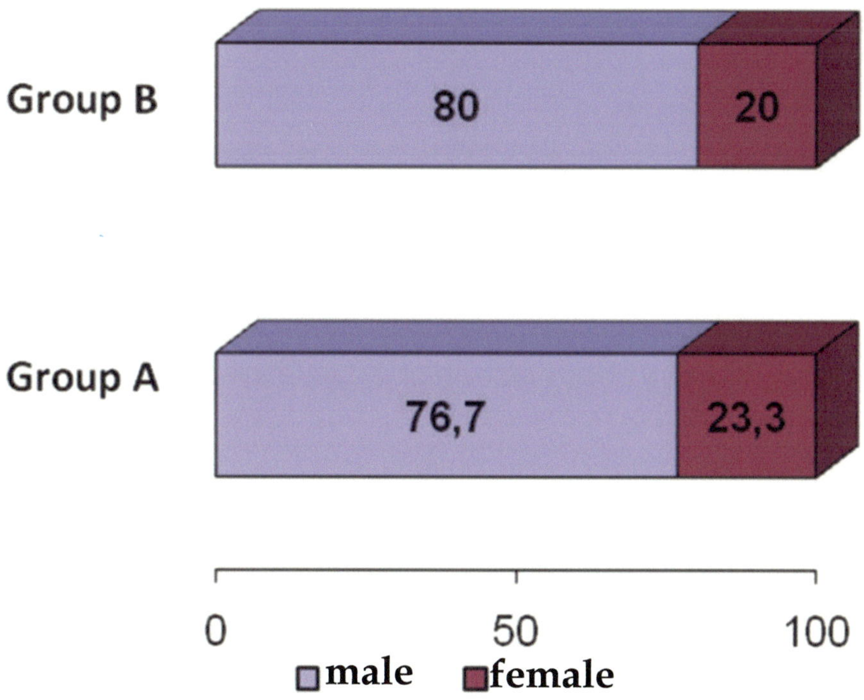

Graph 1. Gender distribution of patients

In group A are recorded 76,7% male pts and 23,3% females. Percentage variation registered among gender categories is statistically significant for p=0,0001. In group B 80,0% pts are male, and 20,0% female. This proportion dissimilarity is also statistically significant for p=0,0000. The diversity recorded among genders between two examinated groups is statistically irrelevant for p>0,05, confirming similarity i.e. equal presence of genders among two studied groups of patients (Graph 1).

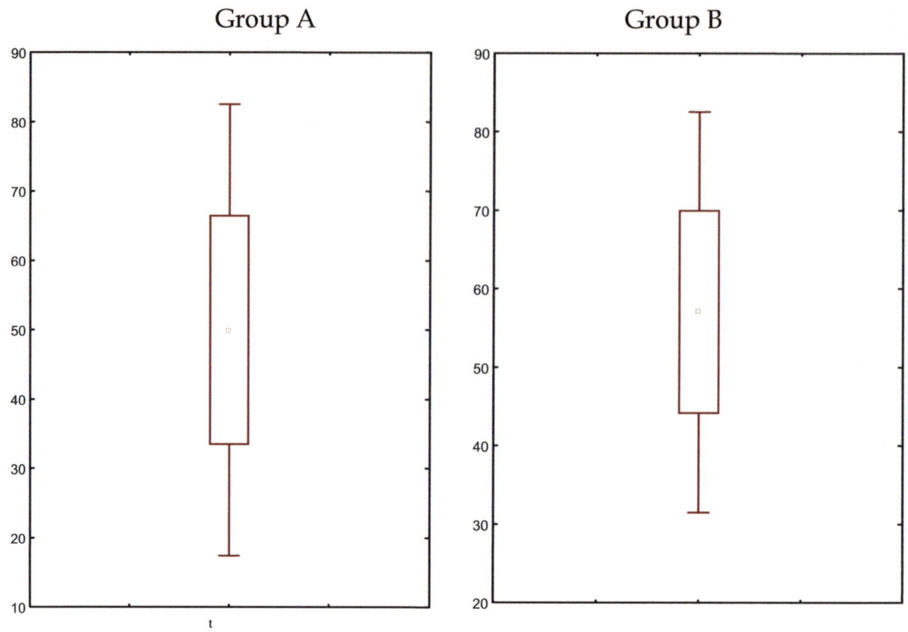

Graph 2. Average age of patients

The average age of patients in group A is 49,96±16,6 years, minimum 17, maximum 74 years. The average age of patients in group B is 57,03±13,0 years, minimum 26, maximum 78 years. The recorded difference in average age of patients among two studied groups is statistically insignificant for p=0,0714 (Graph 2).

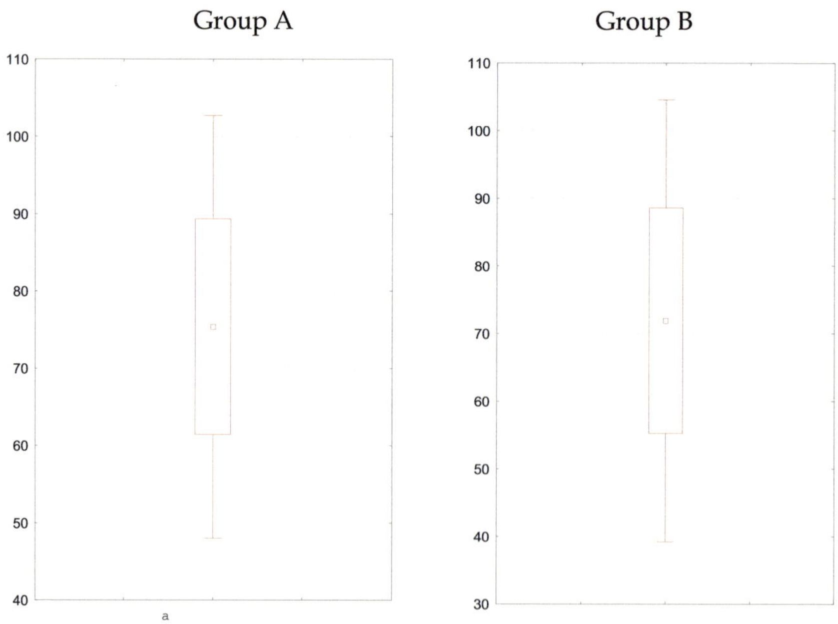

Graph 3. Average body weight of patients

The average body weight of patients in group A is 75,4±14,0 kg, minimum 53,7, maximum 105 kg. The average body weight of patients in group B is 72,0±16,7 kg, minimum 40, maximum 120 kg. The difference in average body weight recorded between patients from two examinated groups is not statistically important for p=0,359335 (Graph 3).

10.2 Clinical assessment

In group A, ASA 1 status is listed in 36,7% of patients, while in 63,3% pts ASA 2 status is recorded. In group B, 33,3% of patients had ASA 1 status, whereas 66,7% had status ASA 2. The percentage variety registered between the presence of ASA 1 and 2 inside both groups is statistically significant for p<0,05; on the other hand, percentage difference among both groups A and B is statistically insignificant for p>0,05 (Graph 4).

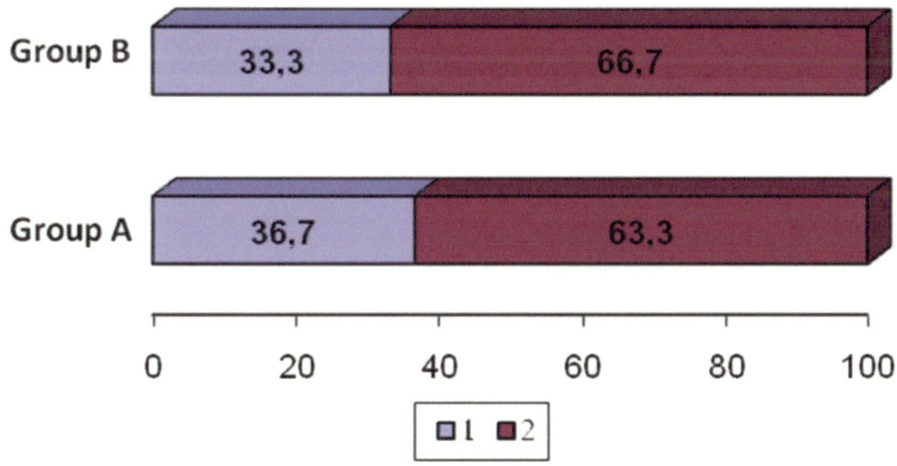

Graph 4. Distribution of patients according to ASA classification

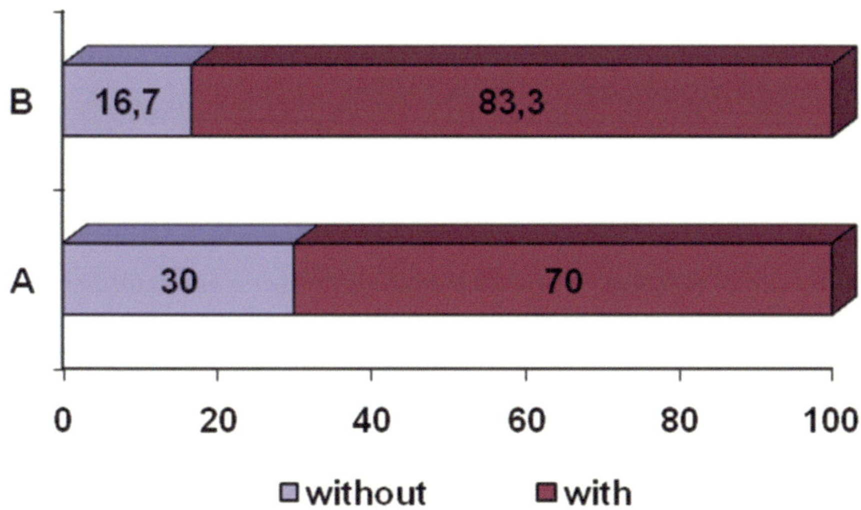

Graph 5. Patients with / without positive medical history in both groups

30,0% of patients in group A don't have positive medical history for co-morbidities, and in group B - 16,7%; the difference is not statistically important for p>0,05. In both groups of patients, the most frequently recorded co-morbidities are smoking, hypertension, diabetes, duodenal ulcer etc. In some patients more than one disorder is listed (Graph 5).

Biochemistry	Rank Sum-A	Rank Sum-B	U	Z	p-level
Hb	916,5	913,5	448,5	0,022177	0,982307
Hct	941,0	889,0	424,0	0,384395	0,700686
Creatinin	872,5	957,5	407,5	-0,628338	0,529783
ALT	1027,5	802,5	337,5	1,663248	0,096264
AST	998,0	832,0	367,0	1,227107	0,219783

Table 1. Mann-Whitney U test for preoperative laboratory data

The average values of laboratory data (hemoglobin, hematocrit, creatinin, ALT, AST) in both studied groups are in the range of referent values. The recorded difference in average values of examinated parameters among two groups of patients is statistically insignificant for p>0,05, according to Mann-Whitney U test (Table 1).

Screening haemostasis	Rank Sum-A	Rank Sum-B	U	Z	p-level
PT	963,5	866,5	401,5	0,71704	0,473347
aPTT	802,0	1028,0	337,0	-1,67064	0,094794
TT	854,5	975,5	389,5	-0,89446	0,371078
PLT	913,5	916,50	448,5	-0,02218	0,982307

Table 2. Mann-Whitney U test for screening haemostasis

The average values of PT, aPTT, TT and PLT from haemostasis in both studied groups are in the range of refferent values. The recorded difference between these average values among two groups is statistically insignificant for p>0,05, according to Mann-Whitney U test (Table 2).

Gas status	Rank Sum-A	Rank Sum-B	U	Z	p-level
PaO2	934,0	896,0	431,0	0,280904	0,778784
PaCO2	979,0	851,0	386,0	0,946203	0,344046
SaO2	890,0	940,0	425,0	-0,369611	0,711673

Table 3. Mann-Whitney U test for preoperative gas status

The average values of PaO2, PaCO2 and SaO2 from preoperative gas status in both studied groups are in extend of refferent values. The recorded differentiation between these values among two groups is not statistically significant for p>0,05, in accordance with Mann-Whitney U test (Table 3).

Graph 6 shows the dispersal of patients from both examinated groups in relation to the value of preoperative intrapulmonary shunt - Qs/Qt.

The average values of FVC and FEV1 in patients from both studied groups are in range of refferent values. The recorded variation between these average values among the two groups is statistically irrelevant for p>0,05, consistent with Mann-Whitney U test (Table 4).

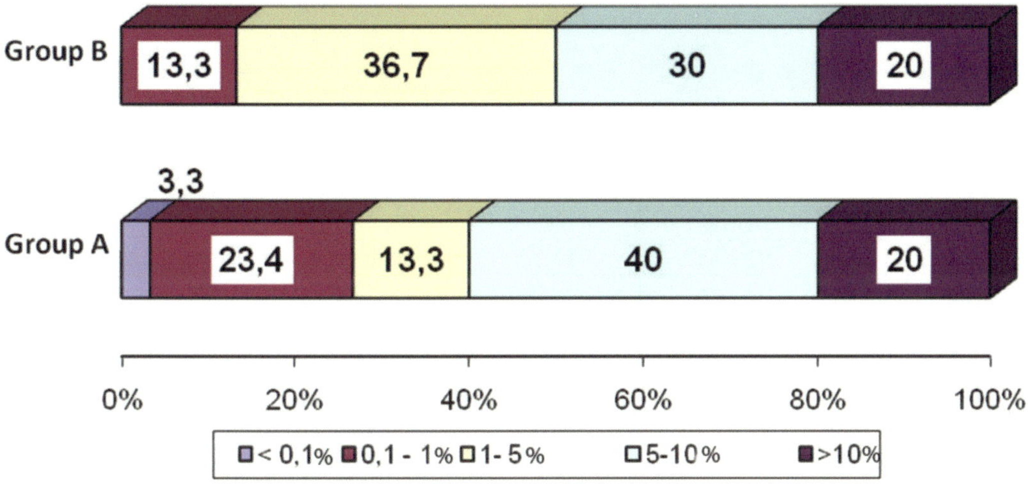

Graph 6. Preoperative value of intrapulmonary shunt (Qs/Qt)

	Rank Sum-A	Rank Sum-B	U	Z	p-level
FVC	850,5	979,5	385,5	-0,95360	0,340289
FEV1	831,0	999,0	366,0	-1,24189	0,214277

Table 4. Mann-Whitney U test for FVC and FEV1

	Rank Sum-A	Rank Sum- B	U	Z	p-level
EF%	465,0	1365,0	0,00	-6,65299	0,000000*

Table 5. Mann-Whitney U test for EF%

The average values of EF% in patients from both examinated groups are in extend of refferent values. The disclosed difference between these parameters among two groups is statistically significant for **p=0,00000***, according to Mann-Whitney U test (Table 5), but without clinical importance.

10.3 Intraoperative monitoring

Average values of HR/min. in both groups show rise during the operative monitoring from T0 to T3. The difference in HR/min. between groups A and B (Mann-Whitney U test) is statistically significant only for T0 and T3 (**p=0,02* and p=0,04***). On the other hand, the differences in these values inside groups A and B (ANOVA test) are statistically insignificant (Tables 6, 7).

Average values of MAP/mmHg in both groups illustrate increase during the operative monitoring from T0 to T2, and then decrease in T3. This difference between groups A and B is statistically irrelevant. Inside groups, the discrepancy of average values of MAP/mmHg is statistically significant only in group A (**p=0,019***).These statistically relevant differences for HR/min. and MAP/mmHg don't have clinical importance (Table 6,7).

Parameters	Rank Sum-A	Rank Sum-B	U	Z	p-level
HR/minT0	1076,500	753,500	288,5000	2,38768	0,016955*
HR/min T1	969,000	861,000	396,0000	0,79836	0,424663
HR/min T2	1020,000	810,000	345,0000	1,55236	0,120576
HR/min T3	1049,000	781,000	316,0000	1,98111	0,047579*
MAP/mmHg T0	787,000	1043,000	322,0000	-1,89241	0,058438
MAP/mmHg T1	916,000	914,000	449,0000	0,01478	0,988204
MAP/mmHg T2	922,000	908,000	443,0000	0,10349	0,917573
MAP/mmHg T3	857,000	973,000	392,0000	-0,85750	0,391171
RR/min T0	915,000	915,000	450,0000	0,00000	1,000000
RR/min T1	986,500	843,500	378,5000	1,05709	0,290473
RR/min T2	973,000	857,000	392,0000	0,85750	0,391171
RR/min T3	942,000	888,000	423,0000	0,39918	0,689761
SAT% T0	1021,000	809,000	344,0000	1,56715	0,117081
SAT% T1	1009,500	820,500	355,5000	1,39713	0,162376
SAT% T2	961,000	869,000	404,0000	0,68008	0,496452
SAT% T3	915,000	915,000	450,0000	0,00000	1,000000
PCO_2/mmHg T0	914,500	915,500	449,5000	-0,00739	0,994102
PCO_2/mmHg T1	953,500	876,500	411,5000	0,56920	0,569221
PCO_2/mmHg T2	912,500	917,500	447,5000	-0,03696	0,970516
PCO_2/mmHg T3	919,000	911,000	446,0000	0,05914	0,952842

Table 6. Mann-Whitney U test for parametres of intraoperative monitoring

Group	Monitoring	SS	df	MS	SS	Df	MS	F	P
A	HR/min	236,425	3	78,8083	17165,177	116	147,97566	0,5326	0,660834
	MAP/mmHg	1422,1588	3	474,0528	16113,43	116	138,9089	3,4127	0,019858*8
	RR/min	369,000	3	123,0000	36,87	116	0,3178	387,0163	0,000000*
	SAT%	429,425	3	143,1417	1745,17	116	15,0445	9,5145	0,000011*
	PCO2 /mmHg	20,852	3	6,9508	106,57	116	0,9187	7,5659	0,000115*
B	HR/min	741,6667	3	247,2222	20349,13	116	175,4236	1,4093	0,243640
	MAP/mmHg	119,4917	3	39,8306	25576,10	116	220,4836	0,1807	0,909345
	RR/min	333,0250	3	111,0083	62,10	116	0,5353	207,3586	0,000000*
	SAT%	408,4250	3	136,1417	1267,57	116	10,9273	12,4589	0,000000*
	PCO2 /mmHg	22,8277	3	7,6092	112,34	116	0,9685	7,8570	0,000081*

Table 7. Analysis of Variance –ANOVA test

The average values of RR/min. in both groups show rise during operative monitoring. The differences in these values are insignificant between groups A and B, and statistically significant inside groups (**p=0,00000***) (Tables 6,7). This difference doesn't have clinical importance for the aims of the study (since respiratory rate during OLV is deliberately increased in all patients, in order to decrease the value of PaCO2).

The average values of SAT% in both studied groups demonstrate fall during the operative monitoring. The difference in these values is statistically irrelevant between groups A and B; however, the dissimilarities inside groups A and B is statisticaly significant for **p=0,000011* and p=0,00000*** (Tables 6, 7), showing decrease in arterial oxygen saturation during OLV in patients from both groups.
The average values of PCO2/mmHg in both groups demonstrate increase during operative monitoring. The differences in these values are statistically insignificant between groups A and B; on the other hand, inside groups A and B, the discrepancy is statisticaly significant for **p=0,000115* and p=0,000081*** (Tables 6, 7). This inequality illustrates the phenomenon of so called *permissive hypercapnia* during OLV (which is expected, inspite of therapeutic increase of RR/min., with intention of maintaining PaCO2 in normal range of values).

10.4 Intraoperative gas analysis and intrapulmonary shunt

The average values of PaO2 in both studied groups show fall during the operative monitoring. The differences in these values between groups A and B are statistically insignificant. Inside groups A and B the dissimilarities are statistically significant for **p=0,0000021*** and **p=0,000000***. The additionally performed post-hoc test for PaO2 in group A and B shows which differences (i.e. measuring times) are statistically relevant **(Tables 8, 9, 10, 12).**

Graphs 7. Parametres from intraoperative gas status.

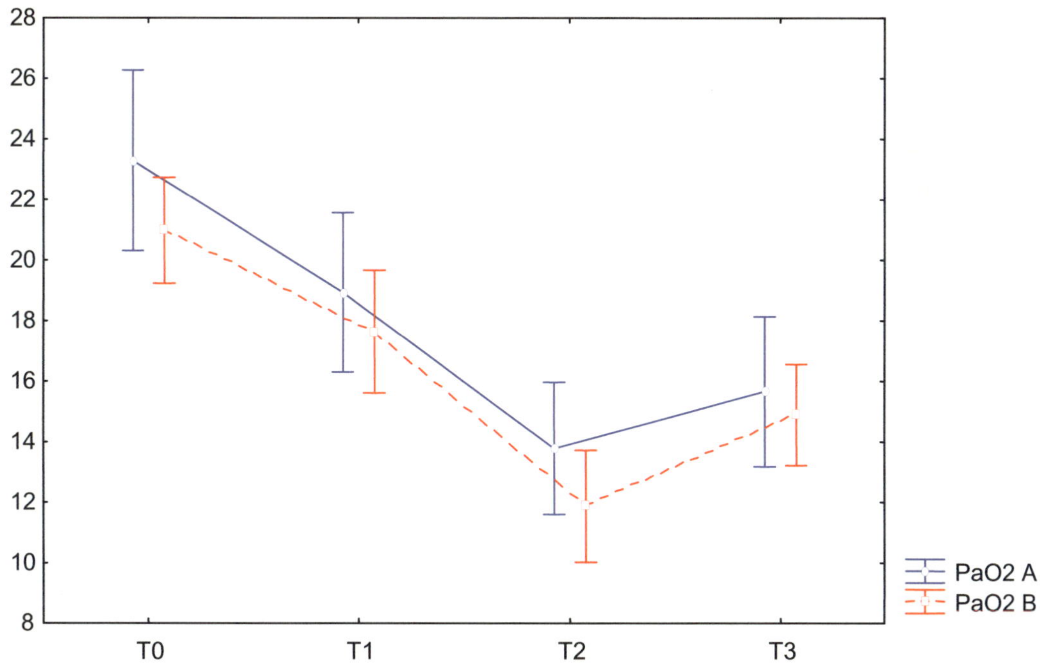

Graph 7a - PaO2 in both groups

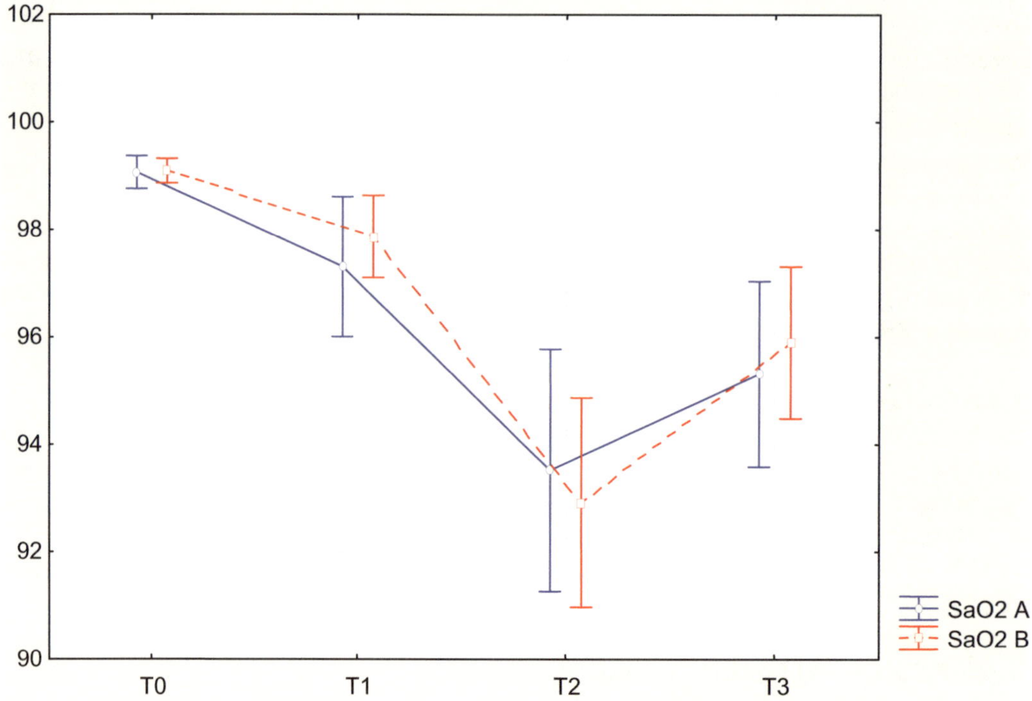

Graph 7b - SaO2 in both groups

Parameters	Rank Sum-A	Rank Sum-B	U	Z	p-level
PaO2 T0	973,000	857,0000	392,0000	0,857497	0,391171
PaO2 T1	961,000	869,0000	404,0000	0,680084	0,496452
PaO2 T2	1019,500	810,5000	345,5000	1,544972	0,122354
PaO2 T3	914,000	916,0000	449,0000	-0,014784	0,988204
SaO2 T0	947,000	883,0000	418,0000	0,473102	0,636141
SaO2 T1	935,000	895,0000	430,0000	0,295689	0,767468
SaO2 T2	978,500	851,5000	386,5000	0,938811	0,347829
SaO2 T3	899,000	931,0000	434,0000	-0,236551	0,813005

Table 8. Mann-Whitney U test

Group	Parameters	SS	df	MS	SS	df	MS	F	p
A	PaO2	1561,721	3	520,5735	5550,851	116	47,85217	10,87879	0,0000021
	SaO2	520,737	3	173,5789	2047,983	116	17,65503	9,83170	0,000008
B	PaO2	1358,527	3	452,8423	2778,338	116	23,95119	18,90688	0,000000
	SaO2	652,413	3	217,4710	1334,600	116	11,50518	18,90201	0,000000

Table 9. Analysis of Variance –ANOVA test

PaO2	T0	T1	T2	T3
T0		0,075231	0,000139*	0,000352*
T1	0,075231		0,024138*	0,265002
T2	0,000139*	0,024138*		0,719175
T3	0,000352*	0,265002	0,719175	

Table 10. Post- hoc - Tukey honest significant difference (HSD) test for Group A - PaO2

SaO2	T0	T1	T2	T3
T0		0,371996	0,000142*	0,004258*
T1	0,371996		0,003861*	0,259930
T2	0,000142*	0,003861*		0,355108
T3	0,004258*	0,259930	0,355108	

Table 11. Post-hoc - Tukey honest significant difference (HSD) test for Group A - SaO2

PaO2	T0	T1	T2	T3
T0		0,045269*	0,000137*	0,000158*
T1	0,045269*		0,000202*	0,135773
T2	0,000137*	0,000202*		0,086017
T3	0,000158*	0,135773	0,086017	

Table 12. Post-hoc - Tukey honest significant difference (HSD) test for Group B - PaO2

SaO2	T0	T1	T2	T3
T0		0,503957	0,000137*	0,002297*
T1	0,503957		0,000137*	0,115369
T2	0,000137*	0,000137*		0,005223*
T3	0,002297*	0,115369	0,005223*	

Table 13. Post-hoc - Tukey honest significant difference (HSD) test for Group B - SaO2

The average values of SaO2 in both groups illustrate decrease during the operative monitoring. The difference between these values among groups A and B is statistically insignificant. Inside groups A and B, the discrepancies are statistically relevant for **p=0,000008*** and **p=0,000000***. The additionally performed post-hoc test for SaO2 in groups A and B demonstrates which differences (i.e. measuring times) are statistically relevant **(Tables 8, 9, 11, 13).**

The acquired statistically significant differences for PaO2 and SaO2 inside the groups A and B show that after some time of OLV initiation (after 10 min.) hypoxia develops, with decrease of the values of PaO2 and SaO2.

The absence of statistically relevant variation for PaO2 and SaO2 among the groups A and B demonstrates that TEA doesn't provoke augmentation of hypoxia during OLV.

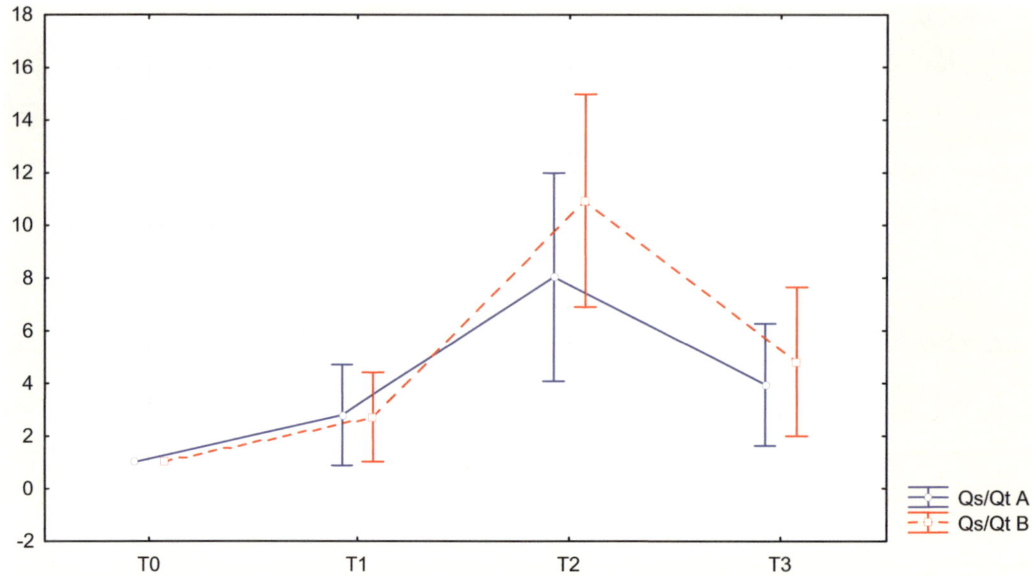

Graph 8. Average intraoperative values of intrapulmonary shunt - Qs/Qt in both groups

Parameters	Rank Sum-A	Rank Sum-B	U	Z	p-level
Qs/Qt T0	915,0000	915,0000	450,0000	0,000000	1,000000
Qs/Qt T1	925,0000	905,0000	440,0000	0,147844	0,882466
Qs/Qt T2	853,5000	976,5000	388,5000	-0,909242	0,363223
Qs/Qt T3	939,0000	891,0000	426,0000	0,354826	0,722720

Table 14. Mann-Whitney U test

Group	Parameters	SS	df	MS	SS	df	MS	F	p
A	Qs/Qt	801,6449	3	267,2150	5133,088	116	44,25076	6,038653	0,000739
B	Qs/Qt	1692,620	3	564,2068	5648,059	116	48,69017	11,58769	0,000001

Table 15. Analysis of Variance -ANOVA test

Qs/Qt	T0	T1	T2	T3
T0		0,725131	0,000563*	0,320393
T1	0,725131		0,014827*	0,907021
T2	0,000563*	0,014827*		0,086875
T3	0,320393	0,907021	0,086875	

Table 16. Post-hoc - Tukey honest significant difference (HSD) test for Group A - Qs/Qt

Qs/Qt	T0	T1	T2	T3
T0		0,776395	0,000137*	0,152861
T1	0,776395		0,000202*	0,648599
T2	0,000137*	0,000202*		0,005223*
T3	0,152861	0,648599	0,005223*	

Table 17. Post-hoc - Tukey honest significant difference (HSD) test for Group B - Qs/Qt

The average values of Qs/Qt in both inspected groups illustrate dynamic trend during the operative monitoring. In group A it begins with the value < 1 in T0, increases in T2, and then decreases in T3. In group B it also starts with a value < 1 in T0, grows up in T2, and then the value drops. The difference between the average values of Qs/Qt recorded among groups A and B is statistically insignificant. On the other hand, the variations in these values inside groups A and B are statistically relevant for **p=0,000739*** and **p=0,000001***. With the additionally performed post-hoc test for Qs/Qt in group A it is evident that the difference is statistically significant **between T0 and T2 and T1 and T2.** The completed post-hoc test for Qs/Qt in group B shows that the dissimilarity is statistically relevant **between T0 and T2, T1 and T2 , as well as T2 and T3 (Tables 14-17).**

The obtained statistically significant differences for Qs/Qt inside groups A and B demonstrate that some time after beginning of OLV (after 10 min.) hypoxia develops, with an increase of the value of intrapulmonary shunt.

The nonexistence of statistically relevant dissimilarity for Qs/Qt among the groups A and B, confirms that TEA neither leads to intensification of hypoxia, nor to an increase of the shunt during OLV.

11. Discussion

OLV creates an obligatory transpulmonary shunt through the atelectatic lung. Passive (gravitation and surgical manipulation) and active (HPV) mechanisms minimize the redirection of blood flow towards the atelectatic lung, thus preventing the fall of PaO2; yet, the most important turn of the blood flow towards the dependent lung is caused by HPV (39).

Hurford et al. in their study (40) tested the hypothesis that during OLV is more likely to come to intraoperative hypoxia if there is bigger pulmonary blood flow in the operated lung before surgery. In their study they examinated 30 patients with previously performed ventilation-perfusion scan preoperatively, who underwent a thoracic procedure in lateral decubitus position with OLV. The percentage of blood flow in the operated lung seen on the preoperative perfusion scan reversely correlated with PaO2, 10 minutes after initiating of OLV (p=-.72). If the percentage of blood flow in the operated lung on the preoperative scan was greater than 45%, the probability for hypoxemia (PaO2 < 75 mm Hg) was bigger. Since the preoperative regional ventilation in these patients was equivalent with the perfusion, also the percentage of preoperative ventilation correlated reversely with PaO2 after 10 min. of OLV initiation (p=-.73). *The arterial gas analyses, pulmonary functional tests and pulmonary volumes, were not associated with the oxygenation during OLV.*

This is opposite of the results of Slinger et al. (41). In their study they discovered that one equation with three variables [PaO2 during intraoperative two lung ventilation in lateral decubitus position, side of surgery and preoperative relation of forced expiratory volume in 1st second (FEV1) and vital capacity (VC)], could be used to predict (p =.73) PaO2 during OLV, using CPAP (continuous positive airway pressure) in non-ventilated lung. However,

Katz et al. (51) agreed with the findings of Hurford et al. (40) that routine preoperative arterial gas analysis and pulmonary functional tests do not anticipate precisely which patients are under risk of developing hypoxia during OLV.
Our results from this study verify that preoperative arterial gas analysis, as well as FVC and FEV1, can't be perceived as confident evidence that the exact patient will develop hypoxia of bigger or smaller extent during OLV.
Previous clinical research studies showed controversial results regarding oxygenation, shunt fraction and hemodynamic parameters during OLV (42, 43, 44, 45).
Spies et al. (42) compared TIVA with propofol (10 mg/kg/h) versus 1 MAC enflurane in patients during thoracotomy. Cardiac output and shunt significantly increased when TLV was converted to OLV, and PaO2 decreased.
Van Keer et al. (43) studied 10 patients who underwent thoracotomy. Their anesthesia was maintained with continuous iv infusion of propofol (10 mg/kg/h). No changes were noticed concerning cardiac output, shunt and PaO2, during TLV (two lung ventilation) and OLV. This fact could be due to methodological differences because all the measurements for the duration of OLV were initiated before opening of the thoracic cavity.
Steegers et al. (44) examined 14 patients who were about to undertake lobectomy, in intravenous general anesthesia with continuous infusion of propofol (6-9 mg/kg/h). The shunt fraction and PaO2 didn't differ during OLV compared with TLV. Their study doesn't include any basic data, like cardiac output. Changes in these hemodynamic parameters would cause secondary alterations in pulmonary circulation.
Kellow et al. (45) studied patients who underwent thoracotomy and noticed significant increase of cardiac index and shunt fraction when TLV was switched to OLV. Nevertheless, interpretation of the shunt fraction is limited as the patients were ventilated with 50% nitrous oxide in oxygen and no PaO2 was measured.
Several studies, including the one of Slinger et al. (46), demonstrated that the beginning of hypoxia is, approximately, about 5-10 min. after initiating of OLV and reaches maximum after 15 min. This matches the time needed for complete absorption of the gases (oxygen and nitrous oxide) from closed cavities, when blood flow is maintained. PaO2 and Qs/Qt usually begin to return towards values existing during TLV about 30 min. after commencing OLV. That is the period required for development of the compensatory mechanism called HPV (hypoxic pulmonary vasoconstriction) and redirection of blood flow away from the atelectatic lung. As a result, the shunt fraction will also decrease.
Our results confirmed the conclusions from the last mentioned studies - that during conversion from TLV to OLV in patient placed in lateral decubitus position throughout thoracotomy / thoracoscopy, it comes to decrease in arterial oxygenation, as well as increase in shunt fraction. Namely, the average values of PaO2 in two examinated groups of patients fall down throughout the operative monitoring (group A from 23,29+/-7,97 kPa in TLV, to 13,78+/-5,84 kPa after 10 min. of OLV, and returns to 15,66+/-6,62 kPa, 30 min. after OLV; and group B – from 20,98+/-4,68 kPa during TLV, to 11,87+/-4,95 kPa, 10 min. after OLV, and returns to 14,88+/-4,45 kPa 30 min. after OLV); the average values of SaO2 in the two groups show decrease during operative monitoring (group A - from 99,06+/-0,81% during TLV, to 93,52+/-6,03%, 10 min. after OLV, and returns to 95,31+/-4,62%, 30 min. after OLV; and group B – from 99,09+/-0,6% during TLV, to 92,92+/-5,2%, 10 min. after OLV, and returns to 95,89+/-3,78%, 30 min. after OLV); also, the average values of Qs/Qt in two examinated groups demonstrate dynamic changes during operative monitoring – in the group A begins with quantity < 1% in T0, increases to 8,03+/-10,59% in T2, and in T3

decreases to 3,94+/-6,21%; in the group B, it begins with value <1% in T0, increases to 10,93+/-10,8% in T2, and in T3 decreases to 4,82+/-7,58%. The statistically significant differences for PaO2, SaO2 and Qs/Qt, inside the groups A and B, show that after a certain time from initiating of OLV (after 10 min.), hypoxia develops with drop of values of PaO2 and SaO2, as well as increase of the quantity of intrapulmonary shunt. The subsequent decrease of Qs/Qt in the fourth measurement (T3), illustrates the development of HPV in this period of time, over and above the decrease of the shunt fraction 30 min. after the beginning of OLV in lateral decubitus position during thoracotomy / thoracoscopy.

Other factors that could reduce PaO2 are cardio-vascular and hemodynamic effects of thoracic epidural anesthesia (TEA): the decline of HR, SAP, stroke volume and cardiac output (CO), as a result of the blockade of sympathetic nervous system. Even more, the systemic consequences from the absorption of local anesthetics could lead to circulatory changes, like reduction of CO (47,48).

The results in our study demonstrated that the average values of HR/min. in both groups showed increase during operative monitoring from T0 to T3 (group A-85,56+/-12,53 to 88,53+/-12,19 and group B -76,16+/-13,15 to 81,6+/-13,49). The difference in average values for HR/min. recorded between groups A and B is statistically significant in T0 and T3 ($p<0,05$), whilst in T1 and T2 it isn't statistically significant ($p>0,05$). Inside the groups A and B, the variation in average values of HR/min. is statistically non-significant ($p>0,05$). But, as it is demonstrated by the comparison of the data from intraoperative arterial gas analysis between the groups A and B, obviously this dissimilarity for HR/min. which is a result of the depth of anesthesia, as well as administration of TEA in group B, doesn't lead to an important difference in arterial oxygenation and shunt fraction between two groups. The other hemodynamic parameter which is intraoperatively monitored in our patients, SAP/mmHg, doesn't differ considerably among two groups, which advocates even more the previous statement - that the mentioned hemodynamic diversity in our patients doesn't have any significance in the process of delivering the conclusions in this study.

The degree of difficulty of the disease in non-dependent lung is also a critical determinant of the quantity of blood flow in non-dependent lung. If this lung is seriously 'diseased', there could be a preoperative fixed reduction of its blood flow, thus its 'collapse' may not cause considerable increase in shunt fraction.

In fact, Hurford et al. (40) in their prospective study provided evidence that the patients who had in affected lung less than 45% of their pulmonary blood flow, had notably smaller risk for development of hypoxia during OLV.

As literature shows, the administration of sodium nitroprussid or nitroglycerin - which is supposed to diminish hypoxic pulmonary vasoconstriction (HPV) in patients with COPD (chronic obstructive pulmonary disease), who have fixed reduction of their pulmonary vascular bed, doesn't initiate enhancement of the shunt. This observation supports the fact that the affected (diseased) pulmonary vasculature is incapable to develop HPV (49, 50). On the other hand, these medicaments augment the shunt fraction in patients with acute regional lung disease, who otherwise have normal pulmonary vascular bed. *Due to this fact, it is more likely that greater degree of shunt through non-dependent lung during OLV will develop in patients who should be subjected to thoracotomy because of non-pulmonary disease.*

This statement was confirmed with our patients also. In three patients with diagnosis Ca esophagi who underwent thoracotomy with intraoperative utilization of OLV (one in group A and two in group B), are recorded values of Qs/Qt during OLV that are very close to the maximal registered ones in two groups of patients. However, this clinical feature could be only understood as higher probability, but not as a rule.

OLV has much less effect on PaCO2 than on PaO2 (52). During clinical use of OLV, the respiratory rate is adjusted in order to maintain a 'safe' level of elimination of CO2, guided by the measurements of capnography (End-tidal CO2) and/or arterial gas analysis. Sometimes the minute ventilation achieved by employing these ventilatory parameters could be minor than the ideal one. The minute ventilation could be limited due to air trapping, not only in patients with COPD, but also in patients with normal preoperative lung function. Controlled hypoventilation is called permissive hypercapnia; furthermore, it is demonstrated as a harmless technique in patients with ARDS (acute respiratory distress syndrome), even with values of pH of 7.15 and of PaCO2 up to 80 mm Hg (10,66 kPa) (53). Maintaining adequate oxygenation (PaO2 > 60 mm Hg, i.e. 8 kPa) is crucial during this period. The secure level of acute hypercapnia for patients under general anesthesia is not known, but the values in this range could be adequate.

In our study, the average (middling) values of PaCO2/kPa in both examinated groups show increase during the operative monitoring (group A and B - from 5,4 to 6,4 kPa). The difference in average values of PaCO2/kPa between two groups (A and B) is not statistically significant (p>0,05), whereas this variation inside the groups A and B is statistically significant (p<0,05). Precisely this difference illustrates the appearance of already mentioned permissive hypercapnia during OLV (which is expected, although RR/min. was increased to facilitate preservation of PaCO2 in normal ranges).

In experimental studies using thoracic epidural anesthesia, TEA didn't inhibit HPV (36, 54). Ishibe et al. (36) demonstrated enhanced response of HPV and improved arterial oxygenation during OLV and TEA in dogs, which was a result of decreased PvO2 and CO owing to the blockade of sympathetic nerve activity. The sensitivity of these variables depends on the extent of lung tissue exposed to hypoxia. In this study the authors used left lower lobe-LLL, which represents approximately one sixth of total lung volume. The hypoxic ventilation reduced the blood flow of LLL and PaO2. The extent of these changes is "realistic", if the pulmonary artery of LLL is supposed to contract maximally. It is obvious that TEA inhibited sympathetic efferent nerve activity in dogs from this study. Because of that, it is probable that TEA-induced changes in systemic hemodynamics resulted in enhancement of HPV, since it is well known that decrease of CO, PAP and PvO2 augment HPV response. However, in this study, the effects of TEA-induced enhancement of HPV on pulmonary hemodynamics and systemic oxygenation were minimal, most probably because the relative extent of hypoxic lung tissue was minor and the intensity of basic HPV response was already near the maximal level before commencement of TEA.

Brimioulle et al. (54) noticed enhancement of HPV during epidural blockade, but without an effect of the previous α- or β-blockade, meaning that all its consequences on pulmonary circulation are connected with sympathetic blockade.

On the contrary, Garutti et al. (55) observed higher shunt fractions (39,5%) and lower values of PaO2 (120 mmHg) during OLV in TEA group, compared with TIVA group in patients who underwent thoracotomy. They concluded that TEA could not be recommended for use in thoracic surgery when OLV is needed (55). Nonetheless, their study has great limitations. CO and PvO2, which are important factors for assessment of the impact of HPV, were not measured. The venous blood for gas analysis used to determine shunt fraction, was taken using central venous catheter (55). TEA was combined with propofol. Kasaba et al. (56) reported that hypotensive effects of propofol are additive to those of epidural anesthesia. Garuti et al. (55) used iv ephedrine only in TEA group when systolic arterial pressure dropped below 100 mmHg. Ephedrine is partial α and β agonist (57). This explains the similarity of compared values of HR and SAP in both groups, but does not make clear the worst oxygenation, because it seems that ephedrine provides an increase of PaO2 without alteration of intrapulmonary shunt during OLV in thoracic surgery. For the reason that copies of β-adrenergic subtype are found in porcine tissue of the lungs and left ventricle (β1: 67/72; β2: 33/28; β3: 2/25) (58), it can't be excluded that augmentation of cardiac output through β-receptor activity could be responsible for increasing the shunt fraction and poorer oxygenation in the study of Garutti et al. (55).

Hackenberg et al. (59), by using multiple elimination of inert gas for analysis of inequality of ventilation/perfusion matching, demonstrated that TEA didn't influenced the development of shunt, before and after induction in general anesthesia.

The reason for the eventual fall of PaO2 while using TEA could be as follows: pulmonary vasculature is innervated by autonomous nervous system. Stimulation of the sympathetic nerves in the lungs causes enhancement of PVR (pulmonary vascular resistance), as a result of the activation of α-receptors in pulmonary vascular bed. The mediator released on the sympathetic nerve endings is norepinephrine (47, 48, 54). The blockade of the sympathetic nervous system with α-adrenergic antagonists or β-adrenergic agonists diminishes HPV, while β-adrenergic antagonists enhance this response. So, maybe the actual factor is the block of the activity of thoracic sympathetic system over pulmonary vascular response.

However, previously mentioned studies, like the one of Ishibe et al. (36), demonstrate that TEA didn't affect the primary pulmonary vascular tone during OLV, but slightly augmented the redistribution of blood flow away from hypoxic lobe and towards other well oxygenated lung areas.

The explanation lies in the fact that most of these studies were not completed under same conditions (for example, anesthetized patients, lateral decubitus position, atelectatic lung tissue).

Our results show that no statistically significant difference exists ($p>0,05$) for Qs/Qt % between the groups A and B in all stages of measurements. This points to the fact that when two anesthetic techniques are compared, the use of combined anesthesia (GA plus TEA with local anesthetics) for thoracic surgery doesn't lead to bigger reduction of PaO2 and greater increase of intrapulmonary shunt during OLV, than intravenous GA.

12. Summary

Based on the experiences of other authors from literature, as well as on our own research, we would provide following recommendations for safe anesthesia during OLV, regarding **the principles of ventilation:**

- OLV should be established in a way that the lungs would inflate adequately, but minimizing the intra-alveolar pressure at the same time, in order to prevent redistribution of pulmonary blood flow towards upper (non-dependent, non-ventilated) lung. It is not easy to accomplish this in practice.
- It seems reasonable to use initial FiO2 of 50%, which could be increased up to 100%, as needed. This can't influence the real shunt in upper lung, but it improves oxygenation throughout alveoli with low Va/Qt relations in lower lung.
- „Over inflation" of one lung (volutrauma) is harmful and leads to acute lung injury. Deflation and inflation of the operated lung, with a possibility of ischemic/reperfusion injury, is also included in lung trauma. Application of very low tidal volumes improves the outcome of mechanically ventilated patients (50, 51, 56).

- Arterial hypoxemia is obviously undesirable, but in spite of everything, it might be better to accept PaO_2 a little lower than preoperative value, than to undertake measures like inflation of the upper lung, which could present an obstacle for surgical intervention and could prolong it (21, 22, 42, 59, 66, 67).

At the end, it could be concluded that:

- In patients subjected to OLV in general anesthesia (GA), hypoxia develops, with decrease in PaO_2 and increase of the value of intrapulmonary shunt, a period of time after initiation of OLV (after 10 min.), with subsequent return of Qs/Qt towards lower values (after 30 min. of OLV), because of the development of compensatory mechanisms (HPV).
- In patients subjected to OLV managed with thoracic epidural anesthesia (TEA) combined with general anesthesia (GA), hypoxia occurs, also, with fall of PaO_2 and increase of the value of intrapulmonary shunt, 10 min. after commencement of OLV, and returning of Qs/Qt towards normal values (approximately), about 30 min. after initiated OLV.
- Thoracic epidural anesthesia (TEA) doesn't lead to augmentation of hypoxia and enhancement of the shunt fraction during OLV.

13. Glossary of terms

1. **LDP** = lateral decubitus position
2. **OLV** = one lung ventilation
3. **TLV** = two lung ventilation
4. **(i)PEEP** = (intrinsic) positive end expiratory pressure
5. **CPAP** = continuous positive airway pressure
6. **Va/Qt** = ventilation/perfusion ratio
7. **Qs/Qt%** = intrapulmonary shunt
8. **PA** = alveolar pressure
9. **Ppa** = pulmonary artery pressure
10. **Ppv** = pulmonary venous pressure
11. **Pisf** = pulmonary interstitial pressure
12. **Ppl** = pleural pressure
13. **PO2** = partial pressure of oxygen (a = in arterial blood, v = in venous blood, A = in the alveoli)
14. **PCO2** = partial pressure of carbon dioxide (a = in arterial blood, v = in venous blood, A = in the alveoli)
15. **FRC** = functional residual capacity
16. **FiO2** = inspired oxygen fraction
17. **PVR** = pulmonary vascular resistance
18. **HPV** = hypoxic pulmonary vasoconstriction
19. **TIVA** = total intravenous anesthesia
20. **MAC** = minimal alveolar concentration
21. **TEA** = thoracic epidural anesthesia
22. **GA** = general anesthesia
23. **FOB** = fiber-optic bronchoscope
24. **ARDS** = acute respiratory distress syndrome
25. **PPPE** = post pneumonectomy pulmonary edema

26. **COPD** = chronic obstructive pulmonary disease
27. **I : E** = inspiration : expiration
28. **ASA** = „American Society of Anesthesiologists“ (classification)
29. **SaO2** = oxygen saturation of arterial blood
30. **AST** = aspartate amino transferase
31. **ALT** = alanine amino transferase
32. **EF** = ejection fraction of the heart
33. **CO** = cardiac output
34. **FEV1** = forced expiratory volume in 1st sec.
35. **FVC** = forced vital capacity
36. **VC** = volume controlled mechanical ventilation
37. **PC** = pressure controlled mechanical ventilation
38. **HR** = heart rate
39. **ECG** = electrocardiography
40. **MAP** = mean arterial pressure
41. **RR** = respiratory rate
42. **SAT%** = oxygen saturation from pulsoximetry
43. **Cc'O2** = oxygen content of pulmonary capillary blood
44. **CaO2** = oxygen content - ml O2/100 ml arterial blood
45. **CvO2** = oxygen content - ml O2/100 ml venous blood
46. **LLL** = lower left lobe
47. **Hb** = hemoglobin
48. **1.39** = Hifner coefficient (1g Hb binds 1.39 ml O2 when totally saturated)
49. **0.0031** = coefficient of oxygen dissolution in plasma
50. **FFP** = fresh frozen plasma
51. **SAGM** = packed erythrocytes
52. **LMWH**=low molecular weight heparin

14. References

[1] Benumof JL. Anesthesia for thoracic surgery. 2nd ed. Philadelphia, WB Saunders, 1995.

[2] Aitkenhead AR, Jones RM (eds). Clinical anaesthesia. Edinburgh: Churchill Livingstone; 1996.

[3] Gothard JWW. Anaesthesia for thoracic surgery, 2nd edn. Oxford: Blackwell Scientific Publications; 1993.

[4] Benumof JL. Mechanism of decreased blood flow to alectatic lung. J Appl Physiol 1979;46:1047- 8.

[5] Domino KB, Wetstein L, Glasser SA, et al. Influence of mixed venous oxygen tension (PvO2) on blood flow to atetectatic lung. Anesthesiology 1983;59:428 -34.

[6] Hambraeus-Jonzon K, Bindslev L, Mellgard AJ, Hedenstierna G. Hypoxic pulmonary vasoconstriction in human lungs: a stimulus-response study. Anesthesiology 1997;86:308 -15.

[7] Cutaia M, Rounds S. Hypoxic pulmonary vasoconstriction: physiologic significance, mechanism, and clinical relevance. Chest 1990;97:706 -18.

[8] Bachand R, Audet J, Meloche R, Denis R. Physiological changes associated with unilateral pulmonary ventilation during operation of the lung. Canad Anaesth Soc J, Nov 1975; 22 (6)

[9] Watanabe S,Noguchi E,Yamda S,et al.Sequential changes of arterial oxygen tension in the supine position during one-lung ventilation.Anesth Analg,2000,90:28-34.
[10] Benumof JL. One-lung ventilation and hypoxic pulmonary vasoconstriction: implications for anesthesic management. Anesth Analg 1985;64:821–3.
[11] Maseda F, Vilchez E, Del Campo JM, et al. Hypoxic pulmonary vasoconstriction during single lung ventilation in the lateral decubitus position and thoracic anaesthesia [abstract]. Br J Anaesth 1995;74:A152.
[12] Kadowitz PJ, Hyman AL. Effect of sympathetic nerve stimulation on pulmonary vascular resistance in the dog. Circ Res 1973;32:221–7.
[13] Kazemi H, Bruecke PE, Parsons ES. Role of the autonomic nervous system in the hypoxic response of the pulmonary vascular bed. Respir Physiol 1972;15:245– 8
[14] Kellow NH, Scott AD, White SA, Feneck RO. Comparison of the effects of propofol and isoflurane anaesthesia on right ventricular function and shunt fraction during thoracic surgery. Br J Anaesth 1995;75:578–582.J Cardiothorac Vasc Anesth 1996;10:860–863.
[15] Aye T, Milne B. Ketamine anesthesia for pericardial window in a patient with pericardial tamponade and severe COPD: [La ketamine utilisee pour l'anesthesie d'une ponction pericardique chez une patiente qui presente une tamponnade et une MPOC severe].Can J Anesth, March 1, 2002; 49(3): 283 - 286.
[16] Weinreich IA, Silvay G., Lumb PD. Continuous ketamine infusion for one-lung anaesthesia. Canad Anaesth Soc J, Sept 1980; 27 (5)
[17] Beck DH, Doepfmer UR, Sinemus C, Bloch A, Schenk MR, Kox WJ. Effects of sevoflurane and propofol on pulmonary shunt fraction during one-lung ventilation for thoracic surgery. Br. J. Anaesth., January 1, 2001; 86(1): 38 - 43.
[18] Westbrook JL, Sykes MK. Peroperative arterial hypoxaemia: the interaction between intrapulmonary shunt and cardiac output. Anaesthesia 1992;47:307–10.
[19] Antman EM, March JD, Green LH, Grossman W. Blood oxygen measurements in the assessment of intracardiac left to right shunts: a critical appraisal of ethiology. Am J Cardiol 1980;46: 265–71.
[20] Berridge JC. Influence of cardiac output on the correlation between mixed venous and central venous oxygen saturation. Br J Anaesth 1992;69:409 –10.
[21] Brodsky JB, Benumof JL, Ehrenwerth J, Ozaki GT. Depth of placement of left double-lumen endobronchial tubes. Anesth Analg 1991;73:570–572.
[22] Brodsky JB, Macario A, Mark BD. Tracheal diameter predicts double-lumen tube size: a method for selecting left double-lumen tubes. Anesth Analg 1996;82:861–864.
[23] Inoue H, Shotsu A, Ogawa J, Kawada S, Koide S. New device for one-lung anaesthesia: endotracheal tube with movable blocker. J Thorac Cardiovasc Surg 1982;83:940–941.
[24] Robertshaw FL. Low resistance double-lumen endobronchial tubes. Br J Anaesth 1962;34:576–579.
[25] de Abreu MG, Heintz M, Heller A, et al. One-lung ventilation with high tidal volumes and zero positive end-expiratory pressure is injurious in the isolated rabbit lung model. Anesth Analg 2003;96:220–8
[26] Tanaka M, Dohi S. The effects of ephedrine and phenilephrine on arterial partial pressure of oxygen during one-lung ventilation. Masui 1994;43:1124 –9.
[27] Chen TL, Lee YT, Wang MJ, Lee JM, Lee YC, Chu SH. Endothelin-1 concentrations and optimisation of arterial oxygenation by selective pulmonary artery infusion of

prostaglandin E1 during thoracotomy. Anaesthesia 1996;51:422–426. Butterworth Heinemann; 1999.

[28] Williams EA, Evans TW, Goldstraw P. Acute lung injury following lung resection: is one lung anaesthesia to blame? Thorax 1996;51:114–116.

[29] Bardoczky GI,Szegedi LL,d' Hollander AA,et al.Two-lung and one-lung ventilation in patients with chronic obstructive pulmonary disease:the effects of position and FiO2.AnesthAnalg,2000,90:35-41.

[30] Ribas J, Jimenez MJ, Barbera JA, Roca J, Gomar C, Canalis E, Rodriguez-Roisin R. Gas Exchange and Pulmonary Hemodynamics During Lung Resection in Patients at Increased Risk: Relationship With Preoperative Exercise Testing. Chest, September 1, 2001; 120(3): 852 - 859.

[31] Fischer LG, Aken HV, Burkle H. Management of Pulmonary Hypertension: Physiological and Pharmacological Considerations for Anesthesiologists. Anesth. Analg., June 1, 2003; 96(6): 1603 - 1616.

[32] Temeck BK, Schafer PW, Park WY, Harmon JW. Epidural anesthesia in patients undergoing thoracic surgery. Arch Surg 1989; 124:415– 8.

[33] Yeager MP, Glass DD, Neff RK, Brinck-Johnsen T. Epidural anesthesia and analgesia in high-risk surgical patients.Anesthesiology 1987;66:729 –36.

[34] Wattwil M, Sundberg A, Arvill A, Lennquist C. Circulatory changes during high thoracic epidural anaesthesia-influence of sympathetic block and systemic effect of the local anaesthetic. Acta Anaesthesiol Scand 1985;29:849 –55.

[35] O'Connor CJ. Thoracic epidural analgesia: physiologic effects and clinical applications. J Cardiothorac Anesth 1993;7:595– 609.

[36] Ishibe Y, Shiokawa Y, Umeda T, et al. The effect of thoracic epidural anesthesia on hypoxic pulmonary vasoconstriction in dogs: an analysis of the pressure-flow curve. Anesth Analg 1996;82:1049 –55.

[37] Chow MY, Goh MH, Boey SK, Thirugnanam A, Ip-Yam PC. The Effects of Remifentanil and Thoracic Epidural on Oxygenation and Pulmonary Shunt Fraction During One-Lung Ventilation. J Cardioth Vasc Anesth, 2003; 17(1):69-72.

[38] Garutti I, Cruz P, Olmedilla L, Barrio JM, Cruz A, Fernandez C, Perez-Peña JM. Effects of Thoracic Epidural Meperidine on Arterial Oxygenation During One-Lung Ventilation in Thoracic Surgery. J Cardioth Vasc Anesth, 2003; 17(3):302-305.

[39] Benumof JL. One-lung ventilation and hypoxic pulmonary vasoconstriction: implications for anesthetic management. Anesth Analg 1985; 64: 821-3.

[40] Hurford WE, Kolker AC, Strauss WH. The use of ventilation/perfusion scans to predict oxygenation during one-lung anesthesia. Anesthesiology 1987; 67: 841.

[41] Slinger PD, Hickey DR. The interaction between applied PEEP and auto-PEEP during one-lung ventilation. J Cardiothorac Vasc Anesth 1998; 12: 133-136.

[42] Wang JY, Russell GN, Page RD, et al. Comparison of the effects of sevoflurane and isoflurane on arterial oxygenation during one-lung ventilation. Br J Anaesth 1998; 81: 850.

[43] Abe K, Shimizu T, Takashina M, et al. The effects of propofol, isoflurane and sevoflurane on oxygenation and shunt fraction during one-lung ventilation. Anesth Analg 1998; 87: 1164.

[44] Kellow N, Scott AD, White SA, Feneck RO. Comparison of the effects of propofol and isoflurane anesthesia on right ventricular function and shunt fraction during thoracic surgery. Br J Anaesth 1995; 75: 578-82.
[45] Berridge JC. Influence of cardiac output on the correlation between mixed venous and central venous oxygen saturation. Br J Anaesth 1992;69:409 –10.
[46] Slinger P, Triolet W, Wilson J. Improving arterial oxygenation during one-lung ventilation. Anesthesiology 1988; 68: 291-295.
[47] Wattwil M, Sundberg A, Arvill A, Lennquist C. Circulatory changes during high thoracic epidural anaesthesia-influence of sympathetic block and systemic effect of the local anaesthetic. Acta Anaesthesiol Scand 1985; 29: 849 –55.
[48] O'Connor CJ. Thoracic epidural analgesia: physiologic effects and clinical applications. J Cardiothorac Anesth 1993; 7: 595- 609.
[49] Holmgren A, Anjou E, Broman L, Lundberg S. Influence of nitroglycerin on central hemodynamics and Va/Qc of the lungs in the postoperative period after coronary bypass surgery. Acta Med Scand 1982; S562: 135.
[50] Parsons GH, Leventhal JP, Hansen MM, Goldstein JD. Effect of sodium nitroprusside on hypoxic pulmonary vasoconstriction in the dog. J Appl Physiol 1981; 51: 288.
[51] Katz JA, Laverne RG, Fairley HB, Thomas AN. Pulmonary oxygen exchange during endobronchial anesthesia: effect of tidal volume and PEEP. Anesthesiology 1982; 56: 164-171.
[52] Kerr JH, Smith AC, Prys-Roberts C, Meloche R. Observations during endobronchial anesthesia I: ventilation and carbon dioxide clearance. Br J Anesth 1973; 45: 159-167.
[53] Feihl F, Perret C. Permissive hypercapnia. How permissive should we be? Am J Respir Crit Care Med 1994; 150: 1722-1737.
[54] Brimioulle S, Vachiery JL, Brichant JF, et al. Sympathetic modulation of hypoxic pulmonary vasoconstriction in intact dogs. Cardiovascular Research 1997; 34: 384-92.
[55] Garutti I, Quintana B, Olmedilla L, et al. Arterial oxygenation during one-lung ventilation: combined versus general anesthesia. Anesth Analg 1999; 88: 494-9.
[56] Kasaba T, Kondou O, Yoshimura Y, et al. Hemodynamic effects of induction of general anesthesia with propofol during epidural anesthesia. Can J Anaesth 1998; 45: 1061-5.
[57] Vansal SS, Feller DR. Direct effect of ephedrine isomers on human beta-adrenergic receptor subtypes. Biochem Pharmacol 1999; 58: 807-10.
[58] Mc Neel RL, Mersmann HJ. Distribution and quantification of beta1-, beta2-, and beta3-adrenergic receptor subtype transcripts in porcine tissues. J Anim Sci 1999; 77: 611-21.
[59] Hachenberg T, Holst D, Ebel C, et al. Effect of thoracic epidural anesthesia on ventilation-perfusion distribution and intrathoracic blood volume before and after induction of anesthesia. Acta Anesthesiol Scand 1997; 41: 1142-8.

4

Thoracic Critical Care

Seyed Mohammad Reza Hashemian and Seyed Amir Mohajerani
Chronic Respiratory Disease Research Center (CRDRC),
NRITLD,
Masih Daneshvari Hospital,
Shahid Beheshti University of Medical Sciences, Tehran,
Iran

1. Introduction

1.1 Ventilator associated pneumonia

Ventilator associated pneumonia (VAP) is one of the sub-types of nosocomial acquired pneumonia occur in patients admitted to ICU who are under ventilator assistant mechanical ventilation occurring more than 48 h after patients have been intubated and received mechanical ventilation. Between 250,000 and 300,000 cases per year occur in the United States solely, which is an incidence rate of 5 to 10 cases per 1,000 hospital admissions[1]. The incidence of VAP increases with the duration of mechanical ventilation higher in day 10 compare to day five[2], and it is associated with high mortality rates (0-50%) in ICU patients, and pneumonia accounts for second cause of death in ICU patients[3], although Using various scoring systems for the mortality prediction along with the guideline-based medicine have helped decrease in VAP mortality rates[4,5]. Although mortality of viral VAP is not determined in ICU patients, the scoring systems provide an acceptable clinical index for such cases [46]. The misuse of insufficient dose or inappropriate antibiotic will lead to outgrow multi drug resistant serotypes of bacterial VAP and induce higher mortality[6]. This high mortality rate also depends on the type of underlying disease, with highest mortality attributable to VAP in patients with trauma or acute respiratory distress syndrome[7], and the type of organism affecting the patient. Higher mortality rates have been explored in VAP caused by *Pseudomonas aeruginosa (in patients with underlying respiratory problems) 8, Acinetobacter, and Stenotrophomonas maltophilia* than those associated with other organisms[9]. *Bacterial VAP can be* due to colonization and spread of organisms from oropharynx, sinus cavities, nares, dental plaque, gastrointestinal tract, patient-to-patient contact, and the ventilator circuit to the lungs[10]. Essentially, each ICU should have an established protocol in place to initial empirical therapy based on previously accepted guidelines modified by local knowledge of prevalence of resistant serotypes unique to that ICU. Notably, empiric therapy should be both appropriate by using more specific antibiotics and adequate by using correct dose and good penetration to the site of infection[11]. Duration of antibiotics are also been a point of controversy; although 8 days of therapy has been effective in non-resistant organisem, but duration of antibiotic therapy for multiple drug resistant (MDR) organism such as P aeruginosa and Acinetobacter spp, is unknown[12].

On the other hand, a key point in management of MDR VAP is rapid diagnosis of VAP and providing culture and anti-biogram in detecting the responsible organism. The antibiotic duration for patients with MDR VAP remains a controversial issue. Several serum biomarkers have been applied as potential biomarker contributing to guide antibiotic use in patients with VAP caused by MDR pathogens. Previously, pro-calcitonin (PCT) has been broadly used as a marker for community acquired pneumonia (CAP) and VAP[13,14], however it does not incorporate into hospital acquired pneumonia(HAP). Using PCT has shortened duration of anti-microbial treatment in VAP[15] in which patients with MDR VAP whose serum PCT concentrations are less than 0.5 ng/mL or decreased by 80% or more, compared with the first peak concentration, antibiotics may be terminated 3 days after initiation[16]. On the other hand usefulness of other bio-markers such as C reactive proteins(CRP) have yielded to conflicting data's[17], probably due to acute phase reactant release in ICU patients such as IL-6 and TNF-α which stimulate CRP release to surmountable amounts.

Our current data on epidemiology, pathogenesis, clinical importance, and risk factors of viral VAP and viral pneumonia in ICU has many pitfalls due to some challenges[18]. First, the diagnosis of viral VAP in critically ill patients requires a high clinical suspicion combined with bedside examination, radiographic examination, and microbiologic analysis of respiratory secretions. Besides, the presence of indolent viral VAP in a critically ill patient makes diagnosis more challenging and increases the mortality rate of patients. It is important to investigate these viral markers in VAP to probe them earlier and estimate their role in increasing mortality rate. ICU patients assumed as immunocompetent are also at risk for Herpes simplex virus (HSV) and cytomegalovirus (CMV) VAP[19]. Although CMV reactivation assumed to increase morbidities like increased length of stay in the ICU but impact on mortality particularly in patients with low CMV-DNA plasma levels is in doubt[20]. Currently there is increasing tendency to CMV infection among ICU patients. One simple explanation is that any bacterial colonization in ICU patients promotes the release of immunomodulatory cytokines and lead to reactivation of CMV[21], and reactivation from the latency induces CMV infection. Because of nonspecific signs and symptoms ICU patients are rarely monitored routinely for active CMV infection, the development of active CMV infection could remain under-diagnosed in critically ill patients.

The 2009 H1N1 influenza virus pandemic has highlighted another challenge faced by intensivists in managing severe influenza A, especially for those at high risk of severe respiratory disease in ICUs[44]. Thus, intensivists should consider performing rapid diagnostic tests and specific scoring for drug resistance genotyping for high risk patients especially in tertiary care centers[45].

2. Hyperglycemia and hypoglycemia in ICU

Essentially, ICU admitted patients encounter a profound hyperglycemia due to stress hormone surge, corticosteroid usage, and inhibition of insulin release of sepsis or trauma induced mediators[22]. Hyperglycemia could harm ICU patients by increase susceptibility to sepsis and increase mortality of critically ill patients[23]. It is supposed to have a tight control of hyperglycemia in ICU patients although threshold of blood glucose is still controversial. As a matter of fact, glucose monitoring and rout of insulin injection is mainstay of hyperglycemia control in ICU patients. Nonetheless, different studies have suggested various blood glucose levels but majorly 180 mg/dl has considered the safe treatment threshold and 140-180 for target glucose level[24,25,26,27,28]. It is widely assumed that sampling in ICU patients could also be a bottleneck in glucose tight control as catheter sampling is easy but have danger of contamination with IV fluids, whether fingerprints sampling may be inaccurate in patients with edema or anemia[29]. On the other hand, insulin therapy induced hyperglycemia may cause severe neurologic damages while neurologic symptoms of hypoglycemia are difficult to detect in critically ill patients, but they are a real concern[30]. Severe hypoglycemia <40 mg/dl could occurred in almost high proportion of patients in intensive insulin therapy and could majorly increase mortality rates of patients[31,32]. Besides, all the studies with target glucose concentration of 80 to 110 mg/dl showed increased rates of hypoglycemia[33]. Notably, even a blood glucose target of 180 mg/dl or less resulted in lower mortality than did a target of 81 to 108 mg/dl[34].

3. Venous thromboembolism (VTE) and Pulmonary Embolism (PE)

Venous thromboembolism(VTE) is a common and lethal complication in critically ill patients, due to several predisposing factors such as pre morbid conditions (e g, trauma, major surgeries, malignancy, sepsis), invasive interventions like central venous catheterization, and prolonged immobility[35]. The incidence of VTE is reported variously in different studies based on the population, prophylactic interventions and screening methods. Patients in intensive care unit have a higher risk of lower limb deep venous thrombosis (DVT) in comparison with other hospitalized patients which may be undiagnosed in considerable number of cases[36]. On the other hand, VTE could remain unrecognized in the intensive care unit because of the difficulty in eliciting signs and symptoms from intubated, sedated patients. It is likely that quite large number of patients under mechanical ventilation with unexpected episodes of tachycardia, hypotension, or hypoxia may have unnoticed pulmonary embolism (PE) [37] which could be diagnosed based on Geneva score with an acceptable predictive accuracy in low and intermediate-probability groups[38]. Undiagnosed or barely suspected PE may also lead to delay weaning patients from mechanical ventilation. Intensive care unit patients, who have reduced cardiopulmonary reserve, are prone to have significant complications of PE. Recent data suggest that the duration of therapy and recurrence rate is associated with persistently elevated levels of d-dimer[39]. Long-term treatment of thrombosis with the low-molecular-weight heparin has been shown to be associated with fewer thromboembolic recurrences in ICU patients[40].

4. Management of ICU-associated agitation by dexmedetomidine

Agitated delirium is common complication occurs commonly in patients undergoing mechanical ventilation in ICU, and is often treated with haloperidol despite concerns about its adverse effects such as unpredictable hepatic toxicity and cardiotoxicity41. Inadequate sedation in ICU particularly in intubated patients adversely affects their morbidity and mortality. Use of sedatives during agitation while patient under mechanical intubation precludes further extubation. Other than that agitation in intensive care may be associated with self-extubation, removal of vascular catheters, increased oxygen consumption and failure to cooperate with treatment. Drug of choice should be effective, safe, titrable, rapidly acting agent that has both sedative and analgesic activity, and could prevent anexiety and unpleasant memories. The newly introduced drug, Dexmedetomidine, a novel selective α2-agonist with sedative and anxiolytic properties, have showed particular utility in ICU-associated delirious agitated patients under mechanical ventilation without inducing excessive sedation, with fewer side effects than haloperidol, little interaction with other drugs and easily titrable. Studies have reported the successful use of dexmedetomidine in this context although multi-centric clinical trials may needed to establish those assumptions. Dexmedetomidine is more effective than conventional haloperidol therapy for the treatment of combined agitation and delirium in intubated patients in the ICU; besides Dexmedetomidine reduce the need of extra sedative known to cause agitation. Its administration superiority to traditional sedatives is reliably shown that has reduced ICU length of stay, hastened liberation from mechanical restraint, reduced the need for supplementary sedation, reduced QTc interval prolongation and possibly reduced the need for tracheostomy[42]. In a study in comparing dexmedetomidine and propofol in patients requiring sedation in ICU, dexmedetomidine revealed safer and protect against myocardial infarction[43]. In addition, some studies have proposed that patients who receive a dexmedetomidine bolous have no clinically significant hypotension or increased epinephrine requirement but others not. Dexmedetomidine induce no respiratory depression and should be considered for patient failing spontaneous breathing due to agitation or anxiety. On the other hand, in dose related hypotension and bradycardia bolus dexmedetomidine is not recommended. Besides, clinicians should consider higher starting dose of dexmedetomidine if used as monotherapy.

Medication	Dose	Consideration
Dexmedetomidine	0.2-1.5 mcg/kg/hr	patients failing spontaneous breathing trials secondary to agitation
Haloperidol	2.5-5mg IV q 15 min prn/ 2.5-5 mg PO q6 hr	Caution if baseline QTc >440 msec
Aripiprazole	10-15 mg po daily	Consider when baseline QTc>440 msec
Quetiapine	50-200 mg po q12 hr	Consider if sedative properties desired
Risperidone	0.5-1 mg po q12 hr	Caution baseline QTc >440 msec
Propofol	1 mg/kg loding+1-3mg/kg/h	Consider vasodilation risk

Table 1. Pharmacologic Treatment for Delirium.

5. References

[1] McEachern, R., and G. D. Campbell, Jr. 1998. Hospital-acquired pneumonia: epidemiology, etiology, and treatment. Infect. Dis. Clin. N. Am. 12:761-779.

[2] Cook DJ, Walter SD, Cook RJ, Griffith LE, Guyatt GH, Leasa D, et al. Incidence of and risk factors for ventilator-associated pneumonia in critically ill patients. Ann Intern Med. Sep 15 1998;129(6):433-40.

[3] Baker, A. M., J. W. Meredith, and E. F. Haponik. 1996. Pneumonia in intubated trauma patients. Microbiology and outcomes. Am. J. Respir. Crit. Care Med. 153:343-349.

[4] Hashemian SM, Jamaati HR, Malekmohammad M, Ehteshami Afshar E, Alosh O, Radmand G, Fakharian A. Assessing the Performance of Two Clinical Severity Scoring Systems in the ICU of a Tertiary Respiratory Disease Center. Tanaffos2010; 9(3): 58-64.

[5] Nooraei N, Hashemian SM, Golfam A, Saghebi A, G Radmand. Preoperative Assessment of Mechanical Ventilation Requirement after Surgical Treatment of Esophageal Cancer. Tanaffos 2010; 9(1): 34-41.

[6] NiedermanMS, Craven DE,BontenMJ, et al.Guidelines for the management of adults with hospital-acquired, ventilator-associated, andhealthcare-associated pneumonia. AmJ Respir Crit CareMed2005;171:388–416.

[7] Melsen WG, Rovers MM, Bonten MJ. Ventilator-associated pneumonia and mortality: a systematic review of observational studies. Crit Care Med. Oct 2009;37(10):2709-18.

[8] Jamaati HR, Malekmohammad M, Hashemian SM, Nayebi M, Basharzad N. Ventilator-Associated Pneumonia: Evaluation of Etiology, Microbiology and Resistance Patterns in a Tertiary Respiratory Center. Tanaffos 2010; 9(1): 21-27.

[9] Kunis KA, Puntillo KA. Ventilator-associated pneumonia in the ICU: its pathophysiology, risk factors, and prevention. Am J Nurs.2003;133(8):64AA-64GG.

[10] Staudinger T, Bojic A, Holzinger U, Meyer B, Rohwer M, Mallner F, et al. Continuous lateral rotation therapy to prevent ventilator-associated pneumonia. Crit Care Med. Feb 2010;38(2):486-90

[11] Nicasio AM, Eagye KJ, Nicolau DP, et al. Pharmacodynamic-based clinical pathway for empiric antibiotic choice in patients with ventilator-associated pneumonia. J Crit Care 2010;25:69–77.

[12] ChastreJ WM, Wolff M, Fagon JY, et al. Comparison of 8 vs 15 days of antibiotic therapy for ventilator associated pneumonia in adults: a randomized trial. JAMA 2003;290:2588–98.

[13] Stolz D,SmyrniosN,EggimannP, et al. Procalcitonin for reduced antibiotic exposure in ventilator-associated pneumonia: a randomised study. Eur Respir J 2009; 34:1364–75.

[14] Kopterides P, Siempos II, Tsangaris I, et al. Procalcitonin- guided algorithms of antibiotic therapy in the intensive care unit: a systematic review and metaanalysis of randomized controlled trials. Crit Care Med 2010;38:2229–41.

[15] Bouadma L, Luyt CE, Tubach F, et al. Use of procalcitonin to reduce patients' exposure to antibiotics in intensive care units (PRORATA trial): a multicentre randomised controlled trial. Lancet 2010;375:463–74.

[16] Hochreiter M, Kohler T, Schweiger AM, et al. Procalcitonin to guide duration of antibiotic therapy in intensive care patients: a randomized prospective controlled trial. Crit Care 2009;13:R83.

[17] Povoa P, Coelho L, Almeida E, et al. Early identification of intensive care unit-acquired infections with daily monitoring of C-reactive protein: a prospective observational study. Crit Care 2006;10:R63.

[18] Moradi A, Nadji SA, Tabarsi P, Hashemian SM, Marjani M, Sigaroodi A, Mansouri D, Masjedi MR, Velayati AA. Prevalence of Oseltamivir-Resistant 2009 H1N1 Influenza Virus among Patients with Pandemic 2009 H1N1 Influenza infection in NRITLD.Tanaffos2011; 10(1): 8-11

[19] Hodson EM, Craig JC, Strippoli GF, Webster AC. Antiviral medications for preventing cytomegalovirus disease in solid organ transplant recipients.Cochrane Database Syst Rev. 2008 Apr 16;(2):CD003774.

[20] Heininger A, Haeberle H, Fischer I, Beck R, Riessen R, Rohde F, Meisner C, Jahn G, Koenigsrainer A, Unertl K, Hamprecht K. Cytomegalovirus reactivation and associated outcome of critically ill patients with severe sepsis. Crit Care. 2011 Mar 1;15(2):R77.

[21] Döcke WD, Prösch S, Fietze E, Kimel V, Zuckermann H, Klug C, Syrbe U, Krüger DH, von Baehr R, Volk HD: Cytomegalovirus reactivation and tumour necrosis factor. Lancet 1994, 343(8892):268-269.

[22] Dungan KM, Braithwaite SS, Preiser JC. Stress hyperglycaemia. Lancet 2009; 373:1798-807.

[23] van den Berghe G, Wouters P, Weekers F, et al. Intensive insulin therapy in critically ill patients. N Engl J Med 2001; 345:1359-67.

[24] De La Rosa GDC, Donado JH, Restrepo AH, et al. Strict glycaemic control in patients hospitalised in a mixed medical and surgical intensive care unit: a randomized clinical trial. Crit Care 2008; 12(5):R120.

[25] Preiser JC, Devos P, Ruiz-Santana S, et al. A prospective randomised multi-centre controlled trial on tight glucose control by intensive insulin therapy in adult intensive care units: the Glucontrol study. Intensive Care Med 2009;35:1738-48.

[26] Griesdale DE, de Souza RJ, van Dam RM, et al. Intensive insulin therapy and mortality among critically ill patients: a meta-analysis including NICE-SUGAR study data. CMAJ 2009;180:821-7.

[27] Marik PE, Preiser JC. Toward understanding tight glycemic control in the ICU: a systematic review and metaanalysis. Chest 2010;137:544-51.

[28] Wiener RS, Wiener DC, Larson RJ. Benefits and risks of tight glucose control in critically ill adults: a meta-analysis. JAMA 2008;300:933-44.

[29] Corstjens AM, Ligtenberg JJ, van der Horst IC, et al. Accuracy and feasibility of point-of-care and continuous blood glucose analysis in critically ill ICU patients. Crit Care 2006;10(5):R135.

[30] Kosiborod M, Inzucchi SE, Goyal A, et al. Relationship between spontaneous and iatrogenic hypoglycemia and mortality in patients hospitalized with acute myocardial infarction. JAMA 2009; 301:1556-64.
[31] Van den Berghe G, Wilmer A, Hermans G, et al. Intensive insulin therapy in the medical ICU. N Engl J Med 2006; 354:449-61.
[32] Egi M, Bellomo R, Stachowski E, et al. Hypoglycemia and outcome in critically ill patients. Mayo Clin Proc 2010;85:217-24.
[33] Kavanagh BP, McCowen KC.Glycemic control in ICU. N Engl J Med 2010;363:2540 -6.
[34] Chittock D. R., Yu-Shuo S., Blair D., Dhingra V. Intensive versus Conventional Glucose Control in Critically Ill Patients. N Engl J Med 2009; 360: 1283 - 97.
[35] Tapson V. F. Acute Pulmonary Embolism. N Engl J Med 2008;358:1037-52.
[36] Segal JB, Streiff MB, Hofmann LV, Thornton K, Bass EB.. Management of venous thromboembolism: a systematic review for a practice guideline. Ann Intern Med 2007;146:211-22.
[37] Goldhaber SZ, Visani L, De Rosa M. Acute pulmonary embolism: clinical outcomes in the International Cooperative Pulmonary Embolism Registry (ICOPER). Lancet 1999;353:1386-9.
[38] Jamaati H. R., Hashemian S. M., Malekmohammad M., Bagheri Moghadam A., Kahkouee S., Miri M., Radmand G., Masjedi M. R. Predictive Accuracy of Revised Geneva Score in the Diagnosis of Pulmonary Embolism. Tanaffos 2009; 8 (4): 7 - 1
[39] Palareti G, Cosmi B, Legnani C, et al. d-Dimer testing to determine the duration of anticoagulation therapy. N Engl J Med 2006;355:1780-9
[40] Lee AYY, Levine MN, Baker RI, et al. Low-molecular-weight heparin versus a coumarin for the prevention of recurrent venous thromboembolism in patients with cancer. N Engl J Med 2003;349:146-53.
[41] Fraser GL, Prato BS, Riker RR, Berthiaume D, Wilkins ML: Frequency, severity, and treatment of agitation in young versus elderly patients in the ICU. Pharmacotherapy 2000, 20:75-82.
[42] Dotson B, Peeters MJ: Sedation with dexmedetomidine vs lorazepam in mechanically ventilated patients. JAMA 2008;299:1540.
[43] Venn RM, Grounds RM. Comparison between dexmedetomidine and propofol for sedation in the ICU: patient and clinician perception. British Journal of Anesthesia.2001;87(5):648-90
[44] Moradi A, Nadji SA,Tabarsi P, Hashemian SM, Marjani M,Sigaroodi A, Mansouri D, Masjedi MR, Velayati AA.Prevalence of Oseltamivir-Resistant 2009 H1N1 Influenza Virus among Patients with Pandemic 2009 H1N1 Influenza infection in NRITLD, Tehran, Iran. *Tanaffos* 2011; 10(1): 8-11.
[45] Pereira JM, Moreno RP, Matos R, Rhodes A, Martin-Loeches A, Cecconi M, Lisboa T, Rello J. Severity assessment tools in ICU patients with 2009 Influenza A (H1N1) pneumonia.. Clinical Microbiology and Infection 2010. DOI: 10.1111/j.1469-0691.2011.03736.x

[46] Hashemian SM, Jamaati HR, Malekmohammad M , Ehteshami Afshar E, Alosh O, Radmand G, Fakharian A. Assessing the Performance of Two Clinical Severity Scoring Systems in the ICU of a Tertiary Respiratory Disease Center. *Tanaffos* 2010; 9(3): 58-64.

5

Standardized Monitoring of Post-Operative Morbidity and Mortality for the Evaluation of Thoracic Surgical Quality

Jelena Ivanovic, Tim Ramsay and Andrew J. E. Seely
Ottawa Hospital Research Institute, Canada

1. Introduction

Reliable and reproducible evaluation of quality of surgical care is of utmost importance for governments, hospitals, clinicians, and patients. Given the elective nature of the majority of surgical care, and the immediacy of its impact, surgeons have long built a strong culture and tradition of quality assessment and peer review. Building upon this foundation, there is increasing focus on standardization of means to evaluate surgical quality, developed by associations, institutions, and individual centers.
The overall aim of this chapter is to review these initiatives, focusing on an individual division of thoracic surgery, and its efforts to standardize the evaluation of surgical quality and develop a means to monitor it over time. While the tools developed may or may not be immediately relevant, it is hoped that the reasources and principles outlined are useful in the development of surgical quality assessment programs.

2. Framework for the evaluation of surgical quality

According to Donabedian, assessment about the quality of care can be made from three interrelated components: structure, process, and outcomes. Structure refers to organizational characteristics of the particular health care setting (Donabedian, 1988). Relative to surgery, structural measures include the following: the physical plant, the equipment and supplies, the members of the surgical team and their qualifications, and provider volume (Daley, Henderson, & Khuri, 2001). It is important to note that many structural measures are not readily actionable, which limit their ultimate effectiveness as a means toward quality improvement (Birkmeyer et al., 2004).
Process refers to the perioperative care received by the patient (Donabedian, 1988). In surgery, important process measures include: informed consent, the preoperative preparation of the patient, the choice of the surgical intervention and its execution, use of preoperative checklists, routine postoperative care and efficient clinical handover (Khuri, Daley, & Henderson, 1999). Although process measures are actionable, they are difficult to measure reliably on a routine basis (Birkmeyer et al., 2004).
Finally, outcomes refer to the effects of care on the health status of the patient (Donabedian, 1988). Outcomes measurement, which are inherently patient-centered, have been the most measured, and indeed fundamental to evaluating the quality of surgical care.

In this chapter, emphasis is placed on the evaluation of surgical outcomes, as surgical outcomes are frequently used in many ongoing efforts as measures of the quality of surgical care (Dimick et al., 2003). Specifically, postoperative morbidity and mortality (M&M) rates remain the most frequently measured and reported outcomes (Martin et al., 2002). M&M rates are often the only data provided as a means of comparing surgical techniques or peri-operative management decisions (Martin et al., 2002).

Postoperative mortality is defined either as in hospital mortality, 30-day mortality, or a combination of both (Khuri et al., 1999). Postoperative morbidity, on the other hand, refers to adverse events and complications following surgery (Khuri et al., 1999). Surgical adverse events contribute significantly to postoperative morbidity, yet the measurement and monitoring of these events is often imprecise and of uncertain validity (Bruce et al., 2001).

The use of standardized, valid and reliable definitions is fundamental for the accurate measurement and monitoring of surgical complications (Bruce et al., 2001). In 1992, Clavien and colleagues were to first to introduce an innovative system to grade complications by severity proportional to the effort required to treat the complications (Clavien et al., 1992). This methodology was recently revised and a novel five-tiered classification system was developed with the intent of presenting an objective and reproducible method for reporting complications (Dindo et al., 2004). This system, now known as the Clavien-Dindo classification system, has been used in several surgical specialties and has widespread applicability (DeOliveira et al., 2006; Feldman et al., 1997; Grobmyer et al., 2007; Guillonneau et al., 2002; Kocak et al., 2006; Liu et al., 2009; Mazeh et al., 2009; Stolzenburg et al., 2006; Tamura et al., 2006; Targarona et al., 2000).

In this chapter, the Clavien-Dindo classification system is adapted to the thoracic surgical setting (Dindo et al., 2004). Therefore, the objectives are to describe the development of a classification system to grade presence and severity of thoracic morbidity and mortality (TM&M), which would enable us to compare surgical procedures and subgroups of patients, and simultaneously allow us to evaluate the feasibility of the system over the first two years of its implementation at the Ottawa Hospital, a high-volume, single academic thoracic surgery center. Second, the reliability and reproducibility of the TM&M classification is explored. Lastly, the impact of a standardized classification of post-operative complications on quality assessment in thoracic surgery is discussed.

The objective evaluation of both the presence and severity of thoracic morbidity and mortality and the prospective monitoring of thoracic surgical volume represents an important means of standardizing surgical outcomes, enabling comparisons between centers and surgeons, and represents a crucial component to ensuring continuous quality improvement and the best practice of care.

3. Large-scale quality initiatives

There are several ongoing, large-scale initiatives aimed specifically at measuring and improving surgical outcomes. For example, the National Surgical Quality Improvement Program (NSQIP) (Khuri et al., 1998) and the Society for Thoracic Surgeons (STS) database (Caceres et al., 2010), provide hospitals and cardiothoracic surgeons with information on their risk-adjusted M&M rates.

The NSQIP was created as a program that originated in the Veteran's Administration Hospitals in the United States as a quality improvement tool for surgical care (Khuri et al., 1998). The NSQIP uses clinical information from medical records to risk-adjust hospital mortality rates. One of the advantages of this type of system includes extensive clinical information on over one million patients for risk-adjusted analyses on 30-day outcomes of surgical care. Since the NSQIP has been implemented, marked improvement in surgical quality has been documented - M&M rates have declined, patient satisfaction has improved, and lengths of stay have decreased (Hall et al., 2009).

Similarly, the STS database was developed as an initiative to standardize nationwide outcomes in adult cardiac surgery, and it has currently expanded into general thoracic and congenital cardiac surgery databases (Caceres et al., 2010). Since its inception, the STS database has grown as a powerful source of risk-adjusted outcomes, large scale scientific contributions, and invaluable information for healthcare policy making (Caceres et al., 2010).

The NSQIP and STS database offer inter-institutional benchmarking, however, they are less applicable as a continuous quality improvement measure for an individual surgical program, as understanding and improving the delivery of a particular operation may require measures tailored to that operation (Birkmeyer et al., 2004), such as proper evaluation of the burden of illness of individual complications and subsequent patient impact. Moreover, the tracking of postoperative morbidity is less successful than of mortality due to the lack uniform definitions within the NSQIP and STS database (Grover et al., 1996).

4. Systematic classification of morbidity and mortality following thoracic surgery

Objective analysis and discussion of surgical M&M is the foundation of quality assurance. However, defining and measuring quality is a particularly difficult undertaking (Donabedian, 1988). Mortality is well defined in the literature and is a comparable surgical outcome, whereas morbidity rates have been poorly reported; thus, limiting comparisons among surgeons, procedures, and centers, and within the same center over time (Clavien et al., 1992; Clavien et al., 1994). To enable such comparisons, data on surgical outcomes must be acquired in a standardized and transparent format (Clavien et al., 1992).

Most surgeons depend on regular review of complications at M&M conferences to evaluate experience, analyze complications and receive feedback regarding quality improvement measures undertaken to minimize risk (Murayama et al., 2002). However, data from M&M conferences are neither systematically collected, nor stored in a standardized and reproducible fashion (Antonacci et al., 2008). These shortcomings of traditional methods for quality assurance have partly encouraged a movement toward a new paradigm for improving surgical care quality (Feldman et al., 1997), involving the continuous surveillance and evaluation of surgical adverse events.

Continuous monitoring of surgical M&M: i) allows for benchmarking; 2) identifies areas in need of improvement; 3) improves knowledge transfer; 4) facilitates staff and resident education; 5) enables prospective research; and 6) evaluates effectives of interventions. Clavien and colleagues were the first to introduce an innovative system to grade complications by severity proportional to the effort required to treat the complications (Clavien et al., 1992). This system of reporting serves as a means of judging the completeness of M&M reporting (Martin et al., 2002). Moreover, the Clavien-Dindo classification schema of surgical adverse events is precise, simple, reproducible and can be used to provide information that can assist in the continuous monitoring of surgical quality.

4.1 Development of the Thoracic Morbidity and Mortality (TM&M)

The TM&M system was developed according to the Clavien-Dindo classification schema of surgical adverse events (Dindo et al., 2004) (Table 1). Definitions of surgical adverse events were modified according to complications in patients following thoracic surgery through peer review and questionnaire, and adjusted based on surgeons' experience. A complication was defined as any deviation from the normal postoperative course. For each of the following systems: pulmonary, pleural, cardiac, renal, gastrointestinal, neurological, wound, and other, complications were defined and classified according to their specific gradation. The Common Terminology Criteria for Adverse Events (version 3.0) (Trotti et al., 2003) was also used to refine some definitions.

Grade	Definition
Minor	
Grade I	Any complication without need for pharmacologic treatment or other intervention.
Grade II	Any complication that requires pharmacological treatment or minor intervention only.
Major	
Grade III	Any complication that requires surgical, radiological, endoscopic intervention, or multi-therapy.
Grade IIIa	Intervention does not require general anaesthesia.
Grade IIIb	Intervention requires general anaesthesia.
Grade IV	Any complication requiring ICU management and life support.
Grade IVa	Single organ dysfunction.
Grade IVb	Multi-organ dysfunction.
Mortality	
Grade V	Any complication leading to the death of the patient.

Table 1. Classification of complications following thoracic surgery

4.2 Data collection

Daily data collection of M&M was carried out by a senior thoracic surgical resident and the thoracic surgery research coordinator using the TM&M form. Weekly lists of operative procedures along with related complications were compiled and further validated by attending staff. These complications were then discussed at monthly departmental M&M conferences. A database for complication reporting was developed; data entered included gender, age and preoperative diagnosis. Surgical details entered were type of operation, including whether it was a video assisted or open operation. The grading of complications was prospectively applied to each patient according to severity and effort required to treat the complication.

Descriptive statistical analyses were performed to analyze surgical volume and M&M rates after thoracic surgery. Incidence of complications in different subgroups was analyzed using the Chi-square test or Fisher's exact test. Correlations between complication grade and hospital length of stay was analyzed using analysis of variance (ANOVA). A p value of less than 0.05 was considered significant. Data were analyzed using SAS version 9.2 software.

4.3 Patients

The TM&M classification system was applied to a cohort of 953 consecutive patients undergoing non-cardiac thoracic surgery at the Ottawa Hospital from January 1, 2008 to December 31, 2009. There were 520 male (54.5%) and 433 female (45.5%) patients with a mean age of 61 years (range, 14–95 years). While 592 patients (62.1%) had a malignant disease, the remaining 361 patients (37.9%) had a range of benign lung, esophageal and other thoracic-related diseases.

4.4 Overall grade and severity of thoracic surgical complications

During the study period, a total of 953 patients (mean age 61, range 14-95) underwent a thoracic surgical procedure, of which 369 (29.3%) patients had at least one complication. Grades I and II complications accounted for 4.9% and 63.9% of all complications, respectively. Grade III and IV complications and comprised 21.1% and 7.8% of all complications, respectively. Overall mortality rate (Grade V) was 2.2%.

4.5 Burden of illness of individual complications

The TM&M classification system offers a comprehensive and objective evaluation of the impact of individual complications on patients. Atrial fibrillation (18.8%) and prolonged air leak (18.2%) compromised the majority of grade II complications following pulomonary resection, and thus, require more careful attention. The majority of prolonged air leak complications following pulmonary resection were grade I or II (87%), grade IIIa and IIIb were 9% and 2%, respectively, and Grade IV was 2%. Upon evaluation of all complications secondary to air leak after pulmonary resection, 97% of all atrial fibrillation was Grade II, with 1 patient (3%) experiencing a Grade IVa complication. In addition, since we began evaluating if complications led to prolonged hospital stay or re-admission, we found air leak led to 17% rate of re-admission, and 29% prolonged hospital stay, compared to 2% and 7% for atrial fibrillation. Thus, despite similar incidence after pulmonary resection, we identified air leak as having a significantly greater burden of illness than atrial fibrillation as defined by more severe complications, re-admissions and longer stay.

5. Testing the reliability and reproducibility of the TM&M classification system

Any system that is developed to provide an objective evaluation of the quality of surgical care must be simple, reproducible, and applicable to any surgical specialty at any medical institution. The next section describes how the reproducibility and reliability of the TM&M classification system was evaluated.

5.1 Methods

The Canadian Association of Thoracic Surgeons (CATS) was approached for a multi-center evaluation of the TM&M classification system (n = 95 members). The membership of CATS includes full-time practitioners of general (non-cardiac) thoracic surgery, along with qualified general and cardiovascular surgeons whose practice includes more than 50% thoracic surgery (Darling et al., 2004).

To assess the reproducibility and reliability of the modified classification, an electronic questionnaire was designed with 31-items. The Ottawa Hospital Research Ethics Board approved this study. The questionnaire consisted of three parts including: i) an information sheet with the TM&M classification system along with definitions of the severity grades; ii) 20 case-based questions asking respondents to classify postoperative adverse events in accordance to the proposed classification system; and iii) questions regarding personal judgments about the classification system.

The 20 case-based scenarios were placed randomly with regards to their complication grade. The 20 case-based scenarios were chosen to have an even representation of minor (Grades I – II) and major case examples (Grades IIIa – V). Respondents were asked to choose the most severe grade of complication for each case.

Weighted kappa statistics were calculated to assess the inter-rater reliability among the survey respondents. The level of agreement among the raters was evaluated using the system put forth by Landis and Koch, 1977, in which a kappa value of 0.21 to 0.4 reflects fair agreement, a value of 0.41 to 0.60 reflects moderate agreement, a value of 0.61 to 0.80 reflects substantial agreement, and a value of 0.81 or more reflects almost perfect agreement (Landis & Koch, 1977). Data were analyzed using R statistical software.

5.2 Results

From the 95 members, 52 surveys were completed (54.7%). The majority of respondents were affiliated with a university teaching hospital (78.8%, n = 41) and practiced in Ontario (32.7%, n = 17) or Quebec (15.4%, n = 8). Ontario and Quebec are the most densely populated provinces in Canada with populations of approximately 12.2 million and 7.6 million, respectively. Of the 52 completed surveys, 8 (15.4%) were completed by members practicing outside of Canada. Most surgeons had been in practice for less than 10 years (51.0%, n = 26).

The weighted Kappa statistic assesses agreement between two raters on an ordered scale (Landis & Koch, 1977). With 52 raters, a total of 1326 individual weighted Kappa statistics were calculated for all distinct pairs of raters. Of those 1326 weighted Kappa statistics, 1152 (87.0%) were greater than 0.81, a range which is interpreted as "almost perfect agreement." Furthermore, 173 (13.0%) were in the range between 0.61 and 0.8, interpreted as "substantial agreement." Thus, all of the statistics indicated at least substantial agreement. All results were statistically significant ($p < .0001$).

Respondents were asked to agree or disagree with several statements regarding their personal judgments of the TM&M classification system. Of the 52 respondents, 49 (98.0%) considered the TM&M classification system as straightforward to understand. A total of 48 respondents (94.1%) considered the TM&M classification system as reproducible; that is, different surgeons would tend to agree on the classification of individual patient events. A total 47 respondents (92.2%) considered the TM&M classification system as logical; that is, it accurately reflects the level of severity of adverse events. Lastly, 50 respondents (98.0%) consider the TM&M classification system useful in their patients; that is, it will be helpful to evaluate both presence and severity of surgical adverse events.

6. Impact of a systematic classification of post-operative complications on quality assessment in thoracic surgery

By using the TM&M system as a continuous measure of quality, we have now embarked on several initiatives to further improve complication rates related to thoracic procedures.

6.1 Example of value: Most common complications

6.1.1 Atrial fibrillation

Non-cardiac thoracic surgeries are often complicated by supra-ventricular arrhythmias, with atrial fibrillation representing the most common type of rhythm disturbance. Despite prevention efforts, atrial fibrillation remains one of the primary reasons for prolonged hospital stay, re-admission and additional complications post-pulmonary resection (Ramzan et al., 2011). The use of the TM&M classification system allows for the determination of the severity and burden of illness of a complication, which can lead to initiatives to improve the quality of care.

Using univariate analysis, several prognostic variables were identified for atrial fibrillation through a retrospective chart review of pulmonary resection cases. Logistic regression was used to identify risk factors with the strongest prognostic value for the outcome of atrial fibrillation. Significant variables in the multivariate analysis included age, left ventricular dysfunction, angina pectoris and open or converted surgery. These risk factors are specific to our individual institution over this two year period and may alter over time. However, identification of risk factors will allow for appropriate and targeted management of individuals with increased risk of developing post-operative atrial fibrillation (Ramzan et al., 2011).

6.1.2 Prolonged alveolar air leak

Another frequent complication after pulmonary resection for pulmonary diseases is prolonged alveolar air leak (Bardell & Petsikas, 2003; Irshad et al., 2002). Like atrial fibrillation, prolonged alveolar air leak has a significant clinical impact on patients and resources. Moreover, prolonged alveolar air leak can lead to additional morbidities, such as respiratory infections, empyema, and prolonged need for chest tubes (Brunelli et al., 2004; Brega et al., 2003).

Using the same methodology as outlined above, risk factors for prolonged alveolar air leak were identified and include obstructive pattern on PFT (FEV1<80%, FEV1/FVC<70%), higher pack-year of smoking, self-reported diagnosis of bronchitis, lobectomy (especially right upper lobectomy) and extended lobectomy (Liang et al., 2011). Risk factors can be used to identify patients who would benefit from prevenetive interventions, such as the use of buttressed stapled lines with bovine pericardium (Cerfolio et al., 2001) (Bio-Vascular Dry Peri-Strips, Mineapolis, MN), pleural tents for upper lobectomy, pneumoperitoneum after lower lobectomy, focal seal (genzyme, biosurgery, Cambridge MA), fibrin glue (Stolz et al., 2005) and collagen patch (Malapert et al., 2010). Practice changes could be monitored for efficacy using the TM&M classification system.

6.2 Example of value: Comparison between surgical procedures

Video-assisted thoracic surgery (VATS) is a relatively new technology that has rapidly become the standard of care for uncomplicated pulmonary resection. However, concerns have been expressed regarding the safety and oncologic efficacy of VATS lobectomy (Nicastri et al., 2008). The TM&M tool was utilized for reporting presence and severity of complications during the initiation of a VATS lobectomy learning curve, and compared to open lobectomy controls. The patterns of postoperative morbidity in patients undergoing VATS lobectomy, was analyzed, in order to deduce if there existed an altered number or pattern of adverse events.

A retrospective review of all patients undergoing thoracic surgery for lung cancer at the Ottawa Hospital was conducted to identify those patients who underwent elective pulmonary lobectomy for clinical stage I and II non-small cell lung cancer. All consecutive VATS lobectomies performed in the Ottawa Hospital since January 2006 until August 2010 were age-matched (±5 years) and stage-matched with a control cohort of open lobectomy cases. Data on patient demographics, co-morbidities, pulmonary function, pathological stage, operative procedure and time, blood loss, type and grade of postoperative complications, and hospital length of stay were recorded and analyzed.

In terms of results, there were no fundamental differences in complication rates between the two groups (47.5% for open vs. 43.3 for VATS; $p = 0.52$). There was also no difference in operative mortality between the two groups (3.3% for open vs. 1.7% for VATS; $p = 0.68$). Compared with open lobectomy, VATSlobectomy was associated with shorter mean length of stay (8.2 days for open vs. 7.8 days for VATS; $p < 0.05$). Mean operative time was higher for VATS lobectomy (239.1 minutes for open vs. 273.2 minutes for VATS; $p < 0.05$). Moreover, mean surgical time was also longer for VATS lobectomy (178.2 minutes for open vs. 220.0 minutes for VATS; $p < 0.05$). The amount of blood loss was significantly less following VATS lobectomy (230.6 cc for open vs. 170.3 cc for VATS; $p < 0.05$).

VATS lobectomy may be a safer procedure in particular patients. Also, the efficacy of VATS lobectomy is further amplified considering that VATS lobectomy is associated with a shorter hospital length of stay. However, more research is needed to identify specific complications that have been recognized to have an important impact on outcomes, such as atrial fibrillation. Several studies have demonstrated the frequency of postoperative atrial arrhythmias to be significantly lower after thoracoscopic surgery (Whitson et al., 2008).

6.3 Morbidity & Mortality (M&M) conference

The most widespread strategy for quality assessment in surgery has been the departmental M&M conference. This approach to quality assessment uses peer-review of cases resulting in adverse outcomes to identify inadequate care (Feldman et al., 1997). M&M rounds are an important educational tool for residents in regards to the causes of the most severe complications. M&M conferences also play a role in teaching surgeons how to present and how to take responsibility for issues (Feldman et al., 1997).

Although the historical and educational roles of the M&M conference are unquestionable, case-finding strategies for quality assessment have several limitations including emphasis on outliers and fault-finding, focus on individual performance rather than organizational processes, and focus on individual events rather than patterns of outcomes (Feldman et al., 1997).

Our departmental M&M conference has greatly been enhanced by the improved quality of statistical reporting of all complications, as collecting TM&M data has inherently been a collegial activity. Collecting TM&M requires participation of the senior residents on a daily basis, weekly confirmation by attending staff, and monthly discussion at M&M conferences. The presence and grade of a complication is not always clear; however, frank collegial discussion enhances the validity of the data. The TM&M classification system does not replace the M&M conference; rather it provides additional information, while maintaining individual patient case presentations.

7. Future directions

7.1 Needs assessment

Assessing the degree of involvement and participation in thoracic surgical research as well as surgical quality improvement conducted across Canadian institutions is difficult as there exists no common data collection system and no prior studies. As a pilot investigation, we designed and conducted a membership survey of the Canadian Association of Thoracic Surgeons (CATS) to evaluate the extent of participation in research and quality improvement processes among thoracic surgeons (Ivanovic et al., 2011).

The survey revealed that a high level of interest and participation exists in thoracic surgery research. However, more robust quality improvement processes are needed for thoracic surgical oncology services locally and nationally (Ivanovic et al., 2011). Moreover, the development of a national database is progressively being recognized as fundamental to the practice, review and quality assessment of thoracic oncology services across Canada (Ivanovic et al., 2011). A national thoracic surgery quality improvement database offers a potential means to improve practice effectiveness, standardize surgical outcomes, enhance multidisciplinary communication, promote thoracic research, and allow for the design and implementation of programs to improve surgical quality (Ivanovic et al., 2011). The results of this pilot project have provided a strong foundation of knowledge upon which we can, with time, enhance the monitoring of quality of care, both locally and nationally. The proceeding section describes the first steps of this process.

7.2 Thoracic Surgery Quality Monitoring, Information Management, and Clinical Documentation (TSQIC) System

Handheld computers are increasingly replacing paper methods for collecting patient-reported information. Studies have shown significant advances in the quality of patient care, in terms of legibility, availability, and data quality (Roukema et al., 2006) with the use of handheld computers for data collection. Moreover, extensive research has demonstrated that point-of-care clinical documentation improves communication amongst health care professionals, augments efficiency of care, and enables monitoring of quality of care. It is well known that new-generation handheld computers offer increasing support to surgeons in their daily clinical activity and an increasing potential for future use (Fischer et al., 2003).

In the Ottawa Hospital's Cancer Assessment Clinic, a paper-based documentation system is currently used to document thoracic oncology care. Numerous problems are reported with respect to the length of time spent on documenting, delay in transcription (requiring days to weeks) and the significant costs of transcription, and the low quality of the documentation. These shortcomings lead to inefficient use of clinic time, delays in communication from surgeon to oncologists, and impaired quality of care relating to poor communication. Documentation may be further compromised if it is not immediately carried out.

Building upon research studies demonstrating the value of electronic documentation to address these problems, we introduce the Thoracic Surgery Quality Monitoring, Information Management, and Clinical Documentation (TSQIC) System, a web-based software application accessed on a portable device (i.e. iPad) to perform point-of-care recording and reporting of standardized essential bedside patient information. The TSQIC has already gone through two years of iterative development by the the Ottawa Hospital's division of thoracic surgery, and comprises standardized electronic templates facilitating recording and reporting of essential patient data for all time points throughout the continuum of thoracic surgical oncology care. The time points include referral, initial investigation, past medical history, physician orders and physical exam, pulmonary report, cardiac evaluation, staging, clinical assessment and plan, operation form, peri-operative surgical adverse events, and a minimum of two years follow up post surgery. The TSQIC is a natural extension of the TM&M. In addition to recording peri-operative adverse events, the TSQIC will automatically record essential clinical data relating to quality of care, including wait times. Optimized for an iPad, but accessible through any web-enabled computer, the TSQIC is designed to augment efficiency of clinic time and decrease costs by eliminating the need for transcription. Our eventual goal is to implement the TSQIC system within the Ottawa Hospital's Thoracic Cancer Assessment Clinic and to evaluate its accuracy, completeness, efficiency, rapidity, usability, and overall quality, compared to traditional paper-based documentation.

The TSQIC not only has the capacity to transform clinical documentation, improve efficiency and augment monitoring of quality at a single center, but has potential to be expanded to other disciplines within the Ottawa Hospital, and to other centers across Canada.

8. Conclusion

Quality assurance has been at the forefront for surgeons in all specialties and to this day it remains a primary objective of their professional careers (Gumpert, 1988). Surgeons have advanced a highly refined system of sustaining and improving the quality of their practice through the measurement and evaluation of structure, process, and outcomes of care. The three areas clearly overlap to some degree, as quality assurance is only possible because good structure increases the likelihood of good process, and good process increases the likelihood of good outcome (Donabedian, 1988). To date, most quality improvement initiatives in surgery have focused on measures of morbidity and mortality (Birkmeyer et al., 2004). Therefore, an objective system for monitoring and accurately reporting postoperative morbidity and mortality is fundamental in order to advance performance in thoracic surgery and collect reliable data for benchmarking. Moreover, an objective and standardized system permits comparison of outcomes between surgical procedures, between different institutions, and allows for knowledge transfer for improvement in one's own institution. The implications are wide-ranging, as all disciplines would be empowered to work towards the same goal of improving surgical in-patient outcomes.

The development of the TM&M classification system and the accompanying TM&M database has facilitated systematic monitoring, reporting and evaluation of postoperative complications across all thoracic surgical procedures performed at The Ottawa Hospital.

To test the reproducibility of the TM&M classification system, clinical case examples were created by the thoracic surgical team at the Ottawa Hospital and sent to all members of the Canadian Association of Thoracic Surgeons. The consistency of a surgeons' rating is an important consideration in outcome assessment. These ratings often fall on an ordinal scale, making the kappa coefficient an appropriate measure of reliability for such data (Brenner & Kliebsch, 1996). A high level of agreement was calculated among the 52 survey respondents for the 20 case scenarios, indicating that the TM&M classification system is consistent among surgeons' opinion and can be applied to multifaceted case examples. Through the application of severity grades, the TM&M classification system has provided standardized measures for discriminating what may represent a minor as opposed to major adverse event following thoracic surgery.

The TM&M classification system is also complementary to several ongoing, large-scale programs designed specifically to measure and improve surgical outcomes (Birkmeyer et al., 2004), such as the National Surgical Quality Improvement Program (NSQIP) (Khuri et al., 1998) and the Society for Thoracic Surgeons (STS) database (Caceres et al., 2010). Incorporation of a standardized complication grading system, such as the TM&M, into large organizational databases would allow identification of areas for improvement for surgeons and institutions. It would provide a common denominator for the implementation of quality improvement programs to reduce the incidence of complications following thoracic surgery.

We further plan to utilize this continuous TM&M classification and reporting system as a backbone for prospective monitoring of essential surgical information, upon which to add additional clinical data collection tools. The TM&M classification system provides a strong base with which we can build a system (that is, the TSQIC system) to continuously monitor and improve the overall quality of thoracic surgical care. Expanding the TM&M classification system to include clinical data on all time points on the continuum of care, starting with patient referral to at least a two year follow-up post surgery, would certainly help improve continuous assurance of care.

A prospectively collected, standardized classification system for accurately identifying and grading thoracic surgical complications in all cases is feasible to implement, facilitates objective comparison between surgical procedures, surgeons and centers, and identifies burden of illness of individual complications. Furthermore, the TM&M classification system advocates for a practice of continuous quality improvement, advances the development of quality improvement programs, and facilitates an open forum for ongoing medical education on surgical quality assurance and evaluation.

9. Acknowledgments

The authors would like to gratefully acknowledge the entire division of thoracic surgery at the Ottawa Hospital including: Dr. Sudhir Sundaresan, Dr. Donna Maziak, Dr. Farid Shamji, Dr. Sebastian Gilbert, Dr. James Villeneuve, Dr. Ahmed Alhussaini, Dr. Derar Alshahab, Zeb Khan and Jennifer Threader. The authors would also like to gratefully acknowledge funding from the Department of Surgery at the Ottawa Hospital, Dr. Lorenzo Ferri (McGill University) for his suggestion to initially explore the Clavien-Dindo classification system, and to Dr. Jack Kitts, president and CEO of The Ottawa Hospital for his encouragement of this project. Lastly, the authors would like to thank the entire membership of the Canadian Association of Thoracic Surgeons for their participation in the questionnaire, in addition to their feedback.

10. References

Antonacci, A. C., Lam, S., Lavarias, V., Homel, P., & Eavey, R. D. (2008). A morbidity and mortality conference-based classification system for adverse events: Surgical outcome analysis: Part I. *Journal of Surgical Research, 147*(2), 172-177.

Bardell, T., & Petsikas, D. (2003). What keeps postpulmonary resection patients in hospital? *Canadian Respiratory Journal : Journal of the Canadian Thoracic Society, 10*(2), 86-89.

Birkmeyer, J. D., Dimick, J. B., & Birkmeyer, N. J. O. (2004). Measuring the quality of surgical care: Structure, process, or outcomes? , *Journal of the American College of Surgeons, 198*(4), 626-632.

Brega Massone, P. P., Magnani, B., Conti, B., Lequaglie, C., & Cataldo, I. (2003). Cauterization versus fibrin glue for aerostasis in precision resections for secondary lung tumors. *Annals of Surgical Oncology, 10*(4), 441-446.

Brenner, H., & Kliebsch, U. (1996). Dependence of weighted kappa coefficients on the number of categories. *Epidemiology (Cambridge, Mass.), 7*(2), 199-202.

Bruce, J., Russell, E. M., Mollison, J., & Krukowski, Z. H. (2001). The measurement and monitoring of surgical adverse events. *Health Technology Assessment (Winchester, England), 5*(22), 1-194.

Brunelli, A., Monteverde, M., Borri, A., Salati, M., Marasco, R. D., & Fianchini, A. (2004). Predictors of prolonged air leak after pulmonary lobectomy. *The Annals of Thoracic Surgery, 77*(4), 1205-10; discussion 1210.

Caceres, M., Braud, R. L., & Garrett, H. E.,Jr. (2010). A short history of the society of thoracic surgeons national cardiac database: Perceptions of a practicing surgeon. *The Annals of Thoracic Surgery, 89*(1), 332-339.

Cerfolio, R. J., Bass, C., & Katholi, C. R. (2001). Prospective randomized trial compares suction versus water seal for air leaks. *The Annals of Thoracic Surgery, 71*(5), 1613-1617.

Clavien, P. A., Camargo, C. A.,Jr, Croxford, R., Langer, B., Levy, G. A., & Greig, P. D. (1994). Definition and classification of negative outcomes in solid organ transplantation. application in liver transplantation. *Annals of Surgery, 220*(2), 109-120.

Clavien, P. A., Sanabria, J. R., & Strasberg, S. M. (1992). Proposed classification of complications of surgery with examples of utility in cholecystectomy. *Surgery, 111*(5), 518-526.

Daley, J., Henderson, W. G., & Khuri, S. F. (2001). Risk-adjusted surgical outcomes. *Annual Review of Medicine, 52*, 275-287.

Darling, G. E., Maziak, D. E., Clifton, J. C., Finley, R. J., & Canadian Association of Thoracic Surgery. (2004). The practice of thoracic surgery in canada. *Canadian Journal of Surgery.Journal Canadien De Chirurgie, 47*(6), 438-445.

DeOliveira, M. L., Winter, J. M., Schafer, M., Cunningham, S. C., Cameron, J. L., Yeo, C. J., et al. (2006). Assessment of complications after pancreatic surgery: A novel grading system applied to 633 patients undergoing pancreaticoduodenectomy. *Annals of Surgery, 244*(6), 931-7; discussion 937-9.

Dimick, J. B., Cowan, J. A.,Jr, & Chen, S. L. (2003). Emerging approaches for assessing and improving the quality of surgical care. *Current Surgery, 60*(3), 241-246.

Dindo, D., Demartines, N., & Clavien, P. A. (2004). Classification of surgical complications: A new proposal with evaluation in a cohort of 6336 patients and results of a survey. *Annals of Surgery, 240*(2), 205-213.

Donabedian, A. (1988). The quality of care. how can it be assessed? *JAMA : The Journal of the American Medical Association, 260*(12), 1743-1748.

Feldman, L., Barkun, J., Barkun, A., Sampalis, J., & Rosenberg, L. (1997). Measuring postoperative complications in general surgery patients using an outcomes-based strategy: Comparison with complications presented at morbidity and mortality rounds. *Surgery, 122*(4), 711-9; discussion 719-20.

Fischer, S., Stewart, T. E., Mehta, S., Wax, R., & Lapinsky, S. E. (2003). Handheld computing in medicine. *Journal of the American Medical Informatics Association : JAMIA, 10*(2), 139-149.

Grobmyer, S. R., Pieracci, F. M., Allen, P. J., Brennan, M. F., & Jaques, D. P. (2007). Defining morbidity after pancreaticoduodenectomy: Use of a prospective complication grading system. *Journal of the American College of Surgeons, 204*(3), 356-364.

Grover, F. L., Shroyer, A. L., & Hammermeister, K. E. (1996). Calculating risk and outcome: The veterans affairs database. *The Annals of Thoracic Surgery, 62*(5 Suppl), S6-11; discussion S31-2.

Guillonneau, B., Rozet, F., Cathelineau, X., Lay, F., Barret, E., Doublet, J. D., et al. (2002). Perioperative complications of laparoscopic radical prostatectomy: The montsouris 3-year experience. *The Journal of Urology, 167*(1), 51-56.

Gumpert, J. R. (1988). Why on earth do surgeons need quality assurance? *Annals of the Royal College of Surgeons of England, 70*(2), 85-92.

Hall, B. L., Hamilton, B. H., Richards, K., Bilimoria, K. Y., Cohen, M. E., & Ko, C. Y. (2009). Does surgical quality improve in the american college of surgeons national surgical quality improvement program: An evaluation of all participating hospitals. *Annals of Surgery, 250*(3), 363-376.

Irshad, K., Feldman, L. S., Chu, V. F., Dorval, J. F., Baslaim, G., & Morin, J. E. (2002). Causes of increased length of hospitalization on a general thoracic surgery service: A prospective observational study. *Canadian Journal of Surgery.Journal Canadien De Chirurgie, 45*(4), 264-268.

Ivanovic J, Gilbert S, Maziak DE, Shamji F, Sundaresan S., Ramsay T, and Seely AJE (2011). Assessing the status of thoracic surgical research and quality improvement programs: A survey of the members of the Canadian Association of Thoracic Surgeons. Accepted for publication in *The Journal of Surgical Education* [In press].

Khuri, S. F., Daley, J., Henderson, W., Hur, K., Demakis, J., Aust, J. B., et al. (1998). The department of veterans affairs' NSQIP: The first national, validated, outcome-based, risk-adjusted, and peer-controlled program for the measurement and enhancement of the quality of surgical care. national VA surgical quality improvement program. *Annals of Surgery, 228*(4), 491-507.

Khuri, S. F., Daley, J., & Henderson, W. G. (1999). The measurement of quality in surgery. *Advances in Surgery, 33*, 113-140.

Kocak, B., Koffron, A. J., Baker, T. B., Salvalaggio, P. R., Kaufman, D. B., Fryer, J. P., et al. (2006). Proposed classification of complications after live donor nephrectomy. *Urology, 67*(5), 927-931.

Landis, J. R., & Koch, G. G. (1977). The measurement of observer agreement for categorical data. *Biometrics, 33*(1), 159-174.

Liang S, Ramzan S, Ivanovic J, Zhang H, Threader J, Khan J, Alhussaini A, Villeneuve PJ, Gilbert S, Maziak D, Shamji F, Sundaresan S, Seely AJE. (2011) Documenting the burden of post-operative air leak after pulmonary resection using a novel system to classify severity of post-operative complications. In preparation.

Liu, B., Yan, L. N., Li, J., Li, B., Zeng, Y., Wang, W. T., et al. (2009). Using the clavien grading system to classify the complications of right hepatectomy in living donors. *Transplantation Proceedings, 41*(5), 1703-1706.

Malapert, G., Hanna, H. A., Pages, P. B., & Bernard, A. (2010). Surgical sealant for the prevention of prolonged air leak after lung resection: Meta-analysis. *The Annals of Thoracic Surgery, 90*(6), 1779-1785.

Martin, R. C.,2nd, Brennan, M. F., & Jaques, D. P. (2002). Quality of complication reporting in the surgical literature. *Annals of Surgery, 235*(6), 803-813.

Mazeh, H., Samet, Y., Abu-Wasel, B., Beglaibter, N., Grinbaum, R., Cohen, T., et al. (2009). Application of a novel severity grading system for surgical complications after colorectal resection. *Journal of the American College of Surgeons, 208*(3), 355-361.e5.

Murayama, K. M., Derossis, A. M., DaRosa, D. A., Sherman, H. B., & Fryer, J. P. (2002). A critical evaluation of the morbidity and mortality conference. *American Journal of Surgery, 183*(3), 246-250.

Nicastri, D. G., Wisnivesky, J. P., Litle, V. R., Yun, J., Chin, C., Dembitzer, F. R., et al. (2008). Thoracoscopic lobectomy: Report on safety, discharge independence, pain, and chemotherapy tolerance. *The Journal of Thoracic and Cardiovascular Surgery, 135*(3), 642-647.

Ramzan S, Liang S, Ivanovic J, Zhang H, Threader J, Khan J, Alhussaini A, Villeneuve PJ, Gilbert S, Maziak D, Shamji F, Sundaresan S, Seely AJE. (2011) Documenting the burden of post-operative atrial fibrillation after pulmonary resection using a novel complication classification system. In prepartion.

Roukema, J., Los, R. K., Bleeker, S. E., van Ginneken, A. M., van der Lei, J., & Moll, H. A. (2006). Paper versus computer: Feasibility of an electronic medical record in general pediatrics. *Pediatrics, 117*(1), 15-21.

Stolz, A. J., Schutzner, J., Lischke, R., Simonek, J., & Pafko, P. (2005). Predictors of prolonged air leak following pulmonary lobectomy. *European Journal of Cardio-Thoracic Surgery : Official Journal of the European Association for Cardio-Thoracic Surgery, 27*(2), 334-336.

Stolzenburg, J. U., Rabenalt, R., Do, M., Lee, B., Truss, M. C., Schwaibold, H., et al. (2006). Categorisation of complications of endoscopic extraperitoneal and laparoscopic transperitoneal radical prostatectomy. *World Journal of Urology, 24*(1), 88-93.

Tamura, S., Sugawara, Y., Kaneko, J., Yamashiki, N., Kishi, Y., Matsui, Y., et al. (2006). Systematic grading of surgical complications in live liver donors according to clavien's system. *Transplant International : Official Journal of the European Society for Organ Transplantation, 19*(12), 982-987.

Targarona, E. M., Espert, J. J., Bombuy, E., Vidal, O., Cerdan, G., Artigas, V., et al. (2000). Complications of laparoscopic splenectomy. *Archives of Surgery (Chicago, Ill.: 1960), 135*(10), 1137-1140.

Trotti, A., Colevas, A. D., Setser, A., Rusch, V., Jaques, D., Budach, V., et al. (2003). CTCAE v3.0: Development of a comprehensive grading system for the adverse effects of cancer treatment. *Seminars in Radiation Oncology, 13*(3), 176-181.

Whitson, B. A., D'Cunha, J., Andrade, R. S., Kelly, R. F., Groth, S. S., Wu, B., et al. (2008). Thoracoscopic versus thoracotomy approaches to lobectomy: Differential impairment of cellular immunity. *The Annals of Thoracic Surgery, 86*(6), 1735-1744.

6

Post-Thoracotomy Pain Syndrome

Anand Alister Joseph R., Anand Puttappa and Donal Harney
Mercy University Hospital, Cork, Ireland

1. Introduction

Trauma and surgery have been well recognised as risk factors for developing chronic pain. The first published article on chronic post-surgical pain (CPSP) was in 1998 by Crombie and colleagues. Since then this concept has gained increasing popularity, evidenced by the dramatic increase in number of research publications focussing on post surgical pain states[1,5]. Despite this awareness, post surgical pain still remains poorly recognised and is under estimated as a cause for pain related morbidity. Post thoracotomy pain syndrome is one of such post surgical pain syndrome which remains a challenge to the treating physician both in terms morbidity for the individual and the incurring health costs on the society [2, 3, 5].

Thoracotomy incisions are considered amongst the most painful incisions as it involves a significant amount of trauma and distraction forces on multiple muscle layers, fascia, neurovascular bundles, bone and joints and parietal pleura all of these being pain sensitive structures. This may also involve rib resection if surgically required[4,6]. A chronic pain state, which occurs after such surgical intervention, is called chronic post thoracotomy pain syndrome (PTPS). The International Association for the Study of Pain has defined post thoracotomy pain syndrome as 'Pain that recurs or persists along a thoracotomy incision atleast two months after the surgical procedure'[7].

2. Epidemiology

There are major discrepancies in the reported prevalence of PTPS. This may in part be explained by the differences in study methodology which include but are not limited to the definition of PTPS, patient characteristics and the duration of follow up. PTPS ranges from 5-80% of thoracotomies and 5-33% for video-assisted thoracoscopic surgeries (VATS) [8-18]. In a recent survey following patients after thoracotomies for lung cancer the incidence of PTPS was 33% for thoracotomies and 25% for VATS procedures. Clinically relevant pain was present in 11-18% and severe pain in 4-12%, which depended on the level of physical activity. More than half of these patients reported pain from other parts. There is no clear evidence to suggest sex predominance but it was observed that women tended to report higher levels of pain with concomitant use of simple analgesics. And younger patients reported more pain as compared to the elderly[19]. There is little consensus regarding the impact that the type of surgery has on the clinical outcome in terms of PTPS. Some studies showing there being no convincing difference and others claiming that video-assisted thoracoscopic procedures to be superior[8, 20-23].

3. Pathophysiology

The etiopathogenesis of post-surgical pain syndromes is multifactorial and is yet to be fully elucidated. There still remains a large gap in our knowledge pertaining to the exact mechanisms involved and is a subject of constant debate with new evolving concepts. Post-thoracotomy pain is by and large one of the classical post-surgical pain syndrome.

3.1 Neurogenic mechanisms – neuroplasticity

Neuroplasticity is a relatively new term and as the name denotes it refers to the inherent ability of the central nervous system to adapt, modify and transform itself both structurally and functionally. The central nervous system was once thought to be hard wired but now is viewed as a dynamic processing unit which responds to various stimuli.

Thoracotomies as previously mentioned involves trauma to various structures, most importantly the intercostal nerves. Injury to the intercostal nerves may occur directly as a result pressure on the nerves by surgical retractors or when surgical resection of the rib is performed or indirectly where the entire nerve is subjected to traction forces by the retractors resulting in ischaemia. The other possibilities being impingement from displaced rib fractures and nerve entrapment in scar tissue. The cycle of events which occur in chronic pain patients after nerve injury may be best explained as a maladaptive response where the nervous systems both the peripheral and central nervous systems are altered, becoming dysfunctional and resulting in a neuropathic pain state

3.1.1 Peripheral sensitisation

Nerve damage leads to an inflammatory response with the outpour of inflammatory mediators as the nerve undergoes degeneration. These mediators which include tumour necrosis factor, prostaglandins, histamine, potassium ions , bradykinin and other products of arachidonic acid degradation which are pro-nociceptive results in peripheral sensitisation. This results in a reduction of required magnitude of stimuli to trigger an action potential and thereafter the transmission of pain signals. This is manifested as primary and secondary hyperalgesia which are exaggerated responses in pain perception for the given noxious stimuli and also allodynia which is increased pain sensitivity to non-noxious stimuli. Primary hyperalgesia is an exaggerated response to stimuli at the damaged site and secondary hyperalgesia is that which is perceived in the surrounding undamaged tissue. While primary hyperalgesia is mainly a peripheral neural phenomenon, secondary hyperalgesia is thought to be a mediated within the central nervous system which is referred as central sensitisation.

3.1.2 Central sensitisation

Peripheral sensitisation results in increased activity in the nociceptors and their primary afferent neurons. Persistent exposure of the cell bodies of these neurons in the dorsal horn to noxious stimuli results in a hyper-excitable state called central sensitisation. The dorsal horn of the spinal cord plays a vital role in impulse modulation and transmission; its acts as a gateway between the peripheral nociceptors and the higher centres where pain in perceived. The dorsal horn functions as a gate where pain signals are either dampened or amplified and transmitted to the higher centres. In this dysfunctional state of hyper-excitability in the spinal cord, signal transmission is augmented at the spinal level along with influence from descending pathways resulting in sensitisation. Central sensitisation is therefore described as a pain amplification process of the central pain-processing unit where there is facilitation in pain transmission and widening of receptor field to stimuli. It is also speculated that cortical remapping occurs in persistent pain with the developments of new neural networks and unfolding of dormant synapses as part of the neuromatrix model.

While intercostal nerve injury is assumed to be the most important cause of PTPS, there is conflicting evidence in the literature. There is evidence to support the fact that intercostal nerve damage does occurs during surgery and that surgical factors may affect outcome. The pattern and degree of nerve damage has also being studied by neurophysiological studies of the intercostal nerve during and following surgery. Patients who have significant intercostal nerve damage like those with rib resection and fractures developed neuropathic pain. And those with neuropathic pain features develop significant chronic pain which may be disabling. Despite these facts to support this mechanism of pain, intercostal nerve damage nerve alone cannot be incriminated as the sole cause for chronic pain after thoracic surgery.

3.2 Myofascial pain

It is well recognised that patients with PTPS may have associated shoulder dysfunction. Soft tissue trauma, which includes muscle, fascia and connective tissue, may result in Myofascial pain syndrome.

3.3 Local factors

Tumour recurrence, infection, costochondritis, costochondrol disruption, costovertebral disruption, pleurisy and healing rib fractures may all contribute to ongoing pain after thoracotomy.

1.	Intercostal nerve injury - neuroma
2.	Tumour recurrence
3.	Myofascial pain syndrome
4.	Frozen shoulder
5.	Healing fracture ribs
6.	Costochondritis
7.	Costochondral disruption
8.	Costovertebral disruption
9.	Infection
10.	Pleuritis
11.	Psychological distress

Table 1. Cause of chronic post thoracotomy pain syndrome

4. Clinical presentation

According to the nomenclature suggested by the IASP, any pain along the thoracotomy incision site, which is persistent beyond 2 months, is PTPS.[7] In general, PTPS is largely neuropathic in nature with charctersitic features of neuropathic pain. A thorough assessment is required as with most pain syndromes is to differentaite between neuropathic, visceral and nociceptive pain; all of which aids in the management. In cancer patients, the appearnce of new pain or worsening of pain which was fairly under control may warrant further investigation to rule out disease progression.

4.1 Neuropathic pain

Neuropathic pain is present in majority of these patients and is manifested by an array of symptoms which include allodynia, hyperalgesia, dysaesthesia or parasthesia. Patients describe the pain as a sharp, shooting or stabbing pain along the scar line. They may also report pain along the dermatomal distribution of the affected intercostal nerves as a constant dysesthetic burning type pain. Table 3.

Allodynia	Pain due to a stimulus that does not normally provoke pain.
Hyperalgesia	Increased pain from a stimulus that normally provokes pain
Hyperesthesia	Increased sensitivity to stimulation, excluding the special senses.
Hypoesthesia	Diminished pain in response to a normally painful stimulus
Dysesthesia	An unpleasant abnormal sensation, whether spontaneous or evoked
Paresthesia	An abnormal sensation, whether spontaneous or evoked

Table 2. Definitions of common neuropathic pain terms

4.2 Myofascial pain

Around one third of patients do not report features of neuropathic pain and myofacial pain, with local tenderness and shoulder dysfunction may predominant the clinical picture. Shoulder dysfunction is common and may be due to the division of the serratus anterior and latissimus dorsi muscle. This results in a viscious cycle of pain, lack of movements, muscle deconditioning and frozen shoulder.

4.3 Visceral pain

Visceral pain is usually as vague, constant, dull aching type of pain. The concept of visceral pain in gaining popularity and may account for those patients who do not present as neuropathic pain post thoracic surgery. Steegers et al 2008 found that this is more common with more extensive surgery and pleurectomy suggesting a visceral component to the PTPS.[57]

5. Perioperative risk factors and preventive strategies

Intercostal nerve damage is an important identifiable cause but not the sole pathogenic mechanism for chronic post thoracotomy pain. Researchers have attempted to identify risk factors associated with PTPS and investigate strategies which may reduce the incidence of PTPS. This has led to a number of publications on this topic but most fail to provide definitive evidence mainly due to inconsistencies in study design. The following table enumerates the various possible perioperative factors which may influence the occurrence of PTPS.

Preoperative factors
1. Demographic factors
2. Genetic makeup
3. Preoperative pain
4. Psychosocial factors
Surgical factors
1. Surgical incision: PLT Vs MPLT
2. Video assisted thoracoscopic surgery(VATS)
3. Intercostal Nerve sparing techniques
Anaesthetic factors
1. Anaesthesia
2. Analgesia

Table 3. Perioperative risk factors and preventive strategies

5.1 Preoperative factors

Preoperative preparation and optimisation is an important part in the care of the surgical patient and can have major influence on patient outcomes. Post thoracotomy pain syndrome is one such entity which may be indirectly influenced by preoperative optimisation. It has been shown that poorly controlled acute pain can progress to chronic pain states. Therefore it could be stated that patients who are appropriately optimised prior to surgery would do better after surgery in terms of being able to engage in the rehabilitative process and recover more rapidly thereby reducing the incidence of PTPS . The other important fact in the preoperative period is to appreciate post thoracotomy pain syndrome as one of the most common complications after thoracic surgery and being proactive could reduce its incidence Recognising this fact is vital in the management of these patients as appropriate identification of those at risk and developing management strategies may improve outcomes in terms of pain morbidity.

5.1.1 Demographic factors

Post surgical pain syndromes after mastectomies have been noted to occur less frequently with increasing age. But, factors such as type of tumour, their presentation and response to treatment need to be considered as these vary with age and may influence the incidence. Post herniorrhaphy pain also tends to decrease with increasing age.[24,25,27,28] There is evidence to suggest a gender difference where women may be at a higher risk of developing post surgical pain.[19,28] Currently there is no definitive evidence to suggest that post thoracotomy pain has age or gender preponderance.

5.1.2 Genetics

In clinical practice we observe that there is significant inter-individual variability in the pattern in patient's presentation, progression and response to therapy. It is extremely difficult to predict the response of an individual to a given insult, there may be a role in the underlying genetic makeup of the individual which might explain why some patents are more prone to post surgical pain. The attempt to identify such genes which play a role in pain processing has shown some association with gene polymorphism of catechol-0-methyltransferase (COMT), genetic variants to determine voltage-gated sodium channels and GTP cyclohydrolase and tetrahydrobiopterin-related genes.[29,30,31] Laboratory studies show an association between genetic factors and the development of neuropathic pain after nerve injury.[31] This may suggest that post thoracotomy pain in which nerve damage is a major pathogenic mechanism may be influenced by genetic factors.

5.1.3 Psychological factors

The biopsychosocial approach to pain is a broad multidimensional concept, which incorporates the traditional biomedical model and the psychodynamic model. In chronic pain states the impact of psychological factors (cognition, affect and behaviour) and social factors (social status, employment, litigation) may play an important role in exacerbation and maintaining pain. This impacts the outcome when assessed in terms of quality of life after surgery.[33] A systematic review on premorbid psychosocial status of depression, stress and psychological vulnerability showed a positive correlation between them and the development of chronic post surgical pain. Patients with higher level of depression and stress are at higher risk for development of chronic pain as is those who are psychologically vulnerable.[34] Pain in the perioperative period as a risk factor for the development of emotional numbing as part of a post traumatic stress disorder was found to be significant predictor of pain disability at 6 and 12 months after lateral thoracotomy. Suggesting that de coupling of pain intensity and disability occurs while emotional numbing takes a more important role in pain disability.[35] The correlation between psychosocial factors and the development of chronic pain after surgery is complex and remains challenge to investigate partly due to the inadequacies in measuring these factors.

5.1.4 Preoperative pain

Pre-existing pain and the use of pain medications has shown to correlate well with chronic post operative pain syndromes after hernia, limb amputation and breast surgery.[25, 36-38] Keller et al found a positive correlation with patients on pain medications in the preoperative period with those on pain medications having an incidence as high as 52% compared to 5.5% for those not on pain medications.[39] Most studies on the association between preoperative pain and chronic post thoracotomy pain syndrome have revealed inconsistent results as most studies exclude patients with pre-existing pain morbidity and pain medications.

5.2 Surgical factors

Surgery in general is now well recognised as a risk factor for chronic pain. Patients undergoing thoracic surgery have a high incidence of chronic pain, and as we have already seen that injury to the intercostal nerve has a major role in the pathogenesis of chronic post thoracotomy pain. Various surgical approaches and procedures to minimise nerve injury have been attempted over the years. These techniques will be discussed in the following section.

5.2.1 Thoracotomy: Posterolateral approach Vs muscle sparing surgery

Access to the thorax is either through a median sternotomy, anterior or anterolateral, lateral or posterior lateral, axillary and transverse sternothoracotomy incision. Among these the lateral and posterolateral approach (PLT) is considered to be the gold standard. The primary advantage of this approach is that it facilitates good access to intrapleural structures which include the lungs, oesophagus, chest wall and mediastinum. The main drawback is that of its invasiveness. This approach may involve rib transection or resection to optimise surgical exposure. But it is also the most painful of incisions because of its invasiveness which involves incision of the serratus anterior, latissimus dorsi and trapezius muscles. This results in the development of shoulder girdle dysfunction and pain which is a common occurrence in PTPS.[40]

In an attempt to reduce muscle trauma, a modification of the classic PLT approach called the muscle sparing posterolateral (MPLT) approach is increasingly being used. This approach does not involve the division of the latissimus dorsi muscle and the size of the incisions is smaller but provides optimal exposure for most pulmonary operations. The advantages of this approach is mainly due to the decreased muscle trauma and incision size, which results in decreased operative time, post operative pain, hospital stay and improved shoulder girdle function and cosmesis. The drawbacks being suboptimal exposure for some procedures especially where adhesions are present, a higher level of expertise is required and there is a higher incidence of seroma formation.[41, 42]

Mario Nosotti et al 2010 published a prospectively conducted randomised controlled trial comparing the two techniques in patients undergoing pulmonary lobectomy. This was done with the primary endpoints of pain, analgesic consumption and post thoracotomy syndrome. The incision type influenced the analgesic consumption, hospital stay and shoulder strength positively in those who had a MPLT but the three year PTPS was not affected.[43] The association between the incision type and the subsequent development of PTPS has not been established and there is a lack of well designed prospective studies focussing on this issue.

5.2.2 Video-Assisted Thoracoscopic Surgery (VATS)

Video assisted thoracoscopic surgery is adopted from the well established and increasingly popular laparoscopic surgical technique in an attempt to avoid large surgical incision and thereby conceived as a minimally invasive technique. But in the case of chronic pain morbidity after VATS there is no current evidence to suggest the superiority of this technique with conflicting reports. Conceptually, the avoidance of large thoracotomy incisions would result in lesser trauma to the neurovascular bundle and thus reduced incidence of PTPS. Unfortunately this is not translated clinically and intercostal nerve injury does occur probably by compressive and distractive forces by thoracoscopic manipulation like excessive torquing of the thoracosope which may cause rib fractures and intercostal nerve injury. And in inexperienced hands and patients with adhesions operating time may be prolonged. Moreover multiple ports may be required and extraction of resected segments may require a small thoracotomy incision and small incisions requiring more force to retract the ribs increasing the possibility of nerve damage. It is accepted that VATS surgery is favourable in short terms outcomes of immediate post operative pain scores, opioid consumption and hospital stay but not different in the long term outcome of PTPS.[4,44,45]

5.2.3 Intercostal nerve sparing techniques

Techniques to reduce the injury caused to the intercostal nerves have shown positive results with a trend towards reduced incidence of chronic PTPS. Retraction on the ribs and the use of pericostal sutures can cause significant injury to the intercostal nerves. This may be overcome partially by dissecting out an intercostal flap or by using intracostal sutures as opposed to pericostal sutures. Pericostal sutures which are commonly used suture technique are placed on the top of the 5th rib and 7th rib whereas intracostal sutures involve the drilling of small hole in the underlying rib and closing the thoracotomy wound with sutures through these holes.

Cerfolio et al 2003, in a prospective radomised controlled trial in 280 patients comparing the two suture techniques found that there was reduced pain in the intracostal at 3 months and that these patients reported lesser neuropathic descriptors of burning and shooting type pain.[46]

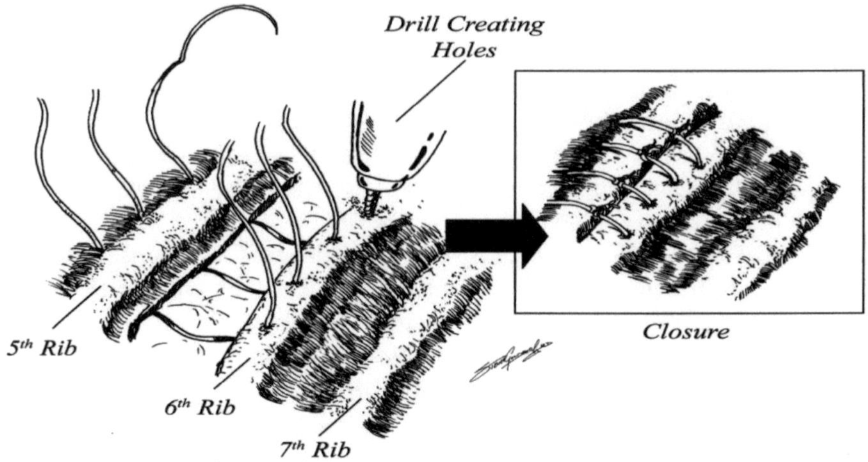

Fig. 1. Intracostal sutures: holes are created in the adjacent ribs and closure is done intracostally excluding the neurovascular bundle in the closure.

Intercostal flap have been long used to cover bronchial stumps but Cerfolio et al investigated the use of this technique for reducing post thoracotomy pain. In the two prospective randomised controlled studies performed by this group one involving a free intercostal muscle (ICM) flap transected anteriorly and the other study which maintained a non-divided ICM flap. Both studies showed a decrease in post thoracotomy pain at 3 months.[47, 48]

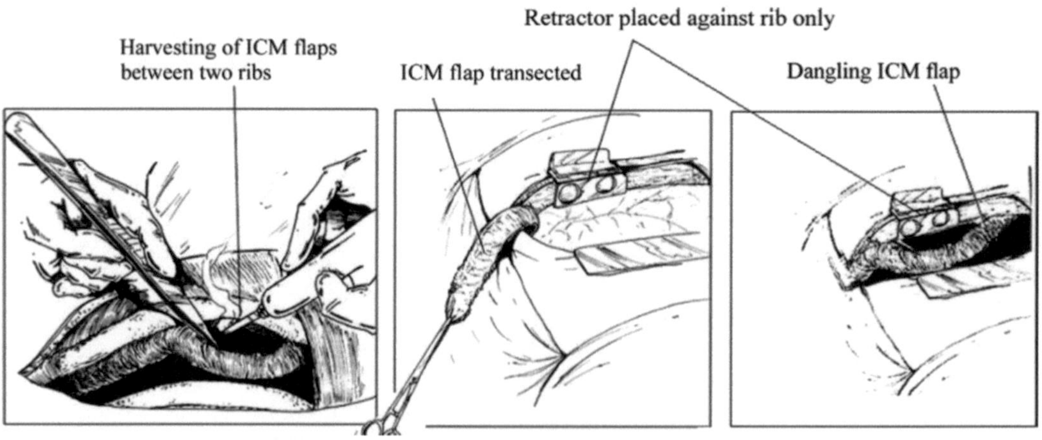

Fig. 2. Intercostal muscle flap (ICM). ICM flap techniques are used to exclude the neurovascular bundle from retraction. Two techniques are shown, the common first step being harvesting of the intercostal muscle flap after which it may be either transacted and excluded or allowed to dangle freely avoiding retraction.

The use of specialised retractors have been studied in animal models which can monitor tissue distractive force and thereby act as a feedback mechanism such that the least amount of force is used in obtaining optimal exposure.[49]

5.3 Anaesthesia and analgesic factors

5.3.1 Anaesthesia

The impact which an anaesthetic technique has on the long term effects of PTPS is unclear. Most studies focus on the analgesic technique used, primarily regional anaesthetic techniques. Remifentanil, which is a pure µopioid receptor agonist, is increasingly being used in anaesthesia; primarily for its rapid onset and offset of action, which is non-reliant on organ metabolism. In a recent publication, Salengros et al 2010 [50] conducted a prospective randomised controlled trial comparing low dose remifentanil and intraoperative thoracic epidural analgesia with high dose remifentanil and post operative epidural analgesia. The patients in the high dose remifentanil group had larger areas of allodynia in the immediate 72 hrs postoperatively and also had a higher incidence of chronic PTPS which was mainly neuropathic in character. This could be explained by either the timing of the epidural or the use of high dose remifentanil. The timing of epidural analgesia has been studied and there is no consensus of its effect on the long term outcome of PTPS. A recent meta-analysis [51] failed to demonstrate that timing of epidural analgesia had any influence on long term outcome. The other possibility is the development of acute opioid induced hyperalgesia (OIH) with the use of remifentanil which is now an established phenomenon. There is good evidence to support OIH from both laboratory and clinical research. This brings to light, as the author concludes stating that even widely accepted anaesthetic practices may have a large impact on long-term outcomes and it is important that we recognise these facts.

5.3.2 Analgesia

Various regional anaesthetic techniques have been used as part of a balanced anaesthetic technique to provide adequate intraoperative and postoperative analgesia. The techniques used include intercostal nerve blocks, interpleural block, cryoanalgesia, paravertebral block and thoracic epidural analgesia. It is considered that adequate analgesia especially during surgery when there is maximal nociceptive input is an important cause for sensitisation both peripheral and central sensitisation, which results is chronic post surgical pain. Establishing a regional anaesthetic technique which abolishes this flow of impulses could reduce sensitisation and thus result in better long term outcomes.[52,53] Practically it remains a challenge to achieve as it is difficult adequately monitor and completely abolish nociceptive input. Moreover the neurohumoral factors which are triggered by the stress of surgery and anaesthesia resulting in the outpour of proinflammatory cytokines leading to hypersensitivity. This may partially explain the discrepancies in the published data on these techniques, where there are both positive and negative outcomes on each technique. Most investigations concentrate on short term endpoints like post operative pain intensity, analgesic requirements, hospital stay and immediate complications with very few analysing the long term occurrence of chronic PTPS. The published data on the use of these techniques are also flawed by methodological inadequacies and very little if any can be extrapolated in terms of chronic pain morbidity.[52, 54-56] But it appears that choosing an appropriate technique which can provide reliable analgesia could help in the improving outcomes.

6. Conclusion

After the above discussion regarding the various factors which influence the occurrence of post thoracotomy pain syndrome, the etiopathogenic mechanisms involved and the possible strategies to improve outcome; it is evident that the management of this clinical condition is challenging and further research is required. There is ongoing interest in this field in thoracic surgery and as previously discussed the broader category of post surgical pain syndromes in which this belongs is increasingly being recognised. Education and creation of a general awareness both in the medical profession and the general public would help up manage this problem more successfully with probably better outcomes.

7. References

[1] Crombie IK, Davies HT, Macrae WA. Cut and thrust: antecedent surgery and trauma among patients attending a chronic pain clinic. Pain 1998; 76:167–71.

[2] Blyth FM, March LM, Cousins MJ. Chronic pain-related disability and use of analgesia and health services in a Sydney community. Med J Aust 2003;179:84–7

[3] Schnabel A, Pogatzki-Zahn E. [Predictors of chronic pain following surgery. What do we know?]. Schmerz 2010;24:517–31; quiz 532–3.

[4] Stephen R. Hazelrigg, MDa,*, Ibrahim B. Cetindag, MDa, James Fullerton, Mdb, Acute and chronic pain syndromes after thoracic surgery,Surg Clin N Am 82 (2002) 849–865

[5] Stephan A. Schug, Esther M. Pogatzki-Zahn. Chronic Pain after Surgery or Injury. IASP Clinical Updates Vol. XIX, Issue 1 January 2011

[6] Peter Gerner,Post-thoracotomy Pain Management Problems,Anesthesiol Clin. 2008 June ; 26(2): 355–vii

[7] Merskey H, Bogduk H. Classification of chronic pain. In: Merskey H, Bogduk H, editors. Descriptions of chronic pain syndromes and definitions of pain terms. Second Edition. Seattle: IASP Press; 1994. pp. 143-144

[8] Landreneau RJ. Prevalence of chronic pain after pulmonary resection by thoracotomy or video-assisted thoracic surgery. J Thorac Cardiovasc Surg 1994; 107(4): 1079–86

[9] Passlick B, Born C, Sienel W, Thetter O. Incidence of chronic pain after minimal-invasive surgery for spontaneous pneumothorax. Eur J Cardio-thorac Surg 2001; 19:355–9.

[10] Lang-Lazdunski L, Chapius O, Bonnet PM, Pons F, Jancovici R. Videothor- acoscopic bleb excision and pleural abrasion for the treatment of primary spontaneous pneumothorax: long-term results. Ann Thorac Surg 2003; 75:960-5.

[11] Landreneau RJ, Pigula F, Luketich JD, Keenan RJ, Bartley S, Fetterman LS, Bowers CM, Weyant RJ, Ferson PF. Acute and chronic morbidity differences between muscle-

sparing and standard lateral thoracotomies. J Thorac Cardiovasc Surg 1996; 112(5): 1346–50.

[12] Passlick B, Born C, Sienel W, Thetter O. Incidence of chronic pain after minimal-invasive surgery for spontaneous pneumothorax. Eur J Cardio-thorac Surg 2001; 19:355–9.

[13] Stammberger U, Steinacher C, Hillinger S, Schmid RA, Kinsbergen T, Weder W. Early and long-term complaints following video-assisted thor- acoscopic surgery: evaluation in 173 patients. Eur J Cardiothoracic Surg 2000; 18:7–11.

[14] Hutter J, Miller K, Moritz E. Chronic sequels after thoracoscopic procedures for benign diseases. Eur J Cardiothoracic Surg 2000;17:687–90.

[15] Perttunen K, Tasmuth T, Kalso E. Chronic pain after thoracic surgery: a follow-up study. Acta Anaesthesiol Scand 1999; 43:563–7.

[16] Dajczman E, Gordon A, Kreisman H, Wolkove N. Long-term post-thoracotomy pain. Chest 1991; 99:270–4.

[17] Katz J, Jackson M, Kavanagh B, Sandler AN. Acute pain after thoracic surgery predicts long-term post-thoracotomy pain. Clin J Pain 1996; 12 (1): 50–5.

[18] Keller SM, Carp NZ, Levy MN, Rosen SM. Chronic post thoracotomy pain, J Cardiovasc Surg 1994; 35(Suppl. 1–6): 161–4

[19] Ochroch EA, Gottschalk A, Troxel AB, Farrar JT,Women suffer more short and long-term pain than men after major thoracotomy,Clin J Pain. 2006 Jun;22(5):491-8

[20] Furrer M, Rechsteiner R, Eigenmann V, Signer C, Althaus U, Ris HB. Thoracotomy and thoracoscopy: postoperative pulmonary function, pain and chest wall complaints. Eur J Cardiothoracic Surg 1997 July; 12(1): 82-7

[21] Maguire MF, Ravenscroft A, Beggs D, Duffy JP. A questionnaire study investigating the prevalence of the neuropathic component of chronic pain after thoracic surgery. Eur J Cardiothorac Surg 2006 May; 29(5): 800-5.

[22] Forster R, Storck M, Schafer JR, Honig E, Lang G, Liewald F. Thoracoscopy versus thoracotomy: a prospective comparison of trauma and quality of life. Langenbecks Arch Surg 2002 April; 387(1): 32-6

[23] K. Wildgaard, J.Ravn, L.Nikolajsen, E.Jackobsen, T. S.Jensen and H. Kehlet, Consequences of persistent pain after lung cancer surgery: a nationwide questionnaire study, Acta Anaesthesiol Scand 2011; 55: 60-68

[24] Aasvang E, Kehlet H. Chronic postoperative pain: the case of inguinal herniorrhaphy. *Br J Anaesth* 2005; 95: 69–76.

[25] Poobalan AS, Bruce J, Smith WC, King PM, Krukowski ZH, Chambers WA. A review of chronic pain after inguinal herniorrhaphy. *Clin J Pain* 2003; 19: 48–54

[26] Katz J, Poleshuck EL, Andrus CL, et al. Risk factors for acute pain and its persistence following breast cancer surgery. *Pain* 2005; 119:16–25.

[27] Kalkman CJ, Visser K, Moen J, Bonsel GJ, Grobbee DE, Moons KG. Preoperative prediction of severe postoperative pain. *Pain* 2003; 105: 415–23

[28] Kehlet H, Jensen TS, Woolf CJ. Persistent postsurgical pain: risk factors and prevention. Lancet 2006;367(9522):1618–25

[29] Pan PH, Coghill R, Houle TT, Seid MH, Lindel WM, Parker RL, Washburn SA, Harris L, Eisenach JC. Multifactorial preoperative predictors for postcesarean section pain and analgesic requirement. Anesthesiology 2006;104(3):417—25

[30] Diatchenko L, Nackley AG, Tchivileva IE, Shabalina SA, Maixner W. Genetic architecture of human pain perception. Trends Genet 2007;23(12):605—13

[31] Max MB, Stewart WF. The molecular epidemiology of pain: a new discipline for drug discovery. Nat Rev Drug Discov 2008;7(8):647—58

[32] Seltzer Z, Wu T, Max MB, Diehl SR. Mapping a gene for neuropathic pain-related behaviour following peripheral neurectomy in the mouse. Pain 2001; 93: 101–6

[33] Thomas Hadjistavropoulos,Kenneth D. Craig, PainPSYCHOLOGICAL PERSPECTIVES, ISBN 0-8058-4299-3

[34] Anke Hinrichs-Rocker, Kerstin Schulz, Imke Järvinen, Rolf Lefering,Christian Simanski, Edmund A.M. Neugebauer, Psychosocial predictors and correlates for chronic post-surgical pain (CPSP) – A systematic review, European Journal of Pain 13 (2009) 719–730

[35] Joel Katz, Gordon J.G. Asmundson, Karen McRae, Eileen Halket, , Emotional numbing and pain intensity predict the development of pain disability up to one year after lateral thoracotomy, European Journal of Pain 13 (2009) 870–878

[36] Liem MS, van Duyn EB, van der Graaf Y, van Vroonhoven TJ.Recurrences after conventional anterior and laparoscopic inguinal hernia repair: a randomized comparison. Ann Surg 2003;237: 136–41 Wright D, Paterson C, Scott N, Hair A, O'Dwyer PJ. Five-year follow-up of patients undergoing laparoscopic or open groin hernia repair: a randomized controlled trial. Ann Surg 2002;235: 333–7

[37] Nikolajsen L, Ilkjaer S, Kroner K, Christensen JH, Jensen TS. The influence of preamputation pain on postamputation stump and phantom pain. Pain 1997; 72: 393 -405

[38] Kroner K, Knudsen UB, Lundby L, Hvid H. Long term phantom breast syndrome after mastectomy. Clin J Pain 1992; 8: 346–50

[39] Keller SM, Carp NZ, Levy MN, Rosen SM. Chronic post thoracotomy pain. J Cardiovasc Surg 1994; 35: 161–4

[40] Robert J Baker, Josef E Fischer, Mastery of Surgery, ISBN: 0-7817-2328-0

[41] Landreneau RJ, Pigula F, Luketich JD, Keenan RJ, Bartley S, Fetterman LS, Bowers CM, Weyant RJ, Ferson PF. Acute and chronic morbidity differences between muscle-sparing and standard lateral thoracotomies. J Thorac Cardiovasc Surg 1996;112(5):1346—50

[42] Kalso E, Perttunen K, Kaasinen S. Pain after thoracic surgery. Acta Anaesthesiol Scand 1992;36:96–100 Khan IH, McManus KG, McCraith A, McGuigan JA. Muscle sparing thoracotomy: a biomechanical analysis confirms preservation of muscle strength but no improvement in wound discomfort. Eur J Cardiothorac Surg 2000;18(6):656—61.

[43] Mario Nosottia, Alessandro Baisib, Paolo Mendognia,*, Alessandro Palleschia, Davide Tosia, Lorenzo Rossoa, Muscle sparing versus posterolateral thoracotomy for

pulmonary lobectomy: randomised controlled trial, Interactive CardioVascular and Thoracic Surgery 11 (2010) 415-419
[44] Iwasaki A, Kawahara K. The role of video-assisted thoracic surgery for the treatment of lung cancer: lung lobectomy by thoracoscopy versus the standard thoracotomy approach. Int Surg 2000;85(1):6—12
[45] Kirby TJ, Mack MJ, Landreneau RJ, Rice TW. Lobectomy—video-assisted thoracic surgery versus muscle-sparing thoracotomy. A randomized trial. J Thorac Cardiovasc Surg 1995;109(5):997—1001
[46] Cerfolio RJ, Price TN, Bryant AS, Sale BC, Bartolucci AA. Intracostal sutures decrease the pain of thoracotomy. Ann Thorac Surg 2003;76(2):407—11
[47] Cerfolio RJ, Bryant AS, Patel B, Bartolucci AA. Intercostal muscle flap reduces the pain of thoracotomy: a prospective randomized trial. J Thorac Cardiovasc Surg 2005;130(4):987—93.
[48] Cerfolio RJ, Bryant AS, Maniscalco LM. A nondivided intercostal muscle flap further reduces pain of thoracotomy: a prospective randomized trial. Ann Thorac Surg 2008;85(6):1901—6
[49] Gil Bolotin, Gregory D Buckner, Nicholas J Jardine, Aaron J Kiefer, Nigel B Campbell, BVetMed, Masha Kocherginsky,Jai Raman and Valluvan Jeevanandam, A novel instrumented retractor to monitor tissue-disruptive forces during lateral thoracotomy The Journal of Thoracic and Cardiovascular Surgery ,Volume 133, Number 4 949
[50] Jean-Corentin Salengros,Isabelle Huybrechts, Anne Ducart ,David Faraoni,Corinne Marsal, Luc Barvais,Matteo Cappello and Edgard Engelman,Different Anesthetic Techniques Associated with Different Incidences of Chronic Post-thoracotomy Pain: Low-Dose Remifentanil Plus Presurgical Epidural Analgesia is Preferable to High-Dose Remifentanil with Postsurgical Epidural Analgesia, Journal of Cardiothoracic and Vascular Anesthesia, Vol 24, No 4 (August), 2010: pp 608-616
[51] Bong CL, Samuel M, Ng JM, et al: Effects of preemptive epidural analgesia on post-thoracotomy pain. J Cardiothorac Vasc Anesth 19:786-793, 2005
[52] Kim Wildgaard , Jesper Ravn , Henrik Kehlet,Chronic post-thoracotomy pain: a critical review of pathogenic mechanisms and strategies for prevention, European Journal of Cardio-thoracic Surgery 36 (2009) 170—180
[53] Peter Gerner, Post-thoracotomy Pain Management Problems *Anesthesiol Clin.* 2008 June ; 26(2): 355–vii
[54] Kissin I. Preemptive analgesia. Anesthesiology 2000 October;93(4):1138–43. [PubMed: 11020772]
[55] Kissin I. Study design to demonstrate clinical value of preemptive analgesia: is the commonly used approach valid? Reg Anesth Pain Med 2002 May;27(3):242–4. [PubMed: 12016595]
[56] Samad TA, Moore KA, Sapirstein A, Billet S, Allchorne A, Poole S, Bonventre JV, Woolf CJ. Interleukin-1beta-mediated induction of Cox-2 in the CNS contributes to inflammatory pain hypersensitivity. Nature 2001 March 22;410(6827):471–5. [PubMed: 11260714]

[57] Monique A. H. Steegers,Daphne M. Snik, Ad F. Verhagen,† Miep A. van der Drift and Oliver H. G. Wilder-Smith, Only Half of the Chronic Pain After Thoracic Surgery Shows a Neuropathic Component, The Journal of Pain, Vol 9, No 10 (October), 2008: pp 955-961

7

Chronic Thromboembolic Pulmonary Hypertension: Effects of Pulmonary Endarterectomy

Coen van Kan[1], Mart N. van der Plas[1], Jaap J. Kloek[2], Herre J. Reesink[1] and Paul Bresser[1,2]
[1]*Department of Respiratory Medicine, Onze Lieve Vrouwe Gasthuis,*
[2]*Department of Cardiothoracic Surgery, Academic Medical Center,*
University of Amsterdam, Amsterdam,
The Netherlands

1. Introduction

Chronic thromboembolic pulmonary hypertension (CTEPH) results from incomplete resolution of the vascular obstruction associated with pulmonary embolism (PE) (Fedullo et al., 2001; Hoeper et al., 2006). This condition is considered to develop in 1-4 % of patients who survive an acute pulmonary embolism (Becattini et al., 2006; Fedullo et al., 2001; Pengo et al., 2004). Given the worldwide incidence of acute PE, approximately 1:1000, this indicates that even in a small country like the Netherlands, CTEPH may be diagnosed in up to 600 patients yearly.

Most CTEPH patients present with gradually progressive exercise intolerance, typically portrayed as exertional dyspnea, fatigue, palpitations and/or on productive cough. In further stages of disease there may be signs of right ventricular failure, chest pain on exertion and syncope. The ensuing progressive right ventricular failure leads to progressive disability and early death (Hoeper et al., 2004) .

If left untreated, CTEPH is a progressive and life-threatening disorder; survival being proportional to the degree of pulmonary hypertension at diagnosis. In CTEPH patients with a mean pulmonary arterial pressure (mPAP) above 30 mmHg at time of diagnosis, 5-years survival is about 30%, whereas in patients with a mPAP above 50 mmHg the 5-years survival may be as low as 10% (Lewczuk et al., 2001; Riedel et al., 1982). Pulmonary endarterectomy (PEA) is the therapy of first choice for CTEPH patients with surgical accessible thrombi (Fedullo et al., 2001; Jamieson et al., 2000, 2003). PEA has been found to improve, and in many cases normalize pulmonary hemodynamics, functional status and long-term survival. PEA, however, does not come without potential risk. Reported peri- and direct postoperative mortality still ranges between 4.4% and 16% even in experienced centres (Archibald et al., 1999; Auger et al., 2007; Condliffe et al., 2008; Jamieson et al., 2000 ; Rubens et al., 2007).

In this chapter we will discuss the pathophysiology of CTEPH. In particular, we will focus on the pathophysiology of the exercise limitation and dyspnea that is observed in these patients. Moreover, the effects of surgical treatment, that is the removal of the obstructing chronic thrombi by pulmonary endarterectomy, on cardiac function and the restoration of exercise tolerance and dyspnea will be discussed.

2. Pathophysiology of CTEPH

Pulmonary hypertension (PH) in general is a progressive and life-threatening disorder. It is pathophysiologically characterized by a gradually progressive increase in the pulmonary vascular resistance. As a consequence, in order to maintain an adequate transpulmonary blood flow, the pulmonary artery pressure will increase. The definition of PH is based on right heart catheterisation measurements; and PH was classically defined as a mean pulmonary artery pressure (mPAP) greater than 25 mmHg at rest or 30 mmHg during exercise. Recently, however, inclusion of exercise-induced PH in the definition has been the subject of debate, leading to it´s exclusion from the most recent guidelines (Kovacs et al., 2009; Galie et al., 2009).
In CTEPH, pulmonary hypertension is considered to be primarily the result of the anatomic loss of pulmonary vascular bed due to the irreversible chronic thromboembolic obstruction. However, the pathophysiology of the disease appears far more complex. Pneumonectomy, for instance, is associated with little, if any, increase in pulmonary artery pressure, even with follow-up to 11 years (Cournand et al., 1950; Smulders et al., 2007). Experimental studies have even indicated that up to a 75% reduction in lung volumes does not cause pulmonary hypertension (Harrison et al., 1957). Nevertheless significant pulmonary hypertension at rest can be observed in CTEPH patients with relatively minor chronic thromboembolic obstruction of the pulmonary vasculature (Jamieson et al., 2000). This indicates that factors other than simple hemodynamic consequences of redirected blood flow are likely to be involved in the pathophysiology of CTEPH.
Concepts of pathogenesis and progression of the disease after the initial pulmonary embolus involve both recurrent thromboemboli and failure to resolve the acute thromboemboli. In the past, abnormalities in coagulation and fibrinolysis pathways have been identified in CTEPH patients, however, the frequency of these defects in such patients were similar to those in the general population. Lupus anticoagulant and antiphospholipid antibodies were shown to be present in 10-20% of patients with CTEPH, which is higher than in patients with acute venous thromboembolism (Auger et al., 1995; Wolf et al., 2000). Bonderman et al. showed increased levels of factor VIII (FVIII) in about 40% of CTEPH patients as compared to both healthy controls and patients with non-thromboembolic pulmonary hypertension (Bonderman et al., 2003). FVIII is a well recognised risk factor for single (O'Donnell et al., 1997) and, in particular, recurrent venous thromboembolism (Kyrle et al., 2000). Furthermore, inherited deficiencies of protein C, protein S and anti-thrombin III were identified in 1-5% of patients (Colorio et al., 2001; Moser et al., 1990). Moreover, other risk factors have been identified in the development of CTEPH, including chronic inflammatory disorders, myeloproliferative syndromes, ventriculo-atrial drains, a history of pacemaker infection, thyroid disease and replacement therapy, and splenectomy (Bonderman et al., 2005, 2009; Jais et al., 2005).
Over time, a gradual hemodynamic and symptomatic decline can be observed in CTEPH patients. Progression of disease may be the consequence of recurrent thromboembolism or in situ pulmonary artery thrombosis. Hemodynamic progression, however, can also be observed in patients without evidence of recurrent thromboembolism, while using adequate oral anticoagulant treatment. Taken together, this indicates that a second pathobiological process is likely to be involved (Lang, 2010). The current understanding is that a hemodynamically significant persistent obstruction of the pulmonary arteries may result in an elevated pulmonary artery pressure and high shear stress in areas which are spared from occlusion; this in combination with a concomitant inflammation, and an imbalance of vasoactive mediators may result in the vascular remodelling that is observed in these

patients (Bauer et al., 2002; Humbert et al., 2004 Humbert et al., 2004; Reesink et al., 2006; Hoeper et al., 2004; Lang, 2010). Histopathologic changes in the microvasculature, similar to those demonstrated in other forms of pulmonary arterial hypertension (PAH), were observed in lung biopsy specimens from CTEPH patients (Moser et al., 1973). The development of this slowly progressive secondary arteriopathy in the non-obstructed pre-capillary pulmonary vessels is likely the cause of the progression of disease that can be observed in CTEPH patients (Fedullo et al., 2011; Hoeper et al., 2006; Lang, 2010). By contributing to the elevated pulmonary vascular resistance, this arteriopathy adversely affects cardiac function and may, in the end, contribute to the progressive hemodynamic instability and increased mortality observed in patients with CTEPH (Riedel et al., 1982).

Advanced CTEPH leads to cardiac remodelling, as characterized by right ventricular (RV) dilatation and hypertrophy, tricuspid regurgitation and leftward ventricular septal bowing (LVSB), with a consequent impact on cardiac function (Fleg et al., 2000; Groepenhoff et al., 2008; Kreitner et al., 2007, 2004; Reesink et al., 2007). We have shown that LVSB is present in the majority of CTEPH patients (Reesink et al., 2007). Early diastolic septal bowing is an ominous sign in patients with pulmonary hypertension. During systole, the pressure in left ventricle (LV) normally exceeds the RV pressure, showing a (positive) curvature away from the LV centre. During early LV diastole, the LV pressure drops to near zero to enable rapid LV filling. The increased RV pressure pushes the septum away from the from the RV centre, causing (negative) LVSB (Marcus et al., 2001). We have shown that the interventricular septal bowing correlates with the severity of pulmonary hypertension in CTEPH patients (Reesink et al., 2007). So, although RV dysfunction is most outspoken, also LV function is significantly impaired these patients. The impairment of the LV function might be attributable to ventricular interaction or ventricular interdependence (also known as the "reversed Bernheim phenomenon"): RV dilatation and hypertrophy shift the interventricular septum leftward, thereby causing decreased LV cavity size, contractility, compliance, and ejection fraction (Alpert et al., 2001). LV diastolic dysfunction, however, may also be caused in part by myocardial hypertrophy of the RV and interventricular septum, as documented in both patients with CTEPH and idiopathic pulmonary arterial hypertension (iPAH) (Hardziyenka et al., 2011; Marcus et al., 2001; Reesink et al., 2007). In iPAH, it was shown that ventricular interaction mediated by interventricular septum bowing caused an impairment of the LV filling and thereby contributed to the decreased stroke volume observed in these patients (Gan et al., 2006). We have recently shown that in (CTE)PH patients also atrophy of the LV free wall may contribute to the impairment of the LV function. In a rat model of right ventricular failure due to pulmonary hypertension, we showed that reduction in LV free wall mass can be, at least in part, explained by myocyte shrinkage due to atrophic remodelling associated with left ventricle underfilling (Hardziyenka et al., 2011).

3. Pathophysiology of exercise limitation in CTEPH patients

In CTEPH, as in pulmonary hypertension in general, exercise is primarily limited by the impairment of cardiac function. As discussed, advanced pulmonary hypertension in CTEPH leads to chronic RV volume overload, cardiac remodelling and dysfunction. The limitation in exercise capacity is in major part caused by the inability of the heart to sufficiently increase pulmonary blood flow due to a decreased RV stroke volume response during exercise (Raeside et al., 2000; Holverda et al., 2006).

Normally, upon exercise cardiac output is elevated by increasing heart rate, stroke volume or both. When stroke volume increases, pulmonary blood flow will increase; pulmonary arterial pressure, however, will not significantly increase due to pulmonary vascular dilatation and recruitment (Bonderman et al., 2011). In PH, however, these mechanisms of lowering pulmonary vascular resistance are lost due to the secondary arteriopathy in the pre-capillary pulmonary vessels. As a result, the pulmonary pressure will rise in order to maintain pulmonary blood flow with a subsequent effect on stroke volume upon exercise. The exercise-associated increase in pulmonary arterial pressure will result in further impairment of RV function, as well as LV underfilling, both leading to a failing stroke volume response to exercise (Raeside et al., 2000). Stroke volume is determined by contractility and the end-diastolic volume (EDV). Holverda and co-workers showed that the failure to increase SV upon exercise in iPAH patients was accompanied by a small increase in RV end diastolic volume (RVEDV) and a decrease in LV end diastolic volume (LVEDV) due to increased LVSB and RV forward failure hampering an adequate LV filling (Holverda et al., 2006). Using exercise studies during cardiac magnetic resonance imaging (cMRI) we found even a negative SV response, i.e. a decrease in SV upon exercise, in CTEPH patients; opposite from the response observed in healthy individuals. The observed maximal SV during exercise, thereby, correlated significantly with exercise capacity as expressed by peak oxygen consumption ($V'O_2$-peak), as well as with the hemodynamic severity of disease at rest.

Next to the decreased RV and LV function, responses related to ventilation-perfusion mismatching caused by the thromboembolic obstruction of the pulmonary vascular bed are also likely to play a significant role in the pathophysiology of the exercise limitation observed in CTEPH patients. (CTE)PH is associated with decreased ventilatory efficiency during exercise (D'Alonzo et al., 1987; Riley et al., 2000; Sun et al., 2001; Wasserman, 2004). As blood flow fails to perfuse the ventilated lung, dead space ventilation increases; to compensate for this increase in death space ventilation the patient's ventilatory requirement must increase. At the same time, the inability to increase cardiac output impairs oxygen transport appropriately in response to exercise, causing a low work rate "lactic acidosis" and exercise-induced hypoxemia, thereby further stimulating the ventilatory drive. Similar to measures of decreased cardiac output, parameters of increased dead space ventilation, were found to be related to the hemodynamic severity of disease in PH patients (Raeside et al., 2000; Van der Plas et al., 2010; Sun et al., 2001; Yasunobu et al., 2005).

The direct relation between exercise limitation and the hemodynamic severity of disease has lead to the use of (non-invasive) exercise testing for both prognostic and diagnostic information in (CTE)PH patients. The most commonly used test to study exercise tolerance in PH patients are the six minute walk test (6-MWT) and the symptom-limited cardio-pulmonary exercise test (CPET).

3.1 Exercise testing

3.1.1 Six minute walk test

The 6-MWT is by far the most popular and most frequently used exercise test in PH clinical practice and research. The 6-MWT is derived from the Cooper test, a 12 minute running test that was developed to evaluate fitness in healthy individuals (Cooper, 1968). The 6-MWT itself is a reproducible, inexpensive, safe, and simple exercise test that requires no exercise equipment or advanced training for technicians. The 6-MWT can be used to evaluate exercise limitation in patients with cardiac and pulmonary diseases (ATS guidelines, 2002). Walking is a daily life activity that can be performed by all but the most severely impaired patients. The 6-MWT measures the distance walked on a flat, hard surface in a period of 6 minutes; the 6-minute walk distance (6-MWD). It evaluates the global and integrated responses of all systems involved during exercise, *i.e.* the pulmonary and cardiovascular system, systemic and peripheral circulation, neuromuscular units and muscle cell metabolism. In contrast to CPET, however, it does not provide specific information on the function of each of the different organs and systems involved in exercise or on the mechanism of the exercise limitation. As the 6-MWT is a self-paced walking test (patients choose their own intensity of exercise and are allowed to stop and rest during the test), it assesses a sub-maximal level of functional capacity. Nevertheless, the 6-MWD has been found to correlate closely with maximal oxygen uptake in various pulmonary and cardiac diseases (Cahalin et al., 1996; Roul et al., 1998). In iPAH patients, the six-minute walk distance (6-MWD) was shown to correlate significantly with hemodynamic severity of disease (Miyamoto et al., 2000). Similarly, we demonstrated in 50 consecutive patients with CTEPH prior to PEA, that the 6-MWD decreases in proportion to New York Heart Association (NYHA) functional class, and correlated strongly with the hemodynamic severity of disease (Figure 1). Compared to the data in iPAH patients, in CTEPH patients, the observed correlations between 6-MWD and pulmonary hemodynamics appeared even more robust (Reesink et al., 2007). Therefore, the 6-MWD is considered a highly useful objective parameter to assess functional limitations and outcome after medical interventions in most CTEPH patients.

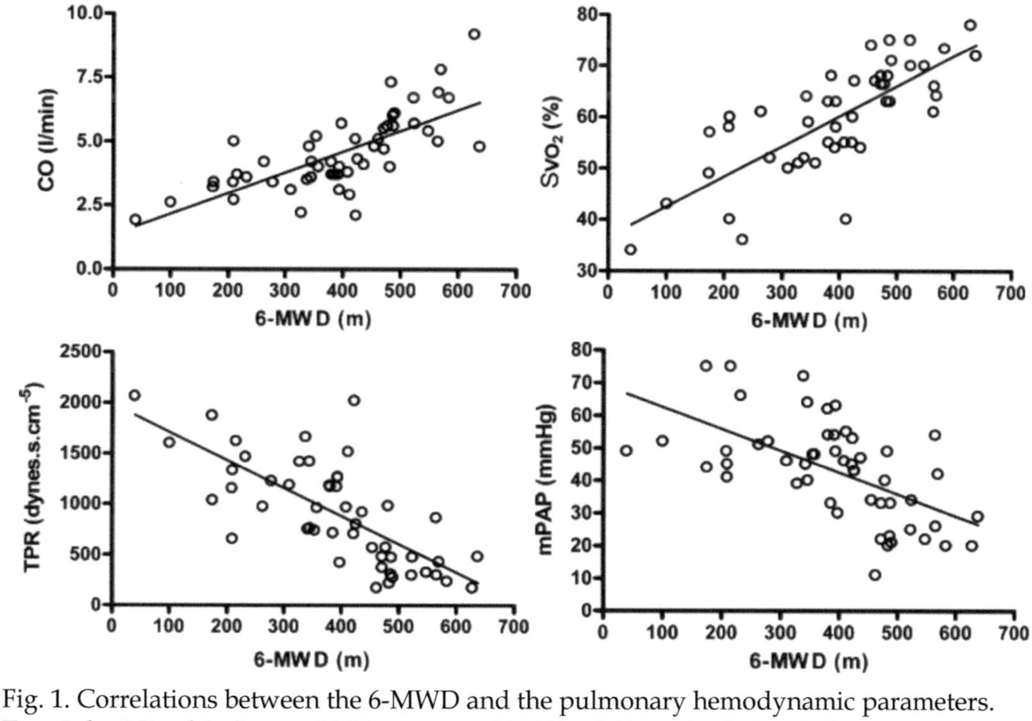

Fig. 1. Correlations between the 6-MWD and the pulmonary hemodynamic parameters. Top right: Mixed SvO_2; n = 46; Pearson r = 0.77; $P < 0.0001$. Top left: CO; Pearson r = 0.76; $P < 0.0001$ Bottom left: TPR; Pearson r = -0.75; $P < 0.0001$ Bottom right: mPAP; Pearson r = -0.62; $P < 0.0001$. *mPAP*, mean pulmonary artery pressure; *6-MWD*, 6-minute walk distance; *TPR*, total pulmonary resistance; *CO*, cardiac output; *SvO_2*, venous oxygen saturation. (Adapted from: Reesink et al., 2007)

The decrease in 6-MWD in patients with CTEPH is assumed to result from reduced maximum aerobic capacity owing to the, already discussed, inability of the heart to increase pulmonary blood flow adequately upon exercise. In the severely impaired CTEPH patients (NYHA stage III and IV), the 6-MWD was shown to reflect maximum aerobic capacity. However, we reported an increasing difference between maximal aerobic capacity and the aerobic capacity attained during 6-MWT, with decreasing severity of disease. In mildly impaired PH patients (NYHA stage II), the 6-MWT did not reflect maximal aerobic capacity. This indicates that mildly impaired PH patients are limited in their 6-MWT for other reasons than their oxygen delivery capacity. Therefore, in this group of patients, the 6-MWD may not be an appropriate parameter to study outcome of medical interventions (Van der Plas et al., 2008).

3.1.2 Cardio pulmonary exercise testing

CPET is considered the gold standard for the evaluation of exercise intolerance in patients with pulmonary and cardiac disease, and is based on the principle that system failure typically occurs while the system is under physical stress (Palange et al., 2007). CPET is based on a symptom-limited incremental exercise protocol in combination with breath-by-breath analysis of cardiopulmonary variables, such as oxygen consumption ($V'O_2$), carbon dioxide output ($V'CO_2$), minute ventilation (V'_E), heart rate (HR) and arterial oxygen saturation. From these variables others can be calculated, like the oxygen pulse (O_2-pulse; $V'O_2/HR$) as derivative of stroke volume, and the ventilatory equivalent of CO_2 ($V'_E/V'CO_2$) as measure of ventilatory efficiency. As such, in contrast to the 6-MWT, CPET requires expensive equipment and well trained technicians. During CPET, workload is typically increased in a stepwise manner, depending on the predicted maximum exercise capacity of the patient; with the prerequisite that maximal effort should be attained in 10-15 minutes. All patients are stimulated to exercise to their personal maximum exercise capability, allowing peak exercise capacity to be determined. As opposed to the 6-MWT, CPET not only evaluates the global and integrated responses of all the organ systems involved during exercise, it also provides specific information on the function of each of the different components determining the exercise capacity. Maximal exercise capacity is determined by the "weakest link" in the interdependent physiological components of the gas transport mechanisms (Wasserman et al., 2004).

In PH, CPET has been shown to be a useful tool to assess the severity of disease and prognosis (Deboeck et al., 2004; Sun et al., 2001; Wensel et al., 2002; Yasunobu et al., 2005). CPET in patients with PH shows a distinct pattern of abnormal responses to exercise, with reductions in peak oxygen uptake ($V'O_2$-peak), O_2 pulse, $V'O_2$ at the anaerobic threshold and an increase in $V'_E/V'CO_2$. This pattern is well validated and has prognostic significance in patients with pulmonary arterial hypertension (D'Alonzo, et al. 1987; Sun, et al. 2001; Wasserman et al., 2004). In CTEPH, most of the patients we studied had by definition a reduced exercise capacity with a decreased peak oxygen uptake ($V'O_2$-peak), i.e. below 84% of the predicted value. On average, $V'O_2$-peak and peak O2-pulse were decreased with increasing severity of PH (Figure 2). $V'_E/V'CO_2$ at anaerobic threshold was increased in almost all patients. $V'O_2$-peak showed a significant inverse correlation with resting mean pulmonary arterial pressure and total pulmonary resistance ($r=-0.625$, $p=0.007$ and $r=-0.676$, $p=0.003$ respectively).

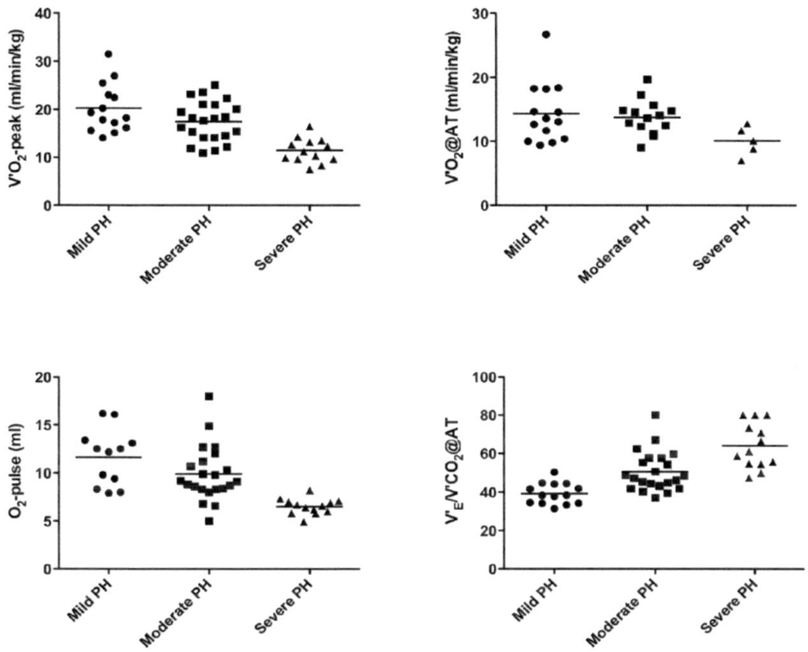

Fig. 2. Characteristic abnormalities of exercise parameters in CTEPH patients (n= 49) with mild PH (mPAP <30 mmHg), moderate PH (mPAP ≥ 30, ≤ 50 mmHg) or severe PH (> 50 mmHg). *$V'O_2$-peak* = peak oxygen uptake. *$V'O_2$*@AT = oxygen uptake at anaerobic threshold; *O_2* –pulse = oxygen pulse; $V'_E / V'CO_2$ = ventilation equivalent for carbon dioxide (unpublished data).

4. Pathophysiology of dyspnea in CTEPH

The one common presenting symptom in patients with CTEPH is dyspnea (Jamieson et al., 2000; Viner et al., 1994). Dyspnea is associated with decreased exercise performance, functional status and quality of life (Wasserman, 2004). Dyspnea includes several qualitatively distinct sensations that can arise from different pathophysiological mechanisms. In general, it is considered to be the result of a complex interaction of signals originating within the central nervous system and a variety of signals from receptors in the upper airway, lungs and chest wall (Manning et al., 1995; Yasunobo et al., 1999).

Dyspnea can be assessed by the NYHA functional classification and the Borg score. NYHA functional class is a doctor reported dyspnea scoring system that quantifies a patient's level of exercise intolerance, expressing the patients (dis)ability to perform everyday activities. The Borg score, on the other hand, is a patient reported quantitative scaling method of the symptomatic dyspnea. Patients rate their own dyspnea on a scale from 0 (no dyspnea) to 10 (absolutely breathlessness) (Borg, 1982).

In CTEPH, dyspnea can be attributed to multiple factors: increased dead space ventilation, hypoxemia, sympathetic overstimulation and/or stimulation of pressure receptors in the pulmonary vascular bed may all give rise to an increased ventilatory demand (Manning et al., 1995). This will contribute to an increase in respiratory motor output with a corresponding increase in the sense of effort, *i.e.* the work of breathing. Increased dead space ventilation, caused by ventilation-perfusion mismatching due to thromboembolic obstruction in the vascular bed might be an attributable factor to the sensation of dyspnea in CTEPH patients (Sun et al., 2001). Dead space ventilation increases, as blood flow fails to perfuse the ventilated lung. To compensate for this increase in dead space ventilation the patient's ventilatory requirement increases, leading to a sensation of dyspnea. Recently, we reported on this relation between dead space ventilation and the experienced dyspnea in fifty-four patients with CTEPH who underwent PEA (Van der Plas, et al. 2010). The dead space ventilation (V_D/V_T), as determined by the Bohr-Enghoff equation, was shown to be increased, and correlated significantly with the hemodynamic severity of disease as well as with patient-reported sensations of dyspnea as assessed by the Borg score and NYHA functional class. Assessment of the expiratory end tidal PCO_2 (PET,CO_2) by capnography showed a significant lower PET,CO_2 compared to the arterial PCO_2 (Pa,CO_2) (3.55 ± 0.43 vs. 4.46 ± 0.42 kPa, $p<0.001$), indicating a parallel origin of the observed dead space ventilation (Figure 3).

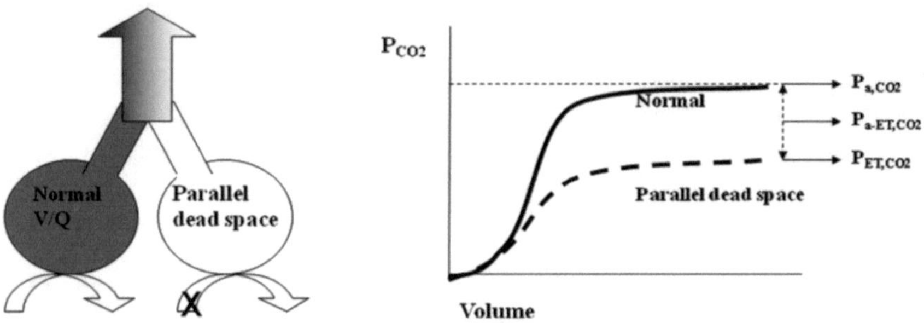

Fig. 3. Model of parallel dead space ventilation. (Adapted from: Van der Plas et al., 2010)

Even more, ventilation itself is stretched beyond the demands of the increased dead space, since patients were relatively hypocapnic, *i.e.* a Pa,CO_2 below the clinical limit of 4.7 kPa. Moreover, Pa,CO_2 correlated inversely with mPAP and TPR. The combination of alveolar hyperventilation and increased (parallel) dead space ventilation is remarkable as it puts an extra ventilatory drive on an already increased effort of breathing. These findings are in unison with reports in patients with iPAH (Meyer et al., 2005; Wessel et al., 1964; Zoia et al., 2002). The alveolar hyperventilation seemed to be only in part hypoxic driven, as administration of 100% oxygen for at least 20 minutes increased but did not normalize Pa,CO_2 (4.50 ± 0.42 kPa vs. 4.58 ± 0.42 kPa). Increased sympathetic activity may play a causative role in the observed alveolar hyperventilation in our patients. Velez-Roa and colleagues found muscle sympathetic nerve activity (MSNA) to be elevated in patients with idiopathic and fenfluramine induced PAH (Velez-Roa et al., 2004). As with Pa,CO_2 in our study, MSNA changed towards normal, but did not normalize by administration of hyperoxia. Increased sympathetic activation has been reported to increase ventilation (Jordan et al., 2000). The presence and cause of increased MSNA in patients with CTEPH and the relation between increased MSNA and alveolar hyperventilation might be subject of further research.

5. Effects of surgical treatment by pulmonary endarterectomy

5.1 Restoration of cardiac function

Pulmonary endarterectomy, first reported in 1958 by Hurwitt and co-workers (Hurwitt et al., 1958), remains the therapy of choice for patients with CTEPH and surgical accessible thrombi (Fedullo et al., 2011). PEA causes an instantaneous and permanent hemodynamic improvement (Corsico et al., 2008; D'Armini et al., 2007; Reesink et al., 2007), which is associated with an improvement in overall cardiac function already shortly after PEA.

The most widely used non-invasive tool in clinical practice to study RV dysfunction is echocardiography. In CTEPH, echocardiographically, restoration of overall RV function shortly after PEA was reported (Menzel et al., 2000; Menzel et al., 2002; Menzel et al., 2002). In fact, improvement of RV geometry and LV diastolic function after PEA was already reported by Dittrich and co-workers in 1988 and 1989 (Dittrich et al., 1988; Dittrich et al., 1989). In addition, reverse RV remodeling, that is improvement of RV dimensions and ejection fraction, was demonstrated in patients with iPAH after lung transplantation (Kasimir et al., 2004; Vizza et al., 1998). The usefulness of echocardiography in this respect, however, is somewhat limited due to its technical limitations (acoustic window) and the absence of a reliable mathematical assumption due to the complex geometry of the RV. In view of these limitations, cardiac MRI is considered a superior imaging technique to quantify the characteristics of RV function and morphology (Helbing et al., 1995; Mayer et al., 1996; Vogel et al., 1997). Using cMRI we and others have shown restoration of RV remodeling after hemodynamically successful PEA (Kreitner et al., 2007, 2004; Reesink et al., 2007). We studied the restoration of RV remodeling in CTEPH patients at least 4 months after PEA (Reesink et al., 2007). After PEA, RV end diastolic and systolic dimensions normalized; RV-SVI and RV-EF improved, but did not fully normalize compared to healthy controls. Also, RV hypertrophy (RV mass) decreased after PEA, but did not fully normalize in all patients. In addition, LVSB, preoperatively present in 15 of the 17 patients studied, normalised after PEA. Moreover, the observed decrease in RV mass and change in LVSB correlated significantly with the observed postoperative hemodynamic improvement. Finally, after PEA, LV end-diastolic volume and the LV-EF, both decreased prior to PEA, normalized (Figure 4 and 5). Recently, Lino and co-workers studied the time course of the restoration of the RV remodeling and showed that it occurs early after PEA. In line with our observations, the parameters of RV remodeling did not fully normalize after a 6-months follow-up period (Iino et al., 2008).

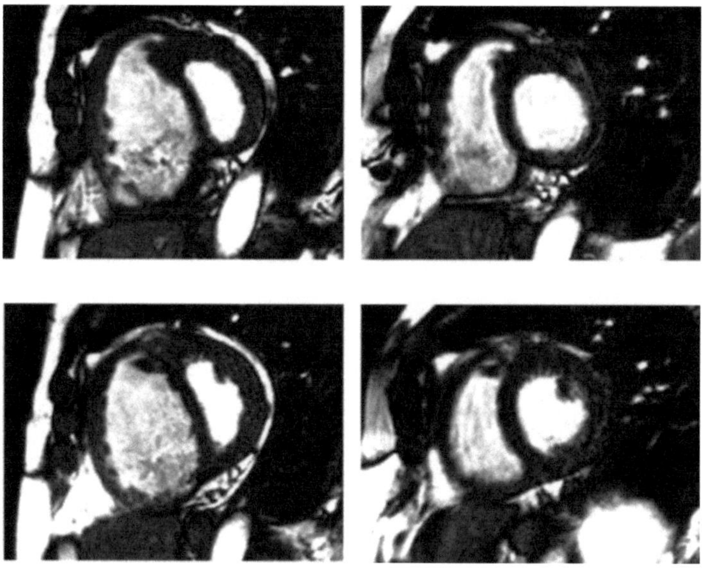

Fig. 4. MRI short-axis cine images at basal (upper panel) and mid-ventricular (lower panel) level, before (A) and after (B) PEA (relative time 55% in the cardiac cycle). Note the encroachment of the interventricular septum into the LV before PEA and the restoration of the septal bowing to normal after PEA. Note also the reversal of RV hypertrophy and the normalization of the RV and LV volumes (Adapted from: Reesink et al., 2007)

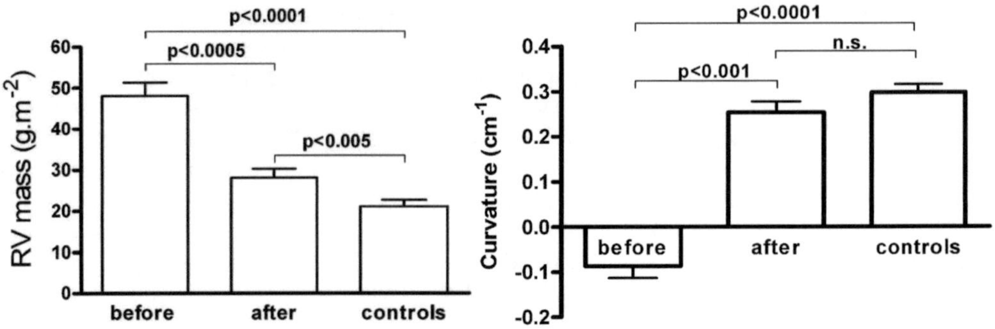

Fig. 5. Left: Right ventricle mass in patients with CTEPH (n = 17) before and after PEA compared with healthy controls (n = 12). Data are expressed as mean ± SEM. Right: Septal bowing (curvature: 1/R) in patients with CTEPH (n = 17) before and after PEA compared with healthy controls (n = 12). Data are expressed as mean ± SE (Adapted from Reesink et al., 2007)

As already extensively discussed, RV dysfunction and LV dysfunction occur in CTEPH patients because both are closely interdependent (Hardziyenka et al., 2011). Decreased RV ejection fraction relates to decreased LV diastolic filling and this may induce LV atrophy. As mentioned, we have observed a significant lower LV free wall mass index as determined by cMRI in CTPEH patients with RV dysfunction. In these patients, after PEA restoration of the LV free wall mass to normal values was observed (Hardziyenka et al., 2011) Recently, we also have reported on our studies on the time course of the restoration of RV systolic and diastolic function after PEA by use of echocardiography (Surie et al., 2011). Two weeks after PEA RV afterload and dimensions had decreased significantly, without further improvement during follow-up. Global RV function, expressed by the myocardial performance index (MPI) (Tei et al., 1996), showed a gradual improvement during the follow-up period. In contrast, 2 weeks after PEA systolic RV function, as assessed by tricuspid annular plane systolic velocity excursion (TAPSE) (Forfia et al., 2006) (Figure 6) and peak tricuspid annular systolic velocity of the RV (Saxena et al., 2006), had worsened, with a subsequent incomplete restoration during follow-up. Also, the diastolic RV function, as determined by the tricuspid-to-annulus ratio (TDI E/E') (Lim et al., 2009) (Figure 6)

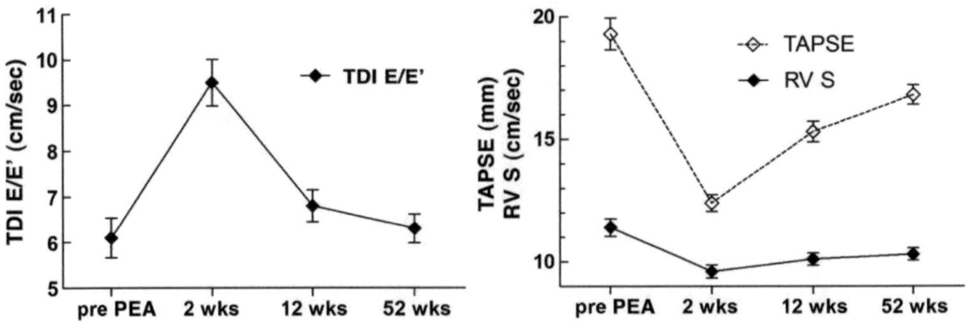

Fig. 6. Time course of restoration of diastolic (TDI E/E'; left) and systolic (TAPSE; right) RV function after PEA (Adapted from: Surie et al., 2011).

showed a similar biphasic response. The observed perioperative dynamics of systolic and diastolic RV function after PEA are in line with studies in patients undergoing coronary artery bypass graft (CABG) surgery for coronary artery disease. The mechanism of the isolated effect on systolic and diastolic RV function remains fully unclear; however, it does not appear solely related to the use of cardiopulmonary bypass (Unsworth et al., 2010). Ischemia, inflammation, and myocardial oedema have been suggested; it can be hypothesized that the hypertrophied and dilated RV in patients with CTEPH might be even more sensitive to ischaemia or other surgery-related injury.

5.2 Restoration of exercise tolerance

5.2.1 Restoration of stroke volume response

Exercise tolerance in patients with CTEPH is limited by an inadequate RV stroke volume response upon exercise. As previously discussed, preoperatively, SV decreases during exercise in patients with CTEPH; moreover, SV during exercise is related to exercise capacity as expressed by $V'O_2$-peak as well as the hemodynamic severity of disease. One year after PEA, we demonstrated restoration of the SV response: change upon exercise in SVI pre-PEA: -2.8 ± 4.6 ml/m^2 vs. change upon exercise SVI post-PEA: 4.0 ± 4.9 ml.m^2 ($p<0.001$; Table 1). The restoration of the SV response was accompanied by an increase in exercise tolerance, and by restoration of cardiac remodelling as assessed by cMRI. However, postoperatively, in some preoperatively more severely affected patients we still observed a negative SV response during exercise, despite (near) normalization in pulmonary hemodynamics.

	Controls		Pre PEA		Post PEA	
	Rest	Exercise	Rest	Exercise	Rest	Exercise
SVI, *ml.m^{-2}*	46.6±7.6	57.9±11.8	35.9±7.4 #	33.0±9.0 *#	35.9±5.2 #	39.9±5.4 *‡#
HR, *min^{-1}*	65±10	94±8	69±12	93±13 *	73±11	97±9.0 *
CI, *l. min^{-1}.m^{-2}*	3.0±0.3	5.4±1.1	2.4±0.4 #	3.0±0.8 *#	2.6±0.5	3.8±0.5 *‡#

Table 1. Stroke volume index (SVI), heart rate (HR) and cardiac index (CI) values at rest and during sub-maximal exercise for healthy controls and CTEPH patients before and after PEA. Data are expressed as mean±SD. * $p<0.05$ compared to resting conditions, ‡ $p<0.05$ post PEA compared to pre PEA, # $p<0.05$ compared with healthy controls (Van Kan et al., unpublished data).

5.2.2 Six-minute walk test

We systematically studied the effects of PEA on the restoration of exercise tolerance by the 6-MWT, and assessed its relation with the hemodynamic improvement observed shortly after surgery. One year after PEA, the 6-MWD had increased significantly, and the change correlated with the observed hemodynamic improvement. Moreover, in patients with normalized pulmonary hemodynamics after PEA, the 6-MWD, expressed as percentage of the predicted value, even tended to normalize (Reesink et al., 2007).

In addition, we studied the time course of the postoperative functional recovery of patients with CTEPH up to 5 years after PEA. Whereas NYHA functional class and sPAP improved within the first 3 months after PEA without further improvement, the 6-MWD showed a gradual improvement over a 2-year follow-up period. Interestingly, the dynamics of functional recovery parallel the observed time course of the restoration of RV systolic and diastolic function. Furthermore, patients with residual pulmonary hypertension after PEA showed a greater improvement in 6-MWD, despite their worse absolute outcome (Van der Plas et al., 2011).

The improvement observed in 6-MWD after PEA can be explained in major part by an increase in maximum aerobic capacity due to the restoration of the SV response upon exercise due to instantaneous decrease in right ventricle afterload. This is supported by our observations that the increase in 6-MWD upon PEA was not associated with a concomitant increase in heart rate; this implicates that PEA improves cardiac output by improving RV SV response and thereby decreasing the need for a chronotropic response. (Van der Plas et al., 2010). A second contributing factor appears decrease in dead space ventilation due to the restoration of pulmonary blood flow. The decrease in dead space ventilation was shown to be associated with an improvement of dyspnea symptoms upon exercise as ventilatory demand decreases (Van der Plas et al., 2010). Another factor, which has been suggested to attribute to the observed long-term improvement of 6-MWD after PEA, might be a long-term restoration of secondary arteriopathy which accommodates greater blood flow and improves gas exchange (Thistlethwaite et al, 2011).

5.2.3 Cardiopulmonary exercise testing

In addition to the restoration of SV response during exercise assessed by cMRI, we also studied the restoration of exercise tolerance in CTEPH patients after PEA by use of CPET. Pre-operatively maximal SV, assessed by cMRI, during exercise correlated with $V'O_2$-peak ($r=0.688$, $p=0.002$) and O_2 -pulse ($r=0.759$, $p<0.001$), and exercise SV correlated inversely with mPAP ($r=-0.719$, $p=0.001$) and TPR ($r=-0.656$, $p=0.001$).
After PEA, we observed a normalization in exercise capacity in 11 out of 13 patients studied. $V'O_2$-peak, peak workload and peak O_2-pulse increased significantly while peak HR and peak V'_E remained unchanged. $V'_E/V'CO_2$ showed a significant decrease, but normalized in 8 out of 13 patients only (Table 2). Changes in $V'O_2$-peak from baseline to 1 year post PEA, correlated significant with the directly after PEA observed changes in mPAP.

Exercise parameters	**Pre PEA**	**Post PEA**
$V'O_2$ –peak, (% predicted)	72.5 ± 13.0	99 ± 13*
Peak workload, (% predicted)	71 ± 23	97 ± 30*
O_2 –pulse, (% predicted)	75 ± 13	95 ± 14*
$V'_E/V'CO_2$	49.8 ± 11.2	32.7 ± 4.0*
Peak HR, (% predicted)	91 ± 8	94 ± 10
Peak V'_E, (% predicted)	98 ± 19	92 ± 14

Table 2. Data are expressed as mean±SD. *$V'O_2$ = oxygen uptake;* O_2 –pulse = oxygen pulse; V'_E = minute ventilation; $V'_E/V'CO_2$ = ventilation equivalent for carbon dioxide; HR = heart rate. * $p<0.05$ post PEA compared to pre PEA (Van Kan et al., unpublished data).

5.3 Effects of pulmonary endarterectomy on dyspnea

Dyspnea can be assessed by using NYHA functional classification and the patient reported Borg score. In a cohort of fifty-four consecutive CTEPH patients both NYHA functional class (Figure 9) and resting Borg scores (Figure 8) improved after PEA. The change after PEA in NYHA functional class and resting Borg scores were independently correlated with the changes observed in absolute dead space and dead space ventilation, as well as with the hemodynamic improvement.
As we have shown, the increase in dead space ventilation in CTEPH patients is significantly correlated with the hemodynamic severity of disease. After PEA, dead space ventilation

decreases, and was shown to normalize in the majority of patients. Hence, although the primary objective of PEA is to lower the right ventricular afterload, normalization of dead space by surgical removal of chronic thromboembolism contributed significantly to the postoperative recovery of the symptomatic dyspnea.

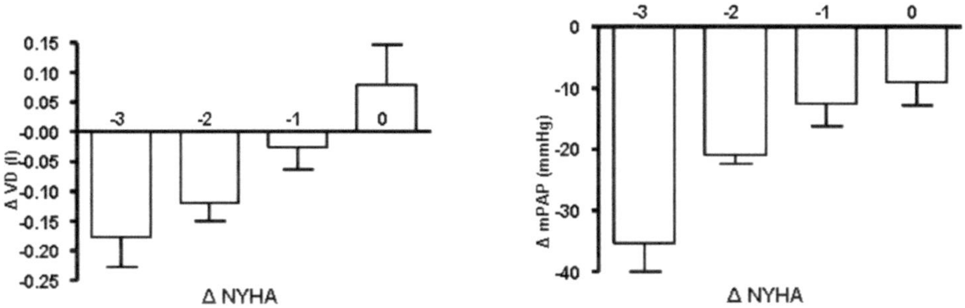

Fig. 8. Change in absolute dead space (Delta V_D) and change in mean pulmonary arterial pressure (Delta mPAP) against changes in NYHA functional class (Delta NYHA) (Adapted from: Van der Plas et al., 2010).

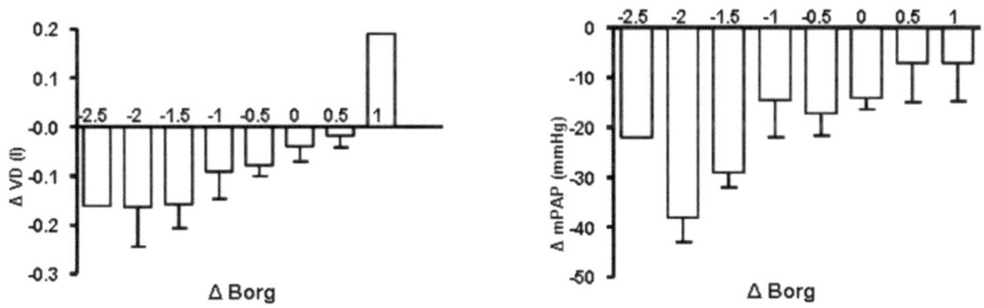

Fig. 9. Change in absolute dead space (Delta V_D) and change in mean pulmonary arterial pressure (Delta mPAP) against changes in Borg score at rest (Delta Borg) (Adapted from: Van der Plas et al., 2010).

6. Future research

In this overview, at least one possibly important factor contributing to the exercise limitation observed in CTEPH patients has not been addressed. The main focus of our studies has been on the cardiac and ventilatory contributing components. However, recently a reduction in respiratory and peripheral muscle strength has been observed in patients with iPAH which may be a determinant of exercise performance as well (Bauer et al., 2007; de Man et al., 2009; Mainguy et al., 2010; Meyer et al., 2005). The underlying mechanisms responsible for muscle weakness in PH patients are not yet known. In COPD and chronic (left) heart failure multiple mechanisms have been suggested to be involved in reduced muscle strength; changes in muscle fibre type ratio, abnormal intracellular Ca^{2+} profile, impaired muscle perfusion, decreased number of mitochondria, decreased oxidative enzymes, electrolyte disturbance, steroid therapy, malnutrition, wasting and cardiac cachexia. Most of these mechanisms do not seem to apply in PH (Meyer et al., 2005). However, we observed an increase in body mass index (BMI) one year after PEA in patients with CTEPH; in 48 consecutive CTEPH patients the BMI increased from 29.7±5.6 preoperatively to 30.8±5.7 at 1 year after surgery ($p=0.001$). Based upon this observation, it might be hypothesized that some form of preoperative malnutrition or wasting may occur in CTEPH patients despite their in itself normal BMI. In COPD and heart failure, weight loss and loss of fat-free mass were shown to be associated with systemic inflammation (Anker et al., 2002; Decramer et al., 2001; Gosker et al., 2000; Anker et al., 2002; Decramer et al., 2001; Gosker et al., 2000). Langer and colleagues found that heart failure due to CTEPH also appears to generate a pronounced systemic inflammatory response with the release of pro-inflammatory and anti-inflammatory cytokines; moreover, PEA resulted in the normalization of preoperatively elevated TNF-alpha levels (Langer et al., 2004). Future research should focus on the clarification of the possible relationship between exercise intolerance, muscle weakness and systemic inflammation induced wasting in (CTE)PH patients. CTEPH patients can serve as an excellent model for these studies, in which the effect of PEA on muscle strength, body composition and systemic inflammation, and the relationships in its changes can be studied.

7. Conclusions

CTEPH results from incomplete resolution of the vascular obstruction caused by pulmonary thromboembolism. Patients typically present themselves with gradually exercise intolerance, portrayed as exertional dyspnea. Exercise is primarily limited by the inability of the right ventricle to sufficiently increase pulmonary blood flow upon exercise. If left untreated, the increased resistance and pulmonary arterial pressure leads to progressive cardiac remodeling with consequent impact on cardiac function. In addition, in CTEPH dead space ventilation is increased due to the vascular obstruction; and dead space ventilation correlates to the patient's experienced dyspnea.

Pulmonary endarterectomy is the therapy of choice for patients with CTEPH and surgical accessible thrombi. PEA causes an instantaneous and permanent hemodynamic improvement, which is (over time) associated with a restoration of parameters of RV and LV remodeling and function. Exercise tolerance increases primarily due to the improvement in stroke volume response. However, full symptomatic recovery also seems to depend on normalisation of dead space ventilation due to the restoration of pulmonary blood flow as a result of the surgical removal of chronic thromboembolism.

8. References

(2002). ATS statement: guidelines for the six-minute walk test. *Am J Respir.Crit Care Med,* Vol.166, No.1, pp. 111-117, ISSN 1073-449X

Alpert, J.S.(2001). The effect of right ventricular dysfunction on left ventricular form and function. *Chest,* Vol.119, No.6, pp. 1632-1633,

Anker, S.D. & Sharma, R.(2002). The syndrome of cardiac cachexia. *Int.J.Cardiol.,* Vol.85, No.1, pp. 51-66,

Archibald, C.J., Auger, W.R., & Fedullo, P.F.(1999). Outcome after pulmonary thromboendarterectomy. *Semin.Thorac.Cardiovasc.Surg,* Vol.11, No.2, pp. 164-171, ISSN 1043-0679

Auger, W.R., Permpikul, P., & Moser, K.M.(1995). Lupus anticoagulant, heparin use, and thrombocytopenia in patients with chronic thromboembolic pulmonary hypertension: a preliminary report. *Am J Med,* Vol.99, No.4, pp. 392-396, ISSN 0002-9343

Auger, W.R., Kim, N.H., Kerr, K.M., Test, V.J., & Fedullo, P.F.(2007). Chronic thromboembolic pulmonary hypertension. *Clin Chest Med,* Vol.28, No.1, pp. 255-69, x, ISSN 0272-5231

Bauer, M., Wilkens, H., Langer, F., Schneider, S.O., Lausberg, H., & Schafers, H.J.(2002). Selective upregulation of endothelin B receptor gene expression in severe pulmonary hypertension. *Circulation,* Vol.105, No.9, pp. 1034-1036, ISSN 1524-4539

Bauer, R., Dehnert, C., Schoene, P., Filusch, A., Bartsch, P., Borst, M.M., Katus, H.A., & Meyer, F.J.(2007). Skeletal muscle dysfunction in patients with idiopathic pulmonary arterial hypertension. *Respir.Med,* Vol.101, No.11, pp. 2366-2369, ISSN 0954-6111

Becattini, C., Agnelli, G., Pesavento, R., Silingardi, M., Poggio, R., Taliani, M.R., & Ageno, W.(2006). Incidence of chronic thromboembolic pulmonary hypertension after a first episode of pulmonary embolism. *Chest,* Vol.130, No.1, pp. 172-175, ISSN 0012-3692

Bonderman, D., Martischnig, A.M., Vonbank, K., Nikfardjam, M., Meyer, B., Heinz, G., Klepetko, W., Naeije, R., & Lang, I.M.(2011). Right ventricular load at exercise is a cause of persistent exercise limitation in patients with normal resting pulmonary vascular resistance after pulmonary endarterectomy. *Chest,* Vol.139, No.1, pp. 122-127,

Bonderman, D., Wilkens, H., Wakounig, S., Schafers, H.J., Jansa, P., Lindner, J., Simkova, I., Martischnig, A.M., Dudczak, J., Sadushi, R., Skoro-Sajer, N., Klepetko, W., & Lang, I.M.(2009). Risk factors for chronic thromboembolic pulmonary hypertension. *Eur Respir.J,* Vol.33, No.2, pp. 325-331, ISSN 1399-3003

Bonderman, D., Jakowitsch, J., Adlbrecht, C., Schemper, M., Kyrle, P.A., Schonauer, V., Exner, M., Klepetko, W., Kneussl, M.P., Maurer, G., & Lang, I.(2005). Medical conditions increasing the risk of chronic thromboembolic pulmonary hypertension. *Thromb.Haemost.,* Vol.93, No.3, pp. 512-516, ISSN 0340-6245

Bonderman, D., Turecek, P.L., Jakowitsch, J., Weltermann, A., Adlbrecht, C., Schneider, B., Kneussl, M., Rubin, L.J., Kyrle, P.A., Klepetko, W., Maurer, G., & Lang, I.M.(2003). High prevalence of elevated clotting factor VIII in chronic thromboembolic pulmonary hypertension. *Thromb.Haemost.,* Vol.90, No.3, pp. 372-376, ISSN 0340-6245

Borg, G.A.(1982). Psychophysical bases of perceived exertion. *Med Sci Sports Exerc.,* Vol.14, No.5, pp. 377-381, ISSN 0195-9131

Cahalin, L.P., Mathier, M.A., Semigran, M.J., Dec, G.W., & DiSalvo, T.G.(1996). The six-minute walk test predicts peak oxygen uptake and survival in patients with advanced heart failure. *Chest,* Vol.110, No.2, pp. 325-332, ISSN 0012-3692

Colorio, C.C., Martinuzzo, M.E., Forastiero, R.R., Pombo, G., Adamczuk, Y., & Carreras, L.O.(2001). Thrombophilic factors in chronic thromboembolic pulmonary hypertension. *Blood Coagul.Fibrinolysis,* Vol.12, No.6, pp. 427-432, ISSN 0957-5235

Condliffe, R., Kiely, D.G., Gibbs, J.S., Corris, P.A., Peacock, A.J., Jenkins, D.P., Hodgkins, D., Goldsmith, K., Hughes, R.J., Sheares, K., Tsui, S.S.L., Armstrong, I.J., Torpy, C., Crackett, R., Carlin, C.M., Das, C., Coghlan, J.G., & Pepke-Zaba, J.(2008). Improved outcomes in medically and surgically treated chronic thromboembolic pulmonary hypertension. *Am J Respir.Crit Care Med,* Vol.177, No.10, pp. 1122-1127, ISSN 1535-4970

Cooper, K.H.(1968). A means of assessing maximal oxygen intake. Correlation between field and treadmill testing. *JAMA,* Vol.203, No.3, pp. 201-204, ISSN 0098-7484

Corsico, A.G., D'Armini, A.M., Cerveri, I., Klersy, C., Ansaldo, E., Niniano, R., Gatto, E., Monterosso, C., Morsolini, M., Nicolardi, S., Tramontin, C., Pozzi, E., & Vigano, M.(2008). Long-term outcome after pulmonary endarterectomy. *Am J Respir.Crit Care Med,* Vol.178, No.4, pp. 419-424, ISSN 1535-4970

Cournand, D.A. & Riley, R.L.(1950). Pulmonary circulation and alveolar ventilation perfusion relationships after pneumonectomy. *J Thorac.Surg,* Vol.19, No.1, pp. 80-116, ISSN 0096-5588

D'Alonzo, G.E., Gianotti, L.A., Pohil, R.L., Reagle, R.R., DuRee, S.L., Fuentes, F., & Dantzker, D.R.(1987). Comparison of progressive exercise performance of normal subjects and patients with primary pulmonary hypertension. *Chest,* Vol.92, No.1, pp. 57-62, ISSN 0012-3692

D'Armini, A.M., Zanotti, G., Ghio, S., Magrini, G., Pozzi, M., Scelsi, L., Meloni, G., Klersy, C., & Vigano, M.(2007). Reverse right ventricular remodeling after pulmonary endarterectomy. *J.Thorac.Cardiovasc.Surg.,* Vol.133, No.1, pp. 162-168,

de Man, F.S., Handoko, M.L., Groepenhoff, H., 't Hul, A.J., Abbink, J., Koppers, R.J.H., Grotjohan, H.P., Twisk, J.W.R., Bogaard, H.J., Boonstra, A., Postmus, P.E., Westerhof, N., van der Laarse, W.J., & Vonk-Noordegraaf, A.(2009). Effects of exercise training in patients with idiopathic pulmonary arterial hypertension. *Eur Respir.J,* Vol.34, No.3, pp. 669-675, ISSN 1399-3003

Deboeck, G., Niset, G., Lamotte, M., Vachiery, J.L., & Naeije, R.(2004). Exercise testing in pulmonary arterial hypertension and in chronic heart failure. *Eur Respir.J,* Vol.23, No.5, pp. 747-751, ISSN 0903-1936

Decramer, M.(2001). Respiratory muscles in COPD: regulation of trophical status. *Verh.K.Acad.Geneeskd.Belg.,* Vol.63, No.6, pp. 577-602,

Dittrich, H.C., Chow, L.C., & Nicod, P.H.(1989). Early improvement in left ventricular diastolic function after relief of chronic right ventricular pressure overload. *Circulation,* Vol.80, No.4, pp. 823-830,

Dittrich, H.C., Nicod, P.H., Chow, L.C., Chappuis, F.P., Moser, K.M., & Peterson, K.L.(1988). Early changes of right heart geometry after pulmonary thromboendarterectomy. *J.Am.Coll.Cardiol.,* Vol.11, No.5, pp. 937-943,

Fedullo, P.F., Auger, W.R., Kerr, K.M., & Rubin, L.J.(2001). Chronic thromboembolic pulmonary hypertension. *N.Engl.J Med,* Vol.345, No.20, pp. 1465-1472, ISSN 0028-4793

Fedullo, P., Kerr, K.M., Kim, N.H., & Auger, W.R.(2011). Chronic thromboembolic pulmonary hypertension. *Am J Respir.Crit Care Med,* Vol.183, No.12, pp. 1605-1613, ISSN 1535-4970

Fleg, J.L., Pina, I.L., Balady, G.J., Chaitman, B.R., Fletcher, B., Lavie, C., Limacher, M.C., Stein, R.A., Williams, M., & Bazzarre, T.(2000). Assessment of functional capacity in clinical and research applications: An advisory from the Committee on Exercise, Rehabilitation, and Prevention, Council on Clinical Cardiology, American Heart Association. *Circulation,* Vol.102, No.13, pp. 1591-1597, ISSN 1524-4539

Forfia, P.R., Fisher, M.R., Mathai, S.C., Housten-Harris, T., Hemnes, A.R., Borlaug, B.A., Chamera, E., Corretti, M.C., Champion, H.C., Abraham, T.P., Girgis, R.E., & Hassoun, P.M.(2006). Tricuspid annular displacement predicts survival in pulmonary hypertension. *Am.J.Respir.Crit Care Med.*, Vol.174, No.9, pp. 1034-1041,

Galie, N., Hoeper, M.M., Humbert, M., Torbicki, A., Vachiery, J.L., Barbera, J.A., Beghetti, M., Corris, P., Gaine, S., Gibbs, J.S., Gomez-Sanchez, M.A., Jondeau, G., Klepetko, W., Opitz, C., Peacock, A., Rubin, L., Zellweger, M., & Simonneau, G.(2009). Guidelines for the diagnosis and treatment of pulmonary hypertension. *Eur.Respir.J.*, Vol.34, No.6, pp. 1219-1263,

Gan, C.T., Lankhaar, J.W., Marcus, J.T., Westerhof, N., Marques, K.M., Bronzwaer, J.G., Boonstra, A., Postmus, P.E., & Vonk-Noordegraaf, A.(2006). Impaired left ventricular filling due to right-to-left ventricular interaction in patients with pulmonary arterial hypertension. *Am.J.Physiol Heart Circ.Physiol,* Vol.290, No.4, pp. H1528-H1533,

Gosker, H.R., Wouters, E.F., van der Vusse, G.J., & Schols, A.M.(2000). Skeletal muscle dysfunction in chronic obstructive pulmonary disease and chronic heart failure: underlying mechanisms and therapy perspectives. *Am.J.Clin.Nutr.,* Vol.71, No.5, pp. 1033-1047,

Groepenhoff, H., Vonk-Noordegraaf, A., Boonstra, A., Spreeuwenberg, M.D., Postmus, P.E., & Bogaard, H.J.(2008). Exercise testing to estimate survival in pulmonary hypertension. *Med Sci Sports Exerc.,* Vol.40, No.10, pp. 1725-1732, ISSN 1530-0315

Hardziyenka, M., Campian, M.E., Reesink, H.J., Surie, S., Bouma, B.J., Groenink, M., Klemens, C.A., Beekman, L., Remme, C.A., Bresser, P., & Tan, H.L.(2011). Right ventricular failure following chronic pressure overload is associated with reduction in left ventricular mass evidence for atrophic remodeling. *J Am Coll.Cardiol.,* Vol.57, No.8, pp. 921-928, ISSN 1558-3597

Harrison, R.W., Buehler, W., Thompson, R.G., Long, E.T., Carlson, R., Charbon, B., & Adams, W.E.(1957). Cardiopulmonary reserve five to fifteen years following fifty per cent or more reduction of lung volume. *Surg Forum,* Vol.7, pp. 209-213, ISSN 0071-8041

Helbing, W.A., Rebergen, S.A., Maliepaard, C., Hansen, B., Ottenkamp, J., Reiber, J.H., & de, R.A.(1995). Quantification of right ventricular function with magnetic resonance imaging in children with normal hearts and with congenital heart disease. *Am.Heart J.*, Vol.130, No.4, pp. 828-837,

Hoeper, M.M., Mayer, E., Simonneau, G., & Rubin, L.J.(2006). Chronic thromboembolic pulmonary hypertension. *Circulation,* Vol.113, No.16, pp. 2011-2020, ISSN 1524-4539

Holverda, S., Gan, C.T.-J., Marcus, J.T., Postmus, P.E., Boonstra, A., & Vonk-Noordegraaf, A.(2006). Impaired stroke volume response to exercise in pulmonary arterial hypertension. *J Am Coll.Cardiol.,* Vol.47, No.8, pp. 1732-1733, ISSN 1558-3597

Humbert, M., Sitbon, O., & Simonneau, G.(2004). Treatment of pulmonary arterial hypertension. *N.Engl.J.Med.,* Vol.351, No.14, pp. 1425-1436,

Hurwit, E.S., Schein, C.J., Rifkin, H., & Lebendiger, A.(1958). A surgical approach to the problem of chronic pulmonary artery obstruction due to thrombosis or stenosis. *Ann.Surg.,* Vol.147, No.2, pp. 157-165,

Iino, M., Dymarkowski, S., Chaothawee, L., Delcroix, M., & Bogaert, J.(2008). Time course of reversed cardiac remodeling after pulmonary endarterectomy in patients with chronic pulmonary thromboembolism. *Eur Radiol.,* Vol.18, No.4, pp. 792-799, ISSN 0938-7994

Jais, X., Ioos, V., Jardim, C., Sitbon, O., Parent, F., Hamid, A., Fadel, E., Dartevelle, P., Simonneau, G., & Humbert, M.(2005). Splenectomy and chronic thromboembolic pulmonary hypertension. *Thorax,* Vol.60, No.12, pp. 1031-1034, ISSN 0040-6376

Jamieson, S.W. & Kapelanski, D.P.(2000). Pulmonary endarterectomy. *Curr Probl.Surg,* Vol.37, No.3, pp. 165-252, ISSN 0011-3840

Jamieson, S.W., Kapelanski, D.P., Sakakibara, N., Manecke, G.R., Thistlethwaite, P.A., Kerr, K.M., Channick, R.N., Fedullo, P.F., & Auger, W.R.(2003). Pulmonary endarterectomy: experience and lessons learned in 1,500 cases. *Ann.Thorac.Surg,* Vol.76, No.5, pp. 1457-1462, ISSN 0003-4975

Jordan, J., Shannon, J.R., Diedrich, A., Black, B., Costa, F., Robertson, D., & Biaggioni, I.(2000). Interaction of carbon dioxide and sympathetic nervous system activity in the regulation of cerebral perfusion in humans. *Hypertension,* Vol.36, No.3, pp. 383-388, ISSN 1524-4563

Kasimir, M.T., Seebacher, G., Jaksch, P., Winkler, G., Schmid, K., Marta, G.M., Simon, P., & Klepetko, W.(2004). Reverse cardiac remodelling in patients with primary pulmonary hypertension after isolated lung transplantation. *Eur.J.Cardiothorac.Surg.,* Vol.26, No.4, pp. 776-781,

Kovacs, G., Berghold, A., Scheidl, S., & Olschewski, H.(2009). Pulmonary arterial pressure during rest and exercise in healthy subjects: a systematic review. *Eur Respir.J,* Vol.34, No.4, pp. 888-894, ISSN 1399-3003

Kreitner, K.F., Kunz, R.P., Ley, S., Oberholzer, K., Neeb, D., Gast, K.K., Heussel, C.P., Eberle, B., Mayer, E., Kauczor, H.U., & Duber, C.(2007). Chronic thromboembolic pulmonary hypertension - assessment by magnetic resonance imaging. *Eur Radiol.,* Vol.17, No.1, pp. 11-21, ISSN 0938-7994

Kreitner, K.F.J., Ley, S., Kauczor, H.U., Mayer, E., Kramm, T., Pitton, M.B., Krummenauer, F., & Thelen, M.(2004). Chronic thromboembolic pulmonary hypertension: pre- and postoperative assessment with breath-hold MR imaging techniques. *Radiology,* Vol.232, No.2, pp. 535-543, ISSN 0033-8419

Kyrle, P.A., Minar, E., Hirschl, M., Bialonczyk, C., Stain, M., Schneider, B., Weltermann, A., Speiser, W., Lechner, K., & Eichinger, S.(2000). High plasma levels of factor VIII and the risk of recurrent venous thromboembolism. *N.Engl.J Med,* Vol.343, No.7, pp. 457-462, ISSN 0028-4793

Lang, I.(2010). Advances in understanding the pathogenesis of chronic thromboembolic pulmonary hypertension. *Br J Haematol.,* Vol.149, No.4, pp. 478-483, ISSN 1365-2141

Langer, F., Schramm, R., Bauer, M., Tscholl, D., Kunihara, T., & Schafers, H.J.(2004). Cytokine response to pulmonary thromboendarterectomy. *Chest,* Vol.126, No.1, pp. 135-141,

Lewczuk, J., Piszko, P., Jagas, J., Porada, A., Wojciak, S., Sobkowicz, B., & Wrabec, K.(2001). Prognostic factors in medically treated patients with chronic pulmonary embolism. *Chest,* Vol.119, No.3, pp. 818-823, ISSN 0012-3692

Lim, H.S., Kang, S.J., Choi, J.H., Ahn, S.G., Choi, B.J., Choi, S.Y., Yoon, M.H., Hwang, G.S., Tahk, S.J., & Shin, J.H.(2009). Is E/E' reliable in patients with regional wall motion abnormalities to estimate left ventricular filling pressure? *Int.J.Cardiovasc.Imaging,* Vol.25, No.1, pp. 33-39,

Mainguy, V., Maltais, F., Saey, D., Gagnon, P., Martel, S., Simon, M., & Provencher, S.(2010). Peripheral muscle dysfunction in idiopathic pulmonary arterial hypertension. *Thorax,* Vol.65, No.2, pp. 113-117, ISSN 1468-3296

Manning, H.L. & Schwartzstein, R.M.(1995). Pathophysiology of dyspnea. *N.Engl.J Med,* Vol.333, No.23, pp. 1547-1553, ISSN 0028-4793

Marcus, J.T., Vonk, N.A., Roeleveld, R.J., Postmus, P.E., Heethaar, R.M., Van Rossum, A.C., & Boonstra, A.(2001). Impaired left ventricular filling due to right ventricular pressure overload in primary pulmonary hypertension: noninvasive monitoring using MRI. *Chest,* Vol.119, No.6, pp. 1761-1765,

Mayer, E., Dahm, M., Hake, U., Schmid, F.X., Pitton, M., Kupferwasser, I., Iversen, S., & Oelert, H.(1996). Mid-term results of pulmonary thromboendarterectomy for chronic thromboembolic pulmonary hypertension. *Ann.Thorac.Surg.,* Vol.61, No.6, pp. 1788-1792,

Menzel, T., Kramm, T., Bruckner, A., Mohr-Kahaly, S., Mayer, E., & Meyer, J.(2002a). Quantitative assessment of right ventricular volumes in severe chronic thromboembolic pulmonary hypertension using transthoracic three-dimensional echocardiography: changes due to pulmonary thromboendarterectomy. *Eur.J.Echocardiogr.,* Vol.3, No.1, pp. 67-72,

Menzel, T., Kramm, T., Mohr-Kahaly, S., Mayer, E., Oelert, H., & Meyer, J.(2002b). Assessment of cardiac performance using Tei indices in patients undergoing pulmonary thromboendarterectomy. *Ann.Thorac.Surg.,* Vol.73, No.3, pp. 762-766,

Menzel, T., Wagner, S., Kramm, T., Mohr-Kahaly, S., Mayer, E., Braeuninger, S., & Meyer, J.(2000). Pathophysiology of impaired right and left ventricular function in chronic embolic pulmonary hypertension: changes after pulmonary thromboendarterectomy. *Chest,* Vol.118, No.4, pp. 897-903,

Meyer, F.J., Lossnitzer, D., Kristen, A.V., Schoene, A.M., Kubler, W., Katus, H.A., & Borst, M.M.(2005). Respiratory muscle dysfunction in idiopathic pulmonary arterial hypertension. *Eur Respir.J,* Vol.25, No.1, pp. 125-130, ISSN 0903-1936

Miyamoto, S., Nagaya, N., Satoh, T., Kyotani, S., Sakamaki, F., Fujita, M., Nakanishi, N., & Miyatake, K.(2000). Clinical correlates and prognostic significance of six-minute walk test in patients with primary pulmonary hypertension. Comparison with cardiopulmonary exercise testing. *Am J Respir.Crit Care Med,* Vol.161, No.2 Pt 1, pp. 487-492, ISSN 1073-449X

Moser, K.M., Auger, W.R., & Fedullo, P.F.(1990). Chronic major-vessel thromboembolic pulmonary hypertension. *Circulation,* Vol.81, No.6, pp. 1735-1743, ISSN 0009-7322

Moser, K.M. & Braunwald, N.S.(1973). Successful surgical intervention in severe chronic thromboembolic pulmonary hypertension. *Chest,* Vol.64, No.1, pp. 29-35, ISSN 0012-3692

O'Donnell, J., Tuddenham, E.G., Manning, R., Kemball-Cook, G., Johnson, D., & Laffan, M.(1997). High prevalence of elevated factor VIII levels in patients referred for thrombophilia screening: role of increased synthesis and relationship to the acute phase reaction. *Thromb.Haemost.,* Vol.77, No.5, pp. 825-828, ISSN 0340-6245

Palange, P., Ward, S.A., Carlsen, K.H., Casaburi, R., Gallagher, C.G., Gosselink, R., O'Donnell, D.E., Puente-Maestu, L., Schols, A.M., Singh, S., & Whipp, B.J.(2007). Recommendations on the use of exercise testing in clinical practice. *Eur Respir.J,* Vol.29, No.1, pp. 185-209, ISSN 0903-1936

Pengo, V., Lensing, A.W.A., Prins, M.H., Marchiori, A., Davidson, B.L., Tiozzo, F., Albanese, P., Biasiolo, A., Pegoraro, C., Iliceto, S., & Prandoni, P.(2004). Incidence of chronic thromboembolic pulmonary hypertension after pulmonary embolism. *N.Engl.J Med,* Vol.350, No.22, pp. 2257-2264, ISSN 1533-4406

Raeside, D.A., Smith, A., Brown, A., Patel, K.R., Madhok, R., Cleland, J., & Peacock, A.J.(2000). Pulmonary artery pressure measurement during exercise testing in patients with suspected pulmonary hypertension. *Eur Respir.J,* Vol.16, No.2, pp. 282-287, ISSN 0903-1936

Reesink, H.J., Marcus, J.T., Tulevski, I.I., Jamieson, S., Kloek, J.J., Vonk Noordegraaf, A., & Bresser, P.(2007a). Reverse right ventricular remodeling after pulmonary endarterectomy in patients with chronic thromboembolic pulmonary hypertension: utility of magnetic resonance imaging to demonstrate restoration of the right ventricle. *J Thorac.Cardiovasc.Surg,* Vol.133, No.1, pp. 58-64, ISSN 1097-685X

Reesink, H.J., Meijer, R.C., Lutter, R., Boomsma, F., Jansen, H.M., Kloek, J.J., & Bresser, P.(2006). Hemodynamic and clinical correlates of endothelin-1 in chronic thromboembolic pulmonary hypertension. *Circ.J,* Vol.70, No.8, pp. 1058-1063, ISSN 1346-9843

Reesink, H.J., Van der Plas, M.N., Verhey, N.E., van Steenwijk, R.P., Kloek, J.J., & Bresser, P.(2007b). Six-minute walk distance as parameter of functional outcome after pulmonary endarterectomy for chronic thromboembolic pulmonary hypertension. *J Thorac.Cardiovasc.Surg,* Vol.133, No.2, pp. 510-516, ISSN 1097-685X

Riedel, M., Stanek, V., Widimsky, J., & Prerovsky, I.(1982). Longterm follow-up of patients with pulmonary thromboembolism. Late prognosis and evolution of hemodynamic and respiratory data. *Chest,* Vol.81, No.2, pp. 151-158, ISSN 0012-3692

Riley, M.S., Porszasz, J., Engelen, M.P., Brundage, B.H., & Wasserman, K.(2000). Gas exchange responses to continuous incremental cycle ergometry exercise in primary pulmonary hypertension in humans. *Eur.J.Appl.Physiol,* Vol.83, No.1, pp. 63-70,

Roul, G., Germain, P., & Bareiss, P.(1998). Does the 6-minute walk test predict the prognosis in patients with NYHA class II or III chronic heart failure? *Am Heart J,* Vol.136, No.3, pp. 449-457, ISSN 0002-8703

Rubens, F.D., Bourke, M., Hynes, M., Nicholson, D., Kotrec, M., Boodhwani, M., Ruel, M., Dennie, C.J., & Mesana, T.(2007). Surgery for chronic thromboembolic pulmonary hypertension--inclusive experience from a national referral center. *Ann.Thorac.Surg,* Vol.83, No.3, pp. 1075-1081, ISSN 1552-6259

Saxena, N., Rajagopalan, N., Edelman, K., & Lopez-Candales, A.(2006). Tricuspid annular systolic velocity: a useful measurement in determining right ventricular systolic function regardless of pulmonary artery pressures. *Echocardiography.,* Vol.23, No.9, pp. 750-755,

Smulders, S.A., Holverda, S., Vonk-Noordegraaf, A., van den Bosch, H.C., Post, J.C., Marcus, J.T., Smeenk, F.W., & Postmus, P.E.(2007). Cardiac function and position more than 5 years after pneumonectomy. *Ann.Thorac.Surg.,* Vol.83, No.6, pp. 1986-1992,

Sun, X.G., Hansen, J.E., Oudiz, R.J., & Wasserman, K.(2001). Exercise pathophysiology in patients with primary pulmonary hypertension. *Circulation,* Vol.104, No.4, pp. 429-435, ISSN 1524-4539

Surie, S., Bouma, B.J., Bruin-Bon, R.A.H., Hardziyenka, M., Kloek, J.J., Van der Plas, M.N., Reesink, H.J., & Bresser, P.(2011). Time course of restoration of systolic and diastolic right ventricular function after pulmonary endarterectomy for chronic thromboembolic pulmonary hypertension. *Am Heart J*, Vol.161, No.6, pp. 1046-1052, ISSN 1097-6744

Thistlethwaite PA, Jamieson SW. Invited commentary. (2011) *Ann Thorac Surg*, Vol.91, No.4 pp. 1100, ISSN21440130.

Tei, C., Dujardin, K.S., Hodge, D.O., Bailey, K.R., McGoon, M.D., Tajik, A.J., & Seward, S.B.(1996). Doppler echocardiographic index for assessment of global right ventricular function. *J.Am.Soc.Echocardiogr.*, Vol.9, No.6, pp. 838-847,

Unsworth, B., Casula, R.P., Kyriacou, A.A., Yadav, H., Chukwuemeka, A., Cherian, A., Stanbridge, R.L., Athanasiou, T., Mayet, J., & Francis, D.P.(2010). The right ventricular annular velocity reduction caused by coronary artery bypass graft surgery occurs at the moment of pericardial incision. *Am.Heart J.*, Vol.159, No.2, pp. 314-322,

Van der Plas, M.N., Duffels, M.G., Ponse, D., Mulder, B.J., & Bresser, P.(2008). Bosentan in mild pulmonary hypertension. *Lancet*, Vol.372, No.9651, pp. 1730

Van der Plas, M.N., Reesink, H.J., Roos, C.M., van Steenwijk, R.P., Kloek, J.J., & Bresser, P.(2010). Pulmonary endarterectomy improves dyspnea by the relief of dead space ventilation. *Ann.Thorac.Surg*, Vol.89, No.2, pp. 347-352, ISSN 1552-6259

Van der Plas, M.N., Surie, S., Reesink, H.J., van Steenwijk, R.P., Kloek, J.J., & Bresser, P.(2011). Longitudinal follow-up of six-minute walk distance after pulmonary endarterectomy. *Ann.Thorac.Surg*, Vol.91, No.4, pp. 1094-1099, ISSN 1552-6259

Velez-Roa, S., Ciarka, A., Najem, B., Vachiery, J.L., Naeije, R., & van de Borne, P.(2004). Increased sympathetic nerve activity in pulmonary artery hypertension. *Circulation*, Vol.110, No.10, pp. 1308-1312, ISSN 1524-4539

Viner, S.M., Bagg, B.R., Auger, W.R., & Ford, G.T.(1994). The management of pulmonary hypertension secondary to chronic thromboembolic disease. *Prog.Cardiovasc.Dis*, Vol.37, No.2, pp. 79-92, ISSN 0033-0620

Vizza, C.D., Lynch, J.P., Ochoa, L.L., Richardson, G., & Trulock, E.P.(1998). Right and left ventricular dysfunction in patients with severe pulmonary disease. *Chest*, Vol.113, No.3, pp. 576-583,

Vogel, M., Gutberlet, M., Dittrich, S., Hosten, N., & Lange, P.E.(1997). Comparison of transthoracic three dimensional echocardiography with magnetic resonance imaging in the assessment of right ventricular volume and mass. *Heart*, Vol.78, No.2, pp. 127-130,

Wasserman, K., ue, D., tringer, W., hipp, B., & ansen, J.(2004). Principles of Exercise Testing and Interpretation. No.4th edn., ISSN 7-7817-4876-3

Wensel, R., Opitz, C.F., Anker, S.D., Winkler, J., Hoffken, G., Kleber, F.X., Sharma, R., Hummel, M., Hetzer, R., & Ewert, R.(2002). Assessment of survival in patients with primary pulmonary hypertension: importance of cardiopulmonary exercise testing. *Circulation*, Vol.106, No.3, pp. 319-324, ISSN 1524-4539

Wessel, H.U., Kezdi, P., & Cucell, D.W.(1964). Respiratory and cardiovascular function in patients with severe pulmonary hypertension. *Circulation*, Vol.29, pp. 825-832,

Wolf, M., Boyer-Neumann, C., Parent, F., Eschwege, V., Jaillet, H., Meyer, D., & Simonneau, G.(2000). Thrombotic risk factors in pulmonary hypertension. *Eur Respir.J*, Vol.15, No.2, pp. 395-399, ISSN 0903-1936

Yasunobo, Y., Oudiz, R.J., & Sun, X.G.(1999). Dyspnea. Mechanisms, assessment, and management: a consensus statement. American Thoracic Society. *Am J Respir.Crit Care Med,* Vol.159, No.1, pp. 321-340, ISSN 1073-449X

Yasunobu, Y., Oudiz, R.J., Sun, X.G., Hansen, J.E., & Wasserman, K.(2005). End-tidal PCO2 abnormality and exercise limitation in patients with primary pulmonary hypertension. *Chest,* Vol.127, No.5, pp. 1637-1646, ISSN 0012-3692

Zoia, M.C., D'Armini, A.M., Beccaria, M., Corsico, A., Fulgoni, P., Klersy, C., Piovella, F., Vigano, M., & Cerveri, I.(2002). Mid term effects of pulmonary thromboendarterectomy on clinical and cardiopulmonary function status. *Thorax,* Vol.57, No.7, pp. 608-612, ISSN 0040-6376

8

Chest Wall Deformities: An Overview on Classification and Surgical Options

Michele Torre[1], Giovanni Rapuzzi[1], Vincenzo Jasonni[1,2] and Patricio Varela[3]
[1]*U. O. Chirurgia Pediatrica, Istituto Giannina Gaslini,*
[2]*Università degli Studi di Genova,*
[3]*Universidad de Chile, Hospital Luis Calvo Mackenna, Clinica Las Condes,*
[1,2]*Italy*
[3]*Santiago Chile*

1. Introduction

Chest wall malformations (CWMs) represent a wide spectrum of anomalies, with a relatively high incidence and a significant impact on the life of patients. Besides a minority of cases with functional respiratory impairment and symptoms, the clinical importance of these anomalies derives primarily from the fact that the majority of children and their parents seek medical advice for psychosocial concerns, sometimes severe, usually due to poor cosmesis and aversion to sports and public exposure. Despite the relatively high incidence, of CWMs are often misdiagnosed or neglected by physicians, thus resulting in a significant delay or mistakes in the diagnostic work up or in the therapeutic management. In the last 12 years, however, since the introduction of the Nuss technique for pectus excavatum (PE) (Nuss et al., 1998), the interest of the scientific community about CWMs has dramatically increased, as well as the number of publications on this topic. A wide range of CWMs exist. Some malformations are very well defined and others are part of a wide spectrum of deformities. Confusion still exists in the literature about CWMs nomenclature and classification. A classification is of paramount importance because of the treatment implications. Other controversial issues are the treatment options: many different surgical techniques or other therapeutic alternatives have been proposed, especially in the last decade, so it can be difficult for a pediatrician or even a surgeon to advise correctly the patients about the possible correction techniques. In this chapter we will propose a simple classification, published few years ago by Acastello (Acastello, 2006), and modified by us, distinguishing CWMs into five types, according to the origin of the anomaly (Table 1). Following this classification, we will go through each of the most important CWMs, with the aim of reviewing and updating this topic, focusing particularly on treatment options.

2. Classification of CWMs

Acastello (Acastello, 2006) classified CWMs in 5 types, depending on the site of origin of the anomaly (cartilagineous, costal, chondro-costal, sternal, clavicle-scapular). We will follow hereafter his classification, with minor modifications regarding PC classification, as explained later in the text (table 1).

2.1 Type I: Cartilaginous anomalies

2.1.1 Pectus excavatum (PE)

PE is the most frequent thoracic malformation, with an incidence of 1/100 to 1/1000 live births, and accounting for around the 90% of all CWMs (Fokin et al., 2009; Lopushinsky & Fecteau, 2008). It is characterized by the presence of a variably deep sternal depression associated to a malformation of the lowest condrosternal joints. Usually it is congenital, but in some cases (around 15%) it appears later during development. In the latter there is a frequent association with malformations of the muscular connective tissue, such as Marfan and Ehlers-Danlos syndrome(Colombani, 2009; Fokin et al., 2009; Kelly, 2008; Kotzot & Schwabegger, 2009; Lopushinsky & Fecteau, 2008). The etiology of PE is not clear, and many hypotheses have been proposed (Kelly, 2008). The role of vitamins or other nutrients deficiencies is probably not influent at all, while a connective tissue disorder and genetic predisposition could play a role. PE shows a familial recurrence in up to 40% of the cases (Kelly, 2008), more rarely we can observe the presence in a PE family of other CWMs such as PC. A study on genetics of PE showed that the most frequent transmission pattern seems to be the autosomal dominant, but there are families with autosomal recessive and X-linked patterns (Creswick et al, 2006). The overgrowth of costal cartilages could be the pathogenetic mechanism leading to the development of PE (Fokin et al., 2009; Haje et al, 1999; Kelly, 2008). Collagen type II disorders have been demonstrated in the costal cartilages in PE (Feng et al, 2001), as well as overexpression or downregulations of some genes playing a role in the metabolism of cartilage and connective tissues, as collagen genes, matrix metalloproteinases, tumor necrosis factor-alpha, and filamin (Fokin et al., 2009).

Type I: cartilagineous	Pectus excavatum (PE) Pectus carinatum (PC) type 1 True PC type 2	
Type II: costal	Simple (1 or 2 ribs) Complex (3 or more ribs)	agenesis, hypoplasia, sovrannumerary, bifid, fused, dysmorphic, rare (always complexes)
	Syndromic (always complex)	Jeune, Jarcho-Levin, Cerebrocostomandibular, others
Type III: condro-costal	Poland Syndrome	
Type IV: sternal	Sternal cleft (with or without ectopia cordis) Currarino Silverman Syndrome	
Type V: clavicle-scapular	Clavicular	Simple or Syndromic
	Scapular	Simple or Syndromic
	Combined	

Table 1. Acastello classification of CWMS according to the site of the defect, modified by us. In the original classification, PC type Currarino Silverman Syndrome was called as superior or type 2 and included in cartilagineous anomalies. We have distinguished superior or type 2 PC into two different anomalies: the true PC type 2, very rare, and the Currarino Silverman syndrome, that we moved into sternal anomalies (see text).

PE patients have often a typical aspect: they are slim and tall, with some degree of joint laxity, rounded shoulders with a kyphotic habit and a "pot belly" (Colombani, 2009). The association with scoliosis or kyphoscoliosis, reported in about 15%-50% of cases (Frick, 2000; Waters et al, 1989), sometimes represents a matter of concern for the patients and families, however spine deformities almost never represent a serious clinical problem and usually do not require any treatment (Waters et al, 1989). Cardiac anomalies are only seldom associated with PE, but mitral valve prolapse is frequent (Kotzot & Schwabegger, 2009). In our experience we observe PE in some neonates with diaphragmatic hernia or children with respiratory obstruction (mostly for hypetrophic tonsils). These particular types of PE are the only ones that can ameliorate significantly or disappear during infancy (Kelly, 2008). In all other cases PE is usually mild at birth but over the years it can become severe, progressing especially during pre - adolescent and adolescent age. When the deformity is very pronounced, patients may manifest dyspnea at exertion, lack of stamina, palpitations and thoracic pain or discomfort (Acastello, 2006; Colombani, 2009; Fokin et al., 2009; Kelly, 2008; Lopushinsky & Fecteau, 2008; Nuss et al., 1998; Williams & Crabbe, 2003). In cases of severe malformations there can be physiological repercussions. Many studies have tried to elucidate the implications of PE on the respiratory and cardiac function (Colombani, 2009; Kelly, 2007, 2008; Williams & Crabbe, 2003). Sternal depression causes a leftward displacement of the heart. In some patients, it is possible to find compression of the right ventricle or atrium with different degrees of dysfunction on the echocardiogram. Inferior cava vein can also be compressed. Lung functional tests can report some degree of dysfunction, more on stress conditions than on rest. Usually the most common pattern of PE patients is a restrictive one, but also obstructive or mixed patterns are not uncommon, while asthma induced by the exercise is rare. The aesthetic consequences greatly affect the self esteem and self image of most of the patients. They are usually extremely shy, withdrawn and not practicing any activity that may imply exposing their chests. Usually they do not go to the swimming pool or beach and they tend to isolate themselves. The thoracic deformity predominates over other physical alterations.

2.1.1.1 Diagnostic assessment and classification

As PE includes a large spectrum of anomalies with different degrees of gravity, it is important to assess the severity in order to select the best treatment. Different indexes have been proposed for this purpose. While we are allowed to calculate some of them during simple patient evaluation, measuring the depth of the excavation by a caliper (Colombani, 2009) or pulvimeter (Fokin et al., 2009), Computerized Tomography (CT) scan is necessary to calculate Haller index (Haller et al., 1987), the most widely accepted one, based on the division between lateral and antero-posterior thoracic diameters. It is recognized that Haller index higher than 3 or 3.25 indicates surgical correction. Another important feature to be considered is if PE is symmetric or asymmetric. The latter, usually more depressed on the right side due to a variable degree of sternal rotation, can be an important factor influencing the final result. In females with asymmetric PE the sternum is usually rotated towards the right side and the right breast is apparently hypoplasic, mimicking a PS and possibly creating some diagnostic difficulties for physicians without large experience in CWMs.
The shape of PE, extremely variable from case to case, is crucial in determining the type of surgical approach and the prognosis of the correction. It is possible to classify morphologically PE as follows (Fokin et al., 2009; Kelly, 2008; Nuss, 2008):

- Grand Canyon (figure 1): It is a severe and deep PE. There is a deep long canal in the sternum. These cases can be corrected with the retrosternal bar, but the correction is extremely difficult, especially when thorax is largely ossified and sternum is extremely rotated (figure 1). A higher complication rate after correction is reported, compared with the other types. In these cases, modified open procedures can be a valid option for correction.

- Punch or cup shape (figure 1): PE is extremely localized, usually on the inferior part of the sternum. It is more often symmetric. This type of PE can be very difficult to correct at any age and sometimes the outcome is partial.
- Saucer type: It can be symmetric or asymmetric. It is an extensive depression, the thorax is usually quite flat and the deep area is along the complete anterior chest.
- Transversal PE (figure 1): The depression is transversal and below the sternum.
- Eccentric PE: The sternal depression is eccentric to midline. It is the highest degree of asymmetric PE.
- PE with flaring chest (figure 1): The main feature of this type of PE (but sometime this is an isolated malformation, without associated PE) is the flaring chest at the level of the last ribs.
- PE-PC: it is a combined malformation with a sunken chest and cartilage protrusion beside the sternum edge.
- Superior PE: this is a very rare PE, localized in the upper part of sternum and cartilage ribs. Lower sternum is normal.

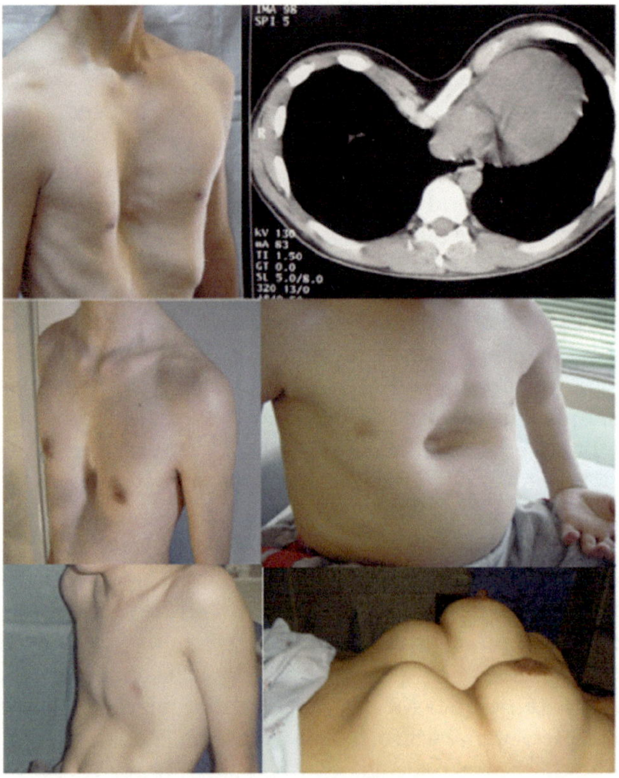

Fig. 1. *First row:* Grand Canyon shape PE (left), Computerized Tomography of the thorax showing Grand Canyon PE with sternal rotation (right); *Second row:* Punch-shaped PE; *Third row:* Transversal PE (left), PE with flaring chest (right)

2.1.1.2 Treatment options

Patients are selected for surgical correction if they demonstrate two or more of the following criteria (Kelly, 2008):

- symptoms;
- history of progression of the deformity;
- paradoxical movement of the chest wall with deep inspiration;
- a chest CT scan with Haller index greater than 3.25;
- cardiac compression;
- cava vein or pulmonary compression identified;
- abnormal pulmonary function studies showing significant restrictive disease;
- cardiac pathology secondary to the compression of the heart;
- history of failed previous repair;
- significant body image disturbance.

The ideal age for correction is a matter of debate (Lopushinsky & Fecteau, 2008; Nuss, 2008). Both open and Nuss procedures are feasible with good results in adult age (Aronson et al., 2007), however it is widely accepted that surgical correction has to be preferably performed in young patients before complete ossification of the thorax, that makes it harder and can jeopardize the final result. Fixing PE in the first years of life is probably unnecessary, and it could carry the risk of relapse (Nuss, 2008) or post-operative severe complications as acquired Jeune syndrome, according to the different techniques (Haller, 1996). A good age for correction with Nuss technique is usually considered from the age of 9 to 15 years of life (Nuss, 2008).

The first description of a PE repair was in 1911 from Meyer (Meyer, 1922). For many years the corrective procedures followed the principle introduced by Sauerbruch (Sauerbruch, 1931) and consisted mainly in resection of costal cartilages and mobilization of the sternum, sometimes with fracture of its anterior body. During the 20's, the resection was accompanied by external sternal traction which lasted for weeks. In 1939 Brown (Brown, 1939) recommended the resection of the ligament between sternum and diaphragm. Later, techniques were modified and standardized. A particular place has to be assigned to the pioneer of the modern era, Ravitch, who described his procedure in 1949 (Ravitch. 1949), consisting in the resection of all deformed costal cartilages without external traction. The modification proposed by Welch (Welch, 1958) preserved the perichondrium in order to facilitate rib regeneration. Another key point was the fixation of the sternum, in order to reduce flail chest and recurrence. It was performed initially with a bone graft (Dorner et al., 1950), later with a steel bar passed posterior to the sternum (Adkins & Blades, 1961). Many means of sternal fixation have been proposed during the following years, some of them absorbable. A totally new concept was introduced by Wada in 1970 (Wada et al., 1970) who described sternal turnover, in which the sternum was completely detached and removed, rotated by 180 degrees, then sutured back to the ribs. Another approach, attempted in mild cases, and proposed for the first time in 1972 by Standford (Stanford et al., 1972), was performed by filling the concavity of PE with some prosthetic material, as Silastic® or other subsequent modifications, as using omental flap (Grappolini, 2008). A revolutionary new technique was proposed by Nuss in 1997, and published after one year (Nuss et al., 1998), consisting of implanting a retrosternal metallic bar which is bent and rotated in 180° in order to obtain an immediate correction of the deformity. This bar is inserted through small lateral incisions and neither costal resections nor sternotomy are required. In Nuss procedure both the approach and the principle were completely new. In fact, although the result of the correction is obtained immediately during operation, the efficacy of Nuss procedure in long term is based on the principle of thoracic cage remodeling under the action of the force determined by the retrosternal bar. For this reason the bar should remain for at least 3 years and then is removed through an outpatient procedure. This bar is fixed to the chest wall muscles and is stabilized via a lateral device that avoids slippage. The technique is simple but requires extreme care and experience. Initially the retrosternal tunnel for the bar was completed blindly, later thoracoscopy was introduced. Thoracoscopy is absolutely necessary, since the bar must pass very close to noble structures such as the heart which is sometimes very attached to the sternum. Other, less adopted, conservative procedures have been described, based on a suction device (Vacuum Bell) (Schier et al., 2005) or magnetic forces (Harrison et al., 2007), and proposed as attempts to correct PE without any surgical maneuver, but results still need to be proved.

Results in all series (Acastello, 2006; Kelly et al., 2007; Lopushinsky & Fecteau, 2008; Nuss, 2008) are usually good in more than 80-90% of cases, depending on the gravity, type of PE and age of correction. The largest experience of 1215 patients is reported by Nuss and colleagues (Kelly et al., 2010), who report a 95.8% surgeon's satisfaction rate, 93% patient's satisfaction rate and a 92% parent's satisfaction rate. It remains to be defined which technique between Nuss procedure and open resections can guarantee better results, however nowadays Nuss procedure is far more used because it is less invasive and does not leave anterior scars. The complications observed both in open and mini-invasive procedures are wound infections, hematomas, bar shifts, pneumothorax, transient Horner syndrome, bleeding from thoracic vessels, overcorrection or mild correction (Acastello, 2006; Haller et al., 1987; Kelly et al., 2010; Lopushinsky & Fecteau, 2008; Nuss, 2008; Park et al., 2004). Complications of an extensive open procedure, particularly at early age, are floating sternum (Prabhakaran et al., 2001) and acquired Jeune syndrome (Haller et al., 1996), while in Nuss procedure pericarditis and allergy to nickel (component of the metal bar) have been reported occasionally (Nuss, 2008). Very few heart lesions and deaths were reported, mainly in cases of procedure done without thoracoscopy (Moss et al., 2001; Nuss, 2008). In case of Nuss bar infection, this can be managed successfully conservatively (Van Renterghem et al., 2005). Recurrence is reported in a range between 2% and 5% (Kelly et al., 2010; Lopushinsky & Fecteau, 2008). In our experience, in case of suboptimal result, one or more lipofilling treatments can improve significantly the final outcome but there are no published series yet. In females with breast asymmetry due to the sternal rotation, Nuss or open procedures alone can correct the breast aspect, but in case some degree of asymmetry persists, breast augmentation can be required, (Rapuzzi et al., 2010).

2.1.2 Pectus carinatum (PC)

PC is the second most frequent malformation. Its incidence is estimated to be 5 times less frequent than PE (Colombani, 2009; Fokin et al., 2009), with a strong male predominance. In some areas of the world, however, PC is almost equally or more frequent than PE (Acastello, 2006; Martinez-Ferro et al., 2008; Peña et al., 1981). The deformity is a protrusion of the sternum and chondrocostal joints (figure 2).

The etiology is unknown, but the pathogenetic mechanism could be the same than for PE, consisting in an overgrowth of the ribs (Haje et al., 1999). The same anomalies in the costal ribs than in PE have been reported in PC patients (Fokin et al., 2009). Familial cases are not uncommon (Fokin et al., 2009; Martinez-Ferro et al., 2008) and in some families it is possible to observe both PC and PE cases (Martinez-Ferro et al., 2008). Connective tissue disorders, Noonan syndrome and cardiac anomalies are seldom associated with PC (Kotzot &

Schwabegger, 2009). PC usually appears later in life than PE, mainly during pre-puberty or puberty, but in some cases it is possible to observe infants or children with this anomaly. PC has the tendency to increase rapidly during the growth spurt. The same symptoms than in PE can be observed, but more frequently some degree of thoracic pain than respiratory complaints (Colombani, 2009). Usually the cardiac and pulmonary function are less implicated than in PE (Fokin et al., 2009), but psychological effects of PC can be severe and they are the fundamental indication to the surgical correction.

2.1.2.1 Diagnostic assessment and classification

PC is classified according to the localization and symmetry into the following types (Colombani, 2009; Williams & Crabbe, 2003):

- Type 1, inferior or Chondrogladiolar (figure 2): It is the most frequent type. The sternal protrusion is located in the inferior or mid sternum. The last ribs can be slightly or severely depressed on lateral aspects. It is more often symmetric.
- Type 2, Superior or Chondromanubrial. In some reports it is called also Currarino-Silverman syndrome (Currarino & Silverman, 1958) or Pouter Pigeon Breast, but there is confusion in the literature regarding superior PC. Actually in our experience we have observed two different anomalies of superior PC that we have to differentiate. The most frequent is a sternal malformation characterized by a premature fusion and ossification of manubrio-sternal joint and the sternal segments, resulting in a high symmetric carinatum chest deformity with a short thick sternum with a depression in the lower third. (figure 2). This anomaly is sometimes described in the literature as Currarino Silverman syndrome or Pouter Pigeon Breast (Currarino & Silverman, 1958). The aspect is of a superior PC with an inferior PE. The sternum on a lateral view is S-shaped. Although this anomaly is included into the cartilagineous anomalies and called type II PC in Acastello classification (Acastello, 2006), we classified it as part of sternal anomalies because of the sternal origin of the anomaly (see table 1).

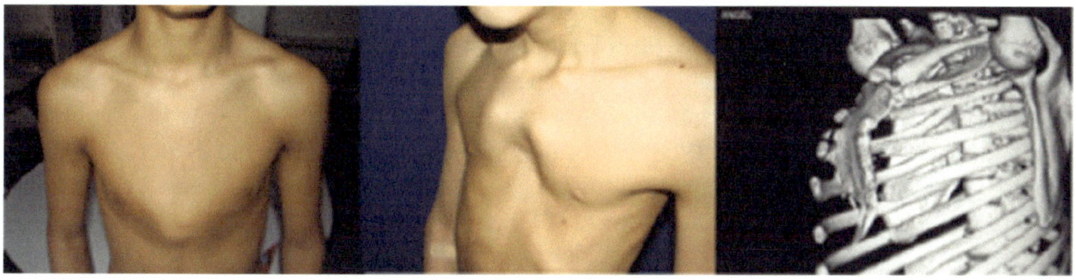

Fig. 2. Type I PC (left image); Type II PC or Currarino-Silverman syndrome (middle image). Lateral Computerized Tomography reconstruction shows S shape of the sternum (right image)

- The second anomaly we have observed in few cases is a superior PC without the typical features of Currarino-Silverman syndrome (figure 3). The sternum has a normal length and is not depressed in the lower third. This anomaly is probably due, similarly to inferior PC, to a cartilage anomaly. We propose to use the term superior PC only for the latter and to include this anomaly in the first category (cartilagineous anomalies) of CWMs classification. This entity is extremely rare in our experience and it has not been described hereto, to the best of our knowledge. The term of superior PC for the description of Currarino Silverman syndrome can be confusing and should be avoided.

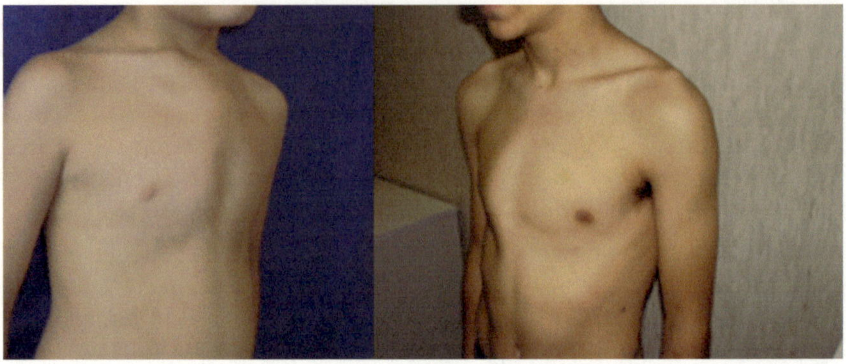

Fig. 3. Superior PC without features of Currarino-Silverman syndrome (left); Unilateral PC (right)

Other types of PC described are:

- Lateral or unilateral PC (Fokin et al., 2009): asymmetric by nature, it consists in a protrusion of some costal cartilages near chondro-sternal joint on one side (figure 3). The sternum can be rotated towards the opposite side.
- Reactive PC (Swanson & Colombani, 2008): this type of PC is a complication of a PE correction, in which in the first months or years after Nuss or open procedure the sternum progressively displaces ventrally. It is more frequent in patients with connective tissue disorders.

To best assess the gravity of PC and the degree of asymmetry, some radiological indexes have been proposed (Egan et al., 2000; Stephenson & Du Bois, 2008), measurable on CT scan, but in clinical practice they are less used than Haller index for PE. CT scan remains the gold standard radiologic evaluation for PC.

2.1.2.2 Treatment options

The standard correction has been performed through costal excision surgery, as for PE. Ravitch in 1952 (Ravitch, 1952) was one of the first who described the surgical technique for PC. While Lester in 1953 (Lester, 1953) proposed the resection of the lower third portion of the sternum, Howard (Howard, 1958) introduced the principle of sternal osteotomy, usually required to correct the defect. Osteotomy on the anterior sternal plate can be performed transversally or, in case of asymmetric PC, in an oblique fashion. Recently, some modifications to the Ravitch and Welch procedure were proposed (Del Frari & Schwabegger, 2011; Fonkalsrud & Anselmo, 2004), attempting to reduce the invasiveness of this approach, by reducing the extent of muscle and cartilage resection. The best treatment for PC type 2 and Currarino Silverman syndrome remains the open procedure (Brichon & Wihlm, 2010), while the following alternatives, minimally invasive or conservative techniques, have been recently proposed for type 1 PC, with good results:

- The *orthotic brace system*, proposed already in 1992 (Haje & Bowen, 1992) but popularized only recently by different groups approximately at the same time (Banever et al., 2006; Frey et al., 2006; Kravarusic et al., 2006; Rapuzzi et al., 2010, Swanson & Colombani, 2008), is based on the principle of reshaping the thorax during puberty due to thoracic malleability (as in Nuss procedure for PE) by applying a dynamic compression on it. Martinez-Ferro (Martinez-Ferro et al., 2008) added to this system the possibility to measure the pressure necessary to the correction and to regulate it (dynamic compression system, DCS). He observed good results in a large proportion of patients, if the brace is used for most of the time during day and night. A significant proportion of non compliant patients (13.8%) who abandoned the treatment, and some minor complications (hematomas, ulcerations, back pain) in 12.5%, were reported (Martinez-Ferro et al., 2008). Moreover, this approach cannot correct a rigid ossified thorax, so it can be applied only to adolescent patients.

- Intrathoracic compression procedure (Abramson's procedure) (Abramson, 2005): the concept is the same as the orthotic brace, but the system is placed surgically. Through two lateral incisions, a metallic bar is inserted in presternal space under the pectoralis muscles and fixed to lateral stabilizer in order to push back the sternum. It is like a reverse Nuss procedure and it is based again on the same principle of the thoracic malleability. As the previous approach, it has an age limit. It has the advantage of obtaining immediately the result without the need of wearing an external brace. In the Abramson experience, at 5 years the results were good; the bar was removed usually after two years or more (Abramson et al., 2009).
- Thoracoscopic cartilage resection (Kim & Idowu, 2009): described recently, it is performed by resecting under thoracoscopic view uni- or bilaterally, according to the type of defect, the anomalous costal cartilages, without damaging the internal thoracic vessels. It can be associated in severe cases with an intrathoracic compression procedure according to Abramson technique in order to stabilize better the sternum.
- Thoracoscopic complete cartilage resection with perichondrium preservation (CCRPP) (Varela & Torre, 2011): reported by our group, this procedure differences itself from the previous because cartilages are prepared both laterally and medially to the internal thoracic vessels, up to the chondrosternal joints. Internal thoracic vessels are coagulated and cartilages completely excised, leaving the anterior perichondrium intact.
- Mini-invasive submuscular dissection (Schaarschmidt et al., 2006): the pectoralis muscle dissection is performed by subpectoral CO_2 insufflation, the resection of the ribs, the sternal osteotomy and the insertion of trans-sternal steel struts are performed through a vertical pre-sternal incision under endoscopic view. Recently, the same Authors reported some technical variations (Schaarschmidt et al., 2011), abandoning the pre-sternal incision and performing a more extense submuscular dissection and two lateral incisions between the anterior and middle axillary lines. These should allow the creation of a submuscular and presternal tunnel in order to implant a Nuss metal bar presternally. Specific eight-hole stabilizers are though required.
- Minimal access treatment of PC (Hock, 2009): the bar is inserted as in Abramson procedure through two lateral incisions above the sternum, but it passes on both sides into the thoracic cavities; thoracoscopy was not used.

Reactive PC after Nuss procedure can be simply corrected with the withdrawal of the bar; in case of failure or in other cases an open procedure is advised; alternatively a mini-invasive technique can be attempted.

2.2 Type II: Costal anomalies

2.2.1 Dysmorphic cartilaginous type II CWMs (not syndromic)

This group is a spectrum of costal anomalies. Cartilages are malformed and the consequence can be a unilateral or bilateral depression in the thoracic wall. The treatment consists in a cartilage excision.

A rare malformation belonging to this group of malformation is the so called "intrathoracic rib" (figure 4), classified into different types (Kamano et al., 2006):

- *type Ia* is a supernumerary rib articulated with a vertebral body, type Ib is a bifid rib taking origin close to the vertebral body;
- *type II* a bifid rib arising more laterally;
- type III is a not bifid rib depressed into the thoracic cavity.

Flaring Chest consists into an hypertrophy or fusion of the cartilages in the lower costal margin. Open resection of all these malformed cartilages is an option treatment.
Cartilage rib asymmetries are quite frequently seen, they appear like isolated protrusion in the cartilage ribs. In the majority of cases the ribs are fused (figures 4).

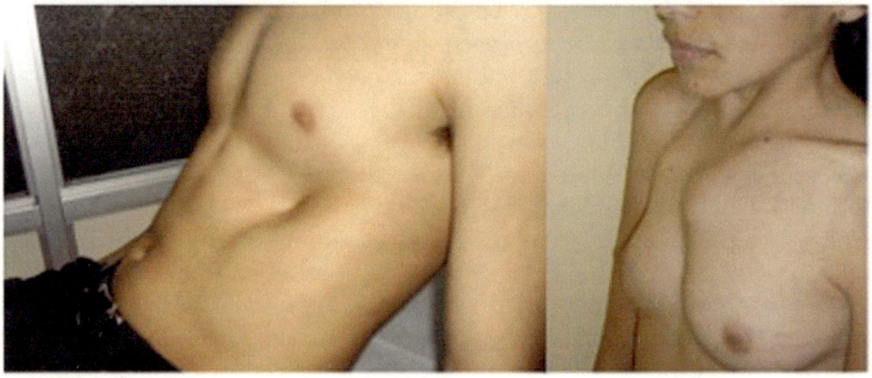

Fig. 4. *Left:* Dysmorphic anomaly of the ribs (type II of Acastello classification); *Right:* Dysmorphic and fused ribs

2.2.2 Syndromic type II anomalies

2.2.2.1 Jeune syndrome

Jeune Syndrome or asphyxiating thoracic dystrophy is an autosomal recessive disorder, originally described by Jeune in 1954 (Jeune et al., 1954) in a pair of siblings. The frequency of the condition is estimated 1/ 100.000 to 1/30.000 live births. Jeune syndrome is characterized by many bone abnormalities, the most pronounced being a long, narrow thorax with a reduced thoracic capacity causing the lungs to not have enough room to expand and grow. Both antero-posterior and lateral thoracic diameters are reduced, so respiratory distress may be severe. Prognosis is poor in patients who have respiratory symptoms during the first months of life, resulting in death during infancy.
All patients have small chests with short, wide and horizontal ribs (figure 5). There is variability in the severity of clinical and radiographic features, and two variants of Jeune syndrome exist:

- Severe variant: It represents the 70% of cases, and it usually is lethal during the infancy. The thorax is extremely small, conversely the abdomen seems prominent; respiratory failure is the rule.
- Mild variant: In 30% of cases ribs are less affected, respiratory symptoms are manageable and survival is prolonged. Renal or liver dysfunctions are present in some cases, and they can lead to death patients affected by this type of malformation.

Surgical repair techniques have typically involved median sternotomy (with graft interposition), resulting in poor outcomes (Philips & van Aalst, 2008). Lateral thoracic expansion, realized by rib incisions and suture in a staggered fashion (Davis et al., 1995), or more recently vertical expandable prosthetic titanium rib (VEPTR) (Waldhausen et al., 2007) are techniques proposed more recently that seem to offer some good results. The mild type of Jeune syndrome may not require any treatment.

2.2.2.2 Cerebrocostomandibular syndrome

Cerebrocostomandibular Syndrome is a rare entity. There is no clinical experience in the world. We have diagnosed one case in the last ten years, the main feature is a lack of development of the rib cage. There are only costal vestiges. There is flail chest and mechanical ventilation is required since birth. In some cases the thoracic cage agenesis is unilateral (figure 5). This defective costal development is also associated with features of the Pierre-Robin anomalad. Cerebral maldevelopment or malfunction is also common (Drossou-Agakidou et al., 1991).

2.2.2.3 Costal agenesis

Costal agenesis is limited to some ribs and is not syndromic. They are rare conditions. Lung herniation occurs. It may require thoracoplasty using the same technique used for PS.

2.2.3 Rare type II CWMs

There is a series of CWMs rarely observed, not included in a standard classification. As they differ each one from the other the treatment must be personalized.

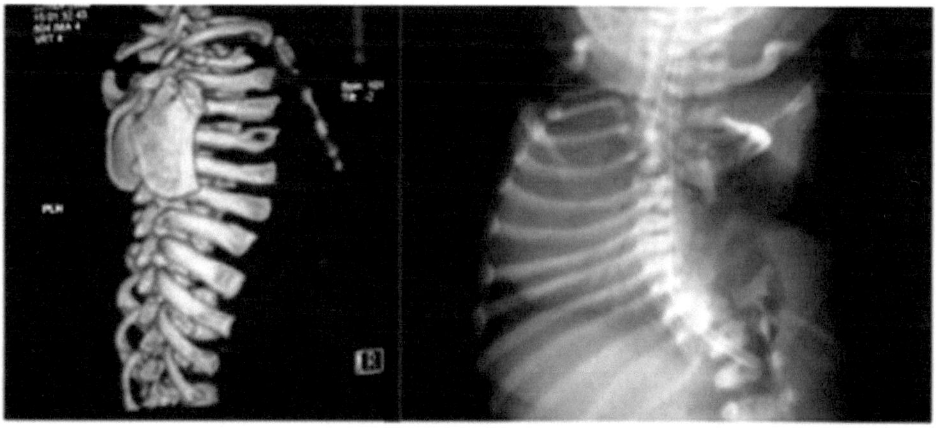

Fig. 5. *Left:* Jeune syndrome (Asphyxiating thoracic dystrophy), type severe. Computerized Tomography reconstruction of the rib cage shows the typical ribs of Jeune syndrome; *Right:* Cerebrocostomandibular syndrome. Unilateral agenesis of thoracic cage shown at thoracic X-Ray

2.3 Type III: Chondrocostal anomalies

2.3.1 Poland Syndrome (PS)

Occurring in approximately 1/30,000 live births (Freire-Maia et al., 1973), PS is characterized by the absence or hypoplasia of the pectoralis major muscle, frequently combined with other ipsilateral abnormalities of the chest wall, breast and upper limb (Kelly, 2008). The defect is essentially unilateral and in two thirds of cases right-sided. There is a male preponderance with a ratio of about 2/1 with females. Very rare bilateral cases have been described (Baban et al., 2009; Karnak et al., 1998). The etiology is unknown, but the most accredited hypothesis is the interruption of the vascular supply in subclavian and vertebral artery during embryonic life (Bavinck & Weaver, 1986), leading to different malformations in the corresponding districts. According to this, PS could be actually interpreted as a sequence.

Alternatevely, paradominant inheritance (Happle, 1999) or the presence of a lethal gene survival by mosaicism (van Steensel, 2004) have been proposed to explain the origin of this anomaly. PS is usually sporadic, but the occurrence of familial cases has raised the hypothesis of a possible transmission with an autosomal dominant pattern; however there is still no evidence of that. Association of PS with other anomalies, as Moebius (Parker et al., 1981), Klippel Feil syndromes and Sprengel anomaly (Bavinck & Weaver, 1986), has been reported.

PS phenotype is extremely variable (Alexander et al., 2002; Shamberger et al., 1989). The thoracic defect is usually evident at birth, but it can be undiagnosed until the child gets older. The pectoral muscle deficiency causes an asymmetric aspect but if there are costal anomalies associated the defect is more evident. In case of rib agenesis, particularly if multiple (the most affected ribs are the third and the forth), lung herniation and paradoxical respiratory movements are always present. Ribs can also be smaller or anomalous. Anomalies like a PE or PC or both can occur, but in less tan 10% of cases they require surgery. Breast region and nipple are frequently involved. A mild degree of breast hypoplasia to a complete absence of mammary gland are constant features. Associated cardiac and renal anomalies, as well as scoliosis, have been reported, but they are uncommon (Alexander et al., 2002). Dextroposition is reported frequently, always associated with left PS, and it seems to be caused by mechanical factors during embryonic life in patients with multiple left rib agenesis (Torre et al., 2010). Patients with PS are asymptomatic, and there are usually no limitations due to the muscle defects. Upper limb is frequently involved, from the classical symbrachydactily to split hand or other defects (Al-Qattan, 2001; Shamberger et al., 1989).

Thoracoplasty finds its main indication in cosmetic reason (Ravitch, 1966). Only rarely it is necessary a thoracoplasty in the infancy. There is no evidence of the utility of thoracoplasty for protection against thoracic traumatic injuries in children with rib agenesis. In case of surgical correction in pediatric age, some options are available, from costal transposition described again by Ravitch in 1966 (Ravitch, 1966), to the repair with absorbable or not absorbable prostheses (Moir & Johnson, 2008; Urschel, 2009). According to some Authors (Acastello, 2006), costal transposition and the consequent stabilization of the thorax could prevent the progression of thoracic deformity, but there is no consensus about this concept. Most Authors (Moir & Johnson, 2008; Urschel, 2009) prefer to wait until puberty and further, in order to correct in one or more times the thoracic flail chest and the pectoral defect. At this age, the most frequent issue in PS is breast and pectoral reconstruction in female patients. Correction with prostheses alone or in association with other surgical procedures (latissimus dorsi or rectal abdominal muscle transposition, lipofilling, or omental flap or other techniques) has been advocated (Urschel, 2009), but the surgical approach has to be tailored on the single case. In males the same techniques can be applied, but the indication to the surgical procedure has to be evaluated case by case, because the esthetical defect is less important. Martinez-Ferro described latissimus dorsi transposition flap using a minimally-invasive approach (Martinez-Ferro et al., 2007). Usually teams including pediatric or thoracic surgeons together with plastic surgeons can treat PS patients with the highest chance to get the best results.

2.4 Type IV: Sternal anomalies

2.4.1 Sternal cleft

A defect in the sternum's fusion process causes the sternal cleft, a rare idiopathic CWM. Acastello et al. found that sternal cleft (SC) accounted for 0.15% of all CWMs (Acastello et al., 2003). The Hoxb gene might be involved in the development of SC (Forzano et al., 2005).
Known from many centuries, these malformations have been classified in many different ways. To our knowledge the clearest classification has been proposed by Shamberger and Welch (Shamberger & Welch, 1990) and includes 4 types:

- Thoracic ectopia cordis: the heart is ectopic and not covered by skin. Usually the heart, in an anterior and kephalic ectopia, has intrinsic anomalies. The sternal defect can be superior, inferior, central (rare) or total. Abdominal wall defects as omphalocele can be associated. Thoracic cavity is hypoplasic, and for this reason the surgical correction is usually not able to save the life to these patients. Isolated survival after surgery has been reported (Dobell et al., 1982).
- Cervical ectopia cordis: much rarer than previous type, the heart is more cranial, sometimes with the apex fused with the mouth. Associated craniofacial anomalies are frequent. Prognosis is always negative.
- Thoraco-abdominal ectopia cordis: the heart is covered by a thin membranous or cutaneous layer. An inferior sternal defect is present. The heart, located into the thorax or into the abdomen, is not rotated as in previous types but intrinsic anomalies are common (Major, 1953). This kind of anomaly is generally found as part of a field defect known as the pentalogy of Cantrell (Cantrell, 1958). Prognosis after surgical repair can be good.
- Sternal cleft is the most common of this group of CWMs, and consists in a congenital malformation of the anterior thoracic wall, arising in a deficiency in the midline embryonic fusion of the sternal valves. The incidence is unknown, and it is more frequent in females (Acastello, 2006).

In sternal anomalies we have included also Currarino Silverman syndrome or Pouter Pigeon Breast, as already described above.
Sternal clefts are classified as being partial (figure 6) or complete (figure 6). The partial deformity can be superiorly or inferiorly located. The rarer inferior variety is often associated with a thoraco-abdominal ectopia cordis, while upper partial cleft (the most common variant) can be an isolated abnormality. The sternal clavicular joints are displaced laterally, but the clavicles have a normal length. There is a bulging of thoracic viscera in the midline across the defect, more evident during forced expiration. The complete form is much less frequent. There is a total lack of fusion; it produces an even bigger paradoxical movement than partial cleft and sometimes respiratory distress.
According to a recent review of the literature, SC is frequently associated with other defects (82%) (Torre et al., 2011). These must be carefully looked for before any surgical procedure, since they can lead to major complications. Some of them are evident on physical examination such as maxillofacial hemangiomas (Fokin, 2000), cleft lip or cleft palate, pectus excavatum, connectival nevi (Torre et al., 2011), supraumbilical raphe, or gastroschisis. Other defects must be ruled out, such as cardiac defects, aortic coarctation, eye abnormalities, posterior fossa anomalies, and hidden haemangiomas.

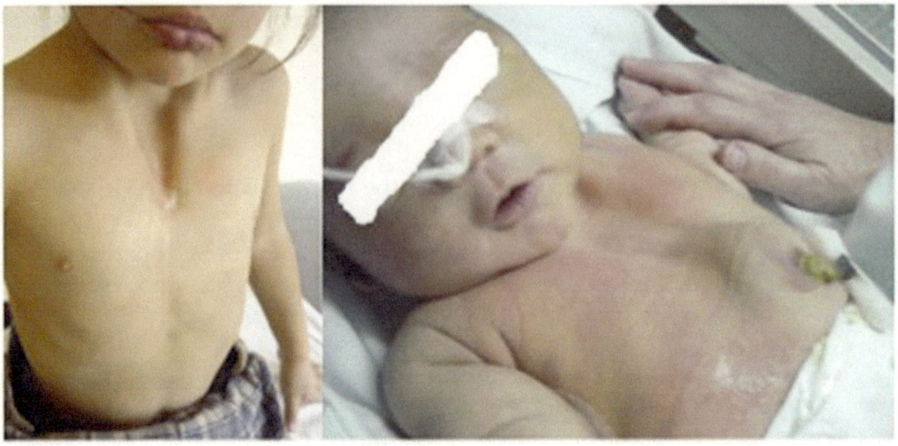

Fig. 6. Partial sternal cleft in a 4-year-old patient not operated at birth; Total sternal cleft in a newborn (right)also part of clinical conditions like PHACES syndrome (Metry et al., 2009), sternal malformation/vascular dysplasia, midline fusion defects, or Cantrell's pentalogy.

There is consensus that ideally correction of sternal clefts should take place during the neonatal period or in the first months of life (Acastello, 2006; Domini et al., 2000; Torre et al., 2008), to re-establish the bony protection of the mediastinum, prevent paradoxical visceral movement with respiration, eliminate the visible deformity and allow the normal growth of thoracic cage. The reason for preferring an early surgical approach is that primary closure is easier and there is no need of a big procedure, maybe necessary at older ages. In fact, after the first few years of life, primary closure requires sterno-clavicular disarticulation, sternal isolation, inferior sternal osteotomy and medialization of the neck muscles after separation of their sternoclavicular attachments laterally (Acastello et al., 2003). As it can bring the risk of a circulatory impairment due to cardiovascular compression, in some cases primary sternal suture can be impossible and prosthetic or autologous closure (De Campos et al., 1998) can be preferable because less invasive. Partial thymectomy can be useful to reduce the pressure on thoracic vessels (Torre et al., 2008). Many prosthetic materials have been described for sternal cleft repair (Domini et al., 2000). In our experience we have closed an upper cleft in one 8 year old female with an artificial bone tissue with an excellent outcome. Complications are not frequent, but PE can occur later in life in patients operated for sternal cleft. In case of prosthetic repair, there is an increased risk of infections and recurrence.

2.5 Type V: Clavicle-scapular anomalies

These anomalies usually are field of interest of orthopedic surgeons more than pediatric surgeons. We do not have experience of this type of CWMs.

2.6 Other anomalies

2.6.1 Post operative surgical deformities

This category includes cases in which thoracic deformity is due to the correction of a previous CWMs. We have experience of few cases of this kind of anomaly (figure 7). They were due to early multiple cartilage resections during an open correction of a PE and finally resulted, after many years, in a thoracic deformity that required an open revision procedure. As discussed above, the optimal age for pectus repair is controversial (Lopushinsky &

Fecteau, 2008; Nuss, 2008). Repair in early childhood is easier but cases of restrictive growth patterns of the chest wall have been reported. Jeune syndrome or acquired asphyxiating thoracic dystrophy is associated with open repair in children less than 4 years with extensive resection of five or more ribs (Haller et al., 1996) and damage to the cartilage growth centers (Robicsek et al., 2009). These children present with an extremely narrow chest. For these reasons most Authors postpone open surgical repair after 10 years of age (Lopushinsky & Fecteau, 2008; Nuss, 2008).

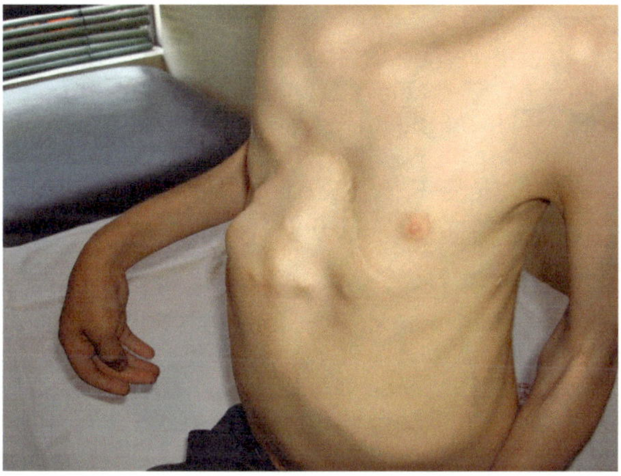

Fig. 7. Post surgical deformity in a 6-year-old boy operated of PE when he was one year old

3. Conclusions

CWMs are a large spectrum of anomalies. Etiology and genetic implication of CWMs are still largely unknown. Precise identification of the single malformation, its classification and an accurate diagnostic assessment, are the first fundamental steps in the modern approach. We have adopted the modified classification of Acastello, based on the origin of the anomaly. Identification of familial cases, possible associated syndromes and anomalies, clinical symptoms and psychological implications have to be considered. Among the therapeutic armamentarium, nowadays classical techniques and new approaches make us able to choose the more appropriate for the single patient, according to the surgeon's experience and preference but in particular tailoring the treatment on the individual clinical and psychological needs. A multidisciplinary approach is advisable in order to manage CWMs in all their complexity.

4. References

Abramson H. (2005) A minimally invasive technique to repair pectus carinatum. Preliminary report. *Arch Bronconeumol*, Vol. 41, No. 6, pp. 349-351

Abramson H, D'Agostino J & Wuscovi S. (2009) A 5-year experience with a minimally invasive technique for pectus carinatum repair. *J Pediatr Surg*, Vol. 44, No. 1, pp. 118-124.

Acastello E, Majluf F, Garrido P, Barbosa LM & Peredo A. (2003) Sternal cleft: a surgical opportunity. *J Pediatr Surg* Vol. 38, No. 2, pp. 178-183.

Acastello E. (2006) *Patologias de la pared toracica en pediatria.* Editorial El Ateneo, Buenos Aires

Adkins PC & Blades BA. (1961) Stainless steel strut for correction of pectus excavatum. *Surg Gynecol Obstet,* Vol. 113, pp. 111-113.

Alexander A, Fokin MD & Robicsek F. (2002) Poland's syndrome revisited. *Ann Thorac Surg,* Vol. 74, No. 6, pp. 2218-2225

Al-Qattan MM. (2001) Classification of hand anomalies in Poland's syndrome. *Br J Plast Surg,* Vol. 54, No. 2, pp. 132-136

Aronson DC, Bosgraaf RP, van der Horst C & Ekkelkamp S. (2007) Nuss procedure: pediatric surgical solution for adults with pectus excavatum. World J Surg, Vol. 31, No. 1, pp. 26-29.

Baban A, Torre M, Bianca S, Buluggiu A, Rossello MI, Calevo MG, Valle M, Ravazzolo R, Jasonni V & Lerone M. (2009) Poland syndrome with bilateral features: case description with review of the literature. *Am J Med Genet* Vol. 149A, No. 7, pp. 1597-1602.

Banever GT, Konefal SH, Gettens K & Moriarty KP. (2006) Nonoperative correction of pectus carinatum with orthotic bracing. *J Laparoendosc Adv Surg Tech,* Vol.16, No. 2, pp. 164-167.

Bavinck JNB & Weaver DD. (1986) Subclavian artery supply disruption sequence: hypothesis of a vascular etiology for Poland, Klippel-Feil and Mobius anomalies. *Am J Med Genet* 1986, Vol. 23, No. 4, pp.. 903-918.

Brichon PY & Wihlm JM. (2010) Correction of a severe pouter pigeon breast by triple sternal osteotomy with a novel titanium rib bridge fixation. *Ann Thorac Surg,* Vol. 90, No. 6, pp. e97-9

Brown AL. (1939) Pectus excavatum (funnel chest): anatomic basis; surgical treatment of the inicipient stage in infancy; and correction of the deformity in the fully developed stage. *J Thorac Surg,* Vol. 9, pp. 164-184.

Cantrell JR, Haller JA & Ravitch MM. (1958) A syndrome of congenital defects involving the abdominal wall, sternum, diaphragm, pericardium, and heart. *Surg Gynecol Obstet,*Vol. 107, No.5, pp. 602-614.

Colombani P. (2009) Preoperative assessment of chest wall deformities. *Semin Thorac Cardiovasc Surg,* Vol. 21, No.1, 58-63.

Creswick HA, Stacey MW, Kelly RE, Gustin T, Nuss D, Harvey H, Goretsky MJ, Vasser E, Welch JC, Mitchell K & Proud VK. (2006) Family study on the inheritance of pectus excavatum. *J Pediatr Surg,* Vol. 41, No. 10, pp.1699-1703.

Currarino G & Silverman FN. (1958) Premature obliteration of the sternal sutures and pigeon-breast deformity. *Radiology,* Vol. 70, No.4, pp.532-540.

Davis JT, Ruberg RL, Leppink DM, Mc Coy KS & Wright CC. (1995) Lateral thoracic expansion for Jeune's asphyxiating dystrophy: a new approach. *Ann Thorac Surg,* Vol. 60, No.3, pp. 694-696.

De Campos JR, Filomeno LT, Fernandez A, Ruiz RL, Minamoto H, Werebe Ede C & Jatene FB. (1998) Repair of congenital sternal cleft in infants and adolescents. *Ann Thorac Surg,* Vol. 66, No.4, pp.1151-1154.

Del Frari B & Schwabegger AH. (2011) Ten-year experience with the muscle split technique, bioabsorbable plates, and postoperative bracing for correction of pectus carinatum: The Innsbruck protocol. *J Thorac Cardiovasc Surg,* Vol. 141, No. 6, pp. 1403-9

Dobell AR, Williams HB & Long RW. (1982) Staged repair of ectopia cordis. *J Pediatr Surg,* Vol. 17, No. 4, pp. 353-358.

Domini M, Cupaioli M, Rossi F, Fakhro A, Aquino A & Lelli Chiesa PL. (2000) Bifid sternum: neonatal surgical treatment. *Ann Thorac Surg,* Vol. 69, No. 1, pp. 267-269.

Donnelly LF, Frush DP, Foss JN, O'Hara SM & Bisset GS. (1999) Anterior chest wall: frequency of anatomic variations in children. *Radiology*, Vol. 212, No. 3, pp. 837-840.

Dorner RA, Keil PG & Schissel DJ. (1950) Pectus excavatum. *J Thorac Surg*, Vol. 20, No.3, pp. 444-53

Drossou-Agakidou V, Andreou A, Soubassi-Griva V & Pandouraki M. (1991) Cerebrocostomandibular syndrome in four sibs, two pairs of twins. *J Med Genet*. Vol. 28, No. 10, pp. 704-7.

Egan JC, Du Bois JJ, Morphy M, Samples TL & Lindell B. (2000) Compressive orthotics in the treatment of asymmetric pectus carinatum: a preliminary report with an objective radiographic marker. J Pediatr Surg Vol. 35, No. 8, pp. 1183-1186.

Feng J, Hu T, Liu SW, Zhang S, Tang Y, Chen R, Jiang X & Wei F. (2001) The biochemical, morphologic, and histochemical properties of the costal cartilages in children with pectus excavatum. *J Pediatr Surg*, Vol. 36, No. 12, pp. 1770-1776.

Fokin AA. (2000) Cleft sternum and sternal foramen.. *Chest Surg Clin N Am*, Vol. 10, No. 2, pp. 261-276.

Fokin AA, Steuerwald NM, Ahrens WA & Allen KE. (2009) Anatomical, histologic and genetic characteristics of congenital chest wall deformities. *Semin Thorac Cardiovasc Surg*, Vol. 21, No. 1, pp. 44-57.

Fonkalsrud EW & Anselmo DM. (2004) Less extensive techniques for repair of pectus carinatum: the undertreated chest deformity. *J Am Coll Surg*, Vol. 198, No. 6, pp. 898-905.

Forzano F, Daubeney PE & White SM. (2005) Midline raphe, sternal cleft, and other midline abnormalities: a new dominant syndrome? *Am J Med Genet A*, Vol. 135, No. 1, pp. 9-12.

Freire-Maia N, Chautard EA, Opitz JM, Freire Maia A & Quelce-Salgado A.(1973) The Poland syndrome - clinical, and genealogical data, dermatoglyphic analysis, and incidence. *Hum Hered*, Vol. 23, No. 2, pp. 97-104.

Frey AS, Garcia VF, Brown RL, Inge TH, Ryckman FC, Cohen AP, Durrett G & Azizkhan RG. (2006) Nonoperative management of pectus carinatum. *J Pediatr Surg*, Vol. 41, No. 1, pp. 40-45.

Frick SL. (2000) Scoliosis in children with anterior chest wall deformities. *Chest Surg Clin N Am*, Vol. 10, No. 2, pp. 427-436.

Grappolini S, Fanzio PM, D'Addetta PGC, Todde A & Infante M. (2008) Aesthetic treatment of pectus excavatum: a new endoscopic technique using a porous polyethylene implant. *Aesth Plast Surg*, Vol. 32, No. 1, pp. 105-110.

Haje SA & Bowen JR. (1992) Preliminary results of orthotic treatment of pectus deformities in children and adolescents *J Pediatr Orthop*, Vol. 12, No. 6, pp. 795-800.

Haje SA, Harcke HT & Bowen JR. (1999) Growth disturbance of the sternum and pectus deformities: imaging studies and clinical correlation. *Pediatr Radiol*, Vol. 29, No. 5, pp. 334-341.

Haller JA, Kramer SS & Lietman SA. (1987) Use of CT scans in selection of patients for pectus excavatum surgery: a preliminary report. *J Pediatr Surg*, Vol. 22, No. 10, pp. 904-906.

Haller JA, Colombani PM, Humphries CT, Azizkhan RG & Loughlin GM. (1996) Chest wall constriction after too extensive and too early operations for pectus excavatum. *Ann Thorac Surg*, Vol. 61, No. 6, pp. 1618-1624.

Happle R. (1999) Poland anomaly may be explained as a paradominant trait. *Am J Med Genet*, Vol. 87, No. 4, pp. 364-365.

Harrison MR, Estefan-Ventura D & Fechter R. (2007) Magnetic mini-mover procedure for pectus excavatum: development, design and simulations for feasibility and safety. *J Pediatr Surg*, Vol. 41, No. 1, pp. 81-86.

Hock A. (2009) Minimal access treatment of pectus carinatum: a preliminary report. *Pediatr Surg Int*, Vol. 25, No. 4, pp. 337-342.

Howard R. (1958) Pigeon chest (protrusion deformity of the sternum) *Med J Aust*, Vol. 45, No. 20, pp. 664-666.

Jeune M, Carron R, Beraud C & Loaec Y. (1954) Polychondrodystrophie avec blocage thoracique d'évolution fatale. *Pediatrie*, Vol. 9, No. 4, pp. 390-392.

Kamano H, Ishihama T, Ishihama H, Kubota Y, Tanaka T & Satoh K. (2006) Bifid intrathoracic rib: a case report and classification of intrathoracic ribs. *Intern Med*, Vol. 45, No. 9, pp. 627-630.

Karnak I, Tanyel FC, Tunçbilek E, Unsal M & Büyükpamukçu N. (1998) Bilateral Poland anomaly. *Am J Med Genet* , Vol. 75, No. 5, pp. 505-507.

Kelly RE, Lawson ML, Paidas CN & Hruban RH. (2005) Pectus excavatum in a 112-year autopsy series: anatomic findings and effect on survival. *J Pediatr Surg*, Vol. 40, No. 8, pp. 1275-1278.

Kelly RE, Shamberger RC, Mellins R, Mitchell KK, Lawson ML, Oldham K, Azizkhan RG, Hebra AV, Nuss D, Goretsky MJ, Sharp RJ, Holcomb GW 3rd, Shim WK, Megison SM, Moss RL, Fecteau AH, Colombani PM, Bagley TC & Moskowitz AB. (2007) Prospective multicenter study of surgical correction of pectus excavatum: design, perioperative complications, pain, and baseline pulmonary function facilitated by internet-based data collection. *J Am Coll Surg*, Vol. 205, No. 2, pp. 205-216.

Kelly RE. (2008) Pectus excavatum: historical background, clinical picture, preoperative evaluation and criteria for operation. *Semin Pediatr Surg*, Vol. 17, No. 3, pp. 181-193.

Kelly RE, Goretsky MJ, Obermeyer R, Kuhn MA, Redlinger R, Haney TS, Moskowitz A & Nuss D. (2010) Twenty-one years of experience with minimally invasive repair of pectus excavatum by the Nuss procedure in 1215 patients. *Ann Surg*, Vol. 252, No. 6, pp. 1072-81.

Kim S & Idowu O. (2009) Minimally invasive thoracoscopic repair of unilateral pectus carinatum. *J Pediatr Surg* Vol. 44, No. 2, pp. 471-474.

Kotzot D & Schwabegger AH. (2009) Etiology of chest wall deformities - genetic review for the treating physician. *J Pediatr Surg*, Vol. 44, No. 10, pp. 2004-2011.

Kravarusic D, Dicken BJ, Dewar R, Harder J, Poncet P, Schneider M & Sigalet DL. (2006) The Calgary protocol for bracing of pectus carinatum: a preliminary report. *J Pediatr Surg*, Vol. 41, No. 5, pp. 923-926.

Lester CW. (1953) Pigeon breast (pectus carinatum) and other protrusion deformities of the chest of developmental origin. *Ann Surg*, Vol. 137, No. 4, pp. 482-489.

Lopushinsky SR & Fecteau AH. (2008) Pectus deformities: A review of open surgery in the modern era. *Semin Pediatr Surg*, Vol. 17, No. 3, pp. 201-208.

Major JW. (1953) Thoracoabdominal ectopia cordis: report of a case successfully treated by surgery. *J Thorac Surg* Vol. 26, No. 3, pp. 309-317.

Martinez-Ferro M, Fraire C, Saldaña L, Reussmann A & Dogliotti P. (2007) Complete videoendoscopic harvest and transposition of latissimus dorsi muscle for the treatment of Poland syndrome: a first report. *J Laparoendosc Adv Surg Tech*, Vol. 17, No. 1, pp. 108-113.

Martinez-Ferro M, Fraire C & Bernard S. (2008) Dynamic compression system for the correction of pectus carinatum. *Semin Pediatr Surg*, Vol. 17, No. 3, pp. 194-200.

Metry D, Heyer G, Hess C, Garzon M, Haggstrom A, Frommelt P, Adams D, Siegel D, Hall K, Powell J, Frieden I & Drolet B. (2009) Consensus statement on diagnostic criteria for PHACE syndrome. *Pediatrics*, Vol. 124, No. 5, pp. 1447-1456.

Meyer L. (1922) Fur chirurgischen bedhandlung der angeborenen trichter-brust. *Klin Vochenschr*, Vol. 1, pp. 647.

Moir CR & Johnson CH. (2008) Poland's syndrome. *Semin Pediatr Surg*, Vol. 17, No. 3, pp. 161-166.

Moss L, Albanese C & Reynolds M. (2001) Major complications after minimally invasive repair of pectus excavatum: case reports. *J Pediatr Surg*, Vol. 36, No. 1, pp. 155-158.

Nuss D, Kelly RE, Croitoru DP & Katz ME. (1998) A 10 year review of a minimally invasive technique for the correction of pectus excavatum. *J Pediatr Surg*, Vol. 33, No. 4, pp. 545-552.

Nuss D. (2008) Minimally invasive surgical repair of pectus excavatum. *Semin Pediatr Surg*, Vol. 17, No. 3, pp. 209-217.

Park HJ, Lee SY & Lee CS. (2004) Complications associated with the Nuss procedure: analysis of risk factors and suggested measures of prevention of complications. *J Pediatr Surg*, Vol. 39, No. 3, pp. 391-395.

Parker DL, Mitchell PR. & Holmes GL. (1981) Poland-Moebius syndrome. *J Med Genet*, Vol. 18, No. 4, pp. 317-320.

Peña A, Perez L, Nurko S & Dorenbaum D. (1981) Pectus carinatum and pectus excavatum: Are they the same disease? *Am Surg*, Vol. 47, No. 5, pp. 215-218.

Philips JD & van Aalst JA. (2008) Jeune's syndrome (asphyxiating thoracic dystrophy): congenital and acquired. *Semin Pediatr Surg*, Vol. 17, No. 3, pp. 167-172.

Poland A. (1841) Deficiency of the pectoralis muscles. *Guys Hosp Rep*, Vol. 6, pp. 191.

Prabhakaran K, Paidas C, Haller JA, Pegoli W & Colombani PM. (2001) Management of a floating sternum after repair of pectus excavatum. *J Pediatr Surg*, Vol. 36, No. 1, pp. 159-164.

Rapuzzi G, Torre M, Romanini MV, Viacava R, Disma N, Santi PL & Jasonni V. (2010) The Nuss procedure after breast augmentation for female pectus excavatum. *Aesthetic Plast Surg*, Vol. 34, No. 3, pp. 397-400.

Ravitch MM. (1949) The operative treatment of pectus excavatum. *Ann Surg*, Vol. 129, No. 4, pp. 429-444.

Ravitch MM. (1952) Unusual sternal deformity with cardiac symptoms operative correction. *J Thorac Surg*, Vol. 23, No. 2, pp. 138-144.

Ravitch MM. (1966) Atyipical deformities of the chest wall - absence and deformities of the ribs and costal cartilages. *Surgery*, Vol. 59, No. 3, pp. 438-449.

Robicsek F, Watts LT & Fokin AA. (2009) Surgical repair of pectus excavatum and carinatum. *Semin Thorac Cardiovasc Surg*, Vol. 21, No. 1, pp. 64-75.

Sauerbruch F. (1931) Operative beseitigung der angeborenen trichterbrust. *Deutsche Zeitschr Chir*, Vol. 234, pp. 760.

Schaarschmidt K, Kolberg-Schwerdt AK, Lempe M & Schlesinger F. (2006) New endoscopic minimal access pectus carinatum repair using subpectoral carbon dioxide. *Ann Thorac Surg*, Vol. 81, No. 3, pp. 1099-1104.

Schaarschmidt K, Lempe-Sellin M, Schlesinger F, Jaeschke U & Polleichtner S. (2011) New Berlin-Buch "reversed Nuss," endoscopic pectus carinatum repair using eight-hole stabilizers, submuscular CO2, and presternal Nuss bar compression: first results in 35 patients. *J Laparoendosc Adv Surg Tech A*, Vol. 21, No. 3, pp. 283-6.

Schier F, Bahr M & Klobe E. (2005) The vacuum chest wall lifter; an innovative, nonsurgical addition to the management of pectus excavatum. *J Pediatr Surg*, Vol. 40, No. 3, pp. 496-500.

Shamberger RC, Welch KJ & Upton J III. (1989) Surgical treatment of thoracic deformity in Poland's syndrome. *J Pediatr Surg*, Vol. 24, No. 8, pp. 760-765.

Shamberger R & Welch K. (1990) Sternal defects. Pediatr Surg Int Vol. 5, pp. 156-164.

Stanford W, Bowers DG, Lindberg EF, Armstrong RG, Finger ER & Dibbel DG. (1972) Silastic implants for correction of pectus excavatum. A new technique. *Ann Thorac Surg*, Vol. 13, No. 6, pp. 529-536.

Stephenson JT & Du Bois J. (2008) Compressive orthotic brace in the treatment of pectus carinatum: the use of radiographic markers to predict success. *J Pediatr Surg*, Vol. 43, No. 10, pp. 1776-1780.

Swanson JW & Colombani PM. (2008) Reactive pectus carinatum in patients treated for pectus excavatum. *J Pediatr Surg*, Vol. 43, No. 8, pp. 1468-1473.

Torre M, Rapuzzi G, Guida E, Costanzo S & Jasonni V. (2008) Thymectomy to achieve primary closure of total sternal cleft. *J Pediatr Surg*, Vol. 43, No. 12, pp. e17-20.

Torre M, Baban A, Buluggiu A, Costanzo S, Bricco L, Lerone M, Bianca S, Gatti GL, Sénès FM, Valle M & Calevo MG. (2010) Dextrocardia in patients with Poland syndrome: Phenotypic characterization provides insight into the pathogenesis. *J Thorac Cardiovasc Surg*, Vol. 139, No. 5, pp. 1177-1182.

Torre M, Rapuzzi G, Carlucci M, Pio L & Jasonni V. (2011) Phenotypic spectrum and management of sternal cleft: literature review and presentation of a new series. *Eur J Cardiothorac Surg*. 2011 Jul 5. [Epub ahead of print]

Urschel HC. (2009) Poland syndrome. *Semin Thorac Cardiovasc Surg*, Vol. 21, No. 1, pp. 89-94.

Van Renterghem KM, von Bismarck S, Bax NM, Fleer A & Höllwarth ME. (2005) Should an infected Nuss bar be removed? *J Pediatr Surg*, Vol. 40, No. 4, pp. 670-673.

van Steensel MA. (2004) Poland anomaly: Not unilateral or bilateral but mosaic. *Am J Med Genet*, Vol. 125A, No. 2, pp. 211-212.

Varela P & Torre M. (2011) Thoracoscopic cartilage resection with partial perichondrium preservation in unilateral pectus carinatum: preliminary results. *J Pediatr Surg*, Vol. 46, No. 1, pp. 263-6.

Wada J, Ikeda K, Ishida T & Hasegawa T. (1970) Results of 271 funnel chest operations. *Ann Thorac Surg*, Vol. 10, No. 6, pp. 526-532.

Waldhausen JH, Redding GJ & Song KM. (2007) Vertical expandable prosthetic titanium rib for thoracic insufficiency syndrome: a new method to treat an old problem. *J Pediatr Surg*, Vol. 42, No. 1, pp. 76-80.

Waters P, Welch K, Micheli LJ, Shamberger R & Hall JE. (1989) Scoliosis in children with pectus excavatum and pectus carinatum. *J Pediatr Orthop*, Vol. 9, No. 5, pp. 551-556.

Welch KJ. (1958) Satisfactory surgical correction of pectus excavatum deformity in childhood. *J Thorac Surg*, Vol. 36, No. 5, pp. 697-713.

Williams AM & Crabbe DC. (2003) Pectus deformities of the anterior chest wall. *Pediatr Respir Rev*, Vol. 4, No. 3, pp. 237-242.

9

Pectus Excavatum: A Historical Perspective and a New Metal-Free Procedure

Akira Masaoka and Satoshi Kondo
Department of Oncology, Immunology and Surgery,
Nagoya City University Graduate School of Medical Sciences,
Japan

1. Introduction

1.1 Epidemiology and etiology/pathogenesis

Pectus excavatum (PE) is a most frequent deformity at the anterior chest wall. Its incidence is about 1:400 in live births. Male to female ratio is 4:1. Various theories have been proposed to explain pathogenesis of PE.

Brown (Brown, 1939) described that the force producing the depression is diaphragm acting primarily in the anteroposterior direction through its attachment to the sternum. He pointed out a membranous structure beneath the sternum, and denominated it substernal ligament.

On the other hand, Sweet (Sweet, 1944) thought that the substernal ligament is not important structure, and stated "it seems almost as though the sternum is pushed down against spine by unusually long, inward curving costal cartilages".

This idea evoked sympathy of many surgeons, and the overgrowth of cartilages theory for PE became the leading theory, because of significance of theoretical background for the surgeon's act to resect the overgrown cartilages.

However, recently, Nakaoka and colleagues (Nakaoka et al., 2009, 2010) measured the length of the 5th and 6th costal cartilages and ribs in PE patients from reconstructed images of 3-dimensional computed tomography (CT). He calculated the C/R ratio, defined as the quotient of the costal cartilage length divided by the adjacent rib length, and compared it between the PE patients and the healthy controls. As the result, he found that the C/R ratio in the PE patients were not longer than that in the healthy controls at any level, so concluded that the overgrowth of costal cartilages is not the pathogenesis of PE.

PE patients often show characteristic figure, such as lanky shape, and thin thorax, and associate sometimes Marfan syndrome or Noonan syndrome. These findings suggest hereditary origin of PE.

Creswick and colleagues (Creswick et al., 2006) analysed 34 families and assumed autosomal dominant inheritance in 14 families, autosomal recessive inheritance in 4 families, and X-chromosomal inheritance in 6 families. However, many family members had additional connective tissue traits, that is, systemic connective tissue diseases can not be ruled out.

Marfan syndrome occurs in 1:5,000 to 10,000 of population. It is genetic disease, which is caused by mutation in the Fibrillin 1 gene localized on the long arm of chromosome 15.

On the other hand, Noonan syndrome is a common autosomal dominantly inherited disorder caused by mutations in various genes (PTPN 11, KRAS, SOS1, RAF1). Incidence is 1:1,000 to 2,500 (Kotzot & Schwabegger, 2009).
However, causative genes of isolated (non syndromic) PE are not yet determined. PE can be an isolated malformation or dysmorphic feature or only one symptom of a genetic syndrome. The research of responsible gene relating with PE is yet on the start line.

1.2 Symptomatology

PE is a deformity of the thorax characterized by depression of the sternum. The cephalic border of the depression situates usually at the conjunction of manubrium and sternal body. The sternal body leans sharply to the depth, deepest just before its junction with the xiphoid. The lower costal cartilages bend inward to form depression.
In infant, a paradoxical inward motion of the lower sternum is conspicuous on inspiration. PE becomes fixed at child age (2~3 years). Eguchi and colleagues (Eguchi et al., 1993) observed natural course of the PE deformity in 25 patients (average 2.5 years). Mean period of observation was 3.2 years. Ten patients (40%) progressed, 14 (56%) did not change, and one (4%) patient improved. In the progressed patients, 5 patients showed asymmetrical progression. These results suggest some clinical implications, i.e., 1) decision of operative indication should be delayed until schoolchild age at least, 2) asymmetry starts already at child age.
Usually, deformity is going to progress together with growth. At puberty, growth of the thorax spurts. The characteristic of progression in this term is reinforce of asymmetry, characterizing deeper depression at right side and torsion of the sternum. Such asymmetric deformity is considered to be resulted from existence of heart in left side.
PE deformity is not common in all patients. There are some types with typical different features. Nuss (Nuss, 2008) expressed as cup shape, saucer shape and Grand Canyon shape. Cup shape means a localized, narrow depression (Fig. 1). Saucer shape is a wide and flat depression (Fig. 2). Grand Canyon shape means asymmetric type with deepest at right side (Fig. 3). Moreover, each patient shows different grade. In order to express objectively the characteristic of each patient, various deformity indices of PE have been proposed.
Introduction of computerized tomography (CT) enhanced such trend. Haller and colleagues (Haller et al., 1987) set transverse diameter/anterior-posterior diameter as an index. The anterior-posterior diameter means a distance between sternum and spine at the deepest depression level. He stated that this index was 4.42±0.76 in PE patients and 2.56±0.35 in normal subjects, and useful in judgment of operative indication.

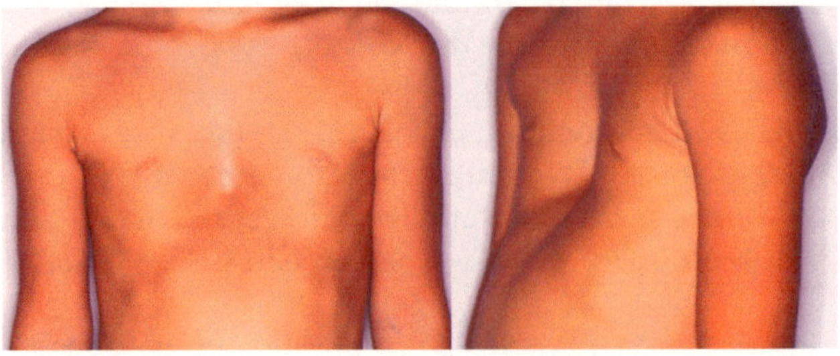

Fig. 1. Cup shape depression

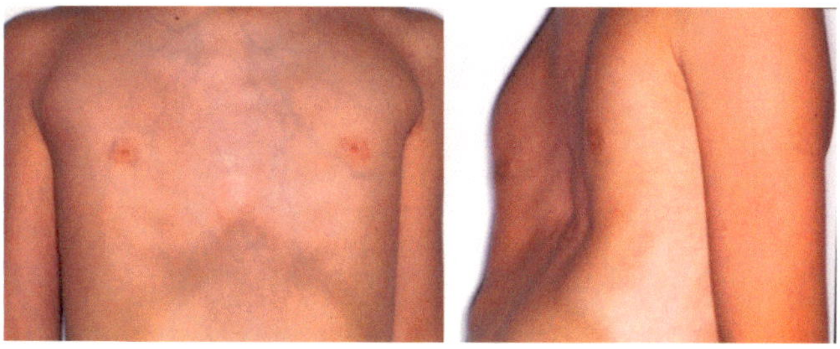

Fig. 2. Saucer shape depression

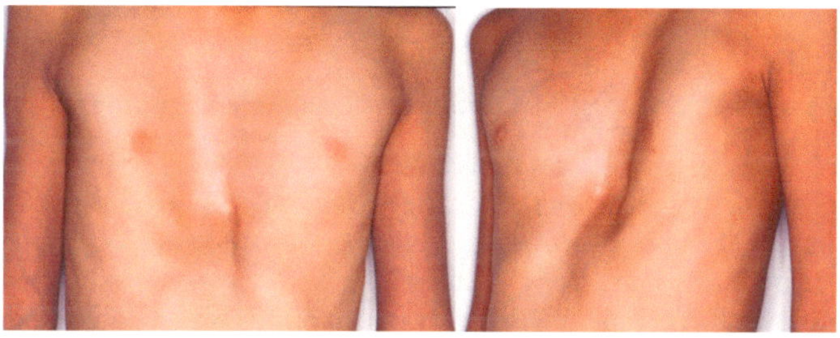

Fig. 3. Grand Canyon shape depression

Nakahara and colleagues (Nakahara et al., 1987) set 3 indices; degree of depression, degree of asymmetry, and degree of flatness (Fig. 4). These indices serve to define the diagnosis, to decide operative indication, and evaluate the effects of operation.

Masaoka and colleagues (Masaoka et al., 2011) proposed 3 other indices; steepness index, excavation volume index, and asymmetry index. These are defined as shown in Fig. 5. This system has properties described below.

1. Three indices express the morphological characteristic in PE straight, respectively. Steepness index represents cup shape, excavation volume index saucer shape, and asymmetry index Grand Canyon shape configuration.
2. Excavation volume index and asymmetry index are defined two-dimensionally, in order to quantify more exactly.

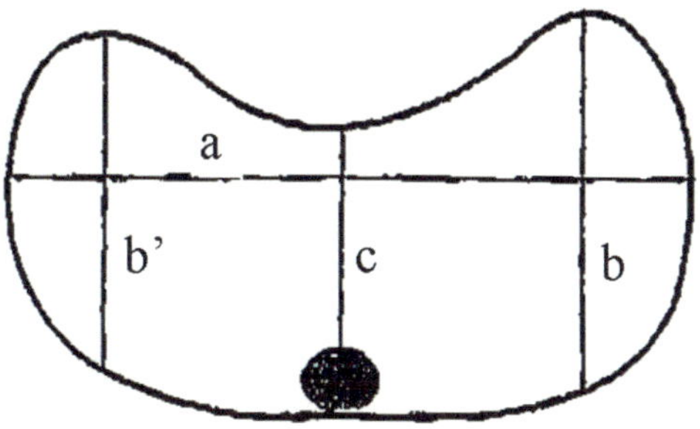

$$\text{Haller's index} = \frac{a}{c}$$

$$\text{degree of depression} = \frac{b}{c}$$

$$\text{degree of asymmetry} = \frac{b'}{b}$$

$$\text{degree of flatness} = \frac{a}{b}$$

Fig. 4. Deformity indices (Nakahara et al., 1987)

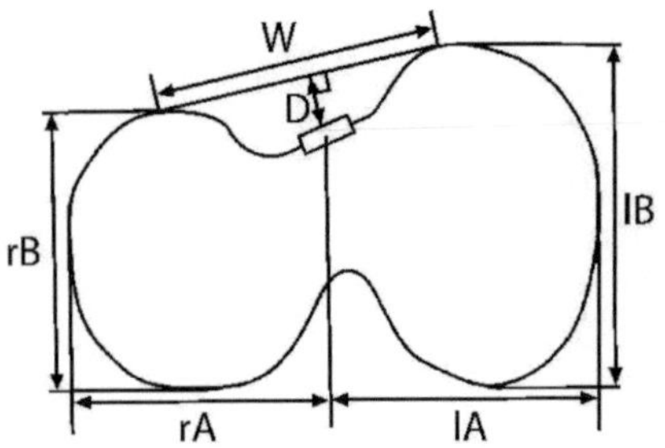

$$\text{steepness index} = \frac{D}{W}$$

$$\text{excavation volume index} = \frac{D \times W}{lA \times lB + rA \times rB}$$

$$\text{asymmetry index} = \frac{lA \times lB}{rA \times rB}$$

Fig. 5. Deformity indices (Masaoka et al., in press)
(Reprinted with permission from *Eur J Cardiothorac Surg* 2011, in press)

PE is a symptomatic disease. Kelly (Kelly, 2008) investigated medical history of 327 PE patients (Table 1). Various symptoms with high percentages are listed up. Representatives are exercise intolerance, lack of endurance, shortness of breath, chest pain etc. Marfan syndrome (4.6%) and Ehlers-Danlos syndrome (2.8%) are associated with PE. Additionally, association of various psychological disturbances is pointed out, such as self-consciousness about chest, withdrawal from social and sports activities, depression even to suicide.

Condition	Number	Percentage
Exercise intolerance	211	64.5
Lack of endurance	205	62.7
Shortness of breath	203	62.1
Chest pain with exercise	167	51.1
Family history of PE	140	42.8
Chest pain without exercise	104	31.8
Asthma	70	21.4
Scoliosis	69	21.1
Cardiac abnormalities	65	19.9
Frequent or prolonged URI	44	13.5
Palpitations	37	11.3
Pneumonia	28	8.6
Fainting/dizziness	27	8.3
Marfan syndrome	15	4.6
Family history of PC	13	4.0
Ehlers-Danlos syndrome	9	2.8
Family history of Marfan syndrome	8	2.4
Patient adopted	4	1.2
Patient has identical twin	3	0.9
Family history of Ehlers-Danlos syndrome	2	0.6
Sprengel deformity	2	0.6

Abbreviations: PC, pectus carinatum; URI, upper respiratory infection.
Table 1. Medical history of 327 patients (Kelly, 2008)
(Reprinted with permission from *Semin Pediatr Surg* 2008; 17;189)

1.3 Physiology

PE causes compression of lung and heart, which might result in impairment of respiratory and circulatory function. The impairment of these functions is sometimes too modest to be evaluated by usual function tests preoperatively, in spite of existence of subjective symptoms.
In order to recognize relationship between the results of the examinations and PE deformity, it is important to confirm, 1) difference between those of the PE patients and the healthy controls, 2) relationship with the severity of deformity, and 3) improvement by surgical repair. Clinically, the results of such examinations could be parameters to evaluate the effects of surgeries.

1.3.1 Respiratory function

Since 1950's, many papers on this topic have been published. In early years, measurement of conventional standard pulmonary volumes by spirometer was only one tool. Thereafter, flow-volume curve by pneumotachograph, TLC (Table 2) and RV by nitrogen washout, or body plethysmograph, and various work load tests were adopted. However, there are various opinions concerning what is the representative parameter expressing decreased pulmonary function due to PE deformity.

TLC	total lung capacity
RV	residual volume
MVV	maximal ventilation volume
FVC	forced ventilatory capacity
FEV	forced expiratory volume
FEV_1	forced expiratory volume in 1 second
$FEF_{25\%\sim75\%}$	forced expiratory flow from 25% exhalation to 75% exhalation
RV	right ventricle
RVSD	right ventricle short distance
PWC	physical work capacity
SV	stroke volume

Table 2. List of abbreviations

In early years, MVV was thought to be a most reliable parameter to assess the reduced pulmonary function. Haller and colleague (Haller & Loughlin, 2000) pointed out significant difference of TLC, FVC, and RV between the PE patients and the matched controls. Nuss and colleague (Nuss & Kelly, 2008) stated that FVC, FEV_1, $FEF_{25\%-75\%}$ reduced in the PE patients, comparing with the age-, height-matched predictive values. Which spirometrical parameter is definitely different between the PE patients and the controls are not agreed in various papers.
Castile and colleagues (Castile et al., 1982) reported that in the symptomatic PE patients, the measured oxygen uptake increasingly exceeded the predicted value as the work loads approached maximum, different from healthy controls. Haller and colleague (Haller & Loughlin, 2000) did not find difference of O_2 pulse (O_2 consumption/heart rate) after treadmill works between the PE patients and the controls. On the other hand, Malek and colleagues (Malek et al, 2003) reported that the O_2 pulse on maximal exercise testing was significantly lower than the reference value, and furthermore, this limitation was caused by cardiovascular factor, but not ventilatory.
As for the relationship between decreased pulmonary function and severity of deformity, Lawson and colleagues (Lawson et al., 2011), after investigation of 310 PE patients, reported that the percentages of the patients with abnormal FVC, FEV_1, $FEF_{25\%-75\%}$, and TLC data

increased with increasing Haller index. He speculated that the large tidal volume required by exercise causes some of the symptoms by the effects of deformity on rib motion and bellows function.
Comparison of the results of pulmonary function tests in preoperative and postoperative period was performed Cahill and colleagues (Cahill et al., 1984). He pointed out significant improvement of MVV, and improvement in exercise performance as quantified by maximal O_2 consumption. Haller and colleague (Haller & Loughlin, 2000) recognized a higher O_2 pulse in exercising tests in postoperative patients. Nuss and colleague (Nuss & Kelly, 2008) pointed out normalization of FEV_1, TLC, and diffusing lung capacity. Lawson and colleagues (Lawson et al., 2005) found that FVC, FEV_1, and $FEF_{25\%-75\%}$ were lower than normal preoperatively, and small but significant improvement of these 3 parameters after the Nuss surgeries and bar removals.
The above-described data about relationship between pulmonary function and PE deformity from many articles are summarized to be unfixed, because conduct of spirometrical test is difficult in child, and comparison of preoperative and postoperative data is difficult due to growth.

1.3.2 Cardiovascular function

Assessment of the cardiovascular function in PE began with introduction of cardiac catheterization. The hemodynamics measured at rest revealed normal pattern in majority of the early papers. However, Fabricius and colleagues (Fabricius et al., 1957) recognized abnormal high right atrial pressure in 3, and increased right ventricular pressure in one, after examinations of 26 patients.
Introduction of angiocardiography clarified dysmorphology of heart by dislocation or compression, i.e., anterior rotation of right atrium and compression on right lateral wall. CT scan substituted the angiocardiography, and verified noninvasively mitral valve prolapse and sternal imprint on the anterior wall of the right ventricle (Shamberger et al., 1987).
Radioisotope angiography appeared as a substitute of cardiac catheterization or angiography with contrast material. Shamberger and Welch performed this examination in 25 cases, and pointed out enlarged right atrium in 15, enlarged right ventricle in 15, dilated pulmonary artery in 10, delayed pulmonary artery transit time in 11, decreased left ventricular volume in 9, and compression defect in the right ventricle in 8 (Shamberger & Welch, 1988).
On the other hand, cardiac catheterization on exercise added new informations. Bevegard (Bevegard, 1962) performed right heart catheterization in 16 patients and found that the patients with severe PE showed 20% decrease of PWC (Table 2) from the supine position to the sitting position, similar to that of the normal subjects. But, increase of SV from rest to exercise was only 18.5%, much less than the 51% increase in the normal subjects. This finding could be an evidence of the exercise-induced symptoms in the PE patients.
Peterson and colleagues (Peterson et al., 1985) assessed cardiac volume and output with radionuclide angiography in 13 patients, and compared those data in preoperative and postoperative period. He found that the right ventricular ejection fraction at rest decreased after repair, which could be attributed to the increase of the right ventricular and diastolic volume index after operation. However, cardiac index did not increase significantly after operation at rest or during exercise.
Recently, cardiovascular resonance imaging was introduced to this field. Saleh and colleagues (Saleh et al., 2010) examined this test in 30 patients, and found reduction of RV ejection fraction and RVSD both at end diastole and systole.

In summary, compression of the right heart leads to diminished stroke volume, and in accordance with the modest decrease of ventilatory activity, leads to diminished cardiopulmonary capacity in severe PE patients. Repair surgery for PE could improve cardiorespiratory function in the patients with impaired function.

2. Corrective surgery for pectus excavatum

2.1 Overview

Surgical correction for PE started at early 20th century, but could not gain successful results. The pioneer to open the curtain to modern era of the corrective surgery for PE was Brown (Brown 1939). Observing inward retraction of the xiphoid in baby's crying, he thought that the retraction is caused by the traction of diaphragm, and speculated that the substance of it could be the substernal ligament and the transverse thoracic muscle which combine the diaphragm with the sternum. Furthermore, he speculated that delay of such condition in infancy could lead to the definite thoracic deformity in adult.

So, he thought up two procedures. The 1st was indicated to infant or little child. The core of the procedure is to dissect the substernal ligament and/or the attachment to diaphragm under a small, vertical incision at level of the xiphoid. He expected that such procedure could prevent to proceed to the definitive PE deformity in adult.

The 2nd was indicated to elder child, adolescent and adult. The core of this procedure is 1) resection of 2cm costo-chondral segments of the 4th~7th ribs near the junction with the sternum, and 2) wedge resection of the sternum on the anterior table at level of junction of the sternal body and the manubrium. Elevation of the sternum is secured by the sutures with wire at the wedge resection site (Fig.6.). He added an external traction by fixation of a wire penetrated the caudal part of the sternum and the 5th costal cartilage with a ladder placed on the anterior chest wall.

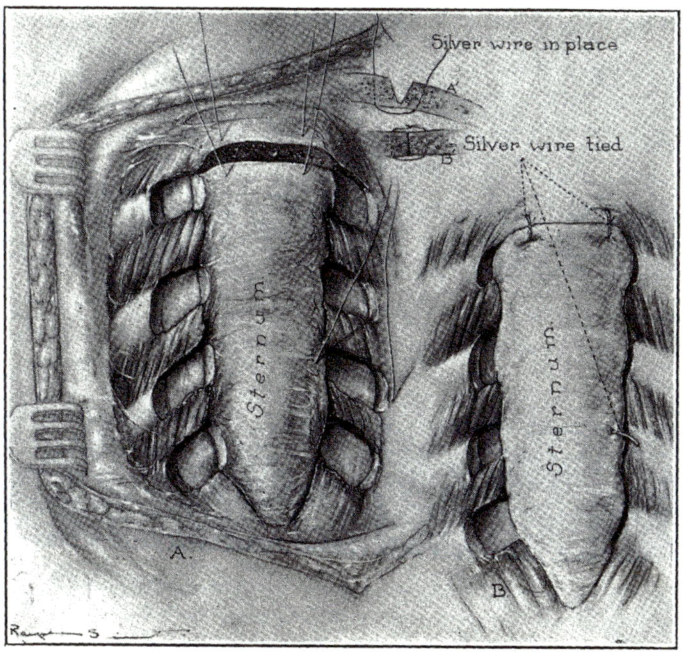

Fig. 6. The 2nd procedure of Brown (Brown, 1939)

The Brown's procedure was took over by Sweet (Sweet, 1944), and led to the Ravitch's procedure, which will be described in the next chapter.
A variety of corrective procedures have appeared, based on various ideas. The sternal turnover method was performed by Wada and colleagues (Wada et al., 1965) in Japan. He made an isolated plastron from the anterior chest wall, and turned it over, and sutured it back in place (Fig. 7.). This procedure had been performed in many cases in Japan, but not in other countries, because it had risk of necrosis of plastron. Laituri and colleagues (Laituri et al., 2010) described that osteo-necrosis or fistula formation occurred in 46% of the patients over 15 years of age in Wada's series. And such complications prompted Taguchi to preserve the internal mammary vessels to maintain the blood flow to the sternum (cited from Laituri et al.). However, despite of such modification, sternal turnover procedure became to be performed infrequently. Recently, Ninkovic and colleagues (Ninkovic et al., 2003) planned revival of the sternal turnover procedure, using technique of vascular surgery to anastomose the internal mammary vessels, i.e., the right internal mammary vessels to the inverted left mammary vessels (Fig. 8.).

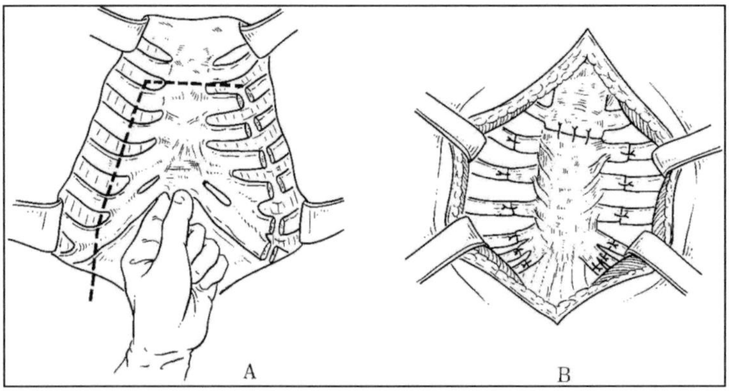

Fig. 7. "Sternoturnover" procedure (Wada et al., 1965)

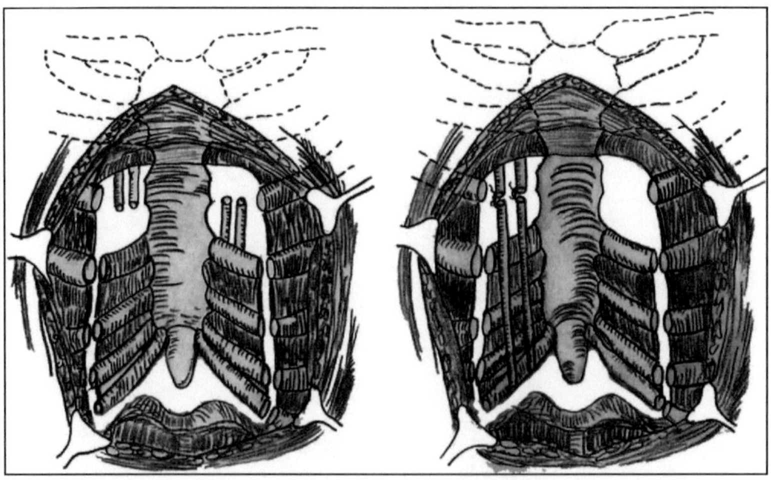

Fig. 8. Ninkovic's modification of "Sternoturnover" (Ninkovic et al., 2003)
(Reprinted with permission from *Plast Reconst Surg* 2003;112:1356)

Proposals from plastic surgeons are various. In 1970, Masson and colleagues (Masson et al., 1970) implanted a preformed silastic implant, with Dacron mesh patches on it, through a transverse incision just below the xiphoid. Although 40 years passed since then, the accumulated cases were not so many. Snel and colleagues (Snel et al., 2009) summed up 75 cases from 5 papers, and showed the long term outcome results of his own 16 patients. Complications occurred in 7 patients (43%); prolonged seroma in 5, in whom explantation of the implant were performed in one, reoperation and repositioning in 2 patients. Two patients underwent explantation of the implants due to pain and discomfort. Satisfactions of the patients were evaluated by 4 grades; excellent 1, good 8, mediocre 3, and poor 1.

Michlits and colleagues (Michlits et al., 2009) performed free fasciocutaneous infragluteal flap in 6 patients. He stated that the patients were satisfied on shape of the corrected PE. However, these plastic surgeries can not release the hearts and lungs from compression. Accordingly, they could not be indicated for symptomatic patients. Moreover, implantations of foreign body do not always provide good results.

In 1998, Nuss and colleagues (Nuss et al., 1998) advocated a new procedure "minimally invasive technique for PE". This proposal invited revolution of corrective surgery for PE. The minimally invasive operation was reinforced with various modifications, and subsequently increased the followers worldwide. Concerning this procedure, detailed description will appear in the 2.3 chapter.

Some new trials originating from new ideas appeared. Harrison and colleagues (Harrison et al., 2010) proposed Magnetic Mini-Mover Procedure (3MP). The 3MP uses a magnetic implant coupled with an external magnet to generate force sufficient to gradually remodel PE deformities. The magnimplant is set at surface of the sternum, and the magnatract is set on the rear table of the external brace, which is worn by the patient (Fig. 9.). The principle of this procedure is that the magnetic gravitation between the magnimplant and the magnatract lifts up the sternum. He performed this procedure in 10 patients, but outcome results were not yet gained. Schier and colleagues (Schier et al., 2005) proposed the vacuum chest wall lifter, which is set at anterior chest wall. Suction with this apparatus is conducted from 30 minutes to 5 hours daily, and repeated for 2 year (Fig. 10.). Reliable outcome results were not yet gained.

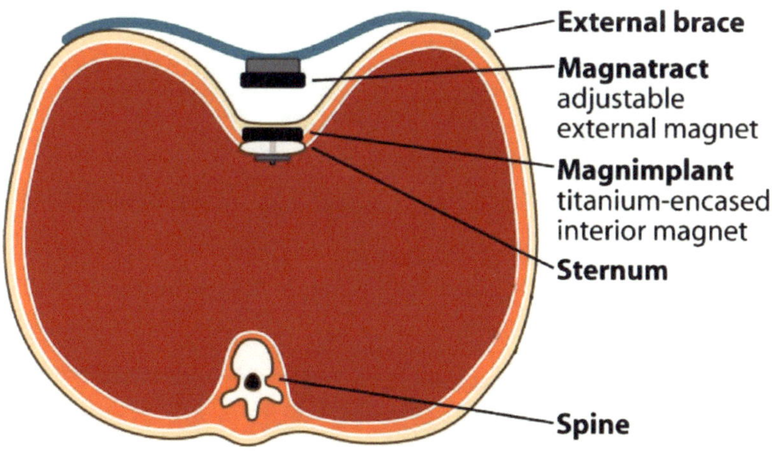

Fig. 9. Magnetic Mini-Mover Procedure (Harrison et al., 2010)
(Reprinted with permission from *J Pediatr Surg* 2010;45:187)

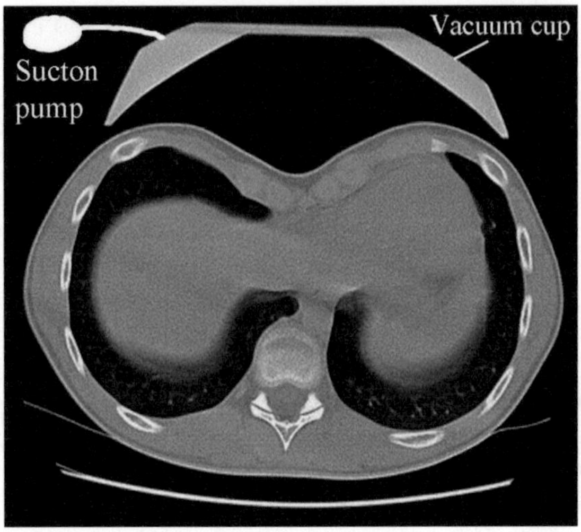

Fig. 10. The vacuum chest wall lifter (Schier, 2005)
(Reprinted with permission from *J Pediatr Surg* 2005;40:497)

2.2 Ravitch's procedure (open repair)

2.2.1 Procedure

In 1949, Ravitch proposed his original procedure for PE. He intended to make free the sternum from all restrictions. In order to carry out his idea, he felt it necessary to divide the xiphi-sternal articulation and substernal ligament and to resect all the deformed costal cartilages for the length of their deformity. Furthermore, to elevate the sternum, he performed a transverse cuneiform osteotomy at the sterno-manubriul junction and sutured it, to maintain the corrected position (Fig. 11.). He did not use the traction apparatus that Brown used. The extensive defect resulting from excision of all of the deformed cartilages was left without sutures of any tissues.

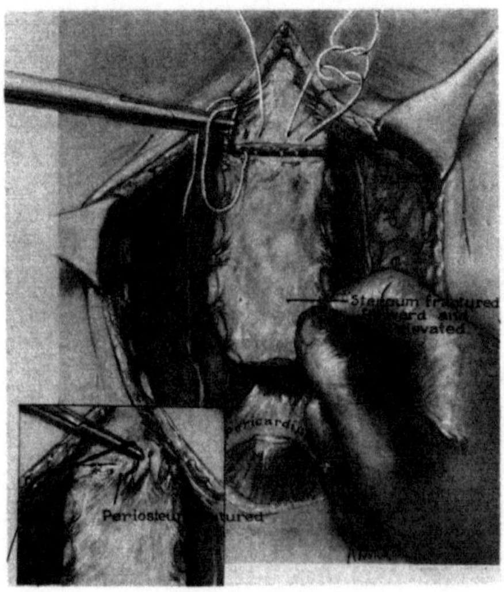

Fig. 11. Original Ravitch procedure (Ravitch, 1949)
(Reprinted with permission from Ann Surg 1949;129:434)

In 1965, Ravitch revised his original procedure; 1) oblique chondrotomy at 2nd or 3rd costal cartilages and overlap suture (Fig. 12 a.), and 2) sternal osteotomy on the rear table of the sternum, instead of the anterior table in the original procedure, and insertion of a small bone graft in the sternal opening (Fig. 12 b.). Such modifications were done, in order to elevate the sternum more effectively and prevent recurrence of depression. At present, the procedure with the above-stated modifications i.e., 3points fixation, is denominated "Ravitch procedure".

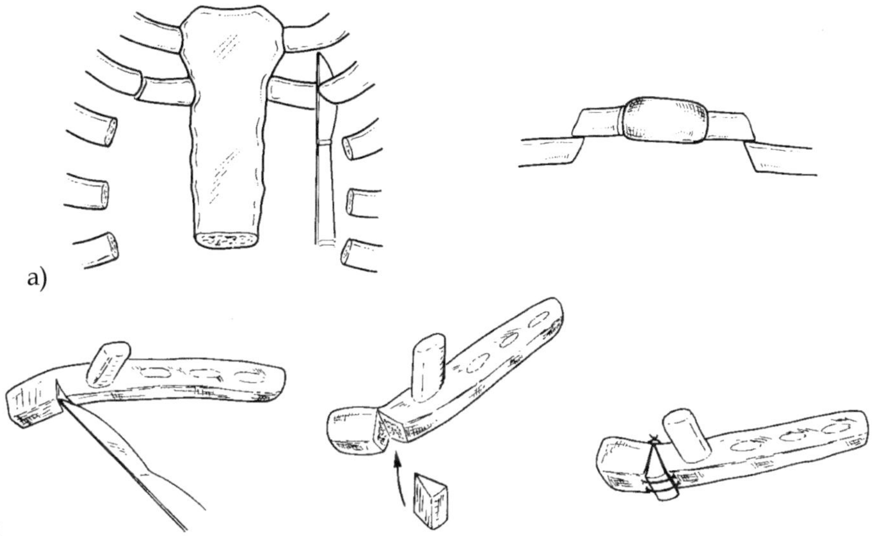

a)

b)

Fig. 12. Modified Ravitch procedure by himself
(Reprinted with permission from *Kokyukigeka 1st ed.*, p. 378, Nanzan-do)

The most faithful successor to Ravitch is Alex Haller Jr. Although he took over the Ravitch procedure in general, he pointed out 2 important problems. The 1st is a fact that support of the anterior chest wall by the Ravitch procedure is not sufficient for children older than 10 years of age, teenagers, and adults. So, he performed placement of a temporary stainless steel strut beneath the sternum, and the strut is anchored bilaterally to the 5th or 6th ribs (Haller et al., 1989). The strut is removed on an outpatient basis, 6~9 months after the primary repair.
The 2nd is a suggestion, that too extensive and too early operation could induce chest wall constriction. The total resections of the deformed costal cartilages in Ravitch procedure resulted to remove growth center activity of costal cartilages. He recognized such severe complication in 12 children, and denominated "aquired Jeune's syndrome" (Haller et al., 1996). He corrected his procedure as follows; 1) exclusion of the children below 4 years of age from indication of the repair, 2) shortening of the resected costal cartilages by 2.5cm.
Fonkalsrud remarked that after the removal of deformed costal cartilages in the Ravitch's procedure, the regenerated cartilages are thin, irregular, and commonly rigid with calcification, even if the perichondrial sheaths are preserved. So, he removed short chips (3~8mm) of the costal cartilages on the medial and the lateral ends of the deformed cartilages (Fonkalsrud, 2004) (Fig. 13.). The remaining costal cartilages are reattached to the sternum and the ribs. Following to a transverse wedge osteotomy on the anterior table of the sternum and fixation of a thin stainless steel Adkins strut was placed posterior to both the sternum and the costal cartilages to elevate the sternum (Fig. 14). He evaluates this procedure as a much less extensive repair.

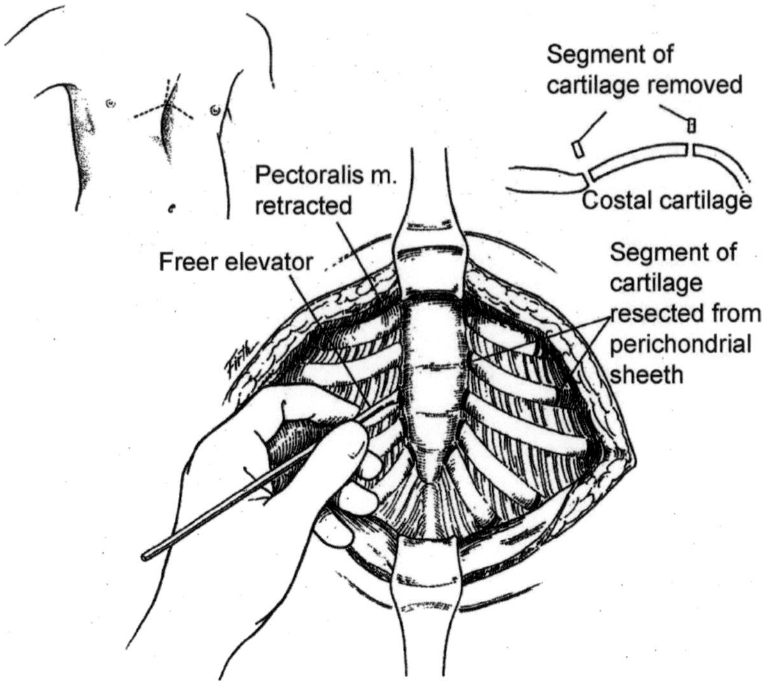

Fig. 13. Fonkalsrud's procedure (I) (Fonalsrud, 2004)
(Reprinted with permission from *Ann Surg* 2004;240:232)

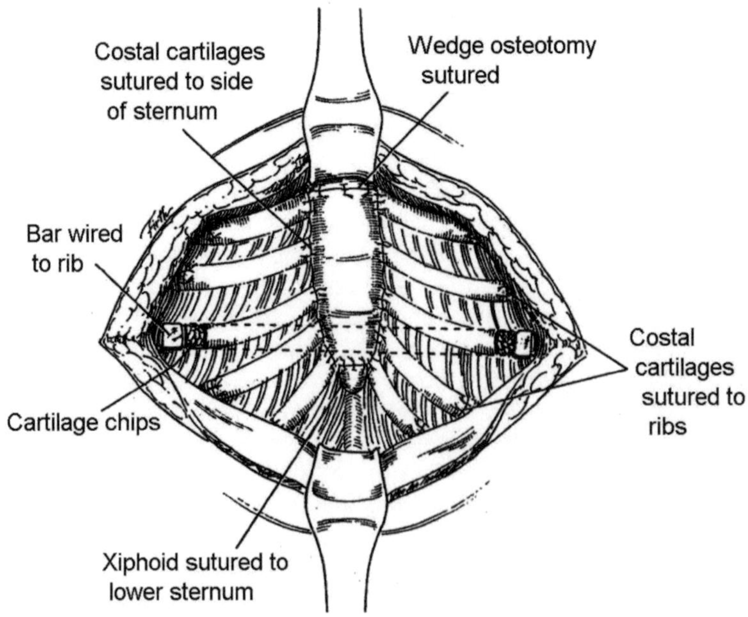

Fig. 14. Fonkalsrud's procedure (II) (Fonalsrud, 2004)
(Reprinted with permission from *Ann Surg* 2004;240:233)

Robicsek hated metal materials supporting the elevated sternum, because they have the potential to leave their original position and wander all over the body. Even if the metal support remains in place, it has possibility to destroy the surrounding organ. So, he thought up a new supporting system using Marlex mesh. After wedge resection of the sternum and resection of the deformed cartilages and detachment of the xiphoid, the sternum is maintained in its corrected position by suturing a sheath of Marlex mesh taut under it (Robicsek, 2000) (Fig. 15.). Concerning the destiny of the implanted material, Robicsek stated that in 2 reoperating cases due to recurrence of depression, he found the area where the mesh was inserted to be a fibrocartilaginous plate with no identifiable traces of the mesh (Robicsek, 2009).

Saxena and Willital (Saxena & Willital, 2007) reported 1,264 open-repair patients with the Willital-Hegemann procedure, which uses 3 struts. The 1st is passed transsternally, with its edges resting anteriorly on the ribs. The other 2 struts are set parasternally with the points of fixation being the 2nd ribs and the lowest ends of the rib cage (Fig. 16.). These struts are removed after 24~36 months. Saxena and colleagues (Saxena et al., 2007) performed the Nuss procedure in 160 patients from 2000~2006 too, and stated the open repair with Willital–Hegemann procedure should be indicated to the severe deformed patients.

Hu and colleagues (Hu et al., 2008) performed open repair in 398 PE patients. His procedure consists of the resections of the deformed costal cartilages and fixation by "arch-shaped" steal strut, which is removed 1 year after the operation.

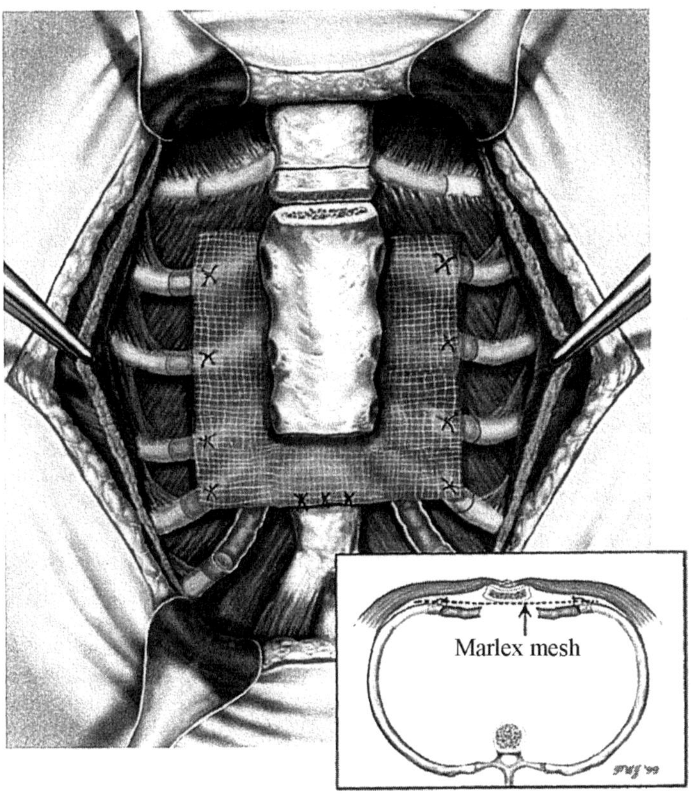

Fig. 15. Robicsek's procedure (Marlex mesh hammock) (Robicsek, 2000)

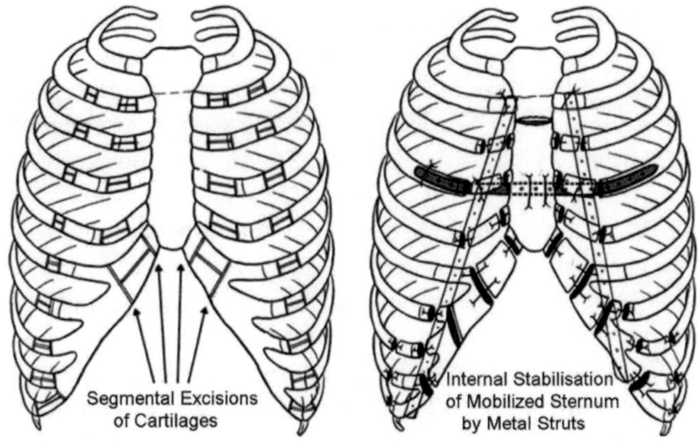

Fig. 16. Saxena & Willital's procedure (Saxena and Willital, 2007)
(Reprinted with permission from *J Thorac Cardiovasc Surg* 2007;134:874)

2.2.2 Complications and outcome results

Table 3 shows large series of the Ravitch repair. However, the complications and the outcome results in them are not completely clear, because these reviews deal not always their complications and outcome results, besides, even if such descriptions are involved, not in uniform style. Ravitch described about 2 cases with staphylococcal infection, one of whom underwent removal of sequester, and stated no other complications except them (Ravitch, 1965).

Haller and colleagues (Haller et al., 1989) stated the morbidity rate was less than 5%, and mean hospital stay was 7 days. Concerning of the outcome results, in early series during evolution of the surgical technique, reoperation occurred in 10% of the patients. However, recent series, revealed only 3 poor results in 352 patients. He stated that, therefore, the operative results with the current technique were quite satisfactory with greater than 95% of the patients having good to excellent results.

Author	Publish	Cases	City (Nation)	Remarks
Ravitch	1965	164	Baltimore (USA)	Original Ravitch
Haller	1989	664	Baltimore (USA)	Strut
Robicsek	2000	800	Charlotte (USA)	Marlex-mesh hammock
Saxena and Willital	2007	1262	Graz (Austria)	Wittel-Hegeman procedure (3 struts)
Hu	2008	398	Sichuan (China)	Strut
Fonkalsrud	2009	912	Los Angeles (USA)	Strut
Masaoka	2011	307	Nagoya (Japan)	Metal-free

Table 3. Large series of Ravitch repair

Robicsek (Robicsek, 2000) stated that mean hospital stay was 3 days, and the important postoperative complications were bleeding from the internal mammary artery, infection, and seroma. However, he did not mention their frequency, as same as outcome results. Saxena and Willital (Saxena & Willital., 2007) stated that the complication rate was 5.7%, and hospital stay decreased from 20.5 days in early series to 6.2 days in recent series. They referred to late results, and indicated 1.4% of major recurrence and 3.6% of mild recurrence. Subjective complaints of the patients before the surgeries were eliminated in 97% of the patients.

Hu and colleagues (Hu et al., 2008) had to perform early removal of metal bar due to its dislodge in 4 patients, and noticed recurrent depression in 3 patients (0.75%), and protrusion of 2nd or 3rd costal cartilages in 5 patients (1.26%). As the final results, normal contour of the costal cage was constructed in 98.74% (393/398). Cardiac function recovered to the healthy level of the same age.
Fonkalsrud (Fonkalsrud, 2009) showed 8% of complication rate. Recurrence occurred in 5 patients from series I (17%), 15 patients from series II (4.3%), 7 patients from series III (3%), and 4 patients from series IV (1.3%), and total 22 patients (2.4%) underwent reoperations. The reoperation rates have decreased in the learning curve. Satisfaction of the patients or parents was evaluated as very good or excellent by 94.2% of all patients.
Complications in our 307 patients of early series before the current procedure, which will be described in the 2.5 chapter, were 34 (11.0%). The list of each complication is shown in Table 4.

Series	Seroma	Wound complications	Pneumothorax	Pleural effusion	Pulmonary complications	Others	Total (%)
I (n=27)	2	Dehiscence 2	1		Pneumonia 1	Paradoxical breathing 1	7 (25.9)
II (n=23)	1		2		Atelectasis 1		4 (17.4)
III (n=117)	1	Wound necrosis 1	2	1	Atelectasis 1	Ventilatory insufficiency 1 Early recurrent of PE 1	8 (6.8)
IV adult type (n=52)	1	Wound infection 1 Osteomyelitis of sternum 1 Bleeding 1		1	Pulmonary edema 1 Atelectasis 1	Sudden death 1 Respiratory insufficiency 2 Pericardial effusion 1	11 (21.1)
IV child type (n=88)			4				4 (4.5)
Total (n=307)	5	6	9	2	5	7	34 (11.0)

Table 4. Complications in early series of us

2.3 Nuss procedure

2.3.1 Procedure

In 1998, Nuss et al. proposed a new procedure – minimally invasive technique –, and assessed their 10 years results. The essence of this procedure is correction of thoracic cage by a metal bar inserted posterior to the sternum without incision or resection of costal cartilages.

His idea was originated from observation of the thoracic deformity in the adult patients with chronic emphysematous lungs – barrel shaped thorax. He thought that, if this configuration of chest wall can occur long after their skeleton has matured and calcified, it should be possible to remodel the chest wall in children whose ribs and cartilages are still soft and pliable without having to resort to rib cartilage incision, resection, or sternal osteotomy. Detail of this procedure is as follows.

1. Preoperatively, a proper length meal bar is selected, and bent into proper convexity.
2. A transverse incision 2.5cm long was made in each lateral chest wall between the anterior axillary and posterior axillary lines.
3. A skin tunnel was raised anteriorly, and 50cm long Kelly clamp is inserted along an intercostal space, and advanced slowly across the mediastinum immediately under the sternum until it emerged on the opposite side (Fig. 17A.).
4. Two strands of umbilical tape were pulled through the track (Fig. 17B.). One strand serves to guide the Kelly clamp from another side.
5. When the track was deemed wide enough, a steel bar is pulled beneath the sternum using the umbilical tape for traction with the convexity facing posteriorly (Fig. 17C.).
6. When the bar is in position, it is turned over with a vice grip so that the convexity faces anteriorly (Fig. 17D.).
7. The bar is secured with heavy sutures to the lateral chest wall muscles.
8. If the bar is unstable, a 2~4cm cross bar is attached to one or both ends of the bar.

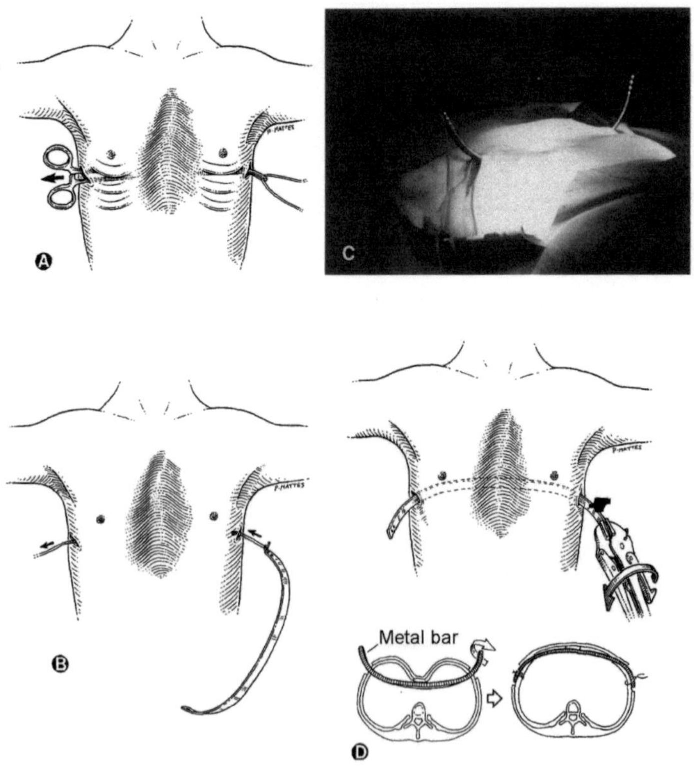

Fig. 17. Nuss procedure (Nuss et al., 1998)
(Reprinted with permission from *J Pediatr Surg* 1998;33:548)

Thereafter, he modificated the original procedure, in order to avoid the injuries to vessels and bar shifts. Modifications are as follows: 1) use of thoracoscopy to secure the insertion of introducer, 2) use of introducer (large metal rod) to secure the tunnel making, 3) fixation of the bar with stabilizer and fixing suture (Fig. 18.). The bar is stabilized by wiring a stabilizer to the left end of the bar and by placing sutures of polydioxanone (PDS) around the bar and underlying ribs on the right end. 4) Use of two or more bars in the patients with unacceptable configuration after use of one bar.

Park and colleagues (Park et al., 2010) added 3 modifications; one of those is the crane technique. This technique involves elevating the depressed sternum before introducer insertion and lifting the wire suture along with the sternum by an operating table-mounted retractor system (Fig. 19.). This technique serves to alleviate the pressure on the bar, and to prevent internal organ injury during the passage of the introducer. The other is the morphology-tailored bar shaping system named "terrain contour matching". Each patient has distinctive terrain characteristics. Park planned to shape the bar as matched to the patient's thorax, and to compress the crest of the depression by the negative momentum of the lever action, during rotation of the bar (Fig. 20.).

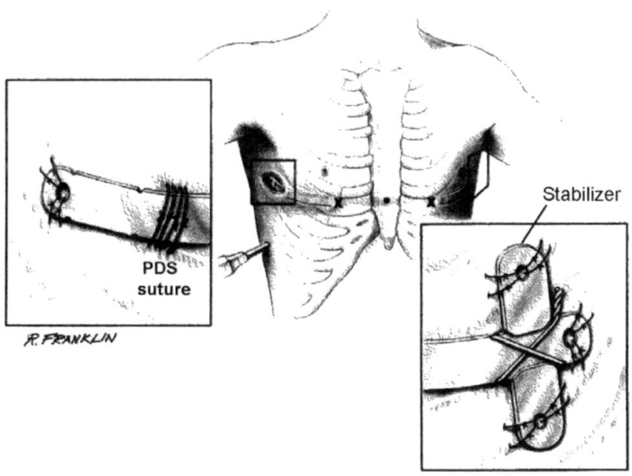

Fig. 18. Modification of Nuss procedure by Nuss (Nuss, 2005)
(Reprinted with permission from *Jpn J Thorac Cardiovasc Surg* 2005;53:339)

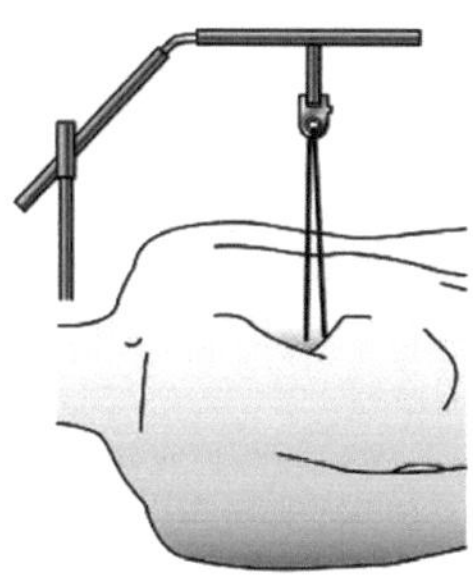

Fig. 19. Park's modification – crane technique – (Park et al., 2010)
(Reprinted with permission from *J Thorac Cardiovasc Surg* 2010;139:381)

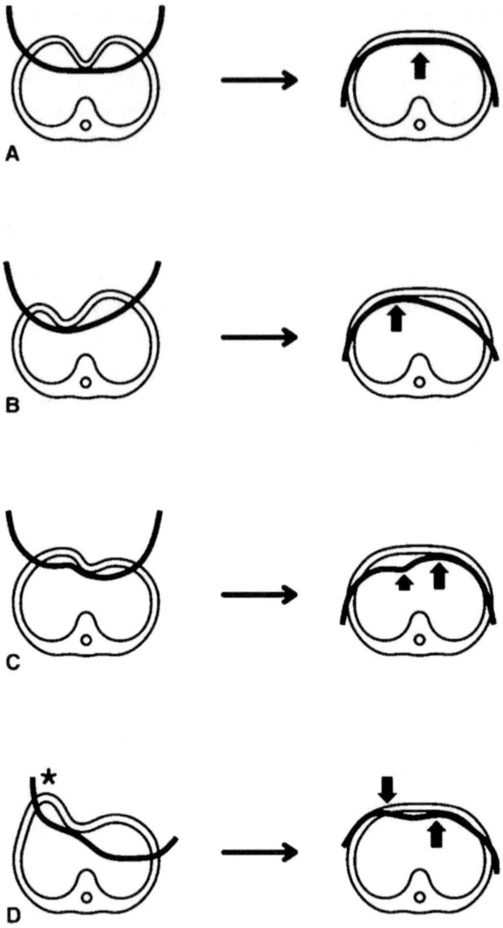

Fig. 20. Park's modification – terrain contour matching – (Park et al., 2010)
(Reprinted with permission from *J Thorac Cardiovasc Surg* 2010;139:382)

The 3rd is the multipoint fixation of the bar. This technique consisted of fixation of the bar, not only at end of the bar, but also at hinge point. The fixation is performed by "through-the-skin" technique, i.e., the needle stick is made directly through the overlying skin, passed around the rib, and passed back through the skin. The sutured wires are grabbed via a subcutaneous dissection. The retrieved sutures are passed through the end-hole of the bar and tied. This technique was developed, to prevent displacement of the bar.

Pilegaard and Licht (Pilegaard & Licht, 2008) proposed to use absorbable stabilizer in order to avoid chronic pain and necessity of removal. However, as it break easier than the one of metal, further research is needed.

2.3.2 Complications and outcome results

Table 5 shows large series of the Nuss repair.

The latest report about postoperative complications after the Nuss repair in the Nuss's institute is shown in Table 6 and Table 7 (Kelly et al., 2010). In the line-up of the early complications, the majority is mild one, but hemothorax includes injury of internal mammary vessels. In the late complications, the majority is one concerning with the bar. The bar displacements occurred in 64 patients (5.7%), in whom 45 patients required repositioning. Kelly and colleagues (Kelly et al., 2010) stated that the bar displacement rate was 12% in the patients without stabilizer, 6% in the patients with wired stabilizer, and with the addition of pericostal sutures placed around the bar and underlying ribs, it dropped to 2%. It should be paid attention that bar allergy is found in 3.1%.

Author	Publish	Cases	City (Nation)	Remark
Dzielicki	2006	461	Gliwice (Poland)	Modified Nuss
Olbrecht	2008	244	Baltimore (USA)	Modified Nuss
Pilegaard	2009	507	Aorhus (Denmark)	Modified Nuss (Absorbable stabilizer)
Park	2010	1170	Ansan (Korea)	Park modification
Kelly (Nuss)	2010	1215	Norfolk (USA)	Modified Nuss

Table 5. Large series of Nuss repair

Pneumothorax with spontaneous resolution	64.7% (n=727)
Pneumothorax with chest tube	4.0% (n=45)
Horner's syndrome	15.5% (n=174)
Drug reaction	3.2% (n=36)
Suture site infection	1.0% (n=11)
Pneumonia	0.5% (n=6)
Hemothorax	0.5% (n=6)
Pericarditis	0.5% (n=5)
Pleural effusion (requiring drainage)	0.3% (n=3)
Death	0%
Cardiac perforation	0%

Table 6. Early postoperative complications of primary surgical patients (Kelly et al., 2010) (Reprinted with permission from *Ann Surg* 2010;252:1076)

Bar displacements—total	64/1123 (5.7%)
Bar displacements requiring revision	45/1123 (4.0%)
Overcorrection (none required surgery)	41/1123 (3.7%)
Bar allergy (3 required bar removal)	35/1123 (3.1%)
Recurrence	11/1123 (1.0%)
Bar infection—total	6/1123 (0.5%)
Bar infection—required early removal	3/1123 (0.3%)
Hemothorax (post-traumatic)	4/1123 (0.4%)
Lactosorb stabilizer inflammation	4/1123 (0.4%)

Table 7. Late postoperative complications (Kelly et al., 2010) (Reprinted with permission from *Ann Surg* 2010;252:1076)

Park and colleagues (Park et al., 2010) reported decrease of the complications, comparing the results of 1999~2002 and 2006~2008, as follows: total complications (57/335, 17.0% vs 33/394, 7.5%) pneumothorax (25/335, 7.5% vs 3/394, 0.8%), bar displacement (13/335, 3.8% vs 2/394, 0.5%). The reoperation rate also decreased (17/335, 5.1% vs 3/394, 0.8%).

Pilegaard and colleagues (Pilegaard et al., 2008) noticed in his series of 383 patients, pneumothorax in 178 (49%), bleeding in 2, pleural effusion in 4, seroma in 11, and deep infection in 8. Seven patients were reoperated because of the bar dislocation (1.8%). In another 13 patients, the stabilizer was removed because of pain.

However, the most important and characteristic complication in the Nuss procedure is massive hemorrhage due to injury of heart or great vessels (Bouchard et al., 2009; Aydemir et al., 2011). This complication is sometimes life-threatening and requires an emergency operation. It might occur during the initial operation, or in the late period of the postoperative course, or during bar removal (Jemielity et al., 2011; Haecker et al., 2009). Despite of various measures, this complication has occurred still.

Mean hospital stay is about 3 days, and the bar is removed after 2~4years, in most institutes performing the Nuss procedure.

The outcome results in the latest paper of the Nuss group are shown in Table 8. Evaluation was made, based on grades of satisfaction of the patients or the parents. Excellent results were gained in 85.3% (Kelly et al., 2010). They compared the preoperative and the postoperative pulmonary function data, and pointed out improvement in FVC (88% to 92%, $p<0.001$), FEV_1 (83% to 88%, $p=0.01$), and $FEF_{25\%-75\%}$ (81% to 87%, p=not significant). They performed echocardiogram in the preoperative patients, and found mitral valve prolapse (MVP) in 216 patients (18%). Forty-four patients with preoperative MVP underwent echocardiogram after surgery, and 20 (44%) had resolution of the MVP.

Park and colleagues (Park et al., 2010) evaluated the operative results by CT indices: The Haller index changed from 6.05±11.82 to 2.76±0.49 ($p<0.001$); the depression index changed from 1.95±1.71 to 1 ($p<0.001$); and the asymmetry index changed from 1.08±0.05 to 1.02±0.02 ($p<0.001$).

Total number of primary patients	1123
Total number with bar removed	790
• Excellent result	674 (85.3%)
• Good result	83 (10.5%)
• Fair result	11 (1.4%)
• Poor result	6 (0.8%)
• Recurrence requiring re-do operation	11 (1.4%)
• No return	5 (0.6%)

Table 8. Results after bar removal median follow-up 854 days post bar removal (Kelly et al., 2010)
(Reprinted with permission from *Ann Surg* 2010;252:1076)

2.4 Pros and cons for both procedures

The Nuss procedure has merits, such as minimal operative wound, lesser operation time, and lesser blood loss, but simultaneously some demerits, such as frequent occurrence of complications, burden of bar(s) for a long time, and necessity of operation for removal of the bar(s).

On the other hand, the open procedure has merits, such as safety and certainly of manipulation under direct vision, and demerits, such as longer operative time, and larger operation wound.

However, there are only few papers comparing the results of both procedures, because the institutes performing both procedures are limited. Fonkalsrud and Hebra (Fonkalsrud et al., 2002) compared 68 Nuss and 139 open repairs in UCLA and South Carolina University, and concluded that the open repair needed longer operating time, but decreased hospital stay, complication rates, and use of pain medications.

Nasr and colleagues (Nasr et al., 2010) reviewed 9 papers performing both procedures, and showed no difference with respect to overall complication and patient's satisfaction. However, the rate of reoperation was higher in the Nuss Procedure.

On the other hand, Robicsek argued against the Nuss procedure (Robicsek & Hebra, 2009). He asserted, how the two 3~4cm cuts (plus the hole for the videoscope) are shorter than the wound of the open repair, and how the Nuss repair is called "minimally invasive", in which a metal bar (or bars) is driven through both pleural cavities, passed by the width of a hair between the heart and the sternum and left there for long time, and then 2 years later the same procedure is performed in "reverse". Furthermore, he was worried, how the Nuss bars may affect the costal cartilages of the growing child?

Hebra argued that the "minimally invasive" implies achievement of correction without the large incisions and the removal of bone or cartilage, and frequent occurrence of the complications was related to early experience, so the Nuss procedure has eliminated majority of complications by refinement of the procedure.

2.5 Metal-free procedure

As described above, all institutes of the Nuss repair and almost institutes of the Ravitch repair use metal bar. Certainly, it can keep configuration of the thorax more rigidly than the other materials.

However, it has some shortcomings; 1) possibility to injure the surrounding organs by compression, 2) displacement requiring reoperation, 3) necessity of removal, 4) pain due to long time burden, 5) growth inhibition of the thorax, 6) metal allergy and 7) possibility of recurrence of depression after removal.

The bar is left at the thoracic wall during 2~4 years in the Nuss procedure, and during 6~12 months in the Ravitch procedure. The longer the duration of bar burden is, the higher the incidence of complications increases.

Accordingly, the metal-free procedures for PE have been tried in some institutes. Hayashi and Maruyama (Hayashi & Maruyama, 1992) used autologous rib with preserved anterior intercostalis branch of the internal mammary artery in 3 cases. The sternoturnover procedure has been performed in minimal cases of limited institutes (Iida et al., 2010; Ninkovic et al., 2003).

On the other hand, trials using artificial materials to support the elevated sternum have been performed, too. Lane-Smith and colleagues (Lane-Smith et al., 1994) used tubular

Dacron vascular graft, which usually 10mm in width, was sutured to the 4th or 5th ribs. Robicsek and colleagues (Robicsek et al., 2009) used Marlex sheet as a hammock, as described earlier. Although Robicsek and colleagues performed this procedure in many patients, outcome results are not shown. Länsman and colleagues (Länsman et al., 2002) tried bioabsorbable polylactide plate as a strut, but this procedure was not performed continuously.

Masaoka and colleagues (Masaoka et al., 2011) developed a new procedure without metal bar, which reconstructs the bony thorax with support of the bridge constructed by autologous costal cartilages. Core of this procedure is as follows.

1. Subperichondrial transection of abnormally deformed 3rd~7th costal cartilages at 1cm lateral to the sternum bilaterally.
2. Removal of about 1cm long deformed cartilages lateral to the cut points. The 8th cartilages are shortened by several centimeters, in order to prevent protrusion of costal arch.
3. Transverse transection of the sternum at level of the lower border of the 4th rib.
4. Ligations and transections of the bilateral aa. et vv. thoracia interna.
5. Isolation of the sternum from the mediastinal structures and pleura. At that time, attention should be paid to preservation of the cranial parts of the internal thoracic vessels.
6. Transection of 4th to 2nd intercostal muscles.
7. Transverse osteotomy on the rear table of the sternum at the 2nd rib level, and gentle fracture to sternal elevation.
8. The caudal part of the sternum is detached from the 5th to 7th intercostal muscle bundles just at the margin of the sternum.
9. The caudal part of the sternum is resected transversely in width corresponding to the 5th costal cartilage, in order to shorten the overlong sternum.
10. The 4th or 5th costal cartilage is attached to the contralateral one at midline, in somewhat tense condition. This bridge contributes as a strut supporting the sternum. Selection of the 4th or 5th costal cartilage depends on the level of the sternum having contact with the bridge, i.e., caudal part of sternum.
11. Anteriorly to the bridge, both ends of the sternum are sutured by five 1-0 absorbable threads.
12. a) In cases, in which the bridge is constructed with the 5th costal cartilage, the 3rd, 4th and 6th costal cartilages on vertebral side are trimmed up in suitable manner, and sutured to the same cartilages on sternal side by two 1-0 absorbable threads.
13. b) In cases, in which the bridge is constructed with the 4th costal cartilages, the 5th costal cartilages on vertebral side sutured to the 6th costal cartilages on sternal side. Similarly, the 6th costal cartilages on vertebral side are sutured to the 7th costal cartilages on sternal side (Fig. 21.)
14. The 7th costal cartilages are resected 2-3cm and sutured to the sternum. Thus, the bridge of the 4th or 5th cartilages supports the caudal part of the sternum and the 6th and 7th costal cartilages.
15. The separated bundles of the 2nd, 3rd, 4th intercostal muscles are sutured to the same bundles again.
16. The 6th and 7th intercostal muscles and perichondria are sutured to the reconstructed sternum.

Fig. 22. shows the resected area. This procedure was performed in 181 child patients. About 23 years follow-up revealed complication rate of 2.8% (5/181), reoperation rate of 0.5% (1/181). Mean operation time is 180.6±40.6 min, and mean blood loss is 133.6±84.8 ml. Mean hospital stay is 11.47±2.2 days. Patient can go to school 2 weeks after operation. Participation in sporting activity is allowed after 1 month, and competitive sports are resumed after 3 months.

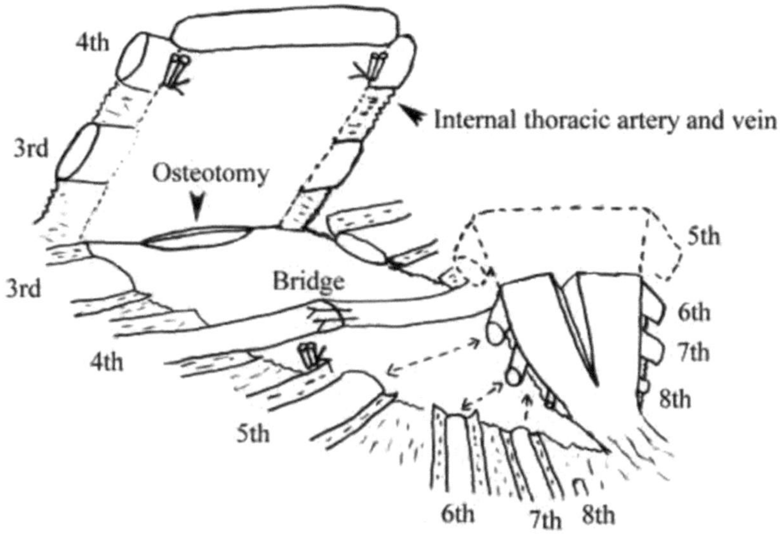

Fig. 21. Metal-free procedure (Masaoka et al., in press)
(Reprinted with permission from *Eur J Cardiothorac Surg* 2011, in press)

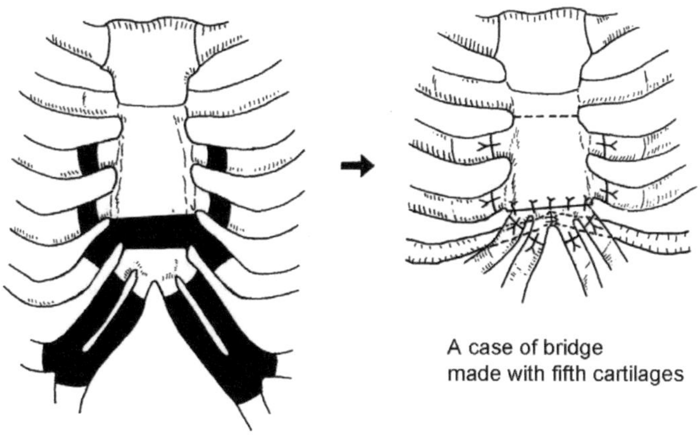

Fig. 22. Metal-free procedure.
The black area is resected.

Evaluation of correction in this operation was done by the deformity indices; Haller's, steepness, excavation volume, and asymmetry index. Table 9 shows preoperative and postoperative data. All indices improve strikingly.

Index	Preoperative	Postoperative	*P*-value
Haller's	5.547±1.835	4.090±1.410	0.0000
Steepness	0.208±0.048	0.064±0.056	0.0000
Excavation volume	0.098±0.031	0.038±0.036	0.0000
Asymmetry	1.105±0.171	1.053±0.126	0.0001

Table 9. Comparison of preoperative and postoperative indices (Masaoka et al., in print) (Reprinted with permission from *Eur J Thorac Cardiovasc Surg* 2011, in press)

The cartilages grow together with the growth of bony thorax, and continue to support sternum. The reconstructed thoracic configurations have been kept satisfactorily during 111±51.7 months after operations in 133 patients, excluding early postoperative (<3 years) and drop-out patients.

This procedure is indicated only to children (<15 years), because of malleable character of their thorax.

Longer operation time, more bleeding and longer hospital stay are shortcomings of this procedure. However, abandon of metal bar could provide benefits that would overcome these drawbacks.

3. Conclusion

Throughout the history of corrective surgery for pectus excavatum, numerous procedures have been proposed, in whom 2 procedures survived and have been performed world-wide with some modifications – Ravitch and Nuss procedure–. Almost all institutes, whether Ravitch or Nuss, use metal bar to maintain configuration of the thorax. The use of metal bar has many drawbacks, i.e., frequent complications, pain, necessity of removal of bar, growth inhibition, metal allergy and possibility of recurrence of depression after removal.

A new metal-free procedure was proposed, in order to eliminate these shortcomings. Correction of thoracic configuration by this procedure was evaluated as excellent. This procedure is recommended as a standard operation for PE of children.

4. Acknowledgement

We appreciated the careful secretarial work by Ms Mitsuko Tenpaku in preparing this manuscript.

5. References

Aydemir B, Sokullu O, Hastaoglu O, Bilgen F, Celik M, Dogusoy I. Aorta-to-right ventricular fistula due to pectus bar migration. *Thorac Cardiovasc Surg.* 2011 Feb;59(1):51-2.

Bevegard S. Postural circulatory changes at rest and during exercise in patients with funnel chest, with special reference to factors affecting the stroke volume. *Acta Med Scand.* 1962 Jun;171:695-713.

Bouchard S, Hong AR, Gilchrist BF, Kuenzler KA. Catastrophic cardiac injuries encountered during the minimally invasive repair of pectus excavatum. *Semin Pediatr Surg.* 2009 May;18(2):66-72.

Brown AL. Pectus excavatum (funnel chest) anatomic basis; surgical treatment of the incipient stage in infancy; and correction of the deformity in the fully developed stage. *J Thorac Surg*. 1939;9:164-184.

Cahill JL, Lees GM, Robertson HT. A summary of preoperative and postoperative cardiorespiratory performance in patients undergoing pectus excavatum and carinatum repair. *J Pediatr Surg*. 1984 Aug;19(4):430-3.

Castile RG, Staats BA, Westbrook PR. Symptomatic pectus deformities of the chest. *Am Rev Respir Dis*. 1982 Sep;126(3):564-8.

Creswick HA, Stacey MW, Kelly RE Jr, Gustin T, Nuss D, Harvey H, Goretsky MJ, Vasser E, Welch JC, Mitchell K, Proud VK. Family study of the inheritance of pectus excavatum. *J Pediatr Surg*. 2006 Oct;41(10):1699-703.

Eguchi T, Sasaki S, Hara F, Kondo S, Masaoka A. Natural course of thoracic deformity in pectus excavatum. *Shonika* 1993;34:61-65. (In Japanese)

Fabricius J, Davidsen HG, Hansen AT. Cardiac function in funnel chest; twenty-six patients investigated by cardiac catheterization. *Dan Med Bull*. 1957 Dec;4(8):251-7.

Fonkalsrud EW, Beanes S, Hebra A, Adamson W, Tagge E. Comparison of minimally invasive and modified Ravitch pectus excavatum repair. *J Pediatr Surg*. 2002 Mar;37(3):413-7.

Fonkalsrud EW. Open repair of pectus excavatum with minimal cartilage resection. *Ann Surg*. 2004 Aug;240(2):231-5.

Fonkalsrud EW. 912 open pectus excavatum repairs: changing trends, lessons learned: one surgeon's experience. *World J Surg*. 2009 Feb;33(2):180-90.

Haecker FM, Berberich T, Mayr J, Gambazzi F. Near-fatal bleeding after transmyocardial ventricle lesion during removal of the pectus bar after the Nuss procedure. *J Thorac Cardiovasc Surg*. 2009 Nov;138(5):1240-1.

Haller JA Jr, Kramer SS, Lietman SA. Use of CT scans in selection of patients for pectus excavatum surgery: a preliminary report. *J Pediatr Surg*. 1987 Oct;22(10):904-6.

Haller JA Jr, Scherer LR, Turner CS, Colombani PM. Evolving management of pectus excavatum based on a single institutional experience of 664 patients. *Ann Surg*. 1989 May;209(5):578-82; discussion 582-3.

Haller JA Jr, Colombani PM, Humphries CT, Azizkhan RG, Loughlin GM. Chest wall constriction after too extensive and too early operations for pectus excavatum. *Ann Thorac Surg*. 1996 Jun;61(6):1618-24; discussion 1625.

Haller JA Jr, Loughlin GM. Cardiorespiratory function is significantly improved following corrective surgery for severe pectus excavatum. Proposed treatment guidelines. *J Cardiovasc Surg (Torino)*. 2000 Feb;41(1):125-30.

Harrison MR, Curran PF, Jamshidi R, Christensen D, Bratton BJ, Fechter R, Hirose S. Magnetic Mini-Mover Procedure for pectus excavatum II: initial findings of a food and drug administration-sponsored trial. *J Pediatr Surg*. 2010 Jan;45(1):185-91; discussion 191-2.

Hayashi A, Maruyama Y. Vascularized rib strut technique for repair of pectus excavatum. *Ann Thorac Surg*. 1992 Feb;53(2):346-8.

Hu TZ, Li Y, Liu WY, Wu XD, Feng JX. Surgical treatment of pectus excavatum: 30 years 398 patients of experiences. *J Pediatr Surg*. 2008 Jul;43(7):1270-4.

Iida H, Sunazawa T, Ishida K, Doi A. Surgical repair of pectus excavatum not requiring exogenous implants in 113 patients. *Eur J Cardiothorac Surg*. 2010 Feb;37(2):316-21.

Jemielity M, Pawlak K, Piwkowski C, Dyszkiewicz W. Life-threatening aortic hemorrhage during pectus bar removal. *Ann Thorac Surg*. 2011 Feb;91(2):593-5.

Kelly RE Jr. Pectus excavatum: historical background, clinical picture, preoperative evaluation and criteria for operation. *Semin Pediatr Surg*. 2008 Aug;17(3):181-93.

Kelly RE Jr, Goretsky MJ, Obermeyer R, Kuhn MA, Redlinger R, Haney TS, Moskowitz A, Nuss D. Twenty-one years of experience with minimally invasive repair of pectus excavatum by the Nuss procedure in 1215 patients. *Ann Surg*. 2010 Dec;252(6):1072-81.

Kotzot D, Schwabegger AH. Etiology of chest wall deformities--a genetic review for the treating physician. *J Pediatr Surg*. 2009 Oct;44(10):2004-11.

Laituri CA, Garey CL, St Peter SD. Review of the technical variants in the repair of pectus excavatum. *Eur J Pediatr Surg*. 2010 Jul;20(4):217-21.

Lane-Smith DM, Gillis DA, Roy PD. Repair of pectus excavatum using a Dacron vascular graft strut. *J Pediatr Surg*. 1994 Sep;29(9):1179-82.

Länsman S, Serlo W, Linna O, Pohjonen T, Törmälä P, Waris T, Ashammakhi N. Treatment of pectus excavatum with bioabsorbable polylactide plates: preliminary results. *J Pediatr Surg*. 2002 Sep;37(9):1281-6.

Lawson ML, Mellins RB, Tabangin M, Kelly RE Jr, Croitoru DP, Goretsky MJ, Nuss D. Impact of pectus excavatum on pulmonary function before and after repair with the Nuss procedure. *J Pediatr Surg*. 2005 Jan;40(1):174-80.

Lawson ML, Mellins RB, Paulson JF, Shamberger RC, Oldham K, Azizkhan RG, Hebra AV, Nuss D, Goretsky MJ, Sharp RJ, Holcomb GW 3rd, Shim WK, Megison SM, Moss RL, Fecteau AH, Colombani PM, Moskowitz AB, Hill J, Kelly RE Jr. Increasing severity of pectus excavatum is associated with reduced pulmonary function. *J Pediatr*. 2011 Aug; 159(2):256-61.e2.

Malek MH, Fonkalsrud EW, Cooper CB. Ventilatory and cardiovascular responses to exercise in patients with pectus excavatum. *Chest*. 2003 Sep;124(3):870-82.

Masaoka A, Kondo S, Sasaki S, Hara F, Mizuno T, Yamakawa Y, Kobayashi T, Fujii Y. Thirty years experience of open repair surgery for pectus excavatum −Development of a metal-free procedure−. *Eur J Cardiovasc Surg* 2011 (in press)

Masson JK, Payne WS, Gonzalez JB. Pectus excavatum: use of preformed prosthesis for correction in the adult. Case report. *Plast Reconstr Surg*. 1970 Oct;46(4):399-402.

Michlits W, Windhofer C, Papp C. Pectus excavatum and free fasciocutaneous infragluteal flap: a new technique for the correction of congenital asymptomatic chest wall deformities in adults. *Plast Reconstr Surg*. 2009 Nov;124(5):1520-8.

Nakahara K, Ohno K, Miyoshi S, Maeda H, Monden Y, Kawashima Y. An evaluation of operative outcome in patients with funnel chest diagnosed by means of the computed tomogram. *J Thorac Cardiovasc Surg*. 1987 Apr;93(4):577-82.

Nakaoka T, Uemura S, Yano T, Nakagawa Y, Tanimoto T, Suehiro S. Does overgrowth of costal cartilage cause pectus excavatum? A study on the lengths of ribs and costal cartilages in asymmetric patients. *J Pediatr Surg*. 2009 Jul;44(7):1333-6.

Nakaoka T, Uemura S, Yoshida T, Tanimoto T, Miyake H. Overgrowth of costal cartilage is not the etiology of pectus excavatum. *J Pediatr Surg*. 2010 Oct;45(10):2015-8.

Nasr A, Fecteau A, Wales PW. Comparison of the Nuss and the Ravitch procedure for pectus excavatum repair: a meta-analysis. *J Pediatr Surg*. 2010 May;45(5):880-6.

Ninkovic M, Schwabegger A, Gardetto A, Moser-Rummer A, Rieger M, Ninkovic M, Rainer C. Free sternum turnover flap for correction of pectus excavatum deformity. *Plast Reconstr Surg*. 2003 Oct;112(5):1355-61.

Nuss D, Kelly RE Jr, Croitoru DP, Katz ME. A 10-year review of a minimally invasive technique for the correction of pectus excavatum. *J Pediatr Surg*. 1998 Apr;33(4):545-52.

Nuss D. Recent experiences with minimally invasive pectus excavatum repair "Nuss procedure". *Jpn J Thorac Cardiovasc Surg*. 2005 Jul;53(7):338-44.

Nuss D. Minimally invasive surgical repair of pectus excavatum. *Semin Pediatr Surg*. 2008 Aug;17(3):209-17.

Nuss D, Kelly RE Jr. Minimally invasive surgical correction of chest wall deformities in children (Nuss procedure). *Adv Pediatr*. 2008;55:395-410.

Park HJ, Jeong JY, Jo WM, Shin JS, Lee IS, Kim KT, Choi YH. Minimally invasive repair of pectus excavatum: a novel morphology-tailored, patient-specific approach. *J Thorac Cardiovasc Surg*. 2010 Feb;139(2):379-86.

Peterson RJ, Young WG Jr, Godwin JD, Sabiston DC Jr, Jones RH. Noninvasive assessment of exercise cardiac function before and after pectus excavatum repair. *J Thorac Cardiovasc Surg*. 1985 Aug;90(2):251-60.

Pilegaard HK, Licht PB. Early results following the Nuss operation for pectus excavatum--a single-institution experience of 383 patients. *Interact Cardiovasc Thorac Surg*. 2008 Feb;7(1):54-7.

Pilegaard HK, Licht PB. Can absorbable stabilizers be used routinely in the Nuss procedure? *Eur J Cardiothorac Surg*. 2009 Apr;35(4):561-4.

Ravitch MM. The Operative Treatment of Pectus Excavatum. *Ann Surg*. 1949 Apr;129(4):429-44.

Ravitch MM. Technical problems in the operative correction of pectus excavatum. *Ann Surg*. 1965 Jul;162:29-33.

Robicsek F. Surgical treatment of pectus excavatum. *Chest Surg Clin N Am*. 2000 May;10(2):277-96.

Robicsek F, Watts LT, Fokin AA. Surgical repair of pectus excavatum and carinatum. *Semin Thorac Cardiovasc Surg*. 2009 Spring;21(1):64-75.

Robicsek F, Hebra A. To Nuss or not to Nuss? Two opposing views. *Semin Thorac Cardiovasc Surg*. 2009 Spring;21(1):85-8.

Saleh RS, Finn JP, Fenchel M, Moghadam AN, Krishnam M, Abrazado M, Ton A, Habibi R, Fonkalsrud EW, Cooper CB. Cardiovascular magnetic resonance in patients with pectus excavatum compared with normal controls. *J Cardiovasc Magn Reson*. 2010 Dec 13;12:73.

Saxena AK, Castellani C, Höllwarth ME. Surgical aspects of thoracoscopy and efficacy of right thoracoscopy in minimally invasive repair of pectus excavatum. *J Thorac Cardiovasc Surg*. 2007 May;133(5):1201-5.

Saxena AK, Willital GH. Valuable lessons from two decades of pectus repair with the Willital-Hegemann procedure. *J Thorac Cardiovasc Surg*. 2007 Oct;134(4):871-6.

Schier F, Bahr M, Klobe E. The vacuum chest wall lifter: an innovative, nonsurgical addition to the management of pectus excavatum. *J Pediatr Surg*. 2005 Mar;40(3):496-500.

Shamberger RC, Welch KJ, Sanders SP. Mitral valve prolapse associated with pectus excavatum. *J Pediatr*. 1987 Sep;111(3):404-7.

Shamberger RC, Welch KJ. Cardiopulmonary function in pectus excavatum. *Surg Gynecol Obstet*. 1988 Apr;166(4):383-91.

Snel BJ, Spronk CA, Werker PM, van der Lei B. Pectus excavatum reconstruction with silicone implants: long-term results and a review of the English-language literature. *Ann Plast Surg*. 2009 Feb;62(2):205-9.

Sweet RH. Pectus excavatum: Report of two cases successfully operated upon. *Ann Surg*. 1944 Jun;119(6):922-34.

Wada J, Ikeda T, Iwa T, Ikeda K. Sternoturnover: An advanced new surgical method to correct funnel chest deformity. *J Int Coll Surg*. 1965 Jul;44:69-76.

10

Surgical Management of Primary Upper Limb Hyperhidrosis – A Review

Geesche Somuncuoğlu
Department of Thoracic Surgery, Schillerhoehe Hospital, Gerlingen, Germany

1. Introduction

Sweating is a physiological and vital condition to control thermoregulation of the skin (Rajesh et al., 2003). Hyperhidrosis is defined as an excess of sweating beyond the amount needed to cool down elevated body temperature (Kreyden & Burg, 2000).

Primary hyperhidrosis as a disease seems trivial to general public because of its falsely perceived rarity (Eisenach et al., 2005). Furthermore, although not life-threatening (Reisfeld et al., 2002), it is evident that it can lead to severe psychologic, social and occupational dysfunction (Shargall et al., 2008). Nowadays primary hyperhidrosis is being recognized increasingly and its treatment options are gaining widespread attention (Eisenach et al., 2005). Although medical therapies have been the main treatment options for many years, surgical interventions have recently been proven to be an important therapeutic alternative. This shift has corresponded with the evolution of minimally invasive surgical techniques (Grondin, 2008), the main topic of this issue.

2. Classification and causes of hyperhidrosis

Hyperhidrosis can be classified either by pathogenesis in a primary (idiopathic) and a secondary (symptomatic) form or by localisation and extension in a localised and a generalised form (Fig. 1).

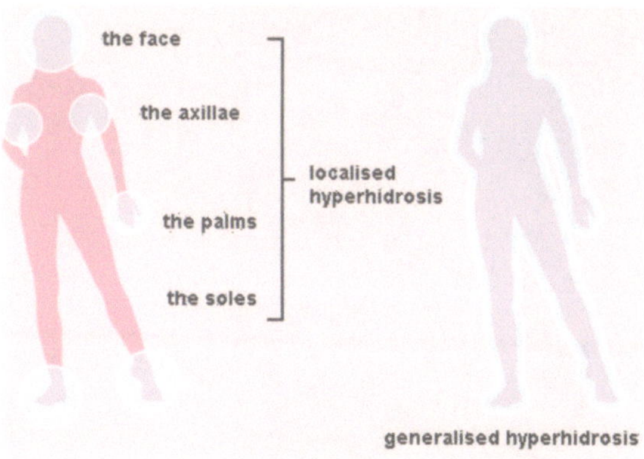

Fig. 1. Classification of hyperhidrosis by localisation and extension

Secondary hyperhidrosis appears to be more generalised and is triggered by an underlying disease process like infectious, endocrine or neurologic disorders (Eisenach et al., 2005; Kreyden & Burg, 2000; Shargall et al., 2008) (Table 1). Therapy of choice is treating the basic disease.

Category	Disorders
Infectious	Influenza, tuberculosis,
Endocrine	Hyperthyroidism, diabetes, menopause, obesity
Malignancy	Leukemia, lymphoma
Neurologic	Spinal cord injury, parkinson´s disease
Drugs	Corticosteroids, antibiotics, antidepressants
Psychogenic	Panic disorder, stress, pain

Table 1. Causes of secondary hyperhidrosis

The cause of primary hyperhidrosis, mostly affecting local parts of the body, is still unknown (Duarte & Kux, 2008). There seems to be a genetic predisposition in autosomal dominant fashion with variable penetrance, in 25-50% of cases a positive family history can be detected (Eisenach et al., 2005). The disease tends to begin in early childhood and becomes worse at puberty. It affects males and females equally (Shargall et al, 2008). The exact pathophysiology also remains unknown. There appears to be an overactive response of the eccrine glands to both heat and emotional stimuli, mediated through the sympathetic nervous system (Lee et al., 1999; Shargall et al., 2008) (Fig. 2). Therefore mostly affected areas are where eccrine glands are concentrated like the palms, the axillae, the face and the soles. Nearly half of diseased people suffer from an axillary manifestation (Schlereth et al., 2009). Overall the estimated prevalence of primary hyperhidrosis might be as high as 0,6-1% of the Western population, 2,8% of the US population and even 3% of the Asian population. Asia is also considered as an endemic area (Eisenach et al., 2005).

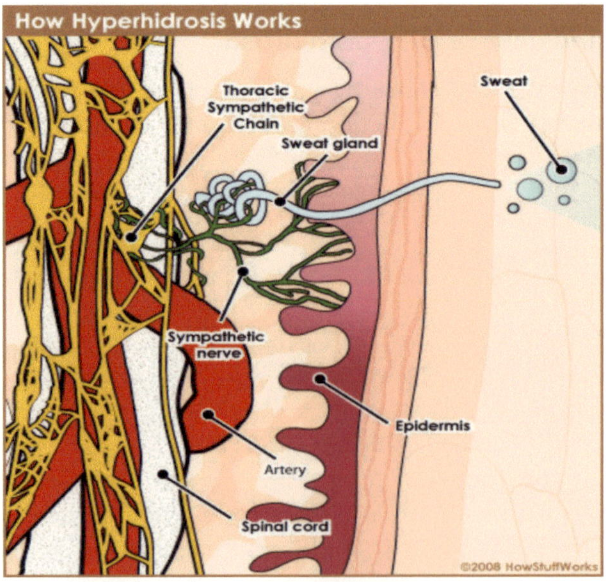

Fig. 2. Innervation of the eccrine glands by the sympathetic nervous system

3. Diagnosis and patient evaluation

A substantial part of the diagnosis of hyperhidrosis can be achieved by obtaining a patients history, followed by a physical examination. Once secondary causes of hyperhidrosis have been ruled out by additional laboratory tests, dermatologists have several techniques to stratify the severity of sweating like gravimetric testing, the Minor starch-iodine test and the ninhydrin test. Quality-of-life assessments may support the categorization of primary hyperhidrosis as a serious medical condition (Eisenach et al., 2005; Solish et al., 2008).

4. Treatment of primary hyperhidrosis

Primary hyperhidrosis is treated symptomatically. There are lots of therapeutic options classified in nonsurgical and surgical treatment. Generally, therapy should be particular to each individual patient and chosen based on disease location, disease severity and expectations for improvement (Gee & Yamauchi, 2008). Dermatologists suggest following a graduated scheme like the guidelines elaborated by the German Society of Dermatology (Wörle et al, 2007).

4.1 Nonsurgical treatment

The initial treatment for primary hyperhidrosis should always be nonsurgical. It includes topical treatments such as aluminium chloride, iontophoresis, oral medications such as anticholinergics and botulinum toxine (Reisfeld & Berliner, 2008). Unfortunately, a lot of cases do not respond sufficiently to these treatment regimes and effects are usually transient (T.S. Lin, 2001). Nonsurgical therapy options are mostly practised by dermatologists, they are listed below (Table 2).

Therapy option	Example	Indication	Mechanism/Specifics
Psycho-vegetative influence	Autogenic training, hypnosis, psychotherapy	Generalised adjuvant	Psychovegetative damping avoids activation of the reduced threshold of the eccrine glands
Medications: - Topical	Antiperspirants (aluminium chloride hexahydrate)	Axillary	Blocking the lumen of the eccrine duct
- Systemic	Anticholinergics, psychotropics, betablockers	Generalised	Anticholinergic, chemical psychovegetative damping Caution: Side effects
Physical therapy	Iontophoresis	Palmar plantar	Exact mechanism unknown: Ionic current causes a temporary block of the eccrine duct
Botulinum toxin (BTX)	Local intradermal injection	Axillary palmar plantar	Chemical block: Inhibits the release of acetylcholine at the cholinergic synapse Caution: Effect decreases within 6 months

Table 2. Nonsurgical therapy options

4.2 Surgical treatment

Surgery should be reserved to severe hyperhidrosis and should only be contemplated when less invasive nonsurgical options have failed to provide adequate treatment (Naunheim, 2000). It includes local surgical axillary procedures such as excision, curettage or liposuction of the sweat glands and thoracoscopic sympathectomy (Baumgartner, 2008) (Table 3).

Therapy option	Procedure	Indication	Specifics
Excision of sweat glands (En-bloc-resection of dermis and subcutis)	Radical excision: several techniques with plastic skin suture	Axillary therapy-refractory	Caution: Scarring, contractures
Subcutaneous Excision of sweat glands (limited resection via tiny incisions)	- Curettage - Liposuction	Axillary therapy-refractory	Caution: Hematoma, infection
Sympathetic block	Thoracoscopic sympathectomy: Detailed description follows below		

Table 3. Surgical therapy options

4.2.1 Thoracoscopic sympathectomy

The rationale for sympathectomy in the management of primary hyperhidrosis is based on interrupting the transmission of impulses from the sympathetic nervous system to the eccrine sweat glands (Reisfeld et al., 2002). Object of surgery is the sympathetic trunk, a series of ganglia which are located in a line lateral and parallel to the vertebral bodies of the spinal column. The thoracic portion of the sympathetic trunk contains 12 ganglia, where the input is switched over to the effector (Naunheim, 2000). Sweat glands are innervated segmentally, that means a certain ganglion level can be ascribed to a certain localisation of hyperhidrosis (C.C. Lin & Telaranta, 2001). During the surgical procedure on the sympathetic trunk, the ganglia, lying in front of the heads of the ribs and covered by a thin layer of parietal pleura, are readily apparent with the lung retracted caudaly (Shargall et al., 2008) (Fig. 3).

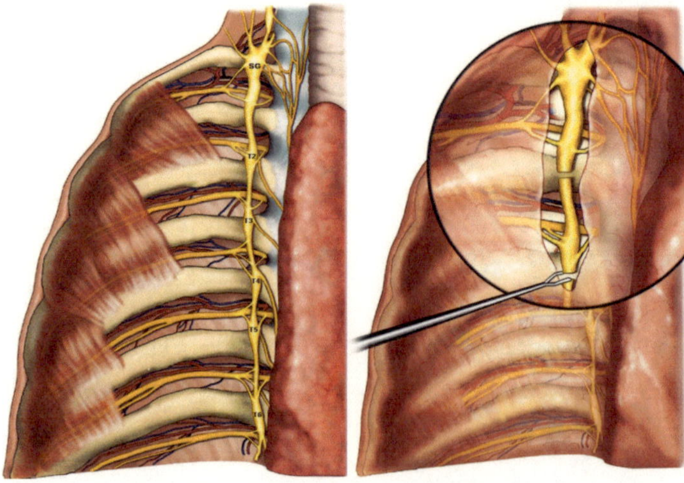

Fig. 3. Anatomy of the sympathetic trunk and applied surgical procedure

4.2.1.1 Surgical approaches and techniques

The first open surgical approaches occurred nearly a century ago (Baumgartner, 2008). These aggressive approaches were associated with significant patient morbidity and a protracted recovery period (Dewey et al., 2006). They often required a moderate to large sized incision in the chest which demanded cutting muscles and separating ribs to expose the sympathetic chain (Naunheim, 2000). Over the past decade, endoscopic sympathectomy, requiring three or two small thoracal incisions, replaced open procedures (Fig. 4). Today magnification and high resolution, attained with videoassisted thoracoscopic surgery, allows a detailed representation of anatomical structures which reduces risk of complications (Zacherl et al., 1999) (Fig. 5). Meanwhile further advances, utilizing microinstrumentation called needlescopic surgery or using a uniportal access, enable procedures done on an outpatient basis with minimal risk of surgical trauma and excellent cosmetic results (Dewey et al., 2006; Lee et al., 2000).

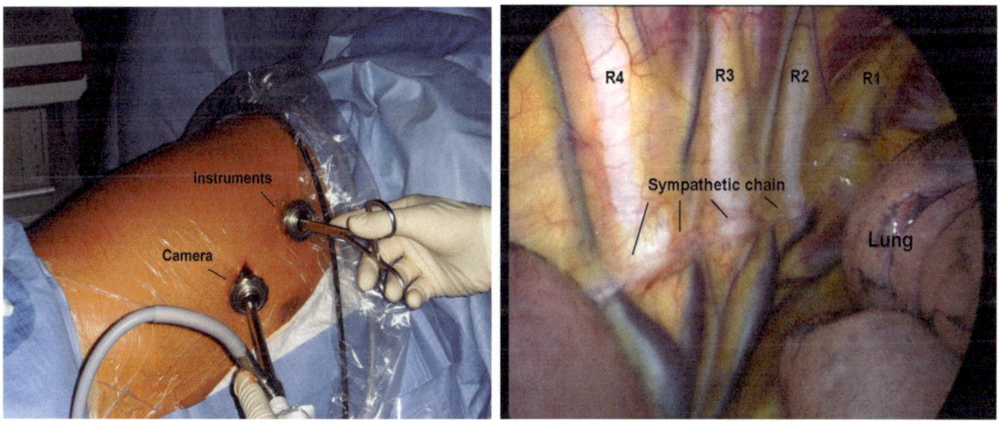

(a) (b)

Fig. 4. (a) Example for a biportal access. (b) View via videothoracoscope (R=rib)

A short overview of the historical development of sympathetic surgery and its application as to primary hyperhidrosis is listed in the table below (Table 4).

Year	History
1889,1896	First open cervical sympathectomies for epilepsy by Alexander and Ionnesco
1920	First open thoracal sympathectomies for hyperhidrosis by Kotzareff
1942	First thoracoscopic sympathectomies for different pathologies by Hughes
1944	Further thoracoscopic sympathectomies for different pathologies by Goetz and Marr
1954	Further thoracoscopic sympathectomies for different pathologies by Kux and Wittmoser
1992	First videoassisted thoracoscopic surgery for posttraumatic pain syndrome by Chandler
1993	Further videoassisted thoracoscopic surgery for hyperhidrosis by Claes and Drott presented at the First International Symposium on Thoracoscopic Sympathectomy, Boras, Sweden

Table 4. Milestones in the history of sympathetic surgery and the therapy of hyperhidrosis

Today much controversy and unanswered questions remain concerning the ideal thoracoscopic sympathetic operation (Baumgartner, 2008). What is the best technique of intervention: Should the sympathetic chain or ganglion be resected (sympathectomy), transected (sympathicotomy) or should only the rami communicantes be divided (selective sympathicotomy or ramicotomy)? Sympathectomy represents an aggressive approach, inducing a high rate of compensatory sweating (CS) (Lee et al., 1999). This unrequested side effect, specified below, could be considerably reduced by the nowadays commonly used sympathicotomy (Fig. 6). Another decrease of CS could be ascribed to ramicotomy, a limited technique first described by Wittmoser (Wittmoser, 1992) (Fig. 7). Due to the high rate of recurrence of preoperative symptoms, this approach is actually no longer used (Gossot et al., 2003).

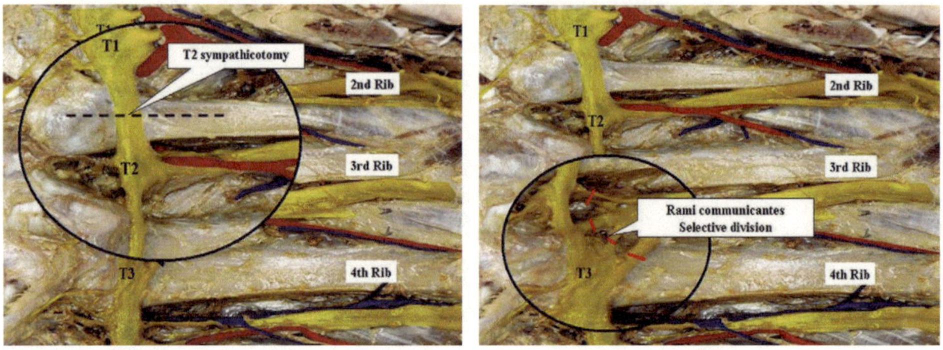

(a) (b)

Fig. 5. (a) Sympathicotomy. (b) Ramicotomy

Which instrument should be utilised to dissect the sympathetic trunk: Harmonic scalpel, ultrasonic, laser or thermocoagulation? All of them yield similar results (Inan et al., 2008), but due to electrocautery, care should be exercised to avoid heat damage to the adjoining structures (Krasna, 2008). Another recently upcoming procedure is the clamping method, published by Lin and colleagues in 1998 (C.C. Lin et al., 1998) with the potential advantage of reversibility in those patients unhappy with the outcome (Reisfeld et al., 2002) (Fig. 6). But so far, there have been only a mere handful of such reversals done with the surgical clamping technique and these reported reversals met with varied success (Kwong et al., 2008). Neural cell death is supposed to be responsible, when the clips are not removed relatively soon postoperatively (Dewey et al., 2006).

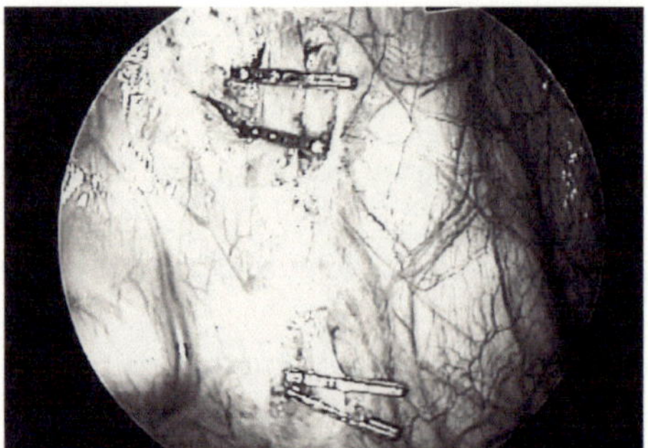

Fig. 6. Clamping method with two clips above and below the third rib

At which level sympathectomy should be performed and what is the correct extent of the procedure? So far, there is no consensus among surgeons, but there seems to be a correlation to postoperative effect and occurrence of side effects. During a long period of time extensive resections from level T2 to T5 were commonly performed (Dewey et al., 2006; T.S. Lin & Fang, 1999; Schmidt et al., 2006). But investigators demonstrated: reducing the extent of sympathectomy leads to a lower incidence of CS (Dumont, 2008). Today surgeons limit the extent of sympathectomy, there is a trend to two-level to the point of single-level surgery. The elected level of intervention is conditioned on the segmentally innervated localisation of hyperhidrosis and is shown in Table 5, based on a review of Krasna in 2008 (Krasna, 2008) (Table 5).

Localisation	Level of intervention
Facial	T2
Palmar	T2, T3
Axillary	T3, T4
Plantar	>T4 (obsolete) L2, L3 (today via endoscopic lumbar extraperitoneal sympathectomy)

Table 5. Localisation of primary hyperhidrosis and related level of intervention

T1 sympathectomy for facial hyperhidrosis is abandoned long time ago due to high risk of Horner´s syndrome. For some time level of choice is T2 ganglia. Although T2 is also seen as centre point of neurologic impulse transmission through the brachial plexus to the hand (Hsia et al. 1999), some investigators suggest preparing lower levels like T3 (Dewey et al. 2006; Kwong et al., 2008; X. Li et al., 2008), because T2 is close to stellate ganglion with a risk of Horner´s Syndrome non-negligible and the fact that higher levels can increase rate of CS (Schmidt et al., 2006). T4 still remains level of choice for axillary hyerphidrosis (Lee et al. 1999; Licht et al. 2005). Isolated plantar hyperhidrosis occurs rarely but rather in combination with palmar or axillary type. As combined manifestation it is often treated by sympathectomy for upper limb hyperhidrosis and leads in 85% of cases to an improvement of plantar symptoms, shown by Reisfeld and colleagues (Reisfeld et al., 2002). Causes of improvement are unknown. Treating plantar hyperhidrosis by preparing lower thoracic levels is no longer practised (Kwong et al., 2008). Today isolated plantar hyperhidrosis is treated at level L2 and L3 by endoscopic lumbar sympathectomy (Loureiro et al., 2008).

4.2.1.2 Complications and side effects

Complications in hyperhidrosis surgery are rare and exceptional. Some can be avoided by experience or by technical improvement of the surgeon, others are unforeseeable. However any complications are less acceptable than for other sorts of thoracic operations because sympathectomy is a functional surgery for young patients in good health (Dumont, 2008).

In 2004 Ojimba and Cameron did a Medline search using the term thoracoscopic sympathectomy and analysed all publications for reported complications (Ojimba & Cameron, 2004) (Table 6): No death has ever been reported in any published series but there are anecdotal reports of nine deaths following thoracoscopic sympathectomy. Five patients died from excessive haemorrhage, three due to incidents of narcosis and one death remained unexplained. Nevertheless, mortality associated with thoracoscopic sympathectomy is a rare condition compared to the high number of surgical procedures. The most common complication is pneumothorax. Up to 75% of patients have some residual gas or air in the thorax at the end of procedure, mostly resolving spontaneously. A temporary tube drainage is only required in 0,4-2,3% of cases, usually either after direct trauma to the lung at the time of trocar insertion, after dissolving adhesions or after rupture of a bulla as a consequence of anaesthesia, if high inflation pressures are used. Apart from the deaths mentioned above, reports of serious intraoperative bleeding are rare. Bleeding usually arises from disrupted intercostal veins or bleeding at the site of trocar insertion. The highest rate of significant bleeding with an incidence of 5,3% was reported by Gossot and colleagues. They also described one laceration of the subclavian artery demanding an immediate thoracotomy (Gossot et al., 2001). Horner´s Syndrome is the mostly feared complication. Occurred by irritation or damage to the stellate ganglion T1, it causes miosis, ptosis and enophthalmus on the same side of the face. Symptoms are often transient and decrease within weeks or months, but can also persist (Kaya et al., 2003). Since introduction of the videothoracoscope, which allows a better view, rate of postoperative Horner´s Syndrome could be significantly reduced (Zacherl et al., 1999). However it is mentioned in almost all series. Gossot and colleagues found three main causes: damage by a direct or indirect current diffusion using diathermy, by excessive traction on the nerve during dissection or misdetermination of the ribs by the surgeon (Gossot et al., 2001). Pain in the form of intercostal neuralgia with dysesthesia at the site of trocar insertion is rarely documented but more frequent than generally recognized. Many centres perform short-stay surgery that may lead to underestimation of pain results. In most series pain resolves within months, but Walles and colleagues could detect a persistence for years (Walles et al., 2008). Further unfrequent complications are wound infection, pneumonia, chylothorax arising from laceration of an accessory thoracic duct (Gossot, 1996), rhinitis caused by increased parasympathetic stimulation of nasal mucosa (Herbst et al., 1994) and cardiopulmonary modification. The latter is recently paid particular attention: In a case report in 2009 O´Connor and colleagues presented a patient with postoperative asystole. After successful resuscitation, permanent bradycardia required a pacemaker treatment (O´Connor et al., 2009). Surveys including pre-, peri- and postoperative measurements of cardiopulmonary function presented: the decreased activity of sympathetic nervous system after sympathectomy is comparable to the effect of a beta-blocker. It reduces heart rate and worsens pulmonary function. But the clinical importance of these findings was not significant (Vigil et al., 2005). However patients suffering from vasovagale syncope or high performance athletes should be advised of possible bradycardia and also asthmatics should be informed about potential deterioration of obstructive lung disease.

More frequently reported complications	Less frequently reported complications
Pneumothorax	Wound infection
Bleeding	Pneumonia
Horner´s Syndrome	Chylothorax
Pain and Dysesthesia	Rhinitis
	Cardiopulmonary modification

Table 6. Overview of possible complications caused by thoracoscopic sympathectomy

Side effects are almost constant and unavoidable. They occur in nearly all series of surgery and therefore they are main topic of numerous articles (Dumont, 2008).

Compensatory sweating (CS) represents the most common side effect. It is defined as a postoperative increased sweating in body regions unaffected by sympathectomy (Lyra et al., 2008) (Fig. 7). The exact mechanism remains poorly understood. It is speculated that a greater amount of sweating elsewhere in the body compensates for the lack of sweating in the treated body area in order to maintain sweating balance of the whole body in a thermoregulatory way (Licht & Pilegaard, 2004). In 2008 Lyra and colleagues tried to study the exact pathogenesis and assumed that sympathetic block causes a dysfunction of control loop with lack of negative feedback to the hypothalamus resulting in CS (Lyra et al., 2008).

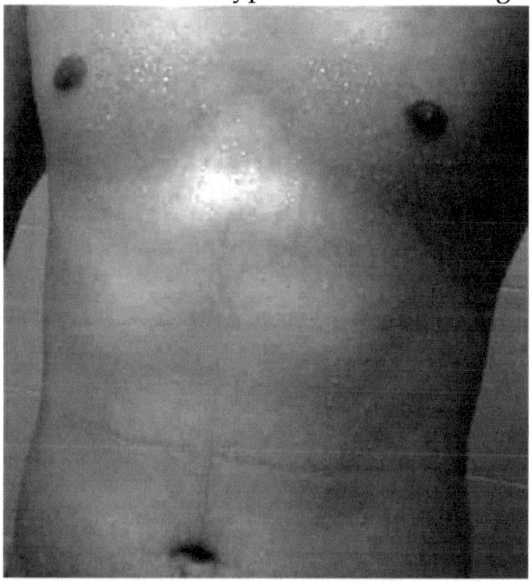

Fig. 7. Patient suffering from compensatory sweating of the thoracic and abdominal parts

The published rates of CS vary widely from 1,2-90% (Dumont, 2008): On the one hand evaluating of CS is subjective and varies according to the patient (Leão et al. 2003). On the other hand most authors do not quantify a severity code. Some investigators only report on patients who have severe CS. They believe that almost all patients develop mild CS after sympathectomy (Ueyama et al., 2004). But also climate plays a decisive role (Lyra et al., 2008). High rates of CS are mostly found in studies of countries with warmer temperatures and humid weather (X. Li et al., 2008). Surgical technique also seems to influence the risk of CS: The lower the level of division and the smaller the extent of sympathectomy, the lower the incidence of CS (Dewey et al., 2006). Treatment options for severe CS are limited: Some investigators try local injection of botulinum toxine in areas where CS is the most severe (Bechara et al., 2006), others use the clamping method with moderate success. At the end of the nineties, Telaranta successfully performed reconstruction with nerve graft by open thoracotomy for a patient suffering from severe CS (Telaranta, 1998). But it is an individual case and a complex procedure. It should be able to avoid CS, because severity does not change over time in 70% of cases (Dumont, 2008). In Taiwan patients suffering from serious CS have already formed a support group based on an internet discussion forum to request the government to take this problem seriously (Hsu & Y.C. Li, 2005). Therefore surgeons are searching for preoperative measurements to determinate postsympathectomy CS. In 2008 Miller and colleagues developed a new technique of a temporary thoracoscopic sympathetic block of the nerve with a local anesthetic that can hopefully predict severity of postoperative CS (Miller & Force, 2008).

Gustatory sweating (GS) is defined as facial sweating when eating certain foods particularly spicy or acidic food (Licht & Pilegaard, 2006) (Fig. 8). This phenomenon has no real explanation, the pathophysiology may be quite complex (Licht et al., 2005). GS is less commonly reported than CS. The reported incidence of GS varies considerably from 0-38% (Dumont, 2008). Except one study published by Licht and Pilegaard in 2006, which analyses the relation between extent of sympathectomy, primary localisation of hyperhidrosis and the incidence of GS (Licht & Pilegaard, 2006), there are only a few investigators dealing with this issue. This occurrence is probably not estimated as very troublesome, both by surgeons and by patients. Furthermore triggers can be easily avoided by patients. Thus treatment options for GS including topical or systemic medications and the injection of botulinumtoxine are rarely performed (Eckardt & Kuettner, 2003).

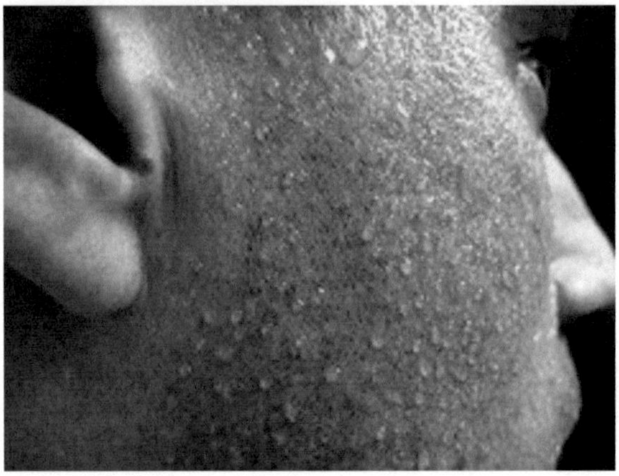

Fig. 8. Patient suffering from gustatory sweating

Due to unforeseeable and unacceptable complications and unavoidable side effects, careful patient selection is important for surgery. Patients should be fully informed before they decide on surgical treatment (Dumont, 2008).

4.2.1.3 Postoperative results and patient satisfaction

Literature suggests: Endoscopic thoracic sympathectomy is a safe and effective therapeutic strategy in patients suffering from severe primary hyperhidrosis with excellent results and high rates of patient satisfaction (Henteleff & Kalavrouziotis, 2008).

Postoperative results seem to depend more on severity and primary localisation of hyperhidrosis than on surgical technique: Best results can be achieved in patients with severe palmar hyperhidrosis (Baumgartner & Konecny, 2007). Patients with isolated axillary hyperhidrosis do not benefit sufficiently from sympathectomy (Gossot et al., 2003; Herbst et al., 1994). One possible explanation for the lower success rate may be that there is a combination of eccrine and apocrine sweat glands in the axilla. The eccrine sweat glands are innervated by sympathetic fibres, but the apocrine glands respond primarily to epinephrine. They are not blocked by sympathectomy and continue to function (Licht et al., 2005; Reisfeld et al., 2002). Therefore local surgical axillary procedures should be recommended as first-line therapy. As already mentioned, isolated plantar hyperhidrosis should be treated by endoscopic lumbar extraperitoneal sympathectomy. Individual reports with positive experiences already exist (Wörle et al., 2007). Also patients with facial hyperhidrosis or blushing do not universally and overwhelmingly benefit by sympathectomy., a case-by-case evaluation is required (Baumgartner, 2008). But patients with severe hyperhidrosis presenting for surgery mostly suffer from combined site hyperhidrosis (Eisenach et al., 2005). Reisfeld requests to establish indication for surgical therapy carefully: Thoracoscopic sympathectomy should only be performed in patients with severe palmar hyperhidrosis, other localisations should only be treated that way if combined with palmar site (Reisfeld et al., 2002).

Short-term studies on sympathectomy can be detected frequently, they continuously present great outcome depending on primary localisation. But unsatisfactory immediate results can occasionally be detected (de Campos et al., 2003). Causes for persistent postoperative sweating are inadequate knowledge and orientation of the surgeon or unrecognised variances of anatomic structures (D.H. Kim et al., 2005; Reisfeld et al., 2002; Yoon et al., 1999) including Kuntz nerve, a communicating sympathetic ramus crossing the second rib (Chung et al., 2002) (Fig. 9). Therefore some authors recommend extension of the sympathectomy line to about three or five centimetres lateral to the sympathetic chain by coagulating the surface of the corresponding rib, a method first described by Linder and colleagues in 1994 (Linder et al., 1994). Adequacy of sympathectomy is also tried to be detected by perioperative use of monitoring device like measuring skin surface temperature or plethysmographic blood flow (Lee et al., 1999; Yoon et al., 1999).

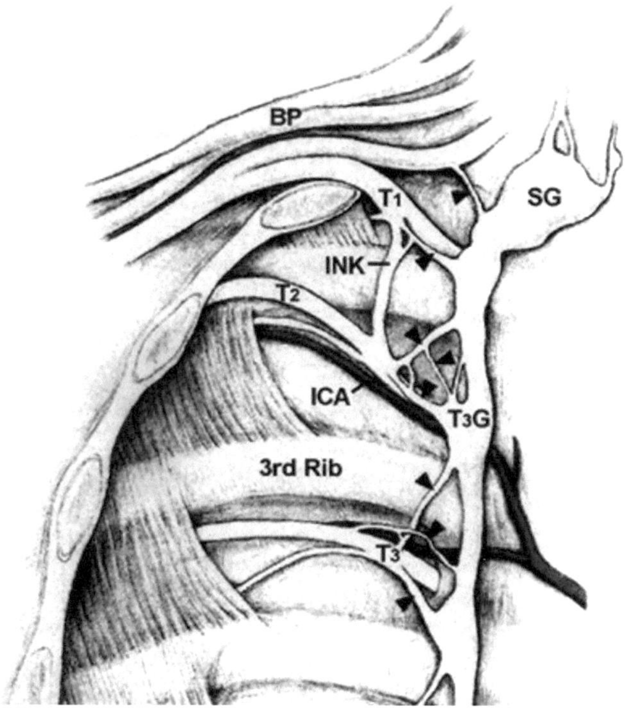

Fig. 9. Anatomy of Kuntz nerve (INK= intrathoracic nerve of Kuntz) and rami communicantes (arrowheads)

Long-term outcomes of more than 10 years are rarely reported (Zacherl et al., 1998). Investigations show that unfortunately results of sympathectomy deteriorate with time (T.S. Lin & Fang, 1999; Walles et al., 2008). This recurrent postoperative sweating may be due to local nerve regeneration but has not yet been proven (Lee et al., 1999).

Today some surgeons offer redo-operations in cause of persistent or recurrent postoperative sweating, also called re-sympathectomies. Usually these procedures can be reperformed by videothoracoscopy, severe pleural adhesions requiring thoracotomy are rarely documented (D.H. Kim et al., 2005; T.S. Lin, 2001). However there is a lack of long-term results too.
Lots of investigators use patient satisfaction as a common parameter to describe overall effectiveness of sympathectomy. Some studies reveal that patient dissatisfaction is primarily associated with persistence or recurrence of preoperative symptoms and to a lesser extent with incidence of side effects (Kwong et al., 2005; Walles et al., 2008). But assessment of surgical result using the conventional method patient satisfaction is imprecise and inaccurate (Leão et al. 2003). Main problem in requesting patient satisfaction, mostly based on patients self-report in questionnaires postoperatively, is subjectivity (Shargall et al., 2008). In some series several quality-of-life measures for assessment of improvements in daily life after treatment of hyperhidrosis are already used to get a more objective point of view (de Campos et al., 2003; Tetteh et al., 2009) (Table 7). In combination with quantitative measurements, which are often not practicable in the clinical setting, a precise evaluation of the effectiveness of sympathectomy would be possible (Cetindag et al., 2008).

General tools	Specific hyperhidrosis tools
- Illness Intrusive Rating Scale (IIRS) - Medical Outcomes Trust Short Form 12 or 36 (SF-12 or SF-36) - State-Trait Anxiety Inventory (STAI) - Symptom Distress Scale (SDS) - Dermatology Life Quality Index (DLQI)	- Hyperhidrosis Impact Questionnaire (HHIQ) - Hyperhidrosis Disease Severity Scale (HDSS)

Table 7. Several tools used for Quality-of-life assessment

5. Conclusion

In literature database hundreds of citations can be identified concerning treatment of primary upper limb hyperhidrosis by thoracic sympathectomy and nearly all investigators suggest that patients can significantly benefit from this procedure.
But fundamental limitations arise: the great majority of currently available studies are retrospective single-centre series. The heterogeneity of study population, the inconsistent definition and terminology of the word sympathectomy, the variety of surgical techniques with the optimal procedure remaining elusive and the lack of uniform measures at both the exposure and outcome levels make comparison and generalisability of these series quite impossible. In future, in addition to standardization, both long-term studies with large numbers of patients and multicentre randomised controlled trials are mandatory to clearly define the role of sympathectomy in treatment of primary hyperhidrosis (Henteleff & Kalavrouziotis, 2008).

6. References

Baumgartner, F. & Konecny, J. (2007). Compensatory hyperhidrosis after sympathectomy: level of resection versus location of hyperhidrosis. *The Annals of Thoracic Surgery*, Vol.84, No.4, (October 2007), pp.1422

Baumgartner, F.J. (2008). Surgical approaches and techniques in the management of severe hyperhidrosis. Review. *Thoracic Surgery Clinics,* Vol.18, No.2, (May 2008), pp. 167-81

Bechara, F.G.; Sand, M., Moussa, G., Sand, D., Altmeyer, P., Hoffmann, K. & Schmidt, J. (2006). Treatment of unilateral compensatory sweating after endoscopical thoracic sympathectomy for general hyperhidrosis with botulinum toxin A. *Dermatologic Surgery,* Vol.32, No.5, (May 2006), pp. 745-48

Cetindag, I.B.; Boley, T.M., Webb, K.N. & Hazelrigg, S.R. (2008). Long-term results and quality-of-life measures in the management of hyperhidrosis. *Thoracic Surgery Clinics,* Vol.18, No.2, (May 2008), pp. 217-22

Chung, I.H.; Oh, C.S., Koh, K.S., Kim, H.J., Paik, H.C. & Lee, D.Y. (2002). Anatomic variations of the T2 nerve root (including the nerve of Kuntz) and their implications of sympathectomy. *Journal of Thoracic and Cardiovascular Surgery,* Vol.123, No.3, (March 2002), pp. 498-501

de Campos, J.R.; Kauffman, P., Werebe Ede, C., Andrade Filho, L.O., Kusniek, S., Wolosker, N. & Jatene, F.B. (2003). Quality of life, before and after thoracic sympathectomy: report on 378 operated patients. *The Annals of Thoracic Surgery,* Vol.76, No.3, (September 2003), pp. 886-91

Dewey, T.M.; Herbert, M.A., Hill, S.L., Prince, S.L. & Mack, M.J. (2006). One-year follow-up after thoracoscopic sympathectomy for hyperhidrosis: outcomes and consequences. *The Annals of Thoracic Surgery,* Vol.81, No.4, (April 2006), pp. 1227-32

Duarte, J.B. & Kux, P. (1998). Improvements in video-endoscopic sympathicotomy for the treatment of palmar, axillary, facial, and palmar-plantar hyperhidrosis. *European Journal of Surgery,* Supplements 580, (1998), pp. 9-11

Dumont, P. (2008). Side effects and complications of surgery for hyperhidrosis. Review. *Thoracic Surgery Clinics,* Vol.18, No.2 (May 2008), pp. 193-207

Eckardt, A. & Kuettner, C. (2003). Treatment of gustatory sweating (Frey's syndrome) with botulinum toxin A. *Head & Neck,* Vol. 25, No.8, (August 2003), pp. 624-28

Eisenach, J.H.; Atkinson, J.L. & Fealey, R.D. (2005). Hyperhidrosis: evolving therapies for a well-established phenomenon. Review. *Mayo Clinical Proceedings,* Vol. 80, No.5, (May 2005), pp. 657-66

Gee, S. & Yamauchi, P.S. (2008). Nonsurgical management of hyperhidrosis. *Thoracic Surgery Clinics,* Vol.18, No.2 (May 2008), pp. 141-55

Gossot, D. (1996). Chylothorax after endoscopic thoracic sympathectomy. Case Report. *Surgical Endoscopy,* Vol.10, No.9 (September 1996), pp. 949

Gossot, D.; Kabiri, H., Caliandro, R., Debrosse, D., Girard, P. & Grunenwald, D. (2001).Early complications of thoracic endoscopic sympathectomy: a prospective study of 940 procedures. *The Annals of Thoracic Surgery,* Vol.71, No.4, (April 2001), pp. 1116-19

Gossot, D.; Galetta, D., Pascal, A., Debrosse, D., Caliandro, R., Girard, P., Stern, J.B. & Grunenwald, D. (2003). Long-term results of endoscopic thoracic sympathectomy for upper limb hyperhidrosis. *The Annals of Thoracic Surgery,* Vol.75, No.4, (April 2003), pp. 1075-79

Grondin, S.C. (2008). Hyperhidrosis. Preface. *Thoracic Surgery Clinics,* Vol.18, No.2, (May 2008), pp. ix-x

Henteleff, H.J. & Kalavrouziotis, D. (2008). Evidence-based review of the surgical management of hyperhidrosis. *Thoracic Surgery Clinics*, Vol.18, No.2, (May 2008), pp. 209-16

Herbst, F.; Plas, E.G., Függer, R. & Fritsch, A. (1994). Endoscopic thoracic sympathectomy for primary hyperhidrosis of the upper limbs. A critical analysis and long-term results of 480 operations. *Annals of Surgery*, Vol.220, No.1, (July 1994), pp. 86-90

Hsu, M.H.; Li, Y.C. (2005). Compensatory sweating after thoracoscopic sympathectomy deserves more attention. *The Annals of Thoracic Surgery*, Vol.80, No.3, (September 2005), pp. 1160, author reply pp.1161

Inan, K.; Goksel, O.S., Uçak, A., Temizkan, V., Karaca, K., Ugur, M., Arslan, G., Us, M. & Yilmaz, A.T. (2008). Thoracic endoscopic surgery for hyperhidrosis: comparison of different techniques. *The Journal of Thoracic and Cardiovascular Surgery*, Vol.56, No.4, (June 2008), pp. 210-13

Kaya, S.O.; Liman, S.T., Bir, L.S., Yuncu, G., Erbay, H.R. & Unsal, S. (2003). Horner's syndrome as a complication in thoracic surgical practice. *European Journal of Cardio-Thoracic Surgery*, Vol. 24, No.6, (December 2003), pp. 1025-28

Kim, D.H.; Paik, H.C. & Lee, D.Y. (2005). Video assisted thoracoscopic re-sympathetic surgery in the treatment of re-sweating hyperhidrosis. *European Journal of Cardio-Thoracic Surgery*, Vol. 27, No. 5, (May 2005), pp. 741-44

Krasna, M.J. (2008). Thoracoscopic sympathectomy: a standardized approach to therapy for hyperhidrosis. Review. *The Annals of Thoracic Surgery*, Vol.85, No.2, (February 2008), pp. 764-67

Kreyden, O.P. & Burg, G. (2000). Die Giftbehandlung von Schweissperlen. Eine Übersicht der Hyperhidrose-Behandlung unter speziellem Blickwinkel der neuen Therapieoption mit Botulinumtoxin A. *Schweizerische Medizinische Wochenschrift*, Vol. 130, No. 29-30, (July 2000), pp. 1084-90

Kwong, K.F.; Hobbs, J.L., Cooper, L.B., Burrows, W., Gamliel, Z. & Krasna, M.J. (2008). Stratified analysis of clinical outcomes in thoracoscopic sympathicotomy for hyperhidrosis. *The Annals of Thoracic Surgery*, Vol. 85, No.2, (February 2008), pp. 390-93, discussion pp. 393-94

Leão, L.E.; de Oliveira, R., Szulc, R., Mari, Jde. J., Crotti, P.L. & Gonçalves, J.J. (2003). Role of video-assisted thoracoscopic sympathectomy in the treatment of primary hyperhidrosis. *Sao Paulo Medical Journal*, Vol.121, No.5, (September 2003), pp. 191-97

Lee, D.Y.; Hong, Y.J. & Shin, H.K. (1999). Thoracoscopic sympathetic surgery for hyperhidrosis. *Yonsei Medical Journal* , Vol. 40, No.6, (December 1999), pp. 589-95

Lee, D.Y.; Yoon, Y.H., Shin, H.K., Kim, H.K. & Hong, Y.J. (2000). Needle thoracic sympathectomy for essential hyperhidrosis: intermediate-term follow-up. *The Annals of Thoracic Surgery*, Vol.69, No.1 (January 2000), pp. 251-53

Li, X.; Tu, Y.R., Lin, M., Lai, F.C., Chen, J.F. & Dai, Z.J. (2008). Endoscopic thoracic sympathectomy for palmar hyperhidrosis: a randomized control trial comparing T3 and T2-4 ablation. *The Annals of Thoracic Surgery*, Vol. 85, No.5, (May 2008), pp. 1747-51

Licht, P.B. & Pilegaard, H.K. (2004). Severity of compensatory sweating after thoracoscopic sympathectomy. *The Annals of Thoracic Surgery,* Vol.78, No.2, (August 2004), pp. 427-31

Licht, P.B.; Jørgensen, O.D., Ladegaard, L. & Pilegaard, H.K. (2005). Thoracoscopic sympathectomy for axillary hyperhidrosis: the influence of T4. *The Annals of Thoracic Surgery,* Vol.80, No.2 (August 2005), pp. 455-59, discussion pp. 459-60

Licht, P.B. & Pilegaard, H.K. (2006). Gustatory side effects after thoracoscopic sympathectomy. *The Annals of Thoracic Surgery,* Vol.81, No.3, (March 2006), pp. 1043-47

Lin CC, Mo LR, Lee LS, Ng SM, Hwang MH (1998): Thoracoscopic T2-sympathetic block by clipping - a better and reversible operation for treatment of hyperhidrosis palmaris: experience with 326 cases. *European Journal of Surgery,* Supplements 580, (1998), pp. 13-16

Lin, T.S. & Fang, H.Y. (1999). Transthoracic endoscopic sympathectomy in the treatment of palmar hyperhidrosis--with emphasis on perioperative management (1,360 case analyses). *Surgical Neurology,* Vol. 52, No. 5, (November 1999), pp. 453-57

Lin, T.S. (2001). Video-assisted thoracoscopic "resympathicotomy" for palmar hyperhidrosis: analysis of 42 cases. *The Annals of Thoracic Surgery,* Vol.72, No.3, (September 2001), pp. 895-98

Linder, A.; Friedel, G. & Toomes, H. (1994). Thermometrically controlled thoracoscopic sympathectomy. *Minimally Invasive Therapy,* Vol.3, (1994), pp. 24

Loureiro, P.; de Campos, J.R., Kauffman, P., Jatene, F.B., Weigmann, S. & Fontana, A. (2008). Endoscopic lumbar sympathectomy for women: effect on compensatory sweat. *Clinics (Sao Paulo),* Vol. 63, No.2, (April 2008), pp. 189-96

Lyra, M.; Campos, J.R., Kang, D.W., Loureiro, P., Furian, M.B., Costa, M.G. & Coelho, S. (2008). Guidelines for the prevention, diagnosis and treatment of compensatory hyperhidrosis. *Jornal Brasileiro de Pneumologia,* Vol.34, No.11, (November 2008), pp. 967-77

Miller, D.L. & Force, S.D. (2008). Temporary thoracoscopic sympathetic block for hyperhidrosis. *The Annals of Thoracic Surgery,* Vol. 85, No.4, (April 2008), pp. 1211-1214, discussion pp. 1215-16

Naunheim, K. (2000). Hyperhidrosis. *Patient information.* Epub. STS.org

O'Connor, K.; Molin, F., Poirier, P. & Vaillancourt, R. (2009). Cardiac arrest as a major complication of bilateral cervico-dorsal sympathectomy. *Interactive CardioVascular and Thoracic Surgery,* Vol.8, No.2, (February 2009), pp. 238-39

Ojimba, T.A. & Cameron, A.E. (2004). Drawbacks of endoscopic thoracic sympathectomy. Review. *British Journal of Surgery,* Vol. 91, No.3 (March 2004), pp. 264-69

Rajesh, Y.S.; Pratap, C.P. & Woodyer, A.B. (2002). Thoracoscopic sympathectomy for palmar hyperhidrosis and Raynaud's phenomenon of the upper limb and excessive facial blushing: a five year experience. *Postgraduate Medical Journal,* Vol. 78, No.925, (November 2002), pp. 682-84

Reisfeld, R.; Nguyen, R. & Pnini, A. (2002). Endoscopic thoracic sympathectomy for hyperhidrosis: experience with both cauterization and clamping methods. *Surgical Laparoscopy Endoscopy & Percutaneous Techniques,* Vol.12, No.4, (August 2002), pp. 255-67

Reisfeld, R. & Berliner, K.I. (2008). Evidence-based review of the nonsurgical management of hyperhidrosis. *Thoracic Surgery Clinics,* Vol. 18, No.2, (May 2008), pp. 157-66

Schlereth, T.; Dieterich, M. & Borklein, F. (2009). Hyperhidrose - Ursache und Therapie von übermäßigem Schwitzen. *Deutsches Aerzteblatt International,* Vol.106, No.3, (2009), pp. 32-37

Schmidt, J. & Bechara, F.G., Altmeyer, P. & Zirngibl, H. (2006). Endoscopic thoracic sympathectomy for severe hyperhidrosis: impact of restrictive denervation on compensatory sweating. *The Annals of Thoracic Surgery,* Vol.81, No.3, (March 2006), pp. 1048-55

Shargall, Y.; Spratt, E. & Zeldin, R.A. (2008). Hyperhidrosis: what is it and why does it occur? Review. *Thoracic Surgery Clinics,* Vol.18, No.2, (May 2008), pp. 125-32

Solish, N.; Wang, R. & Murray, C.A. (2008). Evaluating the patient presenting with hyperhidrosis. *Thoracic Surgery Clinics,* Vol.18, No.2, (May 2008), pp. 133-140

Telaranta, T. (1998). Secondary sympathetic chain reconstruction after endoscopic thoracic sympathicotomy. *European Journal of Surgery,* Supplements 580, (1998), pp. 17-18

Tetteh, H.A.; Groth, S.S., Kast, T., Whitson, B.A., Radosevich, D.M., Klopp, A.C., D'Cunha, J., Maddaus, M.A. & Andrade, R.S. (2009). Primary palmoplantar hyperhidrosis and thoracoscopic sympathectomy: a new objective assessment method. *The Annals of Thoracic Surgery,* Vol.87, No.1, (January 2009), pp. 267-74, discussion pp. 274-75

Ueyama, T.; Ueyama, K., Ueyama, K. & Matsumoto, Y. (2004). Thoracoscopic sympathetic surgery for hand sweating. Review. *Annals of Thoracic and Cardiovascular Surgery,* Vol.10, No.1, (February 2004), pp. 4-8

Vigil, L.; Calaf, N., Codina, E., Fibla, J.J., Gómez, G. & Casan, P. (2005). Video-assisted sympathectomy for essential hyperhidrosis: effects on cardiopulmonary function. *Chest,* Vol. 128, No.4, (October 2005), pp. 2702-05

Walles, T.; Somuncuoglu, G., Steger, V., Veit, S. & Friedel, G. (2008). Long-term efficiency of endoscopic thoracic sympathicotomy: survey 10 years after surgery. *Interactive CardioVascular and Thoracic Surgery,* Vol.8, No.1, (January 2009), pp. 54-57

Wittmoser, R. (1992). Thoracoscopic sympathectomy and vagotomy. In: Cuschieri, A., Buess, G., Perissat, J. *Operative manual of endoscopic surgery.* New York Springer Verlag, (1992), pp. 110–133

Wörle, B.; Rapprich, S. & Heckmann, M. (2007). Definition und Therapie der primären Hyperhidrose. *Journal der Deutschen Dermatologischen Gesellschaft,* Vol.5, No.7, (June 2007), pp. 625-628

Yoon, Y.H.; Lee, D.Y., Kim, H.K. & Cho, H.M. (1999). Reoperation for essential hyperhidrosis. *Asian Cardiovascular & Thoracic Annals,* Vol.7, No.1, (1999), pp. 56-58

Zacherl, J.; Huber, E.R., Imhof, M., Plas, E.G., Herbst, F. & Függer, R. (1998). Long-term results of 630 thoracoscopic sympathicotomies for primary hyperhidrosis: the Vienna experience. *European Journal of Surgery,* Supplements 580, (1998), pp. 43-46

Zacherl, J.; Imhof, M., Huber, E.R., Plas, E.G., Herbst, F., Jakesz, R. & Függer, R. (1999). Video assistance reduces complication rate of thoracoscopic sympathicotomy for hyperhidrosis. *The Annals of Thoracic Surgery,* Vol.68, No.4, (October 1999), pp. 1177-81

11

The Evolution of VATS Lobectomy

Alan D. L. Sihoe
Division of Cardiothoracic Surgery, Department of Surgery,
Li Ka Shing Faculty of Medicine, The University of Hong Kong,
China

1. Introduction

Video-Assisted Thoracic Surgery (VATS) has without doubt been the most significant advance in thoracic surgery over the past half century. No other single innovation has so totally revolutionized the way thoracic surgeons perform their craft, or so greatly improved the surgical experience for patients undergoing thoracic operations worldwide.

In any surgical specialty, patients in the 21st Century are already well aware of the benefits of minimally invasive surgery. Thoracic surgery is no exception. Throughout the world, patients requiring major lung resection surgery are increasingly demanding that they receive VATS. The trend for ever increasing proportions of lung resections being performed with a VATS approach is inexorable. This is true around the globe, from Asia to Europe to North America. It is becoming ever more difficult for thoracic surgeons to justify *not* using a VATS in the face of overwhelming evidence for the benefits of this approach – not only in terms of reducing patient morbidity, but also in improving surgical outcomes.

Yet behind the hype and glamour of VATS today, there are aspects of the approach that even many experienced thoracic surgeons tend to overlook. It is often forgotten that VATS was first used for major lung resection two decades ago. During its infancy, VATS lobectomy was often dismissed as a gimmick or a fad with only limited niche applicability in thoracic surgery as a whole. The story of how VATS lobectomy matured, developed and evolved over the past 20 years to become the mainstream approach it is today contains many lessons for the modern thoracic surgeon. These include: realizing the importance of accurately defining a minimally invasive surgical approach such as VATS; establishing reliable outcome measures to objectively validate its efficacy; and continuing efforts to improving its outcomes and affirm its role in modern clinical practice.

This chapter aims to provide an overview of how VATS lobectomy has evolved over the past two decades from a minor novelty into a fundamental pillar of thoracic surgical practice. The many innovations made and insights gained during the maturation of the VATS approach have had profound influence on how thoracic surgery as a whole is practiced today.

2. Historical background

VATS surgeons worldwide have generally attributed the origination of thoracoscopic therapy to the Swedish physician Hans Christian Jacobaeus (Jacobaeus, 1910; Braimbridge,

2000; Sihoe & Yim, 2008). Towards the end of the 19th century, he first used a modified cystoscope to examine the pleural cavity under local anesthesia. Using a simple candle as a light source, Jacobaeus peered through the rigid tube to look inside the chest. He primarily used this technique of direct thoracoscopy technique to lyse adhesions in order to collapse the lungs as this was the prevailing treatment for tuberculosis at the time. This technique was adopted throughout Europe in the early decades of the 20th century. As this method of direct visualization through a tube has now become forever linked to the term 'thoracoscopy', many VATS surgeons today resolutely refer to modern VATS as 'Video-Assisted *Thoracic* Surgery' and never '*thoracoscopic* surgery' (Lewis, 1996).

The introduction of streptomycin in 1945, and ever improving medical treatment of tuberculosis spelled the end of a period of enthusiasm for traditional therapeutic thoracoscopy. It is only in the last few decades that interest in minimally invasive thoracic surgical therapy was rekindled by two key technological developments. First, the marriage of the rod lens with solid state video systems and micro-cameras in the early 1980s allowed a panoramic view of the hemithorax, instead of the previous tunnel-like vision with direct thoracoscopy. Second, the availability of new endoscopic instruments like the linear mechanical stapler opened up new vistas for a spectrum of diagnostic and therapeutic procedures. From these advances, Video-Assisted Thoracic Surgery (VATS) was born. The video-thoracoscope unit with its own light source provides a well-illuminated, magnified operative view of the thorax, providing very high resolution for details surpassing even that provided by conventional headlight and magnifying loops. Although initially used for simpler diagnostic purposes, the tremendous success of laparoscopic cholecystectomy in the mid-1980s gave impetus to surgeons to apply VATS for therapy of intra-thoracic conditions.

Before long, the potential advantage of the VATS approach for reducing post-operative morbidity and pain began gaining widespread notice. The first major meeting on VATS was held in January 1992 in San Antonio, Texas in conjunction with the Society of Thoracic Surgeons meeting, representing the baptism of a newborn technique (Mack et al, 1993). Over the subsequent years, VATS has become established and developed in many centers in North America, Asia, Europe, Australia and South America (Yim et al, 1998a). Its applications as a diagnostic approach and as a therapeutic modality for benign thoracic diseases have now been firmly incorporated into mainstream thoracic surgery. Throughout the 1990s, VATS gradually became the approach of choice for thoracic procedures such as diagnosis of solitary lung nodules, diffuse pulmonary infiltrates and pleural disease; and simpler therapeutic procedures such as for pneumothorax and excisions of mediastinal lesions. With growing experience with the technique, it was inevitable that more complex pulmonary operations were being performed using VATS.

3. The genesis of VATS lobectomy

For one whole century since the first lung resection was performed in 1891 by Tuffier, the posterolateral thoracotomy - and less frequently the median sternotomy and the clam-shell incisions for bilateral pulmonary procedures - have been the preferred modes of surgical access (Braimbridge, 2000). Unfortunately, although these incisions generally provide good surgical exposure, they are also among the most painful incisions in all of surgery. The trauma of access is often described as worse than that of the procedure itself. It has been reported that 5% to 80% of patients experience significant levels of pain at two months or more after a standard thoracotomy (Rogers & Duffy, 2000; Karmakar & Ho, 2004). This pain can persist in up to 30% of patients at 4 to 5 years after surgery. It has previously been suggested that the pain can result from a combination of skin incision, muscle splitting, rib fracturing, costo-chondral dislocation, pleural injury, diathermy burning, neuroma formation at the wound, and so on. Above all, many surgeons believe that the single most important element is the forcible spreading of the ribs during thoracotomy.

The rationale for VATS pulmonary resection is that by using video technology to minimize the surgical access required, most of these pain-causing elements can be reduced, particularly rib-spreading. The challenge to the first pioneers of VATS lobectomy, however, was how to negotiate the delicate hilar structures - particularly the pulmonary arteries which can easily tear and bleed. Using the small access ports envisaged, innovative strategies or exquisite sill would be required to tackle the structures situated on the medial side of the lobe, often buried by overlying parenchyma and fused fissures.

One of the first to report large series of lobectomies for lung cancer using the VATS approach was Dr Ralph Lewis (Lewis et al, 1992; Lewis, 1995). The technique his group described used 4 ports and explicitly called for the avoidance of rib-spreading. The mediastinal lymph nodes are excised, the fissures divided with endoscopic staplers, and the hilar structures skeletalized. The hilar structures (pulmonary artery, pulmonary vein and lobar bronchus) are then simultaneously stapled in their normal anatomic configuration using two firings of a stapler device. This bold but simple technique permitted efficient resection of a lung lobe in the early days of VATS when the intricate skills needed for conventional isolation-ligation of individual hilar structures via the small incision were still being developed. Even in the early 1990s, in his first 200 consecutive patients using this technique, Lewis claimed impressively short average operating times of 79.5 minutes and length of hospital stay of 3.07 days (Lewis & Caccavale, 2000). There was no mortality and minor complications were only noted in 13% of patients. Importantly, no patient developed a bronchopleural fstula despite the use of simultaneous stapling. After a mean follow-up of 34 months, recurrence-free survival was claimed in 141 out of 171 patients with primary lung cancers (even though less than half had post-operative stage I disease), and 7 deaths were unrelated to neoplasm.

However, despite such promising results, Lewis' simultaneous stapling technique met with considerable skepticism from the more traditional-minded thoracic surgeons' community (Pearson, 2000). Although Lewis and colleagues made a very sound argument that simultaneous stapling was a safe and even historically-proven technique for lobectomy (Lewis, 1995; Lewis & Caccavale, 2000), their approach failed to become established into the mainstream in the face of overwhelming conservatism. Since then, VATS lobectomy has generally conformed worldwide to the strategy of individual isolation-ligation of hilar structures. Nonetheless, Lewis' simultaneous stapling technique has never been discredited on clinical evidence. It can achieve a quick and safe means of removing a lobe, and can still play a part in the surgeon's armamentarium for selected patients when an expeditious lobectomy is required.

The individual isolation-ligation strategy took over as the mainstream for VATS lobectomy subsequently. As the early VATS surgeons tackled the challenge of the hilar structures, the initial instinct was to apply the conventional individual isolation-ligation of open thoracotomy but using smaller wounds. This conventional approach involved dissection of the pulmonary vessels via the interlobar fissure first, then completing the fissures, and finally dividing the bronchus (Roviaro et al, 1993; Kirby et al, 1993; Yim et al, 1996). The advantage of this strategy was that it was immediately familiar for conventional thoracic surgeons – all that was required was getting used to doing the same operation via smaller wounds. The anatomy and intra-thoracic views were essentially familiar, and this made it simpler for surgeons to take the leap into the unfamiliar world of video images. Again, early reported results were encouraging with low mortality and short hospital stays.

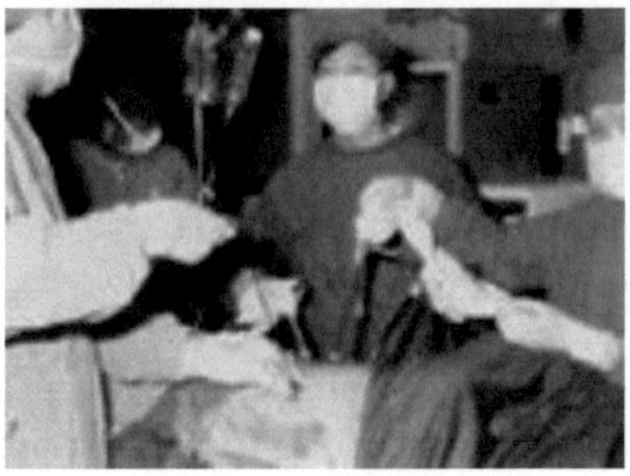

Fig. 1. Professor Anthony Yim was a pioneer of VATS lobectomy in Asia, developing some of the fundamental techniques of this new surgical approach in the 1990s. His work played a pivotal role in establishing VATS lobectomy as a key pillar of modern thoracic surgery. As seen in this early photo from Hong Kong, the basic elements used in the early days of VATS would remain very familiar to the VATS surgeon of today.

However, it was gradually realized that simply copying the open thoracotomy approach (hilum, then fissure, then bronchus) was not necessarily ideal when performing VATS (Roviaro et al, 2000). In particular, the relatively fixed positions of the delicate hilar vessels made them hazardous to isolate and ligate individually. The rigidity of the ribs, the narrowness of the intercostals spaces, and the lack of angulation of the early staplers meant that stapler insertion around the vessels were often difficult - sometimes perilous - undertakings. Some surgeons preferred traditional ligature of the vessels with thread, but this in turn can be limited by the difficulty of intracorporeal knotting through small incisions, especially in patients with deep chests or tight intercostals spaces. The problem is only partly solved with the use of specially designed knot-pushers (Yim & Lee, 1995).

It was only gradually appreciated that the slightly different views and access presented during VATS may require slightly different surgical strategies compared to open thoracotomy. With a conventional postero-lateral thoracotomy, looking straight down into the chest while standing behind the patient made it logically to employ a fissure-first or a posterior-to-anterior dissection strategy. With VATS, where the camera is usually placed at a lower level than the working port(s), this is often more difficult. Instead, working in an anterior-to-posterior direction, tackling vein the artery then bronchus, seemed to work better. The pulmonary vein is almost always easiest to approach first with the video-thoracoscope, with little overlying tissue obscuring it. Once divided, the pulmonary artery branches are usually easy to expose without having to dissect laboriously through often fused interlobar fissures. Indeed, adept use of the video-thoracoscope can make this dissection of the arteries from this more medial aspect of the lobe a much more feasible proposition than with open thoracotomy. Dr Robert McKenna was among the first to advocate such a strategy (McKenna, 1994), and the gradual acceptance of this approach as the mainstream meant that most VATS surgeons nowadays tend to stand anterior to the patient when performing a lobectomy, instead of behind the patient as during a lobectomy via postero-lateral thoracotomy.

By the mid-1990s, the basic technique of VATS lobectomy had become progressively better defined. Certain key concepts were becoming consolidated into the maxim of the VATS surgeon. The ribs were not to be spread. Hilar vessels were to be individually isolated and divided. The sequence of hilar dissection may differ from open surgery. It was also becoming evident that staplers were a quintessential component of a VATS lobectomy, even if conventional ligation and suturing could still be used in some cases. With the key ingredients in place, VATS lobectomy appeared set to take on the thoracic surgery world.

4. The rise and fall of early VATS lobectomy

In establishing any new surgical approach, it is first necessary to demonstrate its safety for patients. With VATS lobectomy, the results of early case series universally ranged from good to excellent. The overall surgical mortality of 0-2% for VATS compared favorably to the conventional technique (Yim et al, 1998a; McKenna et al, 1998; Sihoe & Yim, 2008). Major complications and post-operative morbidity from VATS resections are relatively uncommon (Yim & Liu 1996; Walker, 2000), and minor complication rates are no higher than with open thoracotomy. Tumor implantation following VATS was an early concern (Downey et al, 1996). However, even in a series in which wound protection was not routinely carried out, port site recurrence was noted in only 0.26% (Parekh et al, 2001). This already low figure could be further minimized by routine use of a wound protector, gentle handling of tissue, and copious irrigation of the hemithorax prior to closure (Sihoe & Yim, 2008). Early studies further showed that VATS took similar operating times as open surgery, but consistently produced similar or lower levels of blood loss (Demmy & Curtis, 1999; Sugiura et al, 1999).

In return for equivalent safety as open surgery, VATS delivered the promise of less post-operative pain for patients. Early evidence confiermed that patients who undergo resections via the VATS approach experience less immediate post-operative pain than those having the thoracotomy approach. This has been documented in several large case controlled studies either by objective assessment in terms of analgesic requirements (Yim et al, 1996; Walker et al, 1996), or subjective assessment in terms of pain scoring, usually in the form of a visual analogue scale (Giudicelli et al, 1994; Yim et al, 1996; Demmy & Curtis, 1999). A trend for reduced post-operative analgesic requirement was also seen in early studies comparing VATS with thoracotomy for lobectomy (Kirby et al, 1995; Sugiura et al, 1999). The reduced pain translated into faster recovery, resulting in significantly shorter hospital stays and earlier return to pre-operative work or activities (Demmy & Curtis, 1999; Sugiura et al, 1999).

By the mid to late 1990s, there was already widespread interest in this minimally invasive approach to lung resection surgery. Although relatively few surgeons were actively performing lobectomies this way, the rise of VATS was strikingly reflected in the large volumes of publications in this field. By the turn of the century, the number of papers published in indexed journals on VATS or 'thoracoscopic' lobectomy was being counted in hundreds. It seemed that VATS lobectomy would soon replace open lobectomy in our specialty, so popular was the approach becoming in academic circles. However, this honeymoon period was abruptly brought to a halt.

An early, small, multi-institutional, randomized, prospective study of lobectomy performed through VATS compared to thoracotomy showed no significant benefits for using VATS in terms of pain reduction (Kirby et al, 1995). In another cross-sectional, questionnaire-based study, Landreneau and colleagues reported that the incidence of chronic post-operative pain at one year following VATS was also not different from thoracotomy (Landreneau et al, 1994). Over the years, these studies have been frequently quoted by opponents of VATS to suggest that the benefits of VATS may not extend to the long-term or were not clinically important. Very soon, a number of similar papers followed suit, questioning whether VATS gave patients any real benefit at all. In a separate study comparing VATS and open lobectomy, no statistical differences could be found in the pain assessment after 1 week, nor were any differences detected between groups with respect to respiratory muscle strength or 6-minute walking distance (Nomori et al, 2001). Without doubt, these reports slowed the general acceptance of VATS lobectomy by surgeons in some countries for a number of years. Unsurprisingly, a survey of the General Thoracic Surgery Club members in 1997 showed that the majority considered this application unacceptable (Mack et al, 1997). In that survey, 60% of respondents used VATS less than 20% of the time and 38.1% expressed concern regarding overuse. In particular, several concerns were raised. First, the safety of fine anatomical dissection of the hilum in an essentially closed chest was questioned. Second, there was skepticism over the adequacy of clearance for oncological lung resections with curative intent. Third, although the short term benefits of VATS to patients were intuitively obvious, its long term advantages over conventional surgery remained unclear. Fourth, the relatively high costs of the endoscopic equipments and VATS-related consumables cast doubt on the cost-effectiveness of this.

Clearly, before VATS lobectomy could progress further as a viable surgical option, these concerns needed to be fully addressed. The pleasant surprise was that not only did the subsequent soul-searching by VATS proponents overcome these obstacles, it also revealed a great deal about the fundamental principles of lung cancer surgery itself.

5. Defining VATS lobectomy

When contemplating why some reports of VATS were emerging showing poorer than expected outcomes, it soon became clear that not all those reports were describing the same operation. Careful comparison of published reports confirmed that the 'VATS lobectomy' being reported was not a unified technique, but several variations existed (Yim et al 1998b; Sihoe & Yim 2008). During the initial scramble to become the first to report results with this new surgical technique, this procedure was developed almost simultaneously at different centers, with each unit carrying its own characteristics (Braimbridge, 2000). Not surprisingly, they did so with little consensus over some details of the technique. For example, how long an incision does one allow for a utility "minithoracotomy" before it becomes a "thoracotomy"? How often should one operate through the minithoracotomy as opposed to the video monitor? How much rib spreading can we afford before the benefits of minimal access surgery are lost?

As a result of this lack of standardization in defining the VATS lobectomy procedure, some authors had been loosely applying the term "VATS" to describe any thoracic surgery in which a video-thoracoscope is prepared, often for little more than illumination of the thoracic space while the operation is performed essentially via an open approach (Yim et al 1998b). In some instances, some authors were even tolerating a degree of rib-spreading when performing supposed 'VATS lobectomy' (Nomori et al, 2001). The number and position of ports used also varied considerably between centers. At first, the VATS community was very tolerant of such variations (Sihoe & Yim 2008). After all, the thinking went, how did it matter whether the surgeon was looking at the monitor throughout the operation or frequently chose to peek through the wounds directly? As it turned out, it mattered a great deal.

In a couple of landmark papers, Shigemura and colleagues compared three well-defined surgical approaches for lobectomy: 'complete' VATS (c-VATS) using purely endoscopic techniques with 100% monitor vision without rib-spreading minithoracotomy; 'assisted' VATS (a-VATS) performing the main procedures via rib spreading and using a minithoracotomy (10 cm long) with both monitor and direct vision; and open thoracotomy (20 cm long) with direct vision only (Shigemura et al, 2004 & 2006). In these studies, the average operative time was longer for c-VATS (246 ± 47 minutes) than for a-VATS (169 ± 27 minutes) or open surgery (159 ± 28 minutes) ($P < 0.05$), but estimated blood loss was lower for c-VATS (96 ± 65 mL), and there was no significant difference in the number of dissected lymph nodes. Recovery time objectively analyzed by an accelerometer was shorter in patients undergoing c-VATS than in patients undergoing a-VATS or open surgery ($p < 0.05$). Median length of hospitalization was shorter for patients undergoing c-VATS (11.8 ± 2.7 days) than for patients undergoing a-VATS and open procedures ($P < 0.05$). It was therefore elegantly demonstrated that strict adherence to a completely endoscopic approach could give measurably better outcomes. In effect, it became no longer possible to consider any compromise in technique (as in a-VATS) as acceptable when describing a proper VATS lobectomy.

As a consequence of this realization, VATS surgeons have now applied much stricter definitions when describing VATS lobectomy. The Cancer and Leukemia Group B (CALGB) 39802 trial of the American Society of Clinical Oncology has produced perhaps the most authoritative and accepted definition of the approach thus far (Swanson et al, 2007). In this trial of the safety and feasibility of c-VATS, VATS lobectomy has been defined by the following criteria: no rib spreading; a maximum length of 8 cm of the access incision for removal of the lobectomy specimen; individual dissection of the vein, arteries, and airway for the lobe in question; and standard node sampling or dissection (identical to an open thoracotomy). All specimens were placed in an impermeable bag and removed through the access incision. This definition carries the key points emphasized by the pioneers of VATS lobectomy to reduce surgical access trauma, filtering out 'pseudo-VATS' techniques that gave compromised results (Yim, 2002; Sihoe & Yim, 2008). However, it also allowed enough flexibility for individual surgeons to adapt the approach to their own tastes - as will be discussed below.

Once the definition of VATS lobectomy was re-established, it became once more possible to clearly demonstrate the benefits of the minimally invasive approach over thoracotomy. Since the turn of the century, we have witnessed a second burst of publications espousing the virtues of VATS, no less compelling than the first burst of the early to mid 1990s. A large systematic review of 39 papers involving over 6000 patients compared VATS with thoracotomy with the majority of those papers published since the turn of the century (Whitson et al, 2008). Acknowledging the CALGB definition of VATS lobectomy, this study once more reaffirmed that compared with thoracotomy, VATS lobectomy was associated with significantly shorter chest tube duration, shorter length of hospital stay, and improved survival at 4 years after resection. Furthermore, in a secondary analysis of data from the American College of Surgeons Oncology Group Z0030 randomized clinical trial comparing VATS with open lobectomy for lung cancer, it was also found that VATS gave advantages (Scott et al, 2010). In summary, VATS gave less atelectasis requiring bronchoscopy (0% vs 6.3%, $P = 0.035$), fewer chest tubes draining for longer than 7 days (1.5% vs 10.8%; $P = 0.029$), and shorter median length of stay (5 days vs 7 days; $P < 0.001$).

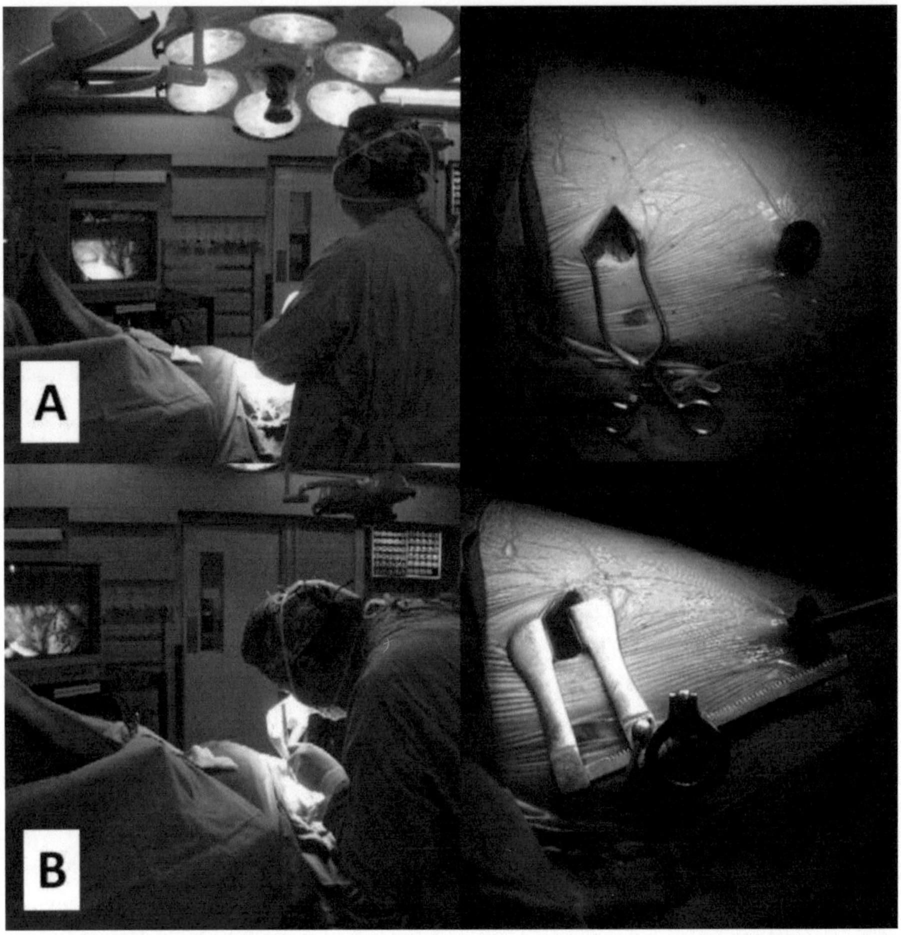

Fig. 2. It is actually not difficult for the casual observer to distinguish whether 'complete' VATS or 'assist' VATS is being performed, even if the wounds appear very similar in size at the end of the operation. In 'complete' VATS (A), the surgeon operates using monitor vision exclusively and can therefore stand comfortably upright throughout the operation. Only gentle skin retraction is occasionally used at the utility port. In 'assisted' VATS (B), the surgeon operates some or most of the time using direct vision via the utility port and consequently is often seen stooping over the patient to 'peek in'. To allow enough room for both direct vision and instrumentation through that port, some degree of rib retraction must typically be used.

It is therefore confirmed that VATS gives clinical advantages once clearly defined. However, this in turn raises the question: 'why?' What is so special about the criteria used for defining VATS that they can significantly impact on outcomes?

Looking at the four listed criteria of the CALGB definition, it is clear that the length of the main incision is not that important. Even when a large number of reports using a large range of wound lengths are considered together, the advantage of VATS over thoracotomy is well maintained (Whitson et al, 2008). Neither is the use of individual isolation-ligation of the hilar structures that important – as evidenced by the excellent results reported by surgeons using a simultaneous stapling technique (Lewis et al, 1992; Lewis, 1995). Even the extent of lymph node dissection is not the critical issue, as similar outcomes in terms of morbidity are seen regardless of how much dissecting is done (Sagawa et al, 2002; Watanabe et al, 2005; Denlinger et al, 2010). What is left of the CALGB criteria is therefore perhaps the most important: avoidance of rib-spreading.

It has been demonstrated that pain or aching can occur in up to 50-70% of patients at two months or more after thoracotomy (Rogers & Duffy, 2000; Karmakar & Ho, 2004). In 5% of these patients, the pain has been described as 'severe and disabling,' and over 40% of patients may still have some degree of pain at one year after surgery. Patients with such post-thoracotomy pain typically describe their pain as being burning, aching, electrical and/or shock-like in quality (Benedetti et al, 1998a; Rogers & Duffy, 2000), and responding poorly to the use of opiates (Benedetti et al, 1998b).These characteristics are the same as those of recognized neuropathic pain syndromes, such as post-herpetic neuralgia and diabetic peripheral neuropathy (Nicholson, 2000; Laird & Gidal, 2000). These all suggest that one of the key mechanisms of post-thoracotomy pain may be neuropathic. Specifically, the rib-spreading during thoracotomy may be causing substantial compression and hence neuropraxic damage to the intercostals nerves. Emerging physiological studies are now gradually confirming this hypothesis (Benedetti et al, 1998a; Rogers et al, 2002; Maguire et al, 2006; Bolotin et al, 2007). In turn, this means that the benefits of VATS over thoracotomy may to a large degree be explained by the eschewing of rib-spreading and intercostals nerve trauma.

This understanding not only helps in lowering morbidity after thoracotomy (such as by increasing use of VATS), but also in improving outcomes after VATS itself. This is because VATS does not absolutely eliminate intercostal nerve trauma as will be discussed below, and this understanding gained by simply appreciating the fundamental definition of VATS may also help in its treatment.

6. Improving the validation of outcomes following VATS lobectomy

Besides honing of the definition of VATS lobectomy, another key factor in the resurgence of this surgical approach since the 1990s has been the improvement in quality of the clinical research published to investigate its worth.

Following from the early success of laparoscopy in abdominal surgery, initial reports on VATS focused on the benefits it promised in terms of reduced pain with the smaller wounds. But how can pain be accurately assessed? Most clinical studies even today use patient self-reporting of levels of pain. The most common self-reporting tools are the Visual-Analog Scale or a simple 10-point numeric score. These are very simple to use and readily understood by both patients and fellow clinicians. However, they are well recognized to be subject to a wide range of confounding variables. For example, these may include patient socio-economic factors, chronic pain or analgesic use pre-operatively, other sources of post-operative satisfaction or dissatisfaction, and so on. The result is both a certain degree of unreliability and considerable variance in the scores collected. The latter in particular may have contributed to some of the more negative findings about VATS in the aforementioned studies of the mid and late 1990s (Landreneau et al, 1994; Kirby et al, 1995; Nomori et al, 2001). Other methods to quantify pain directly are also problematic. More sophisticated pain scores - such as the McGill Pain Scale - have been suggested. However, these are not tailored for use in post-operative patient, and they are often too complex and unwieldy to use in the setting of an acute surgical ward. Counting the use of analgesics is also not ideal. If a standardized post-operative protocol of regular analgesic is used, not enough difference may be shown between VATS and open patients. However, if a very flexible 'as required' analgesic regimen is used the results will again will be confounded by factors such as individual patient pain thresholds and prejudices about taken medications. Early reports describing such results also demonstrated that it is hard to compare results sometimes between different cohorts or studies. For example, does a VATS patient taking two tablets of a non-steroidal anti-inflammatory drug daily have more or less pain than a thoracotomy patient taking a total of 10 tablets of a mild opiate over five days? For all these reasons, early studies reporting the alleged benefits of VATS lobectomy came in for considerable criticism over the years.

Learning from these lessons, VATS surgeons have taken to using surrogate measures of reduced morbidity. If pain is reduced, would this not be reflected in shorter hospital stays and earlier return to work? Again, almost every clinical study on VATS suggests that the minimally invasive approach shortens lengths of stay, but again such results are prone to bias. Although chest drain durations can be crudely regulated by defining drainage volume and air leak cessation criteria triggering removal, lengths of stay are much more subject to confounding variables such as clinician desire to send a VATS patient home or patient keenness or reluctance to leave hospital just days after major surgery. It is already recognized that, for example, that in general, the hospital length of stay in Asian institutions is longer than in North American institutions, reflecting the influence of cultural factors that undermines the usefulness of this outcome measure (Whitson et al, 2008). The same can apply to early reports using return to work to demonstrate the benefit of VATS.

Further efforts to display the morbidity reduction with VATS are now coming to fruition though. One of the methods is to compare pre- and post-operative Quality of Life (QoL). There is increasing realization that post-operative QoL is very important to the cancer patient. It has been shown that patients tend to be more concerned about post-operative functional status and performance in activities of daily living than in abstract survival statistics (Cykert et al, 2000). On a more practical leveler for VATS researchers, many excellent and well-validated QoL assessment tools are widely available. One detailed survey used the EORTC QLQ-C30 and EORTC QLQ-LC13 questionnaires designed to assess QoL in lung cancer patients, supplemented by a self-designed, nine-item surgery-specific questionnaire (Li et al, 2002). The survey was conducted on patients who received lung resections with curative intent for early stage lung cancer either by a VATS approach (median follow-up time of 33.5 months) or by an open thoracotomy approach (39.4 months). Statistically comparable levels of QoL and functional status were noted in both groups, although there was a trend for the VATS group to show better QoL scores and lower incidences of fatigue, dyspnea, coughing, and pain. Since then, an increasing number of papers have confirmed that VATS offers patients better QoL following lobectomy than thoracotomy, providing a much more reliable, quantifiable proof of its advantage (Handy et al, 2010; Rueth & Andrade, 2010).

Another important but often overlooked measure of both post-operative pain and QoL after thoracic surgery is the impairment of shoulder function following thoracic surgery. Shoulder function can be impaired following a thoracotomy by a combination of neurological injury during patient positioning, division of shoulder girdle muscles, direct injury to the long thoracic nerve, and as a result of the significant post-operative pain from the wound. By reducing such surgical trauma and post-operative pain, VATS lung resections may reduce the incidence of post-operative shoulder dysfunction. Previous studies have reported that the strengths of the lattisimus dorsi and serratus anterior muscles may be better preserved following VATS when compared to thoracotomy (Landreneau et al, 1993; Giudicelli et al, 1994). In a prospective study, Li et al reported that short-term shoulder strength and range of movement were significantly better in patients who received VATS pulmonary resection than those who received thoracotomy (Li et al, 2003). Again, such studies provide more objective evidence of morbidity reduction after VATS.

There is emerging evidence that VATS causes less depression of pulmonary function after lung resection surgery than thoracotomy. Kaseda reported that both the forced expiratory volume in one second (FEV1) and forced vital capacity (FVC) values measured at three months post-operatively were significantly preserved relative to pre-operative values in patients who underwent lobectomy by a VATS approach compared to those receiving a thoracotomy approach ($p<0.0001$) (Kaseda et al, 2002). In another similar study, post-operative PaO_2, SaO_2, peak flow rates, FEV1 and FVC were all found to be better on post-operative days 7 and 14 in patients who had VATS rather than thoracotomy for lung resection (Nakata et al, 2000). Blood oxygenation, lung diffusion capacities, 6-minute walk test results, and recovery of vital capacity and cardio-pulmonary function after surgery all tend to be better after VATS than after various forms of open thoracotomy for pulmonary resections(Nagahiro et al, 2001; Nomori et al, 2002 & 2003a).

The most exciting attempt to prove that VATS causes less trauma than thoracotomy have come from studies looking at the impact of surgery on inflammatory and immune markers. There is now a wealth of literature showing that the body's immune function is better preserved following laparoscopic surgery compared to its open counterparts in general abdominal surgery. In thoracic surgery, one study has now demonstrated that patients with clinical stage I lung cancer undergoing VATS lobectomy had significantly reduced post-operative release of both pro-inflammatory (interleukins 6 and 8) and anti-inflammatory cytokines (interleukin 10) into the plasma compared to those having conventional resection (Yim et al, 2000a). Similar findings were also reported in a smaller Japanese study which showed significantly reduced cytokine release (interleukins 6 and 8) into the pleural fluid in the VATS lobectomy group compared to the open group (Sugi et al, 2000a). In a small randomized, prospective study from Edinburgh, it was also shown that VATS lobectomy was associated with a lesser effect on the post-operative fall in circulating T (CD4) cells and natural killer (NK) cells (Leaver et al, 2000). Lymphocyte oxidation was also less suppressed by VATS compared to open surgery. The same group also found that a range of acute phase responses - including C-reactive protein, interleukin 6, tumor necrosis factor, P-selectin, and oxygen free radical activity - were also significantly less amongst the VATS patients (Craig et al, 2001). A separate Hong Kong study found that NK cell levels were suppressed to similar degrees on the first post-operative day following both VATS and thoracotomy lung resections for non-small cell lung cancer, but that T lymphocyte numbers were significantly more reduced following thoracotomy (Ng et al, 2005). The levels of NK cells subsequently rose more quickly in the VATS group. These results suggest that the VATS approach was associated with less, and quicker recovery from, post-operative immunosuppression following lung resection surgery than the thoracotomy approach.

In essence, there is evidence now to believe that VATS is associated with less perturbation in both the humoral and cellular immune functions compared to open surgery, at least in the short term (Walker et al, 2000). So far, there have been no reports demonstrating that VATS pulmonary resection confers a lower incidence of post-operative infection than the open approach. It has also been hypothesized that as immunosurveillance may play an important role in the progression of cancer, surgically induced immunosuppression may predispose to increased tumor growth or recurrence. Whether better preservation of the immune system by VATS may lead to improved long term survival is unclear but certainly deserves further investigation (Yim, 2002).

The ongoing quest to show the advantages of VATS lobectomy over open surgery has succeeded not only in emphatically meeting this primary objective, but also in teaching thoracic surgeons some valuable lessons. The need to find more reliable assessors for peri-operative morbidity has been underscored. This in turn has focused attention on matters important to the patient - such as QoL and post-operative function - rather than just abstract statistics interesting to the surgeon. The extension of the quest to demonstrate less physiological harm to the body using VATS has also begun to highlight the potential oncologic advantage of VATS lobectomy - as will be discussed below.

7. The oncologic efficacy of VATS lobectomy

Critics of the VATS approach for lung cancer research will say - quite rightly - that all the above benefits of VATS are meaningless if the operation cannot fulfill its primary obligation to provide effective oncologic treatment. As mentioned above, the focus of these early doubts on the oncologic efficacy of VATS lobectomy included: whether VATS allowed fine anatomical dissection for individual isolation-ligation of the hilar structures; whether VATS was a cost-effective means of delivering oncologic therapy; and whether VATS gave adequate clearance for oncological lung resections (Mack et al, 1997). The concern over the ability of VATS to allow lobectomy using an individual isolation-ligation strategy has been resoundingly answered by almost two decades of successful surgery around the world.

The question of cost-effectiveness arose because many centers initially baulked at the high consumables costs and potentially longer operating times involved in a typical VATS lobectomy. However, by choosing the right patients for this technique, using mainly conventional instruments, and relying on ligation and suturing in preference to staplers where possible, the consumable costs could be minimized (Yim, 1996). More importantly, VATS promises shorter hospital stays and fewer complications. The savings gained by the shorter stays and having to treat fewer complications tend to offset the higher consumables costs. One study comparing VATS versus open resections for cancer showed that the overall hospital charges were therefore possibly even lower when VATS is used(Nakajima et al, 2000). In experienced hands, VATS major resection could also be as quick an operation as the open approach because less time is needed to open and close the chest. Most centers regularly performing VATS lobectomy no longer find any significant difference in operating times between VATS and open lobectomies (Sihoe & Yim, 2008). Nowadays, the challenge facing VATS lobectomy is ironically not the fear of higher consumables costs, but rather the expectation by patients and/or insurers of lower overall costs - which may even affect compensation for the surgeon in some regions.

The question about whether VATS gives adequate oncologic clearance requires a more complex answer. After all, an anatomic lobectomy is an anatomic lobectomy whether it is done by a minimally invasive or open approach. How is it possible to demonstrate whether a lobe resected by VATS is any more or less a lobe than one removed via thoracotomy? Instead, the battle of the adequacy of VATS is being waged not over the quantity of the lobe itself, but over the amount of lymph node tissue being resected. Opponents of VATS have long suggested that even if a lobe can be removed by VATS, the approach does not allow radical nodal clearance. The debate over the relative merits of lymph node sampling versus lymph node dissection after lung cancer resection is ongoing and beyond the scope of this chapter. However, even if radical nodal dissection is desired, there is now growing evidence that the adequacy of VATS radical lymphadenectomy approaches that of open surgery both in terms of number and mass of nodal tissue removed. In one study, an open thoracotomy immediately after VATS nodal dissection in the same patient could yield only 3% more nodal tissue - an insignificant amount (Sagawa et al, 2002). Two retrospective studies on non-contemporary cohorts of VATS and thoracotomy patients found that VATS gave similar or slightly less nodal tissue, but survival and staging were not affected (Watanabe et al, 2005; Denlinger et al, 2010). In a more recent prospective study of contemporary VATS and thoracotomy cohorts, VATS was confirmed to yield at least as much nodal tissue as thoracotomy regardless of side, lobe or stage of the lung cancer (Sihoe et al, 2011). In addition, VATS gave higher yields at traditionally 'trickier' nodal stations such as the subcarinal nodes (possibly because of the better view VATS afforded in such areas), and the 2-year recurrence-free survival was also higher with VATS. It therefore appears that anatomically-speaking there is no longer a case to suggest VATS is not as oncologically complete as open thoracotomy for lung cancer surgery.

The last bastion of resistance against the adequacy of VATS lobectomy must therefore be long-term survival rates. Ultimately, any quantifiably proven similarity between VATS and thoracotomy intra-operatively must be translated into similar 'cure' rates post-operatively. Thankfully, a large volume of evidence has been accumulated over the past two decades in this regard. These have consistently demonstrated similar survival rates between VATS and open lobectomy patients (Sugi et al, 2000b; Rueth & Andrade, 2010). However, a trend has long been noticed by VATS surgeons for a trend of longer survival amongst VATS patients. Studies from Japan have time and again reported remarkable 5-year survival rates of around 90% for stage IA lung cancer patients receiving VATS lobectomy (Sugi et al, 2000b; Kaseda et al, 2002; Watanabe et al, 2005). In a 2008 systematic review of 39 studies comparing VATS with open lobectomy, patients who underwent VATS lobectomy were finally confirmed to have improved survival versus patients with open lobectomy (88.4% vs 71%; $p = 0.003$) (Whitson et al, 2008). More recently, another similar systematic review reported that 5-year survival was significantly improved for patients who undergo VATS lobectomy for early-stage NSCLC (VATS relative risk, 0.72; $p = 0.04$), further suggesting that VATS lobectomy is at least oncologically equivalent to open lobectomy (Yan et al, 2009).

It is still premature to declare with certainty that VATS gives better survival than open lobectomy. Nonetheless, many surgeons have already begun to speculate over reasons why this phenomenon should be possible. The theory gaining most recent attention is that of the effect of VATS on peri-operative immuno-surveillance. It has been shown that tumor cells may be shed into the circulation during lung cancer surgery (Yamashita et al, 2000). In other surgical specialties, it has been demonstrated that the body's own immune system can help kill or remove such circulating tumor cells - a process often called 'immuno-surveillance' (Shariat et al, 2002; Wu et al, 2002). In theory, if the body's immune function is somehow impaired this may inhibit the peri-operative removal of tumor cells shed during the operation, which can then manifest as subsequent recurrence or metastasis. It has already been mentioned above that studies now show that VATS causing less immune system disruption than open surgery. Therefore, according to this theory, it should be expected that VATS is associated with better long-term survival. At present, this remains fanciful speculation. However, given the impressive speed at which other advantages of VATS are being discovered, it would not be a surprise to see this theory corroborated by new evidence before too long.

8. State of the art

The VATS lobectomy that has established itself as a viable - if not superior - alternative surgical approach to open lobectomy is now practiced widely around the world. In some centers, such as in Hong Kong, VATS lobectomy has been routinely performed for the majority of patients with early stage lung cancer since the mid 1990s (Yim et al, 1996). As said above, other countries have taken up VATS lobectomy at a rather slower pace because of lingering doubts generated by the negative reports of the mid to late 1990s. Nonetheless, over the past several years, major centers several other countries have reached this landmark of over half of all lobectomies being performed using the VATS approach - notably the USA and South Korea. What is most noticeable about the current resurgence of VATS lobectomy compared to the initial rise in the early 1990s is that this time most surgeons are performing the operation according to the same consensus definition of what VATS lobectomy should be. The result is that operations in different centers around the world are now much more similar in the basic characteristics: no rib spreading; a single access incision for specimen retrieval; individual isolation-ligation of the vessels; and systematic nodal dissection. Thankfully, within this broad definition, there remains much scope for variations in the details as individual surgeons adapt their technique to their own preferences - some of which are worth mentioning here. VATS surgeons should never be too proud to refuse adapting the practices of others when they are suitable.

Hong Kong was one of the earliest regions where VATS lobectomy was developed (Yim et al, 1998a). Professor Anthony Yim is undoubtedly the pioneer of this technique in Asia, and his groundbreaking work helped establish its role for lung cancer therapy worldwide. But as mentioned above, in these early days many pioneers strove to replicate open lobectomy via the small VATS incisions. Hence, the sequence of hilar structure dissection was essential unchanged from open surgery (Roviaro et al, 1993; Kirby et al, 1993; Yim et al, 1996). For VATS surgeons in Hong Kong, mediastinal lymph node sampling rather than systematic dissection was the norm, and it was initially deemed acceptable to operate whilst occasionally looking through the main wound. However, these practices soon changed. This author teaches surgical trainees that to operate inside the human chest, the surgeon must place three things inside the patient: his right hand, his left hand, and his pair of eyes. In open thoracotomy, the ribs must be spread apart to permit these three things to enter the patient's chest. With VATS, instruments can replace the right and left hands, and the video-thoracoscope can replace the surgeon's eyes. In this way, rib-spreading can be totally avoided, giving the patient less surgical access trauma. However, if the surgeon still resorts to looking through the wounds to operate, the eyes must once again share access through one of the ports with the hand (or instruments). The only way this can be possible is if there is some rib-spreading, wound enlargement, and/or increasing torquing at the ports (see Figure 2). Any of these can negate the supposed benefits of VATS.

Therefore, since the 1990s, the practice of VATS lobectomy in Hong Kong has evolved. This author now strictly foregoes any form of direct vision through the wounds, and operates exclusively using video monitor visualization. The assistant is reminded to avoid torquing the video-thoracoscope via the camera port. Because of the leverage, even slight torquing could result in significant pressure on the intercostal nerve, causing post-operative neuralgia (Yim, 1995). The rigid plastic camera port can be slid back along the thoracoscope out of the wound after the thoracoscope is inserted into the chest, allowing more flexibility of the thoracoscope in the chest with less torquing at the wound (Sihoe & Yim, 2008). A three-port strategy is used, with two 10mm incisions for the camera and instruments respectively, and a third 4cm utility port in the fourth or fifth intercostals space (with no rib-spreading) for specimen retrieval. Both the surgeon and assistant stand anterior to the patient, and both watch the same video monitor throughout the operation, facilitating camera handling by the assistant (instructions from the surgeon are easier to follow without the hindrance of paradoxical movement or resorting to awkward camera orientations). Dissection is from an anterior-to-posterior direction, typically taking the pulmonary vein first, then pulmonary artery the bronchus. The fissures are taken last of all, and staplers are used in a 'fissureless' technique to minimize post-operative air leak (Nomori et al, 2003b). A systematic dissection at all the ipsilateral mediastinal lymph node stations in routinely carried out in all patients.

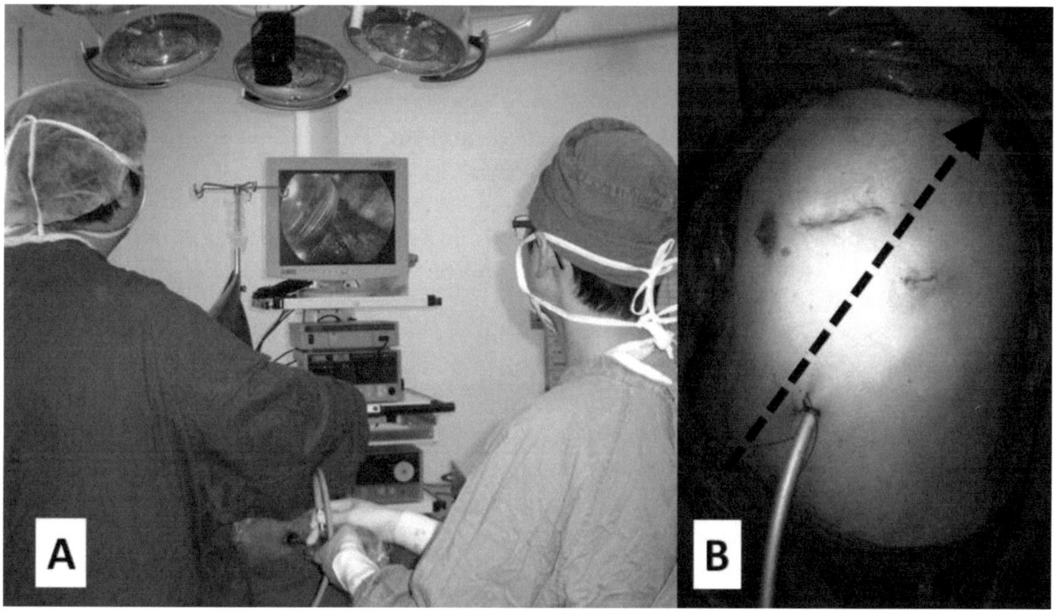

Fig. 3. The photos show the author performing a VATS Left Pneumonectomy (hence the slightly long than usual utility port). (A) Both the surgeon and the assistant stand at the anterior of the patient. (B) The axis of the operation is in an antero-inferior to postero-superior direction as indicated by the arrow. The axis begins at the assistant, goes through the camera port (here used to place the chest drain at the end of the operation), and proceeds straight on to the video monitor. The surgeon 'straddles' the axis anterior to the assistant, with the right and left hands operating comfortably via ports placed either side of this axis. By sharing the same axis and the same monitor, there is better co-ordination between the two throughout the operation and paradoxical camera movements are minimized.

This totally endoscopic c-VATS lobectomy performed in Hong Kong is essentially the same operation found throughout the world nowadays (McKenna et al, 2006; Kim et al, 2010). The basic techniques will be familiar to VATS surgeons from any country: no rib-spreading; surgeon standing anterior to the patient; an anterior-to-posterior strategy; fissureless surgery; and systematic exploration of the nodes. This approach can be summarized as the current state of the art. Certain detail variations exist of course, such as number and size of ports or extent of nodal dissection. However, some VATS surgeons deviate significantly from this basic technique in fine detail (whilst adhering to the same basic principles and definition of VATS lobectomy), and they have achieved success with their modifications. It is worthwhile to consider these variations.

Instead of always standing at the anterior side of the patient, surgeons at several centers in Asia prefer always standing on the right side of the operating table for a VATS lobectomy, regardless of whether the operation is on the right or left lung. In other words, the surgeon would stand anterior to the patient for a left lung operation, but posterior to the patient for a right lung operation. The rationale for this is because for a right-handed surgeon, it is usually ergonomically more comfortable to reach around the patient with the dominant right arm and face the video monitor placed in a more cephalad direction. Proponents of this positioning claim that for the surgeon to stand on the left side of the table, the right arm can be tucked too close to the surgeon's own body for comfortable operating. They claim that by always standing on the right side of the patient, back problems may also be possibly avoided.

Dr Tadasu Kohno of Tokyo, Japan is another leading VATS surgeon in Asia who has developed a rather distinctive strategy for surgeon and assistant positioning (Mun & Kohno, 2008). In this strategy, the surgeon stands posterior to the patient and the camera-holding assistant anterior to the patient. The camera is inserted in the port most anterior on the patient, with the other working ports closer to the surgeon. To ensure the correct orientation of the image on the video-monitor for the surgeon, the camera on the video-thoracoscope is turned so that 'upwards' on the camera and image is towards the anterior of the patient. Because the video-thoracoscope enters the chest via the most anterior camera port, this usually means the camera itself is held almost upside-down by the assistant. The advantage of this strategy is that it best approximates the surgeon's position and views during a traditional open lobectomy via a postero-lateral thoracotomy. This facilitates the transition from open to VATS lobectomy for some surgeons. However, handling the camera in a virtually upside-down position on the opposite side of the operating table from the surgeon requires a very skilled and experienced assistant.

Dr Dominique Gossot of Paris, France also describes an interesting approach to VATS lobectomy (Gossot, 2008). Like Dr Kohno, he also prefers the surgeon standing behind the patient. The peculiar feature of Dr Gossot's technique is that he doesn't create a utility or access port right at the beginning of the operation. He also does not use the more common 3-port strategy. Instead, four to five ports are used to perform the entire operation, with ports sizes ranging from 3mm to 15mm. Only after the lobe has been resected is a utility port created for retrieval of the specimen. It is claimed that by leaving the utility port until the end of the operation, 'use' of this slightly longer incision is only for a brief time and surgical access trauma is minimized. Critics may claim that no rib-spreading is used in modern VATS lobectomy anyway so the size and duration of the utility port does not really contribute significantly to morbidity. Furthermore, whether a shorter duration of having a utility port can ever compensate for having one or two more ports than conventional c-VATS is also debatable. Only time will tell whether any one strategy is better than the others.

These are just a few examples of the many variations on a theme of VATS lobectomy that exist today. Describing them is just meant to illustrate that the strict modern definition of this operation can still accommodate a range of different interpretations. A sage Chinese leader once famously said: "It doesn't matter if the cat is black or white as long as it catches mice". In a similar way, surgeons should be free to experiment with various technique details to find one suiting their own styles, provided the core principles of VATS lobectomy are adhered to and ensure the patient benefits from the minimally invasive approach.

Regardless of the exact details of the operation used, patients today can expect rapid recovery after a VATS lobectomy (Whitson et al, 2008; Yan et al, 2009; Rueth & Andrade, 2010; Scott et al, 2010). Data collected around the world suggest that mortality is no higher than after open lobectomy, and morbidity rates (typically around 15-20%) are usually lower. Chest drain durations average around 4-5 days, and patients are generally discharged around 4-7 days after surgery. For an ultra-major operation that a mere 30 years ago had a mortality rate approaching 10% and a complication rate of almost 60% (Wilkins et al, 1978; Keagy et al, 1985), these modern figures achieved with VATS are commendable.

9. Current challenges, emerging solutions

Despite the current success and popularity of VATS lobectomy, there is no room for VATS surgeons to be complacent. For a start, VATS lobectomy can no longer claim to be the least traumatic mode of curative therapy for lung cancer. Today, ablative therapy (using radio-frequency or microwave energy), stereotactic ('cyberknife') radiosurgery, and stereotactic body radiation therapy (SBRT) all have better claims for that title (Fernando et al, 2005; Pennathur et al, 2009; Crabtree et al, 2010). SBRT is now wholly claimed by Oncologists, and there is no guarantee that surgeons will gain control of ablative and cyberknife therapy. Regardless of the survival rates achievable with these new treatment modalities, to the lay patient they represent an astonishing option that may 'treat' cancer without requiring major surgery. Unless the surgical option is made more palatable for patients, there is no doubt that increasing numbers of patients who are marginally or even completely suitable for surgery may be tempted away from the operating room.

To make VATS lobectomy even better, it is first necessary to appreciate that it is not perfect. First of all, despite the smaller wounds and avoidance of rib-spreading, VATS does not make lobectomy pain-free. It has been found that 52.9% of patients receiving VATS pleurodesis for pneumothorax (in which no rib-spreading is used) experience paresthetic chest wall discomforts which are distinct from classical localized wound pain (Sihoe et al, 2004a). This reported post-operative 'pain' or paresthesia appears characterized by sensations of burning, aching, electrical and/or shock-like in quality - which are all typical of neuropathic pain (Sihoe et al, 2006). In a follow-up study, it was shown that the incidence and nature of the paresthesia remains similar even if the level of surgical trauma is further reduced by performing needlescopic VATS (Sihoe et al, 2005). VATS reduced pain compared to thoracotomy, but was itself still associated with a certain level of neuropathic injury. This injury is most likely caused by the torquing of the video-thoracoscope and instruments at the ports during surgery, and by the placement of a chest tube that is kept for a few days post-operative. Both of these mechanisms contribute to a degree of intercostals nerve trauma. With this in mind, the surgeon can not only attempt to minimize intra-operative torquing and remove chest tubes at the earliest opportunity, but he/she can also use pharmaco-therapy aimed specifically at treating neuropathic pain. At least one study has now shown that use of Gabapentin - a drug previously used to treat trigeminal and post-herpetic neuralgia - may be effective in alleviating post-operative pain after thoracic surgery (Sihoe et al, 2006). The author now frequently prescribes Gabapentin to patients after VATS lobectomy who experience paresthetic discomforts that are distinct from their sharp, localized wound pain.

To combat pain, another strategy has been to make use of 'pre-emptive' analgesia. Some studies now suggest that a painful stimulus can 'sensitize' the central somatosensory pathways, and hence amplify the response to subsequent painful stimuli (Woolf, 1983; Woolf & Salter, 2000; Dahl & Moiniche, 2004). In theory, any treatment given before or during the operation that can prevent the original painful stimulus from activating this sensitization should therefore reduce the subsequent development and severity of post-operative pain. A randomized trial in patients undergoing needlescopic VATS has now demonstrated that giving local anesthesia at the ports sites prior to making the surgical incisions can significantly reduce post-operative pain for up to a week after surgery (Sihoe et al, 2007). In this author's practice, this concept has been combined with the use of regional neural blockade. In VATS lobectomy patients, a bolus paravertebral blockade using bupivicaine is routinely given after induction of general anesthesia and prior to starting the surgical operation.

Besides pain, the most common complication seen after VATS lobectomy today is air leakage. With the reduced pain, earlier mobilization and better preserved lung function after VATS lobectomy, traditionally common respiratory complications such as atelectasis are increasingly rare. Instead, parenchymal air leakage is not something that is directly influenced by the size of the wounds or non-use of rib-spreading. As a result, air leak rates after VATS lobectomy are generally no different than after open lobectomy. Air leakage is not only the most prevalent postoperative complication after a lobectomy today, it is also the single most common reason for an extended length of hospitalization (Abolhoda et al, 1998). Air leaks occur in up to 58% of patients after a lobectomy, and can persist for 5 days or more in 15-18% of patients (Brunelli & Fianchini, 1999; Isowa et al, 2002; Okereke et al, 2005). Traditionally, if a parenchymal air leak is detected on-table, a variety of surgical techniques can be used to repair it. These include suturing, pleural tent creation, and so on. All of these techniques are possible with VATS, but not necessarily easy to perform given the small ports. Surgical sealants were a potentially easy-to-use solution and previous studies have shown that sealants may help reduce air leaks (Tansley et al, 2006; D'Andrilli et al, 2009). However, for a long time there was no effective means of delivery into the chest via the small VATS wounds. Fortunately, the rise of VATS lobectomy has been paralleled by the development of surgical sealant technology. Modern surgical sealants can now be readily aerosolized and delivered via dedicated endoscopic spray applicators. These make them eminently suitable for use in treating on-table air leaks during VATS. In a recent study looking at the endoscopic spray application of fibrin for on-table air leaks detected during VATS lobectomy, use of fibrin sealant significantly reduced air leak incidence, chest drain durations and lengths of hospital stay (Sihoe et al, 2009). A simple and effective solution for VATS lobectomy's last remaining Achilles' heels is therefore now emerging.

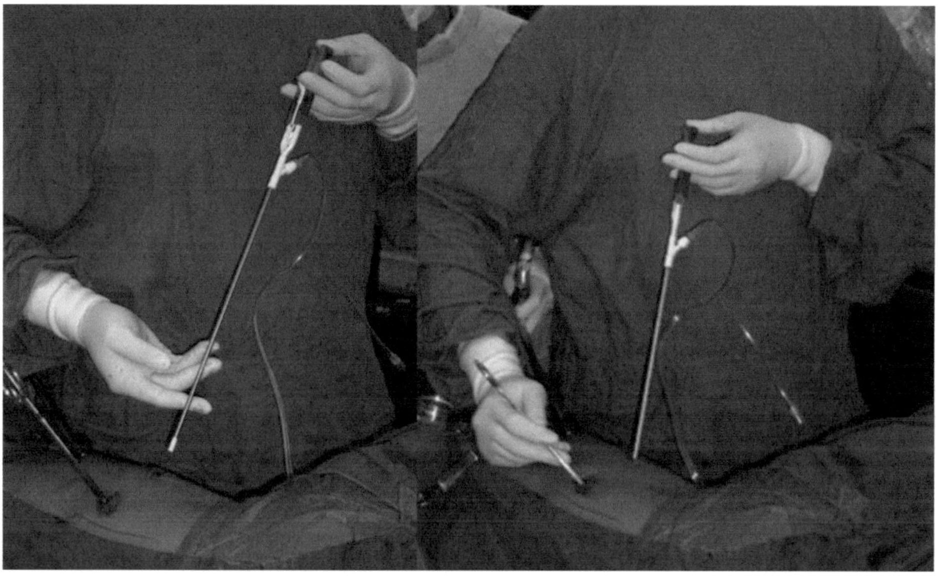

Fig. 4. The latest endoscopic spray applicators allow precise, even and easy delivery of flowable sealants to sites of parenchymal air leak - even via small VATS ports. Evidence is gradually accumulating that support an emerging role for such sealants in selected patients after VATS lobectomy.

It is no use only improving the operation itself if the peri-operative care is not developed to complement the advances. In many traditional thoracic surgery centers, clinical management protocols already exist for how to manage a lung cancer patient who has received lobectomy. In the early days of VATS in Hong Kong, it was noticed that nursing and allied healthcare staff were still managing VATS lobectomy patients according to protocols designed years before for open thoracotomy patients. Mobilization and rehabilitation schedules were slow to take into account the slower recovery of thoracotomy patients, and this meant that VATS patients could not reap the full benefits of the newer minimally invasive approach. Over the past several years, the entire clinical pathway has been re-written in the author's center in Hong Kong to fully complement VATS (Sihoe et al, 2008). The analgesic regime has been revised to reduce the use of opiates - which are both unnecessary given the reduced pain with VATS, and detrimental because the sedation and dizziness caused could delay patient mobilization. In the new VATS pathway, patients are mobilization fully within 24 hours of surgery. Physiotherapy is implemented earlier and more aggressively. Chest drain removal is also expedited. Even post-operative investigations, when a patient opens his/her bowels, and schedules for meeting the patient's relatives are included in the overall clinical pathway package. The literally dozens of items of changes have significantly improved the recovery process of VATS lobectomy patients. Since its implementation, chest drain durations, lengths of hospital stay, rates of complications, and rates of re-admission have all dropped significantly. The lesson learned is that improving operative surgical performance alone must be complemented by appropriate improvements in the ancillary services to bring out the full potential of VATS.

However, in the view of this author, using all the above measures to improve surgical outcomes for the individual patient is not the ultimate goal for VATS. Benefiting the individual patient alone will not ensure the survival of VATS lobectomy in the face of future challenges. Instead, the reduction of morbidity for individual patients must be translated into lowering of thresholds for surgery. If the surgery itself is causing fewer complications and pain, then presumably it can now be offered to patients for whom surgery was previously thought to be 'too high risk'. If this is achieved, then surgery – the only widely established 'cure' for early-stage lung cancer – can reach a larger proportion of the population. 'Marginal' surgical candidates can be offered curative operations instead of compromised therapy (including SBRT) that have only limited chances of achieving tumor eradication.

To this end, some encouraging studies are already emerging. In one study from Hong Kong, VATS lobar and sublobar resection with curative intent was performed in patients with forced expiratory volume in one second on spirometry (FEV1) of <0.8L and/or <50% predicted (Garzon et al, 2006). Patients with such poor lung function would have traditionally been refused any form of curative major lung surgery. However, when VATS was used in this cohort, there was no in-hospital mortality and only a 20% rate of respiratory complications. After a median follow-up of 15 months, only 4% of all patients died of respiratory complications and none of the survivors required home oxygen. In a separate study, VATS and thoracotomy approaches for lung resection with curative intent were compared in lung cancer patients aged over 75 years (Staffa et al, 2010). VATS achieved the same recurrence-free survival rates as open thoracotomy, but at the same time reduced in-hospital complication rates, lengths of post-operative hospital stay, post-discharge complication rates, and also persisting pain at 2 weeks after surgery. Such studies suggest that the list of contra-indications for lung cancer surgery may need to be revised if VATS can be offered. This can potentially offer a hope of effective cure for lung cancer patients previously denied surgery.

10. Future directions

Looking ahead, it is already possible to foresee where the continuing evolution of VATS lobectomy may be headed in the near future. Most of these trends are being driven by rapid technological advances. The rise of Endobronchial Ultrasonography (EBUS) may be one of these (Kurimoto & Miyazawa, 2004). With a minute ultrasound probe positioned at the tip of a flexible bronchoscope, the endoscopist can see 'through' the airway walls into the surrounding mediastinal and hilar structures and attempt biopsy of lymph nodes or other tissues. While EBUS is still predominantly being performed by respirologists, it may still play an important role in thoracic surgery. EBUS can be used for routine mediastinal nodal screening in the operating room immediately prior to embarking on a VATS lobectomy. This approach may overcome the aversion of many thoracic surgeons in offering routine mediastinal screening because of the relative morbidity caused by conventional mediastinoscopy. It is also the strongest argument in favor of surgeons taking responsibility for performing EBUS, as surgeons can offer one-stop staging plus therapeutic surgery in the operating (as opposed to staging by the respirologist and then a separate therapeutic procedure by the surgeon). EBUS may also be useful in patients with suspected N2 nodal metastasis who may be candidates for the strategy of upfront neoadjuvant therapy followed by surgery. If EBUS can confirm the metastasis without needing mediastinoscopy, then the mediastinoscopy can be 'saved' until after the neoadjuvant therapy is completed and used for re-staging purposes.

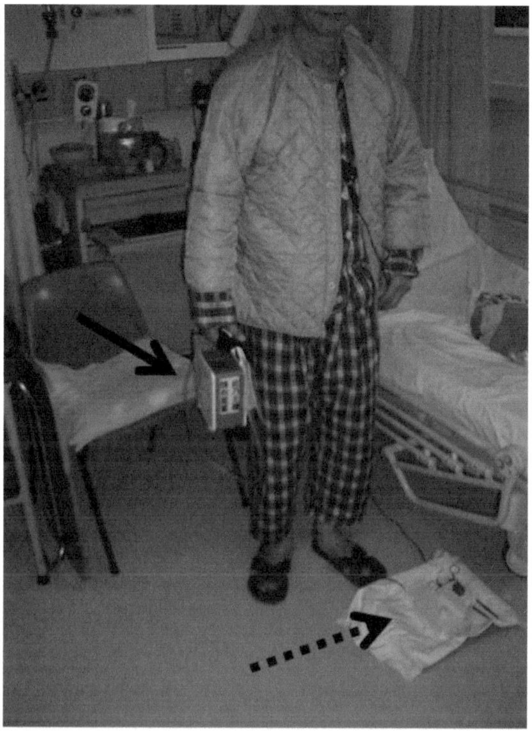

Fig. 5. Using a new portable digital chest drain system (solid arrow), a patient is typically able to mobilize freely within 12-18 hours of a VATS lobectomy. With an inbuilt suction system, the patient's mobility is unrestricted even if suction is required for any reason. When the patient returns to the bedside, the digital drain can simply be placed onto a dock (dotted arrow) which recharges its batteries. Besides promoting post-operative recovery for the patient, the digital drain provides the surgeon an objective, quantified measurement of any air leak via the chest tube. Preliminary clinical evidence suggests that this may improve consistency and hence efficiency of air leak management after VATS lobectomy.

Another emerging technological advance are the new portable digital chest drain systems that have come onto the market over the last few years. Traditional water seal chest drain systems are clumsy and unwieldy. They require attention not to be lifted above the chest level, not to be accidentally tipped over, and not to have the water seal evaporated unnoticed. If suction is required for any reason, connection to an external suction source also effectively ties the patient down like a ball-&-chain restraint. When VATS lobectomy is performed, it is particularly frustrating to see post-operative mobility being restricted not by the surgery but by the use of an old-fashioned chest drain. A modern digital system such as the Medela Thopaz (Medela AG, Switzerland) does away with a water seal altogether, and comes with an inbuilt suction system that maintains a constant, user-set negative pleural pressure without need for any external connection. The result is a compact, portable chest drain that permits complete patient mobility after lobectomy. This complements the early mobility afforded by VATS lobectomy well, and ensures the patient can fully benefit from the minimally invasive approach. An initial survey of patients and nurses on the use of the portable device has already produced preliminary confirmation that chest drain handling and patient mobility are improved compared to conventional water seal systems (Sihoe & Yeung, 2011). Perhaps more importantly, it has also been shown that use of the digital air flow monitor on a digital system such as the Thopaz can accurately and objectively measure post-operative air leaks after lung surgery (Varela et al, 2009). A study from Hong Kong has already demonstrated that the greater consistency in monitoring air leaks can be translated into more decisive, confident post-operative chest drain management resulting in shortened chest drain durations and lengths of hospital stay (Yeung & Sihoe, 2010). The combination of improved patient recovery and more effective air leak management should prove attractive to surgeons looking to maximize the potential of VATS lobectomy in improving outcomes. In the past few years, increasing numbers of abstracts on the use of digital drain systems have been presented at major thoracic surgical conferences in Asia and Europe, reflecting the growing importance of this new technology.

Of course, the one surgical technology capturing the most attention amongst surgeons and the lay public in recent years is undoubtedly that of robot assisted surgery. The da Vinci robotic surgical system (Surgical Intuitive, Mountain View, CA) allows the surgeon at a console to 'remote control' robot limbs inserted into the patient to perform the operation. The purported advantages of using robot assistance include precise tremor-free manipulations, 3D binocular visualization, excellent ergonomics for the surgeon, and the ability of the robotic arms to minimize torquing of the instruments at each working port (Melfi et al, 2002). Early published series have demonstrated the safety and feasibility of robot assisted surgery within the thorax, even for major lung resection (Varonesi et al, 2010). However, good results have so far mainly been reported by a small number of specialist centers with particular experience using robots, and a couple of recognized drawbacks still remain. The first issue is the complete absence of tactile feedback throughout the operation (D'Amico, 2006). For many operations, the visual information can partly compensate for this. However, tactile feedback is often crucial in thoracic surgery, and whether current robotic technology can consistently address this fundamental limitation during the intricate dissections in the course of a lobectomy remains to be fully proven. The other disadvantage of robot assisted surgery is the costs – both of the initial outlay for the advanced hardware and of the bespoke instruments and consumables that must be purchased for each operation. Because of the very low morbidity rates and excellent outcomes with conventional VATS, it may prove difficult – if not impossible – to ever demonstrate any significant superiority of the robot system over VATS. Conceptually, it is hard to see how a robot assisted lobectomy using four ports can ever be convincingly proven to cause less trauma than a typical c-VATS lobectomy using 3 ports. Consequently, for the foreseeable future at least, making a compelling case for robot assisted surgery in terms of cost-effectiveness will very likely prove futile.

In the inevitably upcoming debates over the relative merits of robot assisted surgery and VATS, it is worth making one telling observation. Many (but not all) reports on robot assisted thoracic surgery appear to have originated from centers that are not generally associated with major well-developed VATS lobectomy programs. Even the authors of leading published reports on robot assisted lobectomy acknowledge that their standard approach to lung lobectomy was through thoracotomy, not VATS (Varonesi et al, 2010). Very few of the established VATS lobectomy centers have switched to using the robot. This peculiar phenomenon suggests that for surgeons used to open surgery, the very intuitive and user-friendly robot systems interface may be easier to master than the different set of hand-eye skills demanded by VATS lobectomy. This provides non-VATS surgeons an excellent route into the world of minimally invasive thoracic surgery. However, for those who have mastered VATS lobectomy, the robot systems do not seem to offer any advantage or incentive to switch (Swanson, 2010). Again, only time will tell whether the robot systems are a passing fad or an emerging viable alternative approach to lung surgery as VATS once was.

Whatever the potential of robot systems, there is also another possible (and much simpler) direction for minimally invasive thoracic surgery: needlescopic VATS. In this technique, video-thoracoscopes and instruments of only 2-3 mm diameter are used, requiring much smaller ports than the typical 5-15mm ports used in conventional VATS. The wounds are typically so small that only barely detectable 'pinpoint' scars remain after surgery - leading to term 'needlescopic' VATS. The principle is that if VATS can improve on open thoracotomy by using smaller wounds, then needlescopic VATS should give better outcomes than conventional VATS by using even smaller wounds. Compared to robot assisted surgery, this approach uses far smaller ports and should be much cheaper. Needlescopic VATS has already been used for a variety of diagnostic and simple therapeutic procedures, such as sympathectomy for palmar hyperidrosis (Yim et al, 2000b; Lazopoulos et al, 2002; Sihoe et al, 2004b). More recently, needlescopic VATS has been used for pleurodesis surgery in the management of pneumothorax, achieving equivalent efficacy as conventional VATS but with less pain and faster recovery (Sihoe & Lin, 2011). As mentioned above, some VATS surgeons have already begun using 3-5mm instruments in their lobectomy operations, but only as a supplement to conventional VATS instruments (Gossot, 2008). With the potential benefits of the needlescopic approach, it may just be a matter of time before we witness reports of a totally needlescopic VATS lobectomy.

11. Conclusions

When VATS lobectomy was first conceived during the heyday of minimally invasive surgery, the pioneers had relatively little understanding of how the approach would benefit patients other than that smaller wounds would create less pain. A good number of reports documented that VATS did indeed cause less pain than traditional open surgery via thoracotomy. However, after the initial flurry of promising results, subsequent reports began painting a rather less flattering picture of VATS, suggesting that VATS may not be as advantageous as first hoped. In the quest to address these disappointing results, several important truths emerged. Firstly, the importance of clearly defining what VATS lobectomy is or is not was realized. Thus clearly defined, it became possible to not only reaffirm that complete VATS does improve patient outcomes, but also to better appreciate why VATS does this. Secondly, the use of standardized, objective and reproducible outcome measures are now providing a far more reliable picture of how much VATS can help the patient receiving lung surgery. This has not only established the role of VATS in lung cancer management, but raised the standards of outcome measurement in thoracic surgery as a whole. Thirdly, the pursuit of answers to questions put forth by critics of VATS has trained VATS surgeons to focus on what the key benefits to be gained from minimally invasive surgery really are. This in turn has led to continued efforts to advance those benefits for patients, culminating in many clinical and technological innovations to improve the state of the art.

It behoves the VATS surgeon to learn the lessons of the first two decades of VATS lobectomy. The evolution of VATS is an ongoing process. Challenges to the role of VATS lobectomy will never cease to emerge. Application of the enterprise and diligence of the

VATS pioneers is necessary to constantly test and evolve the practice of thoracic surgery, ensuring it remains as relevant to patients in the future as it is today.

12. References

Abolhoda A, Liu D, Brooks A, Burt M. Prolonged air leak following radical upper lobectomy. An analysis of incidence and possible risk factors. Chest 1998; 113:1507-1510.

Benedetti F, Vighetti S, Ricco C, Amanzio M, Bergamasco L, Casadio C, Cianci R, Giobbe R, Oliaro A, Bergamasco B, Maggi G. Neuorphysiologic assessment of nerve impairment in posterolateral and muscle-sparing thoracotomy. J Thorac Cardiovasc Surg 1998; 115:841-847.

Benedetti F, Vighetti S, Amanzio M, Casadio C, Oliaro A, Bergamasco B, Maggi G. Dose-response relationship of opioids in nociceptive and neuropathic postoperative pain. Pain 1998; 74:205-211.

Bolotin G, Buckner GD, Jardine NJ, Kiefer AJ, Campbell NB, Kocherginsky M, Raman J, Jeevanandam V. A novel instrumented retractor to monitor tissue-disruptive forces during lateral thoracotomy. J Thorac Cardiovasc Surg 2007; 133:949-954.

Braimbridge MV. Thoracoscopy - a historical perspective. In Yim APC, Hazelrigg SR, Izzat MB, et al (eds): Minimal Access Cardiothoracic Surgery. WB Saunders, Philadelphia, USA, 2000, pp 1-10.

Brunelli A, Fianchini A. Prolonged air leak following upper lobectomy: in search of the key. Chest 1999; 116:848.

Crabtree TD, Denlinger CE, Meyers BF, et al. Stereotactic body radiation therapy versus surgical resection for stage I non–small cell lung cancer. J Thorac Cardiovasc Surg 2010; 140:377-386.

Craig SR, Leaver HA, Yap PL, et al. Acute phase responses following minimal access and conventional thoracic surgery. Eur J Cardiothorac Surg 2001; 20:455-463.

Cykert S, Kissling G, Hansen CJ. Patient preferences regarding possible outcomes of lung resection: what outcomes should preoperative evaluations target? Chest 2000; 117:1551-1559.

Dahl JB, Moiniche S. Pre-emptive analgesia. Br Med Bull 2004; 71:13-27.

D'Amico TA. Robotics in thoracic surgery: applications and outcomes. J Thorac Cardiovasc Surg 2006; 131:19-20.

D'Andrilli A, Andreetti C, Ibrahim M, Ciccone AM, Venuta F, Mansmann U, Rendina EA. A prospective randomized study to assess the efficacy of a surgical sealant to treat air leaks in lung surgery. Eur J Cardiothorac Surg 2009; 35:817-821.

Demmy TL, Curtis JJ. Minimally invasion lobectomy directed toward frail and high-risk patients: a case control study. Ann Thorac Surg 1999; 68:194-200.

Denlinger CE, Fernandez, Meyers BF, et al. Lymph node evaluation in video-assisted thoracoscopic lobectomy versus lobectomy by thoracotomy Ann Thorac Surg 2010; 89:1730-1736.

Downey RJ, McCormick P, LoCicero J, et al. Dissemination of malignant tumors after video-assisted thoracic surgery: A report of twenty-one cases. J Thorac Cardiovasc Surg 1996; 111:954-960.

Fernando HC, De Hoyos A, Landreneau RJ, et al. Radiofrequency ablation for the treatment of non-small cell lung cancer in marginal surgical candidates. J Thorac Cardiovasc Surg 2005; 129:639-644.

Garzon JC, Ng CSH, Sihoe ADL, Manlulu AV, Wong RHL, Lee TW, Yim APC. Video-assisted thoracic surgery pulmonary resection for lung cancer in patients with poor lung function. Ann Thorac Surg 2006; 81:1996-2003.

Giudicelli R, Thomas P, Lonjon T, et al. Video-assisted mini-thoracotomy versus muscle sparing thoracotomy for performing lobectomy. Ann Thorac Surg 1994; 58:712-718.

Gossot D. Technical tricks to facilitate totally endoscopic major pulmonary resections Ann Thorac Surg 2008; 86:323-326.

Handy JR Jr, Asaph JW, Douville EC, Ott GY, Grunkemeier GL, Wu Y. Does video-assisted thoracoscopic lobectomy for lung cancer provide improved functional outcomes compared with open lobectomy? Eur J Cardiothorac Surg 2010; 37:451–455.

Isowa N, Hasegawa S, Bando T, Wada H. Preoperative risk factors for prolonged air leak following lobectomy or segmentectomy for primary lung cancer. Eur J Cardiothorac Surg 2002; 21:951.

Jacobaeus HC. Ueber die Möglichkeit die Zystoskopie bei Untersuchung seröser Höhlungen anzuwenden. München Med Wchenschr 1910; 57:2090-2092.

Karmakar MK, Ho AMH. Postthoracotomy pain syndrome. Thorac Surg Clin 2004; 14:345-352.

Kaseda S, Aoki T. Video-assisted thoracic surgical lobectomy in conjunction with lymphadenectomy for lung cancer. J Jap Surg Soc 2002; 103:717-721.

Keagy BA, Lores ME, Starek PJK, Murray GF, Lucas CL, Wilcox BR. Elective pulmonary lobectomy: factors associated with morbidity and operative mortality. Ann Thorac Surg 1985; 40:349-352.

Kim K, Kim HK, Park JS, et al. Video-assisted thoracic surgery lobectomy: single institutional experience with 704 cases Ann Thorac Surg 2010; 89:S2118-S2122.

Kirby TJ, Mack MJ, Landreneau RJ, et al. Initial experience with video-assisted thoracoscopic lobectomy. Ann Thorac Surg 1993; 56:1248-1253.

Kirby TJ, Mack MJ, Landreneau RJ, Rice TW. Lobectomy video-assisted thoracic surgery versus muscle-sparing thoracotomy: a randomized trial. J Thorac Cardiovasc Surg 1995; 109:997-1002.

Kurimoto N, Miyazawa T. Endobronchial ultrasonography. Semin Respir Crit Care Med 2004; 25:425-431.

Laird MA, Gidal BE. Use of gabapentin in the treatment of neuropathic pain. Ann Pharmacother 2000; 34:802-807.

Landreneau RJ, Mack MJ, Hazelrigg SR, et al. Post-operative pain-related morbidity: video-assisted thoracic surgery versus thoracotomy. Ann Thorac Surg 1993; 56:1285-1289.

Landreneau RJ, Mack MJ, Hazelrigg SR, et al. Prevalence of chronic pain after pulmonary resection by thoracotomy or video-assisted thoracic surgery. J Thorac Cardiovasc Surg 1994; 107:1079-1086.

Lazopoulos G, Kotoulas C, Kokotsakis J, et al. Diagnostic mini-video assisted thoracic surgery: effectiveness and accuracy of new generation 2.0 mm instruments. Surg Endosc 2002; 16:1793-1795.

Leaver HA, Craig SR, Yap PL, Walker WS. Lymphocyte responses following open and minimally invasive thoracic surgery. Eur J Clin Invest 2000; 30:230-238.

Lewis RJ, Caccavale RJ, Sisler GE, et al. One hundred consecutive patients undergoing video-assisted thoracic operations, Ann Thorac Surg 1992; 54:421-426.

Lewis RJ. Simultaneously stapled lobectomy: a safe technique for video-assisted thoracic surgery. J Thorac Cardiovasc Surg 1995; 109:619-625.

Lewis RJ. VATS is not thoracoscopy. Ann Thorac Surg 1996; 62:631-632.

Lewis RJ, Caccavale RJ. Video-assisted thoracic surgical non-rib-spreading simultaneously stapled lobectomy. In Yim APC, Hazelrigg SR, Izzat MB, et al (eds): Minimal Access Cardiothoracic Surgery. WB Saunders, Philadelphia, USA, 2000, pp 135-149.

Li WWL, Lee TW, Lam SSY, Ng CSH, Sihoe ADL, Wan IYP, Yim APC. Quality of life following lung cancer resection: video-assisted thoracic surgery versus thoracotomy. Chest 2002; 122:584-589.

Li WW, Lee RL, Lee TW, Ng CS, Sihoe AD, Wan IY, Arifi AA, Yim AP. The impact of thoracic surgical access on early shoulder function: video-assisted thoracic surgery versus posterolateral thoracotomy. Eur J Cardiothorac Surg 2003; 23:390-396.

Mack MJ, Hazelrigg SR, Landreneau RJ, Naunheim KS. The First International Symposium on Thoracoscopic Surgery. Ann Thorac Surg 1993; 56:605-806.

Mack MJ, Scruggs GR, Kelly KM, et al. Video-assisted thoracic surgery: has technology found its place? Ann Thorac Surg 1997; 64:211-215.

Maguire MF, Latter JA, Mahajan R, David Beggs F, Duffy JP. A study exploring the role of intercostal nerve damage in chronic pain after thoracic surgery. Eur J Cardiothorac Surg 2006; 29:873-879.

McKenna RJ. Lobectomy by video-assisted thoracic surgery with mediastinal node sampling for lung cancer. J Thorac Cardiovasc Surg 1994; 107:879-882.

McKenna RJ, Jr, Wolf RK, Brenner M, et al. Is VATS lobectomy an adequate cancer operation? Ann Thorac Surg 1998; 66:1903-1908.

McKenna Jr RJ, Houck W, Fuller CB. Video-assisted thoracic surgery lobectomy: experience with 1100 cases Ann Thorac Surg 2006; 81:421-425.

Melfi FM, Menconi GF, Mariani AM, et al. Early experience with robotic technology for thoracoscopic surgery. Eur J Cardiothorac Surg 2002; 21:864-868.

Mun M, Kohno T. Video-assisted thoracic surgery for clinical stage I lung cancer in octogenarians. Ann Thorac Surg 2008; 85:406-411.

Nagahiro I, Andou A, Aoe M, et al. Pulmonary function, postoperative pain, and serum cytokine level after lobectomy: a comparison of VATS and conventional procedure. Ann Thorac Surg 2001; 72:362-365.

Nakajima J, Takamoto S, Kohno T, Ohtsuka T. Costs of video thoracoscopic surgery versus open resection for patients with lung carcinoma. Cancer 2000; 89:2497-2501.

Nakata M, Saeki H, Yokoyama N et al. Pulmonary function after lobectomy: video-assisted thoracic surgery versus thoracotomy. Ann Thorac Surg 2000 ; 70:938-941.

Ng CS, Lee TW, Wan S, Wan IY, Sihoe ADL, Arifi AA, Yim AP. Thoracotomy is associated with significantly more profound suppression in lymphocytes and natural killer cells than video-assisted thoracic surgery following major lung resections for cancer. J Invest Surg 2005; 18:81-88.

Nicholson B. Gabapentin use in neuropathic pain syndromes. Acta Neurol Scand 2000; 101:359-371.

Nomori H, Horio H, Naruke T, Suemasu K. What is the advantage of a thoracoscopic lobectomy over a limited thoracotomy procedure for lung cancer surgery? Ann Thorac Surg 2001; 72:879–84.

Nomori H, Horio H, Naruke T, Suemasu K. Posterolateral thoracotomy is behind limited thoracotomy and thoracoscopic surgery in terms of postoperative pulmonary function and walking capacity. Eur J Cardiothorac Surg 2002; 21:155-156.

Nomori H, Ohtsuka T, Horio H, et al. Difference in the impairment of vital capacity and 6-minute walking after a lobectomy performed by thoracoscopic surgery, an anterior limited thoracotomy, an anteroaxiallry thoracotomy, and a posterolateral thoracotomy. Surg Today 2003; 33:7-12.

Nomori H, Ohtsuka T, Horio H, Naruke T, Suemasu K. Thoracoscopic lobectomy for lung cancer with a largely fused fissure. Chest 2003; 123:619-622.

Okereke I, Murthy SC, Alster JM, Blackstone EH, Rice TW. Characteri-zation and importance of air leak after lobectomy. Ann Thorac Surg 2005; 79:1167–1173.

Parekh K, Rusch V, Bains M, et al. VATS port site recurrence: a technique dependent problem. Ann Surg Oncol 2001; 8:175-178.

Pearson FG. Commentary. In Yim APC, Hazelrigg SR, Izzat MB, et al (eds): Minimal Access Cardiothoracic Surgery. WB Saunders, Philadelphia, USA, 2000, p 151.

Pennathur A, Luketich JD, Heron DE, et al. Stereotactic radiosurgery for the treatment of stage I non-small cell lung cancer in high-risk patients J Thorac Cardiovasc Surg 2009; 137:597-604.

Rogers ML, Duffy JP. Surgical aspects of chronic post-thoracotomy pain. Eur J Cardiothorac Surg 2000; 18:711-716.

Rogers ML, Henderson L, Duffy JP. Preliminary findings of a neurophysiological assessment of intercostal nerve injury during thoracotomy. Eur J Cardiothorac Surg 2002; 21:298-301.

Roviaro CG, Varoli F, Rebuffat C, et al. Videothoracoscopic major pulmonary resections Ann Thorac Surg 1993; 56:779-783.

Roviaro CG, Varoli F, Vergani C, Maciocco M. Anatomic lung resection. In Yim APC, Hazelrigg SR, Izzat MB, et al (eds): Minimal Access Cardiothoracic Surgery. WB Saunders, Philadelphia, USA, 2000, pp 107-114.

Rueth NM, Andrade RS. Is VATS lobectomy better: perioperatively, biologically and oncologically? Ann Thorac Surg 2010; 89:S2107-S2111.

Sagawa M, Sato M, Sakurada A, et al. A prospective trial of systematic nodal dissection for lung cancer by video-assisted thoracic surgery: can it be perfect? Ann Thorac Surg 2002; 73:900-904.

Scott WJ, Allen MS, Darling G, et al. Video-assisted thoracic surgery versus open lobectomy for lung cancer: a secondary analysis of data from the American College Of Surgeons Oncology Group Z0030 randomized clinical trial. J Thorac Cardiovasc Surg 2010; 139:976-983.

Shariat SF, Lamb DJ, Kattan MW, et al. Association of preoperative plasma levels of insulin-like growth factor I and insulin-like growth factor binding proteins-2 and -3 with prostate cancer invasion, progression, and metastasis. J Clin Oncol 2002; 20:833-841.

Shigemura N, Akashi A, Nakagiri T, Ohta M, Matsuda H. Complete vs assisted thoracoscopic approach. A prospective randomized trial comparing a variety of video-assisted thoracoscopic lobectomy techniques. Surg Endosc 2004; 18:1492-1497.

Shigemura N, Akashi A, Funaki S, Nakagiri T, Inoue M, Sawabata N, Shiono H, Minami M, Takeuchi Y, Okumura M, Sawa Y. Long-term outcomes after a variety of video-assisted thoracoscopic lobectomy approaches for clinical stage IA lung cancer: a multi-institutional study. J Thorac Cardiovasc Surg 2006; 132:507–512.

Sihoe ADL, Au SS, Cheung ML, Chow IK, Chu KM, Law CY, Wan M, Yim APC. Incidence of chest wall paresthesia after video-assisted thoracic surgery for primary spontaneous pneumothorax. Eur J Cardiothorac Surg 2004; 25:1054-1058.

Sihoe ADL, Ho KM, Sze TS, et al. Selective lobar collapse for video-assisted thoracic surgery. Ann Thorac Surg 2004; 77:278-283.

Sihoe ADL, Cheung CS, Lai HK, Lee TW, Thung KH, Yim APC. Incidence of chest wall paresthesia after needlescopic video-assisted thoracic surgery for palmar hyperhidrosis. Eur J Cardiothorac Surg 2005; 27:313-319.

Sihoe AD, Lee TW, Wan IY, Thung KH, Yim AP. The use of gabapentin for post-operative and post-traumatic pain in thoracic surgery patients Eur J Cardiothorac Surg 2006; 29:795-799.

Sihoe AD, Manlulu AV, Lee TW, Thung KH, Yim AP. Pre-emptive local anesthesia for needlescopic video-assisted thoracic surgery: a randomised controlled trial. Eur J Cardiothorac Surg 2007; 31:103-108.

Sihoe ADL, Yim APC. Video-Assisted Pulmonary Resections. In: Thoracic Surgery (3rd Edition). Patterson GA, Cooper JD, Deslauriers J, Lerut AEMR, Luketich JD, Rice TW, Pearson FG (Eds). Elsevier, Philadelphia, USA, 2008, pp 970-988.

Sihoe ADL, Cheng LC, Das SR. Protocol-based post-operative management following lung cancer surgery. Presented at: Hospital Authority Convention 2008, May 2008, Hong Kong.

Sihoe ADL, Lee A, Cheng LC. Aerosolized endoscopic spray application of fibrin for on-table air leaks following lung resection surgery: a case-match study. Presented at: 19th Biennial Congress of the Association of Thoracic and Cardiovascular Surgeons of Asia, October 2009, Seoul, Korea.

Sihoe ADL, Yeung ESL, Cheng LC, Wang E, Wong MP. Lymph node evaluation during lobectomy for lung cancer: complete video-assisted thoracic surgery versus open surgery. Presented at: 2011 Joint Meeting of the Asian Society for Cardiovascular and Thoracic Surgery and the Association of Thoracic and Cardiovascular Surgeons of Asia, May 2011, Phuket, Thailand.

Sihoe ADL, Yeung ESL. Use of a portable digital chest drain system in thoracic surgery: a survey of patients and nurses. Presented at: 2011 Joint Meeting of the Asian Society for Cardiovascular and Thoracic Surgery and the Association of Thoracic and Cardiovascular Surgeons of Asia, May 2011, Phuket, Thailand.

Sihoe ADL, Lin PMF. Needlescopic video-assisted thoracic surgery for primary spontaneous pneumothorax. Presented at: Annual Scientific Meeting 2011 of the International Society for Minimally Invasive Cardiothoracic Surgery, June 2011, Washington, DC, USA.

Staffa J, Lampl B, Sihoe ADL. Lung cancer resection in elderly patients: VATS offers faster recovery. Presented at: 17th European Congress on General Thoracic Surgery, European Society of Thoracic Surgeons, June 2010, Valladolid, Spain.

Sugi K, Kaneda Y, Esato K. Video-assisted thoracoscopic lobectomy reduces cytokine production more than conventional open lobectomy. Jpn J Thorac Cardiovasc Surg 2000; 48:161-165.

Sugi K, Kaneda Y, Esato K. Video-assisted thoracoscopic lobectomy achieves a satisfactory long-term prognosis in patients with clinical stage IA lung cancer. World J Surg 2000; 24:27-30.

Sugiura H, Morikawa T, Kaji M et al. Long-term benefits for the quality of life after video-assisted thoracoscopic lobectomy in patients with lung cancer. Surg Laparosc Endosc 1999; 9:403-408.

Swanson SJ, Herndon JE 2nd, D'Amico TA, et al. Videoassisted thoracic surgery lobectomy: report of CALGB 39802—a prospective, multi-institution feasibility study. J Clin Oncol 2007; 25:4993–4997.

Swanson, SJ. Robotic pulmonary lobectomy: the future and probably should remain so. J Thorac Cardiovasc Surg 2010; 140:954.

Tansley P, Al-Mulhim F, Lim E, Ladas G, Goldstraw P. A prospective, randomized, controlled trial of the effectiveness of BioGlue in treating alveolar air leaks. J Thorac Cardiovasc Surg 2006; 132:105-112.

Varela G, Jiménez MF, Novoa NM, Aranda JL. Postoperative chest tube management: measuring air leak using an electronic device decreases variability in the clinical practice. Eur J Cardiothorac Surg 2009; 35:28-31.

Veronesi G, Galetta D, Maisonneuve P, Melfi F, Schmid RA, Borri A, et al. Four-arm robotic lobectomy for the treatment of early-stage lung cancer. J Thorac Cardiovasc Surg 2010; 140:19-25.

Walker WS, Pugh GC, Craig SR, Carnochan FM. Continued experience with thoracoscopic major pulmonary resection. Int Surg 1996; 81: 255-258.

Walker WS, Leaver HA, Craig SR, Yap PL. The immune response to surgery: Conventional and VATS lobectomy. In Yim APC, Hazelrigg SR, Izzat MB, et al (eds): Minimal Access Cardiothoracic Surgery. WB Saunders, Philadelphia, USA, 2000, pp 152-167.

Walker WS. Complications and Pitfalls in Video Assisted Thoracic Surgery. In Yim APC, Hazelrigg SR, Izzat MB, et al (eds): Minimal Access Cardiothoracic Surgery. WB Saunders, Philadelphia, USA, 2000, pp 341-348.

Watanabe A, Koyanagi T, Ohsawa H, et al. Systematic node dissection by VATS is not inferior to that through an open thoracotomy: a comparative clinicopathologic retrospective study Surgery 2005; 138:510-517.

Whitson BA, Groth SS, Duval SJ, Swanson SJ, Maddaus MA. Surgery for early-stage non-small cell lung cancer: a systematic review of the video-assisted thoracoscopic surgery versus thoracotomy approaches to lobectomy. Ann Thorac Surg 2008; 86:2008-2018.

Wilkins EW Jr, Scannell JG, Craver JC. Four decades of experience with resections for bronchogenic carcinoma at the Massachusetts General Hospital. J Thorac Cardiovasc Surg 1978; 76:364.

Woolf CJ. Evidence for a central component of post-injury pain hypersensitivity. Nature 1983; 306:686-688.

Woolf CJ, Salter MW. Neuronal plasticity: increasing the gain in pain. Science 2000; 288:1765-1769.

Wu Y, Yakar S, Zhao L, Hennighausen L, LeRoith D. Circulating insulin-like growth factor-1 levels regulate colon cancer growth and metastasis. Cancer Res 2002; 62:1030-1035.

Yamashita JI, Kurusu Y, Fujino N. Detection of circulating tumor cells in patients with non-small cell lung cancer undergoing lobectomy by video-assisted thoracic surgery: a potential hazard for intraoperative hematogenous tumor cell dissemination. J Thorac Cardiovasc Surg 2000; 119:899-905.

Yeung ESL, Sihoe ADL. Use of a portable digital chest drain system in thoracic surgery improves consistency in air leak management. Presented at: 20th Annual Congress of the Association of Thoracic and Cardiovascular Surgeons of Asia, October 2010, Beijing, China.

Yan TD, Black D, Bannon PG, McCaughan BC. Systematic review and meta-analysis of randomized and nonrandomized trials on safety and efficacy of video-assisted thoracic surgery lobectomy for early-stage non-small-cell lung cancer. J Clin Oncol 2009; 27:2553-2562.

Yim APC. Minimizing chest wall trauma in video assisted thoracic surgery. J Thorac Cardiovasc Surg 1995; 109:1255-1256.

Yim APC, Lee TW. 'Home-made' knot pusher for extracorporeal ties. Aust NZJ Surg 1995; 65:510-511.

Yim APC. Cost containing strategies in video assisted thoracoscopic surgery: an Asian perspective. Surg Endosc 1996; 10:1198-1200.

Yim APC, Ko KM, Chau WS, et al. Video-assisted thoracoscopic anatomic lung resections: the initial Hong Kong experience. Chest 1996; 109:13-17.

Yim APC, Liu HP. Complications and failures from video assisted thoracic surgery: experience from two centers in Asia. Ann Thorac Surg 1996; 61: 538-541.

Yim APC, Liu H, Izzat MB, et al. Thoracoscopic major lung resection: an Asian perspective. Semin Thorac Cardiovasc 1998; 10:326-331.

Yim APC, Landreneau RJ, Izzat MB, Fung ALK. Is video assisted thoracoscopic lobectomy a unified approach? Ann Thorac Surg 1998; 66:1155-1158.

Yim APC, Wan S, Lee TW, Arifi AA. VATS lobectomy reduces cytokine responses compared with conventional surgery. Ann Thorac Surg 2000; 70:243-247.

Yim APC, Liu HP, Lee TW, et al. 'Needlescopic' VATS for palmar hyperhidrosis. Eur J Cardiothorac Surg 2000; 17:697-701.

Yim APC. VATS major pulmonary resection revisited: controversies, techniques, and results. Ann Thorac Surg 2002; 74:615-623.

12

The Era of VATS Lobectomy

Stefanie Veit
Department of Thoracic Surgery, Schillerhoehe Hospital, Gerlingen, Germany

1. Introduction

Primary lung cancer remains the most lethal of all malignancies. The cornerstone of therapy for early-stage non-small cell lung cancer (NSCLC) is surgical resection by lobectomy with complete systematically lymphadenectomy (Hartwig & D'Amico, 2010). One of the initial reports on video-assisted thoracoscopic lobectomy was published 1994 by Robert McKenna (McKenna, 1994). Since then thoracoscopic techniques to perform major anatomic lung resections evolved dramatically and have gained widespread adoption. But in fact, worldwide only 20% of all lobectomies are done using a thoracoscopic approach (Buffa et al., 2008).
Germany Advantages of thoracoscopic lobectomy compared to open thoracotomy include a lower incidence of complications (Paul et al., 2010), shorter hospitalization (Scott et al., 2010), better pulmonary function (Kaseda et al., 2000), less postoperative pain (McKenna et al. 2006), decreased overall costs (Burfeind et al., 2010; Casali & Walker, 2009) and improved delivery of adjuvant chemotherapy to selected patients (Lee at al., 2011; Petersen et al., 2007). These outcomes suggest that thoracoscopic lobectomy should be considered the gold standard for patients with early-stage NSCLC (Hartwig & D'Amico 2010).

2. Definition

To discuss VATS lobectomy and its results, standardization of the terminology is essential. Thoracoscopic lobectomy is defined as the anatomic resection of an entire lobe of the lung, using a videoscope, an access and work incision. Use of a mechanical retractor or rib-spreader is obsolete. Oncologic and anatomic resection as open thoracotomy lobectomy: individual dissection and stapling of vessels and bronchus and complete hilar and mediastinal lymph node dissection (D'Amico, 2008; McKenna et al., 2006).

3. Indications

You can differentiate between general indications and relative contraindications for VATS lobectomy. General indications are important to consider when starting a VATS lobectomy program. As the skill of VATS surgeons improve during the learning curve constantly relative contraindications diminish. As long as the oncological and correct anatomic resection is not compromised any lobectomy can be performed as a VATS procedure.

3.1 General indications

Clinical stage 1 non-small cell lung cancer is the best indication for thoracoscopic lobectomy. Preferred localisation of these tumors is peripherally in the parenchyma so there is no

interference with blood vessels or bronchus during dissection. Furthermore it is easier to perform a wedge resection for frozen section if a histological result couldn't be achieved before the operation.
Tumors less than 6 cm in diameter do not compromise exposure of the lung in the thoracic cavity. Dissection becomes more difficult and dangerous the larger the tumor appears in the parenchyma. Removal of the lobe or specimen and placing into the protective bag before removal is sometimes strenuous for large tumors.
Elderly patients or patients with a compromised performance status benefit the most from a muscle sparing and no-rib spreading incision. Shorter hospitalization, lower complications and earlier mobilization are important advantages VATS lobectomy can offer this group of patients.

3.2 Relative contraindications

Advanced tumors or advanced clinical stages afford a sophisticated and experienced technique of the surgeon and the whole team. Perioperative complications are more likely to occur in tumors that invade the chest wall, pericardium or diaphragm.
Preoperative chemotherapy and especially radiotherapy destroy the tissue planes for dissection. It affords an advanced skill in thoracoscopic dissection.
Centrally located tumors make thoracoscopic preparation challenging as the great vessels might be harmed and bleeding is a major complication.
Abnormal lymph nodes which are often seen in patients with tuberculosis or other inflammatory diseases in their history might invade vessels or bronchus. In those cases dissection by VATS is often impossible.

4. Technique

There are general operative considerations for VATS lobectomy. The patient is positioned in the lateral decubitus position with flexion at the hip to spread the costal interspaces for the VATS ports. Port site placement is different among VATS surgeons but mostly 3-4 incisions

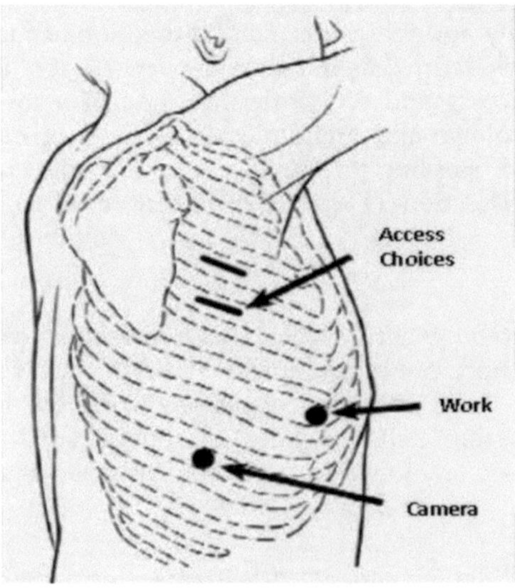

Fig. 1. Incisions for VATS lobectomy

are used. The use of endoscopic tools is essential but often standard instruments can be preferred because of better grasping strength and tactile feedback (Demmy et al., 2005). Use of an angeled scope (30 or 50 degree) for panoramic visualization is needed to provide a range of views and to minimize collision of operative instruments (Hartwig & D'Amico, 2010). Mechanical staplers are used for ligation of vessels, bronchus and parenchyma. To reduce air leaks dissection in the fissure should be avoided. The first step is to start with mobilization of hilar structures and the pulmonary vein. Further dissection follows the landmarks of artery and bronchus. When completing the operation removal of the lobectomy specimen is achieved by using a protective bag to prevent port site recurrences. Complete mediastinal lymph node dissection is either performed before the resection or at conclusion of the lobectomy.

4.1 Right upper lobe

Dissection of the parenchyma is the most difficult issue concerning the right upper lobe (RUL). Even in open thoracotomy it can be difficult to place the mechanical stapler between the parenchyma of middle and upper lobe. After mobilizing the pleura division of superior and middle lobe vein is performed followed by dividing the apical branches (truncus anterior) of the pulmonary artery. The next step is either to divide the upper lobe bronchus or to staple the fissure between upper and middle lobe to gain a better view. After identification and dividing remaining pulmonary artery (PA) branches in the fissure (segment 2) completion of the posterior fissure is done. To prevent torsion suturing or stapling of middle lobe to lower lobe is recommended as well as division of the pulmonary ligament.

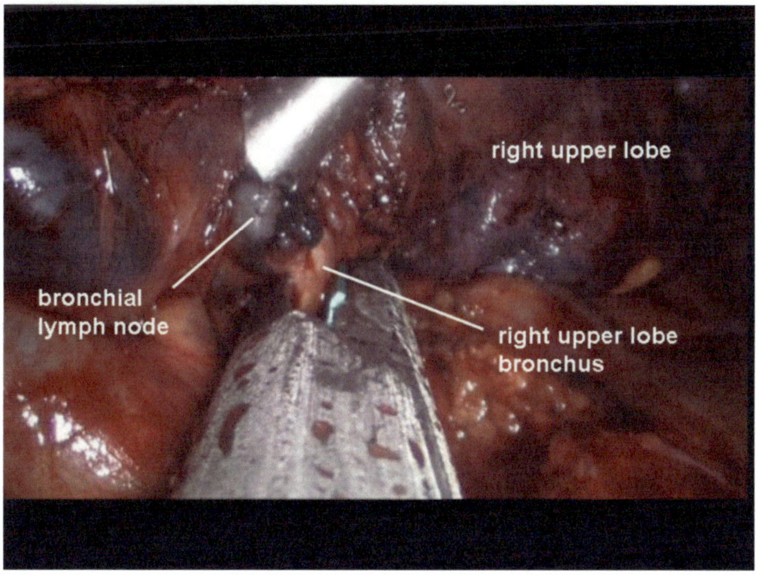

Fig. 2. Division of upper lobe bronchus with mechanical stapler

4.2 Right middle lobe

First step is to mobilize the pleura followed by dividing the middle lobe branch of the superior vein. The next step includes identification of either the middle lobe bronchus or the pulmonary artery branches to the middle lobe. It might be necessary to partially dissect the minor fissure before dividing the arteries or bronchus by stretching the lung to the chest wall. Before dividing the middle lobe arteries creation of a plane along the pulmonary artery should be performed to expose full course of the pulmonary artery. Most cases require dissection of the middle lobe bronchus before the middle lobe arteries. Last step is to complete the fissures and divide the inferior ligament.

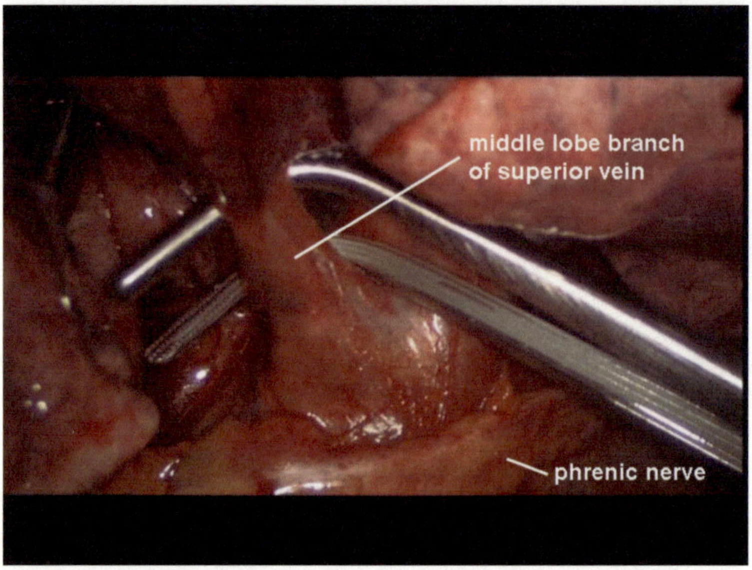

Fig. 3. Division of middle lobe branch of superior vein

4.3 Right and left lower lobe

After mobilizing the pleura division of the inferior ligament is followed by division of the inferior vein. Next step is to identify the pulmonary artery in the major fissure and complete the anterior fissure. Dissection and Division of the pulmonary artery branches to the lower lobe can then be performed. The last step consists of dissecting and dividing the lower lobe bronchus with completion of the posterior fissure. If you cannot identify the pulmonary artery branches in the major fissure you can divide and dissect the bronchus and the pulmonary artery branches from below by stretching the lung to the apex of the thoracic cavity.

4.4 Left upper lobe

Mobilizing the pleura is followed by division of the superior vein. By further mobilizing the pleura along the aorta division of the apical pulmonary artery branches is possible. Next step is to identify the lingular branch of the pulmonary artery in the fissure and staple the anterior fissure. Division of the lingular artery and the remaining pulmonary artery branches to the left upper lobe is required. In many cases division of the left upper lobe bronchus is necessary before dividing the remaining pulmonary artery branches. Last steps are completion of the posterior fissure and dividing the inferior ligament.

All lobectomies are finished by inserting the lobe into a bag and pulling it through the work incision. Air leak check is essential to see if you have to use sealants or suture the air leaks. After confirming reexpansion of the lung a chest tube is inserted and fixed.

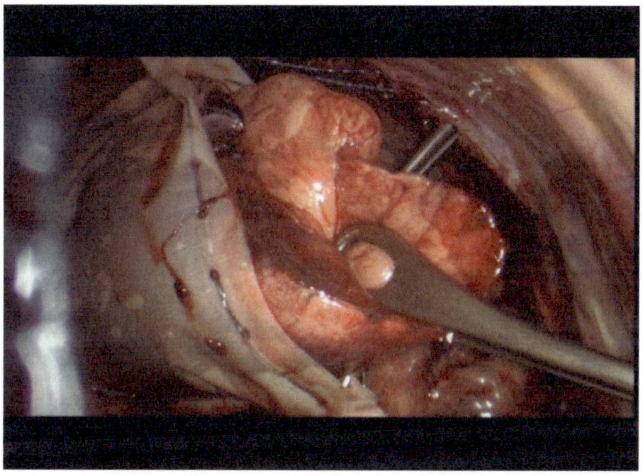

Fig. 4. Insertion of lobe into bag

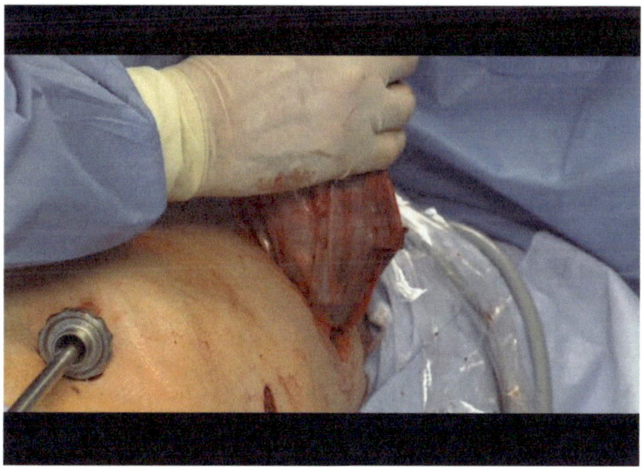

Fig. 5. Pulling lobe through work incision

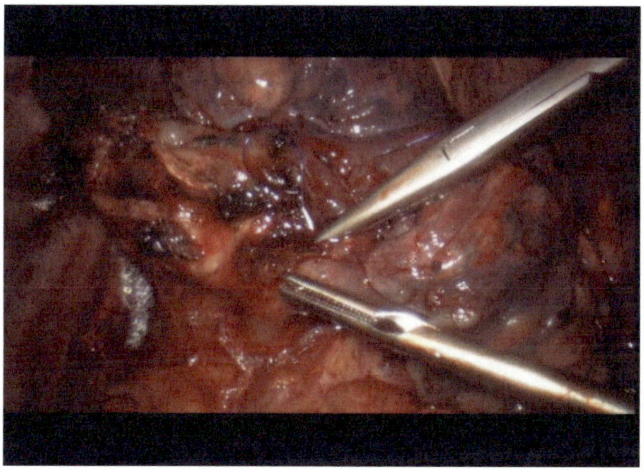

Fig. 6. Suturing parenchyma because of air leak

5. Outcomes

VATS lobectomy has gained international acceptance (D'Amico, 2008; Mahtabifard et al., 2008; McKenna et al., 2007) which contributes to outcomes and good results of thoracoscopic lobectomy when performed in an experienced institution.

5.1 Postoperative length of stay

There are multiple studies that have shown that VATS lobectomy is associated with a short postoperative length of stay (McKenna et al., 2006; McKenna et al., 2007; Paul et al., 2010; Scott et al., 2010). This might be due to the fact that length of chest tube duration is considerably reduced in most of the VATS lobectomy patients (Paul et al., 2010; Scott et al., 2010) Another reason might be that postoperative pain control is easier to manage in VATS lobectomy patients and therefore the hospitalization is shorter and patient recovery faster (Nagahiro et al., 2001).

5.2 Postoperative pulmonary function

Postoperative pulmonary function is better in patients with VATS lobectomy than with thoracotomy (Kaseda et al., 2000). The minimally invasive incision preserves the flexibility of the thorax and therefore ability to breath in the same pattern the patients are used to preoperatively.

5.3 Compliance with adjuvant chemotherapy

One of the most promising advantages associated with VATS lobectomy addresses to the ability of patients to receive and tolerate adjuvant chemotherapy (D'Amico, 2008). Delivery of adjuvant chemotherapy to eligible patients is improved with VATS lobectomy (Lee, J., 2011). Patients undergoing VATS lobectomy had fewer delayed and reduced chemotherapy doses. A higher percentage of patients undergoing thoracoscopic lobectomy received 75% or more of their planned adjuvant regimen without delayed or reduced doses (Petersen et al., 2007).

5.4 Costs

VATS lobectomy is less expensive than conventional lobectomy (Burfeind et al., 2010; Casali et al., 2009). The theatre cost of VATS lobectomy has frequently been cited as a major obstacle to its adoption. Considered only theatre costs this is true but cost analysis through 30 days postoperatively reduced the overall costs of VATS lobectomy. This is due to a significantly shorter stay and therefore by the reduced length of stay related costs (Nakajima et al., 2000).

5.5 Morbidity and mortality

Morbidity and mortality associated with thoracoscopic lobectomy is lower than for conventional thoracotomy and resection (Demmy & Curts, 1999; Onaitis et al., 2006; Paul et al., 2010; Rueth & Andrade, 2010; Scott et al., 2010). Thoracoscopic lobectomy, using a case-matched strategy, showed a reduced specific complication rate in favour for VATS lobectomy (Paul et al., 2010). Patients with thoracoscopic resection had fewer reintubations postopertively. Similar overall cardiovascular morbidity was significantly lower in VATS lobectomy patients, with a significant reduction noted in atrial arrhythmias requiring treatment.

The frequency of blood transfusion was also significantly lower following VATS lobectomy.

5.6 Lymph node dissection

Possible advantages of complete mediastinal lymph node dissection include improvement on local control and survival, so consistently VATS lobectomy is challenged to support the concept that complete mediastinal lymph node dissection can be performed (Flores & Alam, 2008). There are similarities in all studies comparing lymph node dissection by VATS to thoracotomy: the number of lymph nodes resected by VATS tend to be slightly less than in open thoracotomy, but statistically difference cannot be proven (Denlinger et al., 2010; Kondo et al., 1998; Scott et al., 2010; Watanabe et al., 2005). Technically lymph node dissection by VATS is possible (Cassina et al., 1995), concentration and focussing are required. Therefore it might make sense to do the lymph node dissection before performing lobectomy. Another approach is to switch operating and assisting surgeon for lymph node dissection, to guarantee a fresh mind.

5.7 Survival

The true measure of any cancer treatment is survival. A VATS approach does not compromise survival for lung cancer patients. 5-year survival for VATS lobectomy show outcomes that are typically expected for surgical treatment of lung cancer (McKenna et al., 2006; Walker et al., 2003; Yamamoto et al., 2010; Rueth & Andrade, 2010). With no proven difference in stage specific survival VATS lobectomy can be recommended for clinical stage I and II non-small cell lung cancer.

5.8 Complications

There are many series that report VATS lobectomy to be a safe and reasonable procedure. Table 1 shows typical complications after VATS lobectomy. Mortality rates for VATS lobectomy vary from 0% to 2,6% (McKenna et al., 2006; Roviario et al., 2003; Walker et al., 2003).

Major complications		Minor complications	
Readmission	1% - 2%	Atrial fibrillation	3% - 12%
Pneumonia	2%	Air leak	5%
Myocardial infarction	1%	Transfusion	<5%
Empyema	<1%	Serous drainage	<2%
Broncho pleural fistula	<1%	Subcutaneous emphysema	1%
Stroke	<1%	Gastrointestinal	<1%

Table 1. Typical complications after VATS resections

6. Learning and teaching

Among the younger generation of thoracic surgeons there is a strong belief that the routine use of minimal-invasive methods for major pulmonary resection is on its way. To integrate VATS procedures into the curriculum training programs are indispensible. There are many requirements for developing a VATS lobectomy program. The individual surgeon must be experienced with other VATS procedures, such as wedge resections or pleurectomies (Chin & Swanson, 2008). The surgeon must also be familiar with basic video skills like camera work, stapling, dissecting and suturing. The practice should include a minimal number of 50 lobectomies per year (McKenna, 2008).

6.1 Introduction

If the surgeons and the program have the technology and preconditions developing a VATS lobectomy program can proceed (McKenna, 2008). The first surgeons who started VATS lobectomy were pioneers who had to break new ground and develop new technologies.
For practicing thoracic surgeons there are many methods to gain the skill to perform VATS lobectomy. There are many journal articles, lately published atlases and videos in the internet about the technical details of how to perform the operation. Often these steps are not sufficient to learn the technique. Tissue simulators are an alternative (Meyerson et al., 2010) and they might become an integral part of surgical education. There are courses offered by professional societies, industry or practicing surgeons. The observation of the VATS lobectomy procedure is perhaps the most beneficial. The observing surgeon can precisely see the proper placement of the incisions, the use of the instruments and has the ability to ask the operating surgeon questions about the procedure and dissecting steps. Observation should take place over a period of time, not just for one or two days. During subsequent observations you see more troubleshooting aspects of VATS lobectomy and how to handle them in a professional way. In this way the observing surgeon gets a realistic understanding of the operation.

6.2 Learning curve

The learning curve for VATS lobectomy varies considerably as the procedure is still performed at relatively few centers and the learning curve is very shallow (Petersen & Hansen, 2010). To learn VATS lobectomy it might be helpful to switch from a posterolateral thoracotomy to muscle-sparing anterior thoracotomy and, ultimately to VATS lobectomy (Ng et al., 2006). For training reason every operation for operable lung cancer should start thoracoscopically to gain practice step by step (Belgers et al., 2010). In this way all the involved surgeons can learn the correct sequence of the resection. The best way to safely learn VATS lobectomy is to be guided through the operation by a consultant surgeon (Ferguson & Walker, 2006; Petersen & Hansen, 2010). Using this method VATS lobectomy can safely be taught in a surgical institution experienced in VATS lobectomies. The surgical outcome for the training surgeon is comparable to the outcome of the experienced surgeon. The learning curve is reflected in a longer operating time for the training surgeon, which must be taken into account when starting VATS lobectomy programs. In view of the limited number of centres performing VATS lobectomy at high levels, training should be coordinated at a national level to concentrate experience and improve uptake of this technique.

7. Pitfalls of VATS lobectomy – a short troubleshooting guide

7.1 Vessels

If dissection is efficiently done the use of vessel loops enlarges the space behind the pulmonary vessels by pulling on the loop. Before launching the stapler putting the sucker or a right-angled clamp behind the vessel is auxiliary. This maneuver proofs that there is no excess tissue behind the pulmonary vessel. Slightly rotation of the stapler facilitates passage. In difficult cases a common technique is to secure the cut end of a rubber catheter (8F to 14 F) to the anvil of the stapler. This serves to guide the stapler around the pulmonary vessel. For very small vessels (≤5mm) harmonic scalpel or bipolar dissecting instruments can be safely used.

In case of bleeding application of a peanut or ring forceps sponge on the vessel stops bleeding and gives the surgeons a survey where the bleeding exactly comes from. If appropriate use of a clip or 4-0 Prolene is recommended, in more severe bleeding converting to open thoracotomy is unavoidable but safe if the ring forceps sponge is in place.

7.2 Parenchyma

Dissection of the parenchyma is especially difficult on the right side (minor fissure). Marking the fissure with electrocautery is auxiliary to insert the stapler in the right anatomic position. Before dividing any fissure identification of the pulmonary vessels is crucial. For mild adhesions in the fissure application of the harmonic scalpel is recommended, once the anatomic structures are identified application of a stapler is recommended. In case of air leaks in the parenchyma suturing or application of a biological sealant is essential.

7.3 Lymph node dissection

For carinal lymph node dissection dividing the pulmonary ligament is crucial, to create a plane that leads into the carina. For exposure of the carina application of a small lung clamp into the carina and spreading it offers more space in a tiny anatomic compartment. A step which is specially needed on the left side. Dissection of paratracheal lymph nodes starts below the azygos vein. Dividing the azygos vein is possible but not essential. Mobilization of the lymph nodes below the azygos vein facilitates en bloc resection of the paratracheal lymph nodes. By grasping the mobilized lymph node package from above the azygos vein and gradually dissecting along the trachea and superior cava vein completes paratracheal lymph node dissection. For lymph node dissection use of the harmonic scalpel is recommended.

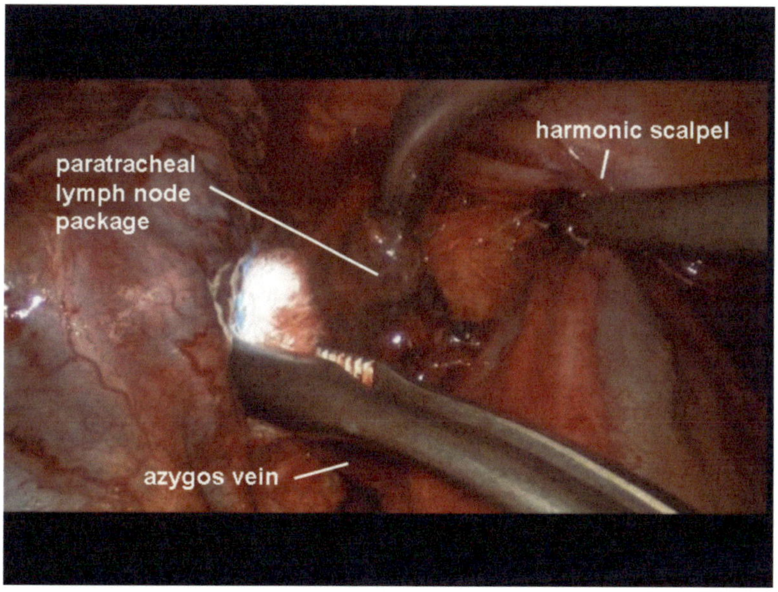

Fig. 7. En bloc nodal dissection paratracheal right

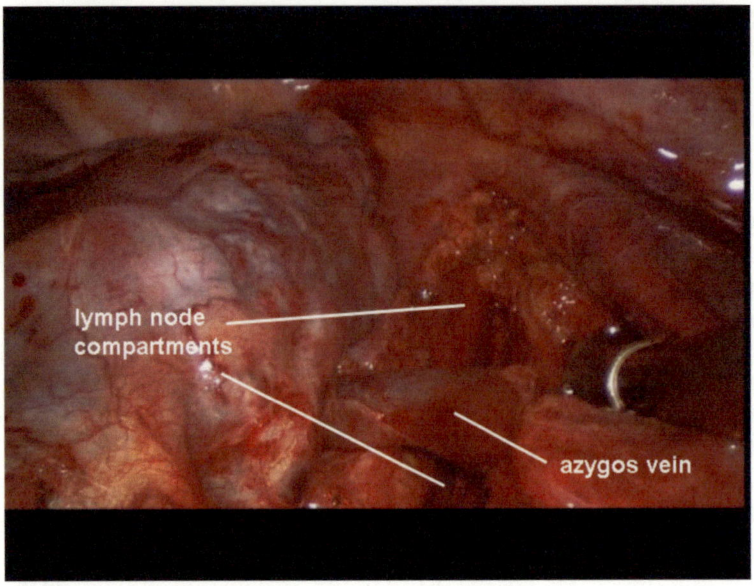

Fig. 8. Right paratracheal region after lymph node dissection

7.4 Extraction sac

Triangulate opening of the extraction sac in a small thoracic cavity is important to get the lobe into the extraction sac. To have no problems with this maneuver fix the sac with four stitches to big lung forceps, insert the forceps with the attached sac, open the forceps and the attached sac opens automatically. This technique avoids triangulate opening of the sac with two extra forceps. Insertion of the small end of the specimen first is auxiliary. Extracting the sac is completed by pulling alternately on one side seam then the other. Rarely a rip osteotomy is required.

8. References

Belgers E.; Siebenga J., Bosch A., van Haren E., Bollen E. (2010) Complete video-assisted thoracoscopic surgery lobectomy and its learning curve. A single center study introducing the technique in The Netherlands. *Interactive Cardiovascular and Thoracic Surgery* Vol. 10, No. 2, pp. 176-180

Boffa D.; Allen M. & Grab J. (2008) The Society of Thoracic Surgeons General Thoracic Surgery database: the surgical management of primary lung tumors. *The Journal of Thoracic and Cardiovascular Surgery* Vol. 135, No. 2, pp. 247-54

Burfeind W.; Jaik N., Villamizar N:; Toloza E., Harpole D., D'Amico T. (2010) A cost-minimisation analysis ofv lobectomy: thoracoscopic versus posterolateral thoracotomy. *European Journal of Cardio-Thoracic Surgery* Vol. 37, No. 4, pp. 827-832

Cassina P.; Julke M., Weder W. (1995) Thoracoscopic medistinal lymph node dissection: an experimental study in pigs. *European Journal of Cardio-Thoracic Surgery* Vol. 9, No. 10, pp. 544-547

Casali G. & Walker W. (2009) Video-assisted thoracic surgery lobectomy: can we afford it? *European Journal of Cardio-Thoracic Surgery* Vol. 35, No. 3, pp. 423-428

Chin C. & Swanson S. (2008) Video-Assisted Thoracic Surgery Lobectomy: Centers of Excellence or Excellence of Centers? *Thoracic Surgery Clinics* Vol. 18, No. 3, pp. 263-268

D'Amico T. (2008) Long-Term Outcomes of Thoracoscopic Lobectomy. *Thoracic Surgery Clinics* Vol. 18, No. 3, pp. 259-262

Demmy T.; Curtis J. (1999) Minimally invasive lobectomy directed toward frail and high-risk paients: a case control study. *The Annals of Thoracic Surgery* Vol. 68, No.1, pp. 194-200

Demmy T.; James T., Scott J., McKenna R., D'Amico T. (2005) Troubleshooting Video-Assisted Surgery Lobectomy *The Annals of Thoracic Surgery* Vol. 79, No. 5, pp. 1744-1752

Ferguson J. & Walker W. (2006) Developing a VATS lobectomy programme - can VATS lobectomy be taught? *European Journal of Cardio-Thoracic Surgery* Vol. 29, No. 5, pp. 806-9

Flores R.; Alam N. (2008) Video-Assisted Thoracic Surgery Lobectomy (VATS), Open Thoracotomy, and the Robot for Lung Cancer. *The Annals of Thoracic Surgery* Vol. 85, No.2, pp. 710-5

Hartwig M. & D'Amico T. (2010) Thoracoscopic Lobectomy: The Gold Standard for Early-Stage Lung Cancer? *The Annals of Thoracic Surgery* Vol. 89, No. 6, pp. 2098-101

Kaseda S.; Aoki T., Hangai N., Shimizi K. (2000) Better pulmonary function and prognosis with video-assisted thoracic surgery than with thoracotomy. *The Annals of Thoracic Surgery* Vol. 70, No. 5, pp. 1644-6

Kondo T.; Sagawa M., Tanita T., Sato M., Ono S., Matsumura Y., Fujimura S. (1998) Is complete systematic nodal dissection by thoracoscopic surgery possible? A prospective trial of video-assisted lobectomy for cancer of the right lung. *The Journal of Thoracic and Cardiovasclar Surgery* Vol. 116, No. 4, pp. 651-2

Lee J.; Cho B., Bae M, Lee C., Park I., Kim D., Chung K. (2011) Thoracoscopic Lobectomy Is Associated With Superior Compliance With Adjuvant Chemotherapy in Lung Cancer. *The Annals of Thoracic Surgery* Vol. 91, No. 2, pp. 344-348

Mahtabifard A; Fuller C. & McKenna R. (2008) Video-Assisted Thoracic Surgery Sleeve Lobectomy: A Case Series. *The Annals of Thoracic Surgery* Vol. 85, No. 2, pp. 729-732

McKenna R. (2008) Complications and Learning Curves for Video-Assisted Thoracic Surgery Lobectomy. *Thoracic Surgery Clinics* Vol. 18, No. 3, pp. 275-280

McKenna R. (1994) Lobectomy by video-assisted thoracic surgery with mediastinal node sampling for lung cancer. *The Journal of Thoraccic and Cardiovascular Surgery* Vol. 107, No. 3, pp. 879-82

McKenna R.; Houck W., Fuller C. (2006) Video-Assisted Thoracic Surgery Lobectomy: Experience With 1,100 Cases. *The Annals of Thoracic Surgery* Vol. 81, No. 2, pp. 421-6

McKenna R.; Mahtabifrad A., Pickens A., Kusuanco D., Fuller C. (2007) Fast-Tracking After Video-Assisted Thoracoscopic Surgery Lobectomy, Segmentectomy, and Pneumonectomy. *The Annals of Thoracic Surgery* Vol. 84, No. 4, pp. 1663-1668

McKenna R.; Wolf R., Brenner M., Fischel R., Wurnig P. (1998) Is lobectomy by video-assisted surgery an adequate cancer operation? *The Annals of Thoracic Surgery* Vol. 66, No. 6, pp. 1903-1907

Meyerson S.; LoCascio F., Balderson S., D'Amico T. (2010) An Inexpensive, Reproducible Tissue Simulator for Teaching Thoracoscopic Lobectomy. *The Annals of Thoracic Surgery* Vol. 89, No. 2, pp. 594-7

Nagahiro I.; Andou A., Aoe M., Sano Y., Date H., Shimizu N. (2001) Pulmonary function, postoperative pain and serum cytokine level after lobectomy: a comparison of

VATS and conventional procedure. *The Annals Thoracic Surgery* Vol. 72, No. 2, pp. 362-5

Nakajima J.; Takamoto S., Kohna T., Ohtsuka T. (2000) Costs of videothoracoscopic surgery versus open resection for patients with lung carcinoma. *Cancer* Vol. 1, No. 89, pp. 2497-501

Ng T.; Ryder B. (2006) Evolution to video-assisted thoracic surgery lobectomy after training: initial results of the first 30 patients. *Journal oft he American College of Surgeons* Vol. 203, No. 4, pp. 551-7

Onaitis M.; Petersen P., Balderson S., Toloza E., Burfeind W., Harpole D., D'Amico T. (2006) Thoracoscopic Lobectomy is a safe and versatile procedure: experience with 500 consecutive patients. *Annals of Surgery* Vol. 244, No. 3, pp. 420-5

Paul S.; Altorki N., Sheng S., Lee P., Harpole D., Onaitis M., Stiles B:, Port J., D'Amica T. (2010) Thoracooscopic lobectomy is associated with lower morbidity than open lobectomy: A propensity-matched analysis from the STS database. *The Journal of Thoracic and Cardiovascular Surgery* Vol. 139, No. 2, pp. 366-378

Petersen R. & Hansen H. (2010) Learning thoracoscopic lobectomy. *European Journal of Cardio-Thoracic Surgery* Vol. 37, No. 3, pp. 516-520

Petersen R.; Pham D., Burfeind W., Hanish S., Toloza E., Harpole D. Jr, D'Amico T. (2007) Thoracoscopic Lobectomy Facilitates the Delivery of Chemotherapy after Resection for Lung Cancer. *The Annals of Thoracic Surgery* Vol. 83, No. 4, pp. 1245-50

Rueth, N.; Andrade R. (2010) Is VATS Lobectomy Better: Perioperatively, Biologically and Oncologically? *The Annals of Thoracic Surgery* Vol.89, No. 6, pp. 2107-11

Roviario G.; Varoli F., Vergani C. Long term survival after video-assisted thoracoscopic surgery lobectomy for stage I lung cancer. *The Annals of Thoracic and Cardiovascular Surgery* Vol. 9, No. 1, pp. 14-21

Scott W.; Allen M., Darling G., Meyers B., Decker P., Putnam J., McKenna R., Landrenau R., Jones D., Inculet R., Malthaner R. (2010) Video-assisted thoracic surgery versus Open lobectomy for lung cancer: A secondary analysis of data from the American College of Surgeons Oncology Group Z0030 randomized clinical trial. *The Journal Of Thoracic and Cardiovascular Surgery* Vol. 136, No. 4, pp. 976-81

Walker W.; Codispoti M., Soon Y., Stamenkovic S., Carnochan F., Pugh G. (2003) Long-term outcomes following VATS lobectomy for non-small cell bronchogenic carcinoma. *European Journal of Cardio-Thoracic Surgery* Vol. 23, No.3, pp. 397-402

Watanabe A.; Koyanagi T., Ohsawa H., Mawatari T., Nakashima S., Takahashi N., Sato H., Abe T. (2005) Systematic node dissection by VATS is not inferior to that through an open thoracotomy: a comparative clinicopathologic retrospective study. *Surgery* Vol. 138, No. 3, pp. 510-7

Yamamoto K.; Ohsumi A., Kojima F., Imanishi N., Matsuoka K., Ueda M., Miyamoto Y. (2010) Long-Term Survival After Video-Assisted Surgery Lobectomy for Primary Lung Cancer. *The Annals of Thoracic Surgery* Vol. 89, No. 2, pp. 353-359

Yim A. (2010) Video-Assisted thoracic Lung Surgery: Is There a Barrier to Widespread Adoption? *The Annals of Thoracic Surgery* Vol. 89, No. 6, pp. 2112-3

13

Video-Assisted Thoracic Surgery Major Pulmonary Resections

Khalid Amer
Consultant Thoracic Surgeon, The Cardiovascular & Thoracic Unit, Southampton General Hospital, United Kingdom

1. Introduction

Video-Assisted Thoracic major pulmonary resections (VMPR) such as lobectomy, pneumonectomy and segmentectomy are rarely performed procedures, but steadily growing in popularity. Less than 4% of all lobectomies performed in the United Kingdom (UK)[1] and less than 5% in the United States [1] and Europe [2] are performed this way. The surgeon's knack, personal preference, and convictions about what constitutes a proper cancer surgery played a role in this reluctance to take up VATS lobectomy [3-7]. The first published series of VATS lobectomy was that of Roviaro et al 1992 from Milan [8]. The technique was already practiced by the American thoracic surgeons and popularised by Kirby, Landreneau and McKenna [9-10], but apparently Roviaro beat them at publishing. Kirby et al (US) published their initial experience with 35 patients undergoing VATS lobectomy in 1993. They have been performing the procedure 2 years prior to publication. 1993 witnessed the publication of several initial experiences with the technique. William Walker presented 11 cases from Edinburgh [11], and Coosemans, Lerut et al from Belgium published their series of four lobectomies [12]. However; it was McKenna who popularised the technique worldwide since his first publication in 1994 followed by publication of the largest series thus far of 1100 cases in 2006 (standing at 2600 cases in 2011 - by personal communication) [1, 10].

The operation is suited for early lung cancer and benign disease, but worry about the oncological feasibility of resection was one of the major criticisms against it. There is enough experience and data around the world to answer the questions of safety and long survival rates. With the advent of High Definition monitors, safer stapling devices and surgical instruments specifically designed for minimal access chest surgery, the procedure is expected to be adopted by new generations of thoracic surgeons. More and more the procedure is getting less invasive, and the literature already includes single port VATS lobectomy [13]. Progress of miniaturising the procedure is attributable to a head surge of similar technology by our peer gastrointestinal surgeons.

---

[1] Page R, Keogh B. First National Thoracic database report 2008. Published by the Society for Cardiothoracic Surgery in Great Britain and Ireland. 2008.P52, http://www.scts.org/documents/PDF/ThoracicSurgeryReport2008.pdf (21 June 2011).

In addition to conventional video-assisted thoracoscopic surgery (VATS), robotic technology with the da Vinci System® has emerged over the past 10 years [14]. Robotic major pulmonary resections proved to be feasible and safe. It requires training of the entire operating room team. The upshot of robotic surgery is the intuitive hand motion that translates the surgeon's movements into scaled, filtered and seamless movements to the robot arms, the 3 dimensional high definition vision with up to X10 magnification and the endowrist instrumentation designed to simulate the dexterity of the human hand inside the chest. The drawbacks are the exorbitant initial cost, the fact that the surgeon works away from the patient, and the loss of tactile feedback from the instruments. Its advantage over VATS is unproven; a longer follow-up period and randomized controlled trials are necessary to evaluate a potential benefit over conventional VATS approach.

VATS lobectomy programme is usually met by scepticism and resistance from the establishment, mainly due to financial and time constraints to meet cancer waiting times. There are problems of training and clinical governance issues but these are not insurmountable. Proper training and acquisition of the necessary skills is a prerequisite to starting such a programme. Safety of the technique is well established, and adherence to proper indications is essential. The technique is not recommended for central lesions, which should be removed by open thoracotomy.

2. Definitions

VATS major Pulmonary Resections (VMPR) relate to lobectomy, pneumonectomy, bilobectomy, segmentectomy and combinations thereof. This excludes procedures such as VATS wedge resection and lung biopsy. Controversy surrounds the definition of what constitutes minimal access surgery, but now there is wide acceptance of the following definition:

- Surgeon operating via monitor, and not looking directly through the wound.
- Strictly no rib spreading.
- Anatomical individual structure dissection, as opposed to simultaneous stapling of structures.
- Less than 5 ports, the aggregate length of which is <10cm (with the advent of 3mm ports this criterion is not mandatory).

3. Best practice evidence

There are three established randomised controlled trials (RCT) comparing VATS lobectomy to open thoracotomy. In 1995 Kirby et al randomized 61 patients with clinical stage I NSCLC to undergo lobectomy by VATS (31patients) or muscle-sparing thoracotomy (30 patients) [15]. The VATS were performed without rib spreading. They concluded that VATS did not increase risks, but did not state superiority of VATS over mini-thoracotomy in terms of length of stay, drain dwell time and postoperative pain. The study is criticised for not comparing VATS to full posterolateral thoracotomy.

The second RCT is the only one examining survival differences between VATS and open lobectomy published by a Japanese group, Sugi et al in 2000 [16]. They randomised 100 patients with clinical stage Ia lung cancer to VATS (48 patients) or open (52 patients) lobectomy and mediastinal lymph node dissection. They concluded no significant

differences in the recurrence or survival rates. The overall 5 years survival rates after surgery were 85% and 90% in the open and VATS groups, respectively.
The third RCT comes from Edinburgh, and was published in 2001 by Craig, Walker et al [17]. It addressed the body immune responses to trauma, randomising 25 patients to open (16 patients) or VATS lobectomy (19 patients). Acute phase indicators were analyzed in patients undergoing surgery for suspected lung cancer. They concluded that VATS lobectomy was associated with less traumatic insult to the patient, and consequently reduced peri-operative changes in acute phase responses. This finding may have implications for peri-operative tumour immuno-surveillance in lung cancer patients.
There has been a number of published case-series, and the most impressive and the largest worldwide is that of McKenna et al [1]. Safety of the technique was proven beyond doubt to be at least equal to open thoracotomy, but benefits in less postoperative pain, shorter hospital stay and quicker recovery were now well established. Walker et al (2003) published long term survival results of VATS versus open thoracotomy [18]. The available evidence suggests that VATS lobectomy for clinical Stage I and II NSCLC is a technically safe procedure which is associated with long-term survival and recurrence outcomes that are at least equivalent to those provided by open thoracotomy.

4. Indications

VMPR is suitable for benign and malignant disease both with intension to cure or prolong the disease free interval. The following is a list of some of the current indications, but it keeps growing:

a. Benign:
   1. Hamartomas
   2. Solitary fibrous tumours
   3. Teratomas
   4. Fibromas / lipomas / leiomyomas
   5. Sclerosing haemangiomas
   6. MALToma (Mucosa associated Lymphoid tumours)
   7. Lung sequestration
   8. A-V malformations leading to haemoptysis
b. Malignant:
   1. Non Small Cell Lung Cancer stage cT1-2 N0-1 M0
   2. Small Cell Lung Cancer (contained disease)
   3. Carcinoid tumours
   4. Solitary or multiple secondaries within one lobe (usual rules apply: control of primary site, enough residual pulmonary reserve, absence of extra-thoracic metastases, and fitness for general anaesthetic).

The distribution of histological findings in our series of 156 patients considered for VATS resection is shown in Table 1.
All presumed lung cancer cases should be discussed in a multidisciplinary meeting. VMPR is designed for early lung cancer, and should be considered as first choice for T1-2, N0-1, M0 lesion on PET/CT. Tumours larger than 5-6 cm across, and central tumours are better removed by open thoracotomy. Resection of Non Small Cell Lung Cancer in the absence of

mediastinal nodes is performed with a curative intent, an axiom supported by the international literature. The controversy arises in operable early cancer in the presence of a histologically proven single station mediastinal node (cT1-3, N2). The current best practice evidence supported by the S9900 trial follow up published in 2010 continues to show that the best treatment for N2 resectable lung cancer would be induction chemotherapy followed by surgery (evidence level 1b) [19]. Multizonal lung cancer is thought to be a systemic disease beyond cure by surgery alone, and is best treated by chemo-radiotherapy. Albain et al (2009) have shown that lobectomy will add little to Chemo-radiotherapy for patients with stage IIIa (N2) non-small-cell lung cancer, at the expense of higher mortality [20].

Malignant 142	Lung cancer - NSCLC Subtypes:		127 (81.3%)
	Adenocarcinoma	86 (55.1%)	
	Squamous Carcinoma	24 (15.4%)	
	Adeno-squamous carcinoma	4 (2.6%)	
	Broncheoloalveolar	4 (2.6%)	
	Large cell	3 (1.9%)	
	Other	6 (3.8%)	
	Lung cancer - Small Cell		3 (1.9%)
	Carcinoid tumour Typical 3 Atypical 3		6 (3.8%)
	Lung cancer - metastatic Breast 1 Kidney 1 Colon 3 Endometrium 1		6 (3.8%)
Benign 14	Inflammatory mass 4 TB granuloma 2 Hamartoma 3 Aspergilloma 1 Benign cyst 1 Other 3		14 (8.9%)

Table 1. Histological types of surgically removed 156 specimens suitable for VATS resection.

5. Contraindications

1. Central tumours. Interpretation of the CT scan must establish clearance to apply stapling devices before embarking on VATS pneumonectomy.
2. Large tumours possibly >5-6 cm, as these will require large incision and rib spreading for retrieval. The surgical specimen should not be divided in pieces to improve retrieval, as histological details or limits of invasions can be lost.
3. CT evidence of clear invasion of central vascular structures by tumour or lymph nodes. Very high experience in VMPR is required to deal with vascular invasion.

VATS pneumonectomy was proven to be feasible and safe [21]. Tumours crossing the fissure from one lobe to the other could either be dealt with by lobectomy and wedge of the neighbouring lobe, or pneumonectomy according to the side. The presence of a thick major fissure is also no longer a contraindication, as the technique of fissure-last dissection is widely practiced [22, 23]. Obese patients with BMI>30 could pose a challenge as the chest wall thickness might be greater that the port length. By the same token, these are the very same patients who would benefit maximally from VATS procedure, as their postoperative rehabilitation is much better compared to open thoracotomy.
As experience with this procedure increases more challenges are taken up by thoracic surgeons. VMPR used to be contraindicated for redo procedure after previous thoracotomy, or cardiac procedure that has breached the pleura. This is not the case anymore, and more surgeons are venturing into the realm of redo surgery by VATS. New indications are being explored for VMPR as the surgeons become more experienced and daring. Currently surgeons are attempting chest wall resections, extrapleural pneumonectomy for mesothelioma and sleeve resections by VATS [24-26].

6. Preoperative investigations

Preoperative investigations should target the following areas:

a. The patient's general fitness for undergoing a 3 hours operation under general anaesthesia.
b. Residual pulmonary reserve after lung resection.
c. Feasibility of VATS resection and extent of resection.
d. Risk assessment and estimation of life quality after surgery.

The following is not an exhaustive list of investigations and should be individually tailored to the patient:

- Pulmonary function tests (lung capacity FEV1, FVC, and gas transfer TLCO)
- Calculated predicted postoperative FEV1 ($PPOFEV_1$) expressed as % predicted
- Calculated predicted postoperative T_{LCO} ($PPOT_{LCO}$) expressed as % predicted
- Fresh CT chest and abdomen, within 4-6 weeks of operation.
- Fusion PET/CT full body within 4 weeks of operation.
- CT/MRI brain to exclude the 10% brain metastases at time of presentation (particularly adenocarcinoma).
- Flexible bronchoscopy possibly performed by the chest physician for histological diagnosis.
- In selected cases CT-guided needle aspiration biopsy should be considered. If this was turned down by the radiologists then a VATS wedge resection and frozen section should be planned. Patients with previously treated extra-thoracic adenocarcinoma pose a special challenge, as frozen section might not be able to determine the original mother organ of adenocarcinoma cells obtained at operation. Currently there is no reasonably quick method of staining for TTF1 marker which is almost pathognomonic of primary lung adenocarcinoma.
- N2 disease suggested by PET/CT should be confirmed histologically by mediastinoscopy, EBUS, EUS, TEMLA (Trans-cervical Extended Mediastinal Lymph Adenectomy) or VATS nodal dissection. Confirmed single station N2 disease should receive neoadjuvant chemotherapy before consideration of VMPR.

- Other studies might be necessary to decide on fitness of patient, such as exercise tolerance test, 6 minute walk test, Shuttle test, quantitative V/Q scan and echocardiography.

7. Technical aspects

7.1 General considerations

The patient should be consented for VMPR by the highest authority, usually the consultant surgeon who will personally perform the procedure. The side of operation must be visibly marked on the patient before going to theatre. The CT scans should be available in theatre for reference, and the side and site of lobe to be removed should be confirmed by the operating team before starting. Prior cross matching of blood is not necessary, but this depends on how quickly blood could be cross matched in case of vascular injury. Under general anaesthesia the operation is usually started by rigid and/or flexible bronchoscopy in the anaesthetic room to ascertain operability and exclude obvious contraindications. The anaesthetist then slips in a double lumen endotracheal tube or bronchial blockers and a single lumen tube, to establish single lung ventilation. The patient is then positioned on the operating table, on the lateral side, operative side up, as for a standard thoracotomy. Breaking the operative table at the torso, or elevating a bridge under the chest opens the intercostal spaces. Early isolation of the lung by the anaesthetist at this stage pays dividend when complete collapse of the lung is welcomed by the operating surgeon. A central venous access and arterial invasive monitoring are not mandatory and are not routinely practiced at the author's institution. After draping the patient, the port sites are chosen and operation started. Co2 insufflation is completely unnecessary as it does not add space and can be life threatening. High intrathoracic pressures can lead to mediastinal shift and cardiac arrest. Space could be at a premium in badly emphysematous lungs due to trapped air, despite good lung isolation by the anaesthetist. Sometimes deliberate digging of holes in the target lobe using diathermy, might improve lung collapse and allow more room for operating. VMPR is usually performed via three port sites, but more minimisation of the technique is making it possible to work through a single port (uniportal approach) [13]. The principle of triangulation of ports is important to observe in our institution, and fencing (scissoring) of instruments is to be avoided. The use of a 0° scope gives a good image but is slightly limited, and might necessitate the camera to be moved from one port to the other. Certainly the vision could be improved by using a 30° scope, but the camera operator should be aware of standardising the orientation of the scope over the camera. If this orientation is not adhered to anatomical disillusion can easily occur, and identification of structures can be erroneous. Anatomical disorientation usually does not occur with the 0° scope, and bendable 0° scopes will probably go a long way. The surgeon, assistant, anaesthetist and scrub nurse should carefully rehearse beforehand their roles in the event of a major uncontrollable vascular injury requiring immediate thoracotomy.

7.2 Different surgical approaches

There are two approaches to VMPR, based on where the surgeon stands in relation to the patient. Each approach has its advantages and disadvantages:

1. The anterior approach: championed by R. McKenna, Cedars Sinai Medical Centre, Los Angeles, California.

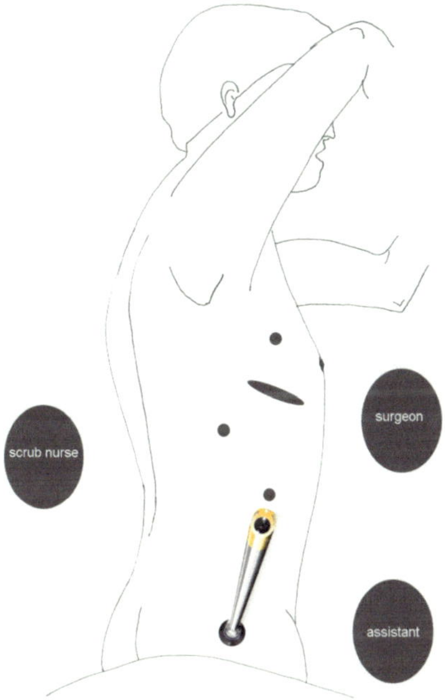

The anterior approach:

- Surgeon stands at the front of the patient, with his assistant (camera operator) to his left on the same side.
- 4 ports are fashioned, the utility port 5-6 cm is fashioned low at the 5th or 6th space.
- 30° scope.
- Direct approach over the hilum.
- Less operative time.

2. The posterior approach (fissure oriented approach), preached by W Walker, Edinburgh Royal Infirmary - UK.

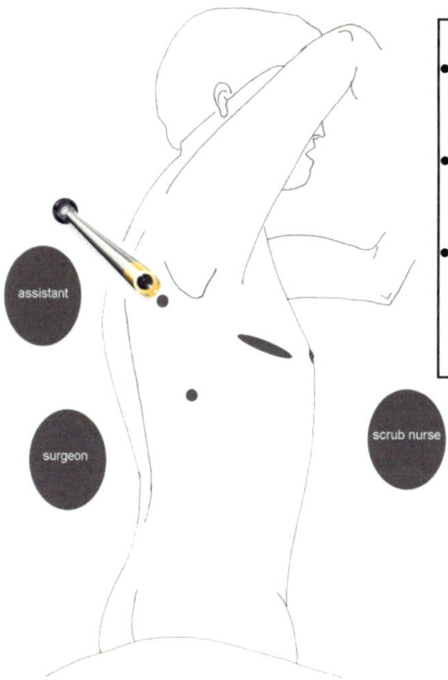

The posterior approach:

- Surgeon stands at the back of the patient, assistant to the left, same side (camera operator).
- 3 ports and the utility port is 4-5 cm at the widest space anteriorly (5th, 6th, or 7th).
- 0° scope introduced from the back top port in line with the axis of the major fissure. Camera is moved from one port to the other.

3. The Southampton approach, practiced by the author, Southampton General Hospital – UK.

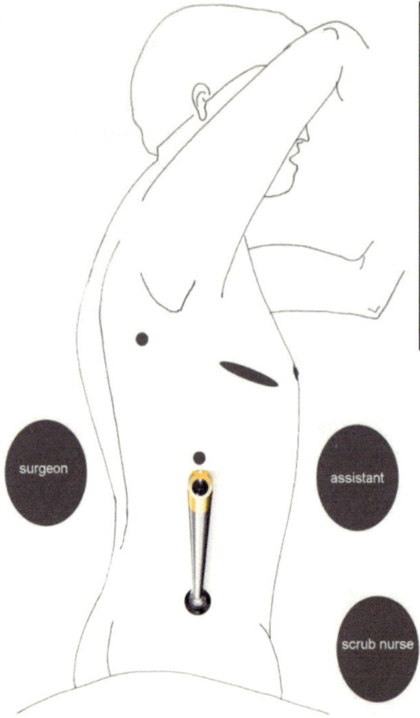

The Southampton approach:

- Surgeon stands at the back of the patient, opposite assistant (camera operator – helper - retractor).
- 2 ports + the utility port; 3-4 cm at the widest space anteriorly (4th, 5th).
- 30° scope introduced from the inferior port in line with the axis of the hilum, and stays there.

Whereas the anterior approach is the widely used internationally, the posterior approach is the one commonly taught in the UK. The Southampton approach is an adaptation of the posterior approach. The anterior approach is the quickest, gives a better view of the anterior hilum and apex, but poor view to the back of the hilum. The view is foreshortened when stapling the fissures and as a result the tip end of the stapling device is not visible, requiring a leap of faith to staple the fissures. Also the view is not optimal for nodal dissection, especially the subcarinal space. Anatomy is viewed from an unfamiliar angle, and the surgeon's brain requires retraining to appreciate structures from different perspective. In case of conversion to thoracotomy, the surgeon has to swap sides, or extend the utility port into an anterior thoracotomy and stay anterior to the patient.

The posterior approach is oriented around the axis of the oblique (major) fissure, and gives also a good view, except for the superior vein. To get a right angle approach of the stapling device to the superior vein, the camera has to swap ports. Dissection usually starts at the centre of the fissure, and the advantage of this approach is lost when the fissure is thick, or does not peel easily.

The Southampton approach keeps the 30° camera at the inferior port, in line with the hilar axis, thus giving good views anterior as well as posterior to the hilum. The anatomical view is exactly as open thoracotomy, at all times. Good access to harvest all groups of nodes when performing Systematic Nodal Dissection (SND), however; a utility port below the 5th space makes access to stations 2-4 at the apex difficult. As lung retraction is essential, it take longer than other approaches.

7.3 Port site fashioning

The ports must be carefully chosen and designed, as this could influence the ease of surgical accessibility. The technique of microthoracotomy is commonly used [Figure 1], whereby the use of a long forceps blades are used to retract the incision, and the muscles over the superior border of the rib are diathermised down to the pleural space. Care must be taken not to diathermise in midspace, as this might lead to nerve injury, and short and long term neuropathic pain would ensue [Figure 2].

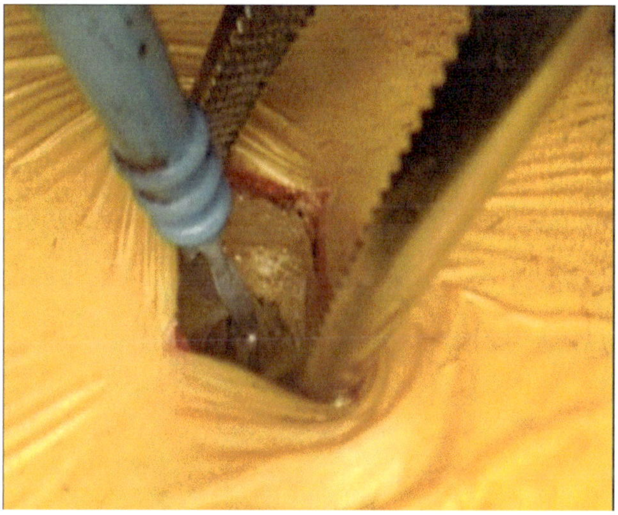

Fig. 1. Microthoracotomy by diathermy 10mm wide.

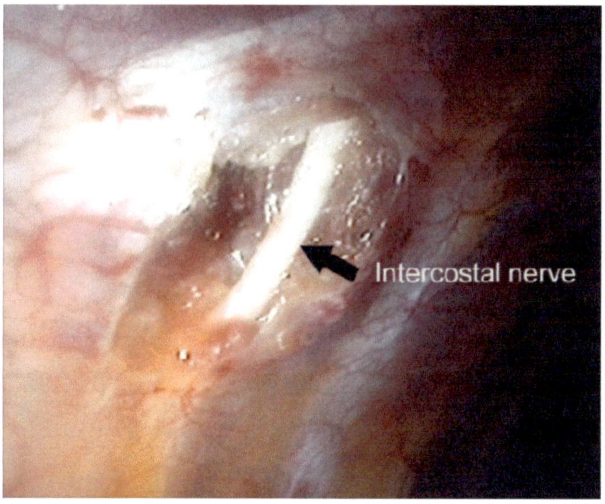

Fig. 2. Midspace diathermy resulting in nerve damage.

We usually start the procedure by fashioning the anterior utility port over the (widest) 4th-5th space, centred over the mid-axillary line. There is advantage in fashioning the utility port first, as this enables finger palpation of the primary tumour site, and early usage of conventional thoracic instruments. The port would be used at the end to retrieve the specimen out of the chest, so it is sensible to open the full 3-4 cm right at the beginning.

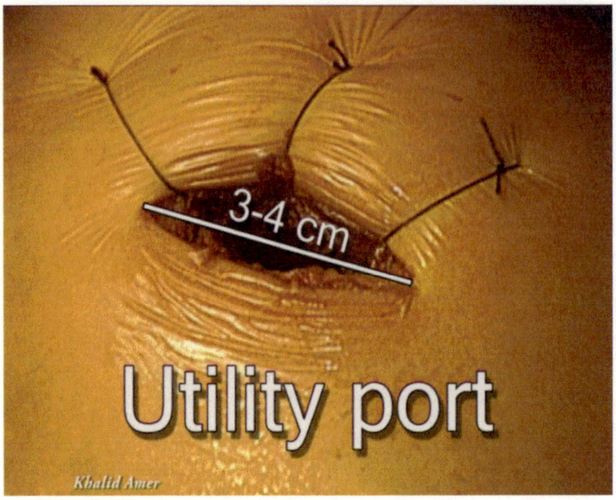

Fig. 3. Utility port kept open by stay sutures.

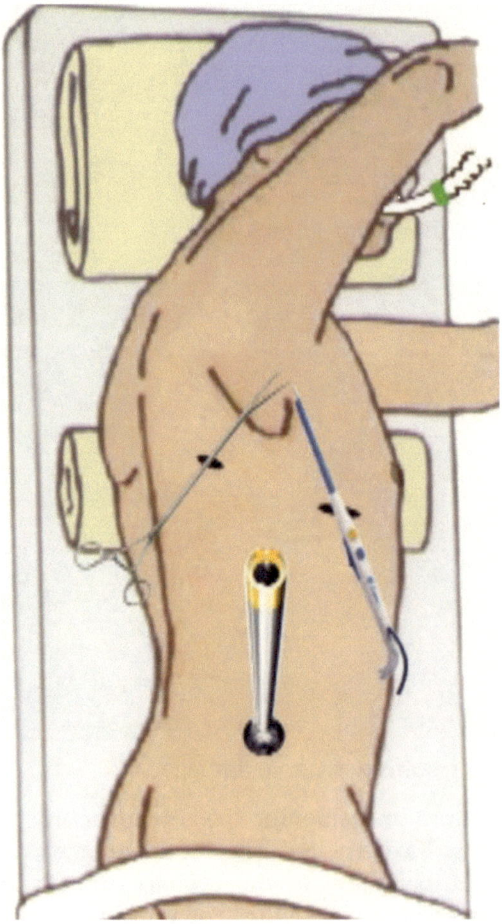

Fig. 4. Fashioning ports for VMPR: the inferior port is dedicated to the camera.

Beyond the skin incision the fibres of latissimus muscles are split in the direction of its fibres, rather than cut. The rib is exposed using the diathermy spatula and the upper border of the rib is cleared of muscle attachment, until the pleura is entered. The port is then kept open at all times by stay silk sutures taken deep to the muscles and over the skin [Figure 3]. This ensures a dry and self retracted port, suitable for accommodating more than one instrument at any given time. Similar silk sutures could be used to keep the other operative ports open, so that instruments could be passed directly without the need for a plastic or metal port. However; the use of such port is recommended for the camera, as this insures the lens will be dry for a longer period. Port site bleeding can be a problem, and may require too frequent cleaning of the camera lens, therefore it is best to construct the camera port site carefully, bloodlessly and first time. The 30° scope is then inserted, and a quick scout for pleural deposits is performed. Having excluded secondary deposits, attention is then paid to creating the inferior port. This is fashioned in line with the hilar axis, over the highest most point in the dome of the diaphragm. The camera scope is then transferred to the inferior port, where it remains for the rest of the operation. The posterior port is fashioned over the auscultatory triangle, one or two finger's breadth from the medial border of the scapula [figure 4].

7.4 The fissures

We define a nice fissure as a fissure that goes all the way from the surface of the lung down to the pulmonary artery. The perivascular sleeve of the artery is clearly visible throughout the length of the fissure; there are no crossing veins and no lymph nodes stuck to the artery. A nice fissure peels easily when two kissing peanuts are dissecting in opposite directions (Bill Walker manoeuvre) [27]. A thick fissure on the other hand goes a short distance from the lung surface, the artery is not seen and the fissure does not peel easily. It would be futile to persevere with dissecting such a fissure, as good time would be wasted, and major bleeding might result in conversion [Figure 5a & 5b]. In such cases the fissure-last technique is adopted [22, 23].

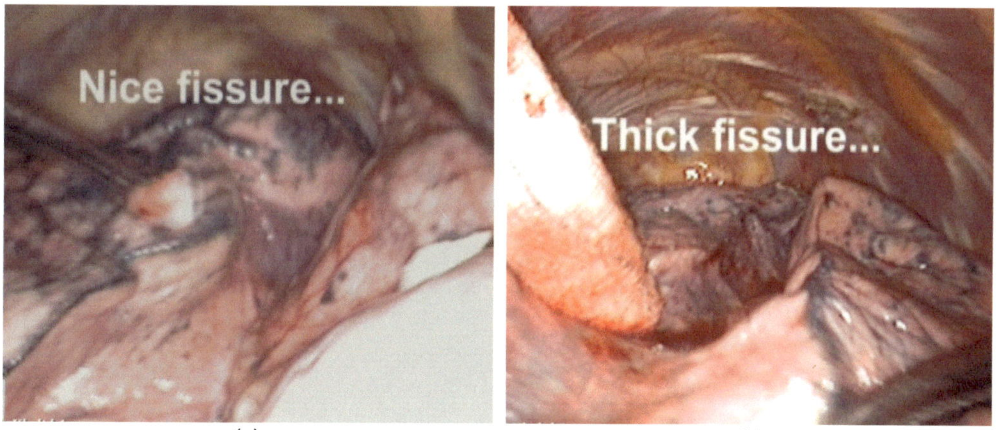

(a) (b)

Fig. 5. (a) Nice major fissure, and (b) Thick or incomplete fissure.

7.5 VATS lobectomy

Right upper lobectomy:

After fashioning the triangulated three ports, the pleural cavity is scrutinised for secondary deposits that might contraindicate proceeding with the operation. The index finger is then introduced via the utility port, to palpate the lesion, helped by a peanut on a Robert to push the lung towards the palpating finger. Sometimes the tumour puckers the surface of the lung and confirmation of the lesion *and* target lobe is obvious. If the target lobe could not be identified at operation, we strongly recommend conversion to open thoracotomy (even if the CT clearly locates the lesion and the lobe!) [Figure 6].

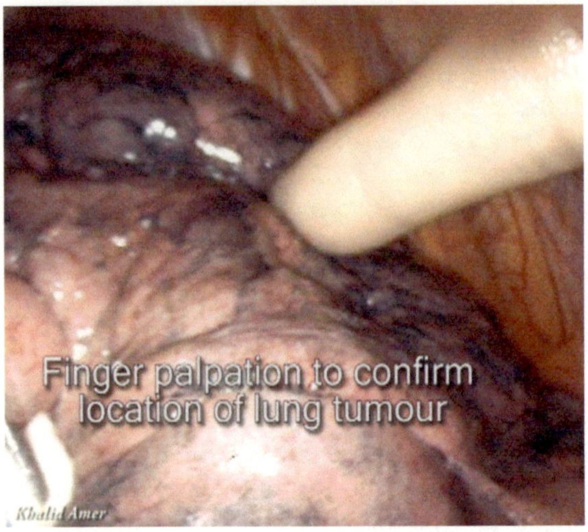

Fig. 6. Early visual and tactile identification of the lesion within the target lobe.

The operation is started at a simple and constant step, and the level of complexity is increased as the operation proceeds. The inferior pulmonary ligament is released, the inferior vein confirmed to arise separately from the main pulmonary vein (sometimes it joins the superior vein in a single trunk as a delayed origin). The anterior hilar pleura is opened lateral to the phrenic nerve and the veins from middle and upper lobe are confirmed. The upper lobe vein is then skeletonised and secured using a stapling device [Figure 7]. It is to be remembered that taking the middle lobe vein by mistake will lead to infarction of the middle lobe later, so ample time must be spent to ascertain the venous anatomy.

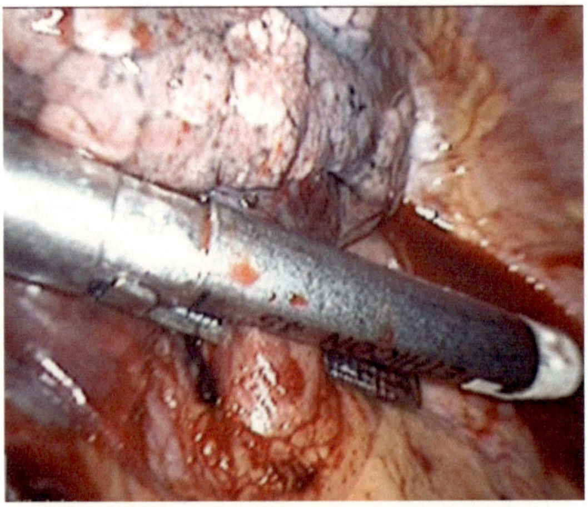

Fig. 7. Stapling the upper lobe vein (part of the superior pulmonary vein) using a 3 row stapling device.

This manoeuvre exposes the pulmonary artery branches. An anterior pulmonary artery branch might lend itself readily to stapling at this stage, but it is usually difficult to secure the Truncus arteriosus (which usually divides into 2 branches). At this stage attention is drawn to the bronchus. The lung is retracted anteriorly and the pleura over the back of the hilum is opened from inferior ligament to Azygos vein. The right main bronchus is exposed, and its division into upper lobe and bronchus intermedius is displayed. Blind dissection around the back of bronchus has to take into account that the truncus artery lies closely behind the bronchus in a blind spot. Opening of curved devices behind the bronchus has to be very gentle, until the tip of the instrument is seen emerging from the other side of the bronchus. The bronchus is then encircled with a vascular sloop and a (green) stapling device is placed perpendicular to the longitudinal axis of the upper lobe bronchus, flush with bifurcation. No matter how clear the anatomy is, the stapling device should not be fired before test inflating the lung, to ensure that the remaining lobes are not obstructed or stapled by mistake. Only then the bronchus is transacted. This manoeuvre exposes the posterior segmental artery and the truncus. Both of which should be skeletonised and secured. Different methods have been used to secure large vessels, ranging from simple endoscopic tying, stapling, clipping or using energy devices, such as ultrasonic or bipolar devices. The choice depends on the diameter of the vessel and what the operator feels comfortable with. If the anterior arterial branch was not encountered earlier on, it might be visible after securing the posterior segmental artery from a posterior view. The lobe by now should be attached to the rest of the lung by the fissures, which are stapled off. If the horizontal fissure is not well developed, incomplete or absent (25% of cases), it might be helpful at the beginning of the operation to staple the lung at an imaginary line between the upper and middle lobes, where the fissure is thought to have existed. This is done at the medial anterior border of the lung, to mark the spot for joining later from a posterior approach, when all structures had been secured. The free lobe is then retrieved in a sturdy Polythene bag. Systematic nodal dissection is performed if it was deferred to this stage.

Right middle lobectomy:

Same as above, but the sequence would be; inferior ligament followed by middle lobe vein, middle lobe bronchus before identifying and tackling the middle lobe artery. All three structures are approached anterior to the hilum. Beware of the delayed origin of the middle lobe bronchus arising from the lower lobe bronchus, as this might be included in a stapling device aimed at freeing the medial part of the oblique (major) fissure.

Right lower lobe:

This could be the trickiest to remove especially if dissection is retrograde, and the fissures were thick. Nevertheless; dissection is started by releasing the inferior ligament and confirming a normal venous drainage of all lobes. The inferior vein is taken next. This exposes the lower lobe bronchus, which must be carefully dissected proximally to satisfy one's self with the take-off of the middle lobe bronchus. Again the stapling device across the bronchus should not be fired unless the middle lobe is seen to inflate fully and easily. It should be resisted to staple the lower lobe bronchus obliquely as a matter of convenience. Enough time must be paid to make sure that the lower lobe bronchus is stapled perpendicular to the longitudinal axis of the bronchus. Oblique stapling could lead to stenosis of the origin of the middle lobe bronchus [figure 8]. It should be remembered that the wall of the bronchus at the stapling line is stiff, and gradually widens from the site of the staples to the full diameter of the bronchus, in a funnel shape profile that practically narrows the lumen by further 2-3 mm. This is usually overlooked, and leads to unexpected stenosis in the postoperative period. An hour-glass anatomy of the origin of the middle lobe leads to twisting of the bronchus as the remaining lobes inflate, and that might lead to complete dynamic obstruction in the postoperative period. The postoperative chest x-ray would reveal a collapsed middle lobe, which fails to re-inflate with aggressive physiotherapy. The middle lobe artery take-off has to be identified before taking the common basal trunk. There could be one trunk dividing into common basal and apical lower arteries, or the apical branch might require separate stapling. Also be wary of a posterior segmental artery to the upper lobe arising from the apical lower branch (delayed branching).

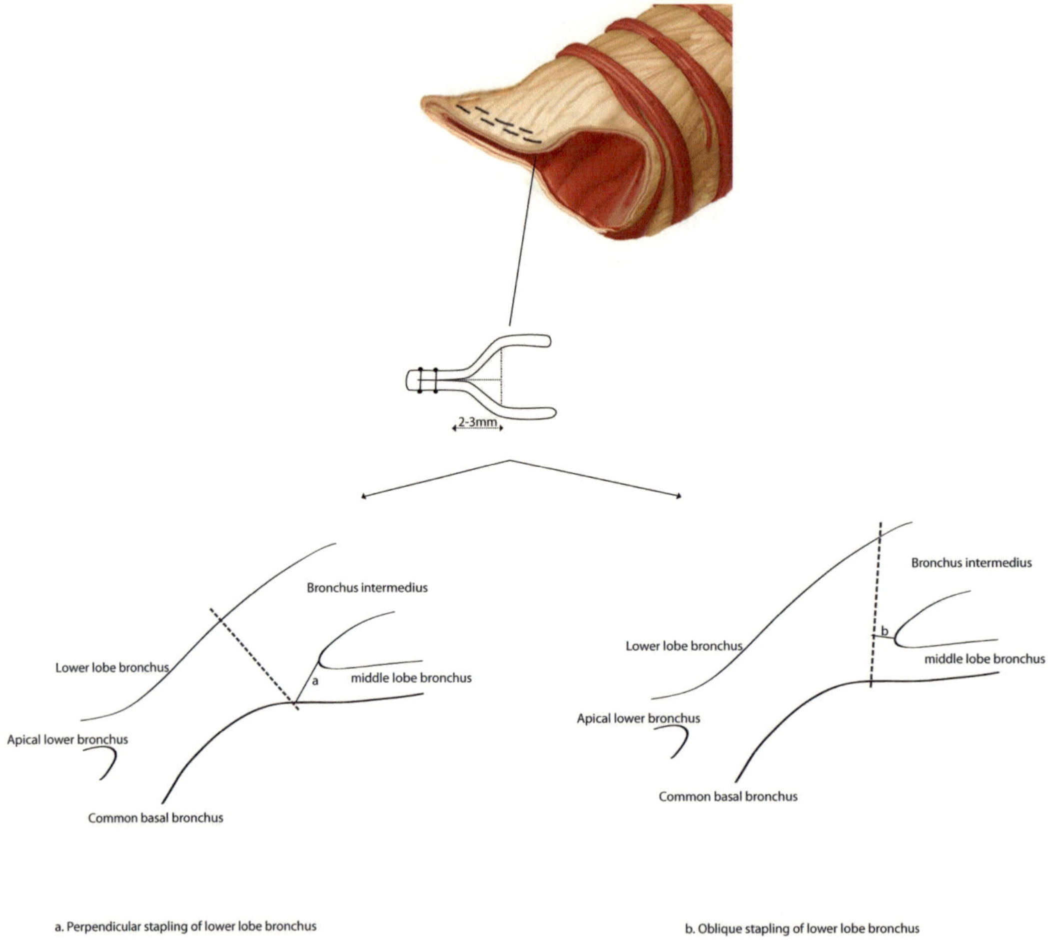

Fig. 8. (a) Perpendicular transverse stapling of lower lobe bronchus resulting in a normal patent orifice of the middle lobe bronchus. (b) Narrowed orifice of middle lobe bronchus as a result of oblique stapling.

Left upper lobectomy:
The sequence of dissection is more or less similar to the right side. Dissection is started with the inferior ligament, and venous anatomy identified. The superior vein is taken either as a

single trunk or for ease of dissection taking the lingular vein first might simplify the dissection. It is recommended to keep the vascular stumps as short as practicable, to avoid clot formation and embolisation. The bronchus is exposed next. It must be further cleared to identify the secondary carina, and subsequently the upper lobe bronchus. Make sure you include the lingular bronchus in the sloop. Again before firing the stapling gun, the lung is inflated to ensure patency of the lower lobe bronchus. Doing this as a matter of routine ensures that no mistake is made, and the left main bronchus is not mistaken for the upper lobe bronchus (it can happen!) [23]. At this stage the lingular arteries (1 or 2) would have lend themselves amenable to stapling. Next the Truncus artery is taken, and the fissure is tackled as before.

Left lower lobectomy:

This is the easiest lobe to remove, and perhaps a good one to start training with. After releasing the inferior ligament the inferior vein is stapled. This exposes the bronchus, which is dissected proximally until the bifurcation is identified and a stapling device is placed across. The lung is inflated and the bronchus transected. Further retrograde dissection identifies the branches of the pulmonary artery, and the arrangement verified. Again there could be one trunk, or two separate branches; common basal and apical lower arteries. These are taken and the fissure completed by stapling, peeling, diathermy or ultrasonic device.

From the previous description, fissure-last technique is the default technique to start with, but in our experience a nice fissure should be taken advantage of. The sequence of dissection could be modified to start with the fissure and deal with the arterial branches first. Previously it was claimed that early venous stapling leads to engorgement of the lung and that might impede dissection. In our experience, it does not make any difference what so ever. In fact it serves the oncological principle of preventing the dissemination of malignant cells resulting from handling the tumour or the target lobe.

VATS segmentectomy:

The same principles apply for removing a segment of a lobe. It is to be remembered that pulmonary arteries are end arteries, i.e. ligation of an artery by mistake leads to infarction of part of the lung. There is quite a lot of shared venous flow, and ligation of veins (apart from the central final tributaries, such as the middle lobe vein) does not lead to infarction. The most important structures to secure are the segmental bronchus and the artery. The vein could be ignored or stapled as part of stapling the fissure. If the fissures are permitting then dissection is started at the centre of the fissure. The arterial pattern is identified and the segmental artery is secured. This usually exposes the bronchus, where it is identified and cross clamped, using a Robert forceps. A fine butterfly needle is connected to a giving-set plastic tube and air is injected into the segmental bronchus, using a bladder syringe, distal to the clamp. This will inflate the anatomical confines of the segment, demarcating the intersegmental plane [28]. Alternatively, the anaesthetist could inflate the upper lung while the segmental bronchus is clamped, and the segment will stay deflated. The first method is preferred by the author, as it keeps the lung deflated and allows space to operate. However; pressurised air from an Oxygen cylinder should not be used, as the danger from massive air embolisation is high [23]. The lung parenchyma is then stapled off the rest of the lung, guided by the intersegmental demarcation.

VATS pneumonectomy:

Very rarely lung cancer allows the performance of a VATS pneumonectomy. The reason for that is by the very same nature of the central lesion that dictates pneumonectomy, makes it unsuitable for VATS technique. Clearance of the 3 major structures; bronchus, artery and vein is usually not possible, and this judgement could be made on scrutinising the CT scan. However; sometime a central tumour at the bifurcation of the secondary carina, crossing the fissure, and resectable only by pneumonectomy, might have sufficient clearance on the main bronchus, artery and vein (possibly intrapericardially). These cases are rare but resectable by VATS [21, 23]. The utility port has to be slightly bigger, but no rib spreading is required. Sturdy Polythene bag is indispensible. Generally speaking central tumours are best dealt with by open operation. The advent of the articulating 3 row stapling devices has given a great boost to the confidence of stapling major vessels such as the main pulmonary artery, which has a thinner wall than the main pulmonary vein.

Retrieval of surgical specimens:

The initial case-series of VATS lobectomy reported port-site seedling, and recommended retrieval within a Polythene bag. It has become our standard practice to exteriorise the resected lobe within a polythene bag for that matter. However, McKenna et al suggested the use of the bag does not completely eliminate this risk [1]. We encountered a single port-site seedling in a series of 200 cases (0.5%) [figure 9]. The patient had a previously resected colonic adenocarcinoma. The adenocarcinoma within the lobe was retrieved in a bag, but none of the nodes. Incidentally all nodes were free from metastases. Port-site metastasis could not be explained merely by mechanical seedling in our case, and humoral spread had to be presumed.

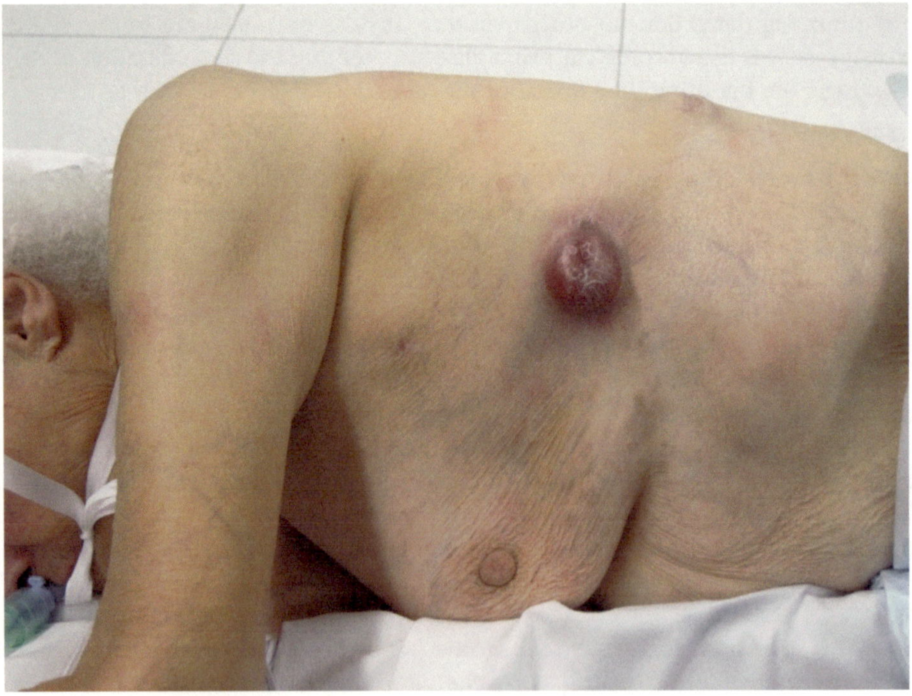

Fig. 9. Port-site seedling 3 months after VATS left upper lobectomy.

Closure:

After retrieval of the specimen and securing haemostasis we routinely test the bronchial stump under water and partial inflation up to 20-30 mm Hg. An extra pleural catheter is inserted under videoscopic guidance, for continuous infusion postoperative analgesia. The chest is closed over a single chest drain, 24-28F with an extra basal hole. We use the camera port for the drain site, and close the utility and posterior ports in layers, after observing the lung expanding satisfactorily. Care must be exercised to close the utility port in proper layers, as mass closure might lead to unsightly ledge or step if the skin is fixed to the deeper tissues. The final resulting scars of the ports are usually pleasing to the patient [Figure 10]

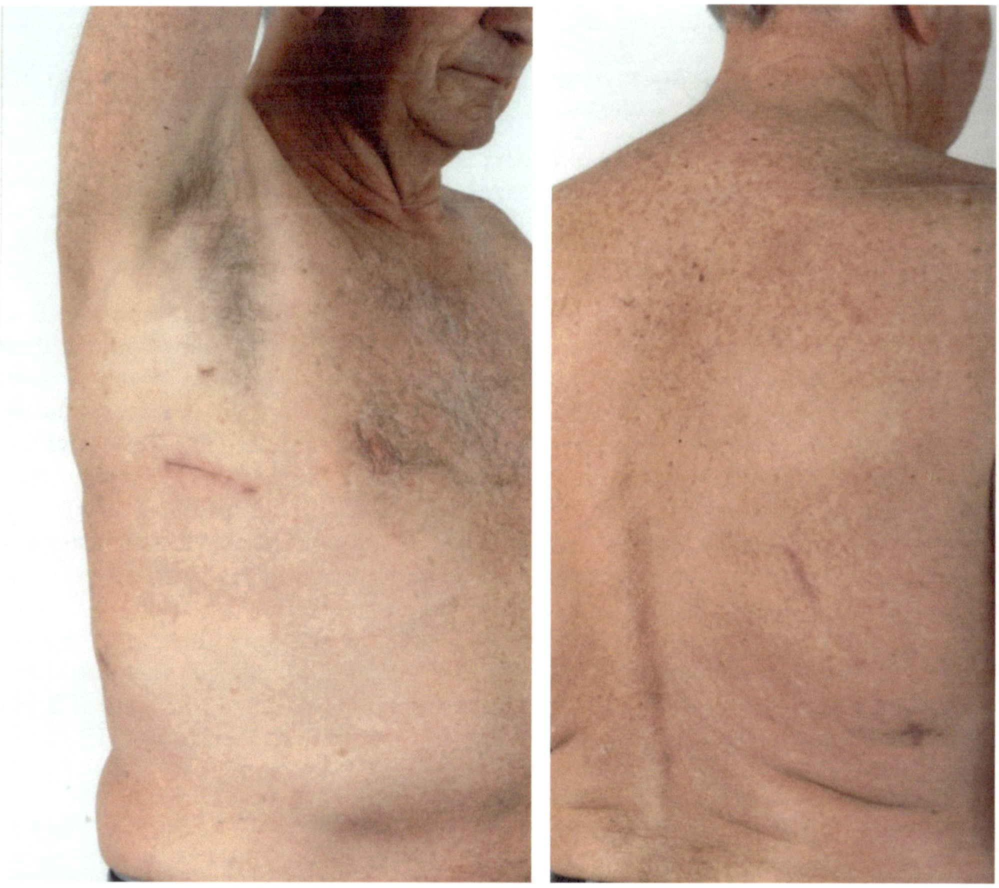

Fig. 10. The cosmetic scars of VATS lobectomy.

8. Surgical operative time

The average time of performing VATS lobectomy + SND is 03:00 hours. Table 2 shows the mean operative time in 133 completed procedures in our unit. There was no statistical difference between the lobes.

Lobe removed	Frequency	Mean operative time (min)	Standard Deviation
RUL	44	232	51.7
RML	9	186	34.3
RLL	23	227	63.5
LUL	35	218	65.5
LLL	18	203	52.7
Right Lower Bilobectomy	2	250	56.1
Pneumonectomy	1	220	
Apical RLL Segmentectomy	1	125	

Legend:
RUL=Right Upper Lobectomy, RML= Right Middle Lobectomy, RLL= Right Lower Lobectomy, LUL= Left Upper Lobectomy, LLL= Left Lower Lobectomy,

Table 2. Completed 133 VATS major pulmonary resections and mean operative times (excluding node dissection time. Not significant by ANOVA test p=0.15)

9. Complications

Table 3 shows the complications encountered in our unit, which are consistent with previously published complications [29]. 62 patients (40%) had no complications during their short hospital stay, whereas 94 patients (60%) had at least one operative or post operative event, including those picked at clinic follow up visits. Air leak remains the most critical factor in postoperative rehabilitation and prolonged LOS [30]. This might out-balance the expenditure, and tip the cost-effectiveness away from VATS lobectomy. A lung sealant could be used to reduce intercostal tube dwell time, and subsequently LOS. Adopting the fissure-last technique has resulted in significant reduction in air leak, as the fissures are nearly always stapled. However, the combination of ferocious air leak and a collapsed lung on the chest x-ray is an indication for re-exploration of the leak site. A Bronchopleural fistula is usually the culprit. Generally speaking there are high post operative incidences when starting a VATS lobectomy programme, but these include the trivia and the serious. The LOS in our series stayed at 4±4 days (range 1-25), and 45% of the patients were discharged on or before the third postoperative day [23].

Bronchial complications:

The technique of fissure-last lobectomy necessitates absolute mastery of the anatomical relations inside the chest, in different angles and perspectives. This can be very tricky at times especially on performing right lower lobectomy. Early in our experience we were tricked twice into removing the middle lobe as a result of anatomical disorientation. The first time the bronchus intermedius was mistaken for the lower lobe bronchus, and in the second instance stapling of the medial part of the oblique fissure failed to identify the delayed origin of the middle lobe bronchus within it. The middle lobe had to be removed in both cases without additional morbidity.

In another case the left main bronchus was mistaken for the left upper lobe bronchus, and thoracotomy was performed to re-implant the lower lobe bronchus into the left main bronchus. Starting with systematic nodal dissection may have predisposed to this complication, as dissection around the subcarinal area skeletonised the left main bronchus, making it easier than the usual to encircle it from an anterior approach. This patient was discharged 5 days later and had no complications on follow up clinic visits. No matter how clear the bronchial anatomy is, the bronchus should never be stapled before inflating the lung and ensuring patency of other lobes.

Bronchopleural fistula (BPF) occurred in two patients, who were treated aggressively by returning to theatre and exploring the air leak via the same port-sites. In both patients a small hole was found proximal to the stapling line, possibly caused by the stapling device. Videoscopic stitching using Vicryl 2/0 controlled the leak and the rest of their hospital stay was uncomplicated. Similar complication was reported before [31]. Two further patients developed ferocious air leak and severe surgical emphysema on the first postoperative day. BPF was suspected and they were both re-explored on the same day via the same port-sites. Apical ruptured bullae were found in both cases and were treated by bullectomy and partial pleurectomy. We now staple incidental bullae prophylactically to safeguard against such a scenario.

Wound complications:

There was one port-site seedling with malignant adenocarcinoma, with evidence of pleural recurrence 3 months after VATS lobectomy [Figure 9]. This was treated by wide surgical excision and radiotherapy. The patient died 24 months later of disseminated disease. Similar dissemination to port-site was reported from the Memorial Sloan-Kettering Cancer Centre, New York [32]. Follow up in clinic detected 7 (4.5%) port-site infections. Only one port-site needed surgical debridement and healing by secondary intension.

Pain control and long term pain:

Compared to thoracotomy, VATS lobectomy was associated with shorter chest tube duration, shorter length of hospital stay, and improved pain control. Open thoracotomy patients required 42% more morphine and 25% more nerve blocks than VATS patients who were 33% more likely to sleep following surgery [1, 31, 33, 34]. At clinic follow up port-site discomfort, paraesthesia and dermatome numbness were common. Complete recovery within 6-8 weeks was the rule. Two (2.1%) out of 156 of our patients experienced prolonged port-site neuralgia. Both were referred to specialised pain clinic and received Gabapentin and Amitriptyline long term. Similar long term pain has been reported before [35]. In our opinion this could be related to inattention at port-site creation. The technique of diathermy microthoracotomy to create bloodless ports must stick to the superior border of the rib [27]. Mid space diathermy can lead to nerve injury [Figure 2]. We now fashion the utility port by avoiding muscle cutting. The latissimus dorsi is separated in the direction of its fibres.

Thromboprophylaxis and Pulmonary embolism:

All patients should receive low molecular weight heparin on the first postoperative day. There were no incidences of in hospital deep vein thrombosis or pulmonary embolism (PE) in our series. At least three patients had thrombotic complications two proving fatal (1.2%) two weeks and 36 days after discharge from hospital. The Edinburgh experience reported one death within 4 postoperative days, and two further deaths within 30 days, all due to pulmonary embolism [31]. This highlights the possibility of hypercoagulability in this cohort of patients. Despite the fast-tracked physiotherapy and early discharge from hospital they should be considered a higher risk for thrombosis compared to open operation. The protracted hospital stay in the latter allows adequate anticoagulation until mobility is resumed. It is not unusual for patients discharged early after VATS lobectomy to reduce their activity and 'take it easy', whilst not covered by thrombo-prophylaxis. Further studies are needed to look into the role of domiciliary low molecular weight heparin and low dose Aspirin.

	Complications	VATS completed N=133
Major	protracted air leak >3 days (range 3-19 days)	13 (9.8%)
	ITU / HDU admission (total)	14 (10.5%)
	For mechanical ventilation	7 (5.3%)
	For inotropic support	4 (3%)
	For CPAP / BIPAP (HDU)	3(2.3%)
	Postoperative bleeding requiring re-exploration	1 (.8%)
	Bronchial complications	5 (3.8%)
	Out of hospital PE	2 (1.6%)
	Sputum retention requiring bronchoscopy under general anaesthesia	4 (3%)
Minor	Pulmonary complications / collapse / consolidation requiring antibiotics	14 (10.5%)
	Atrial fibrillation >24 hrs	7 (5.3%)
	Extra drain / reinsertion of drain	3 (2.3%)
	Pneumothorax, residual air capping after drain removal	19 (14.3%)
	Surgical emphysema	7 (5.3%)

Table 3. Complications for VATS completed major pulmonary resections

Conversion to thoracotomy:
There were 23(14.7%) true conversions to open thoracotomy in our series, for brisk bleeding 13(8.3%), thick fissure 3(1.9%), time constraint 2(1.3%), bad vision 2(1.3%), main bronchus transection 1(0.6%), massive air embolism during segmentectomy 1 (0.6%) and densely adherent nodes 1(0.6%). Our conversion rate of (14.7%) is in keeping with a recent meta-analysis reporting VATS to open lobectomy conversion rate ranging from 0% to 15.7% (median = 8.1%) [33]. Conversion should not be considered as a failure of VATS technique, and certainly should not be counted against the surgeon. It should be regarded as a patient safety necessity. Conversion does not prejudice immediate and long-term outcomes [36]. However; thoracotomy following a successful VMPR for postoperative bleeding is not always mandatory, as bleeding could be controlled videoscopically in most cases.
We cannot over emphasise the golden rule that VATS lobectomy should not be attempted by anyone who is not trained to deal proficiently with sudden brisk bleeding. Moderate bleeding early in our series led to conversion in 3 cases. However, with experience it was possible to salvage 3 major bleedings in excess of 500mls, and continue the VATS lobectomy to completion. Such confidence comes after a sizable experience with bleeding.

10. Disease progression and survival analysis

Table 4 shows the pattern of recurrence in 13(8.3%) patients with primary NSCLC treated by VATS resection. One patient with a negative PET scan was diagnosed with fresh bone metastases two weeks after the operation. She was well 2 year after chemo-radiotherapy and surgical knee replacement. The Kaplan-Meier survival at 1, 2 and 3 years of patients who had VATS resection of NSCLC (all stages) was 85±3.8%, 82.2±4.2% and 73.5±7.0%, respectively [Figure 11]. This compares well to McKenna et al in his large multi-institutional series [1].

Stage	Clinical staging (preoperative)	Pathological staging (postoperative)	Local Recurrence (progression)	Distant Metastases (progression)
Ia	54 (42.5%)	36 (28.8%)	0	3
Ib	48 (37.8%)	55 (43.3%)	4	3
IIa	7 (5.6%)	4 (3.2%)	0	0
IIb	5 (4%)	12 (9.6%)	3	2
IIIa	6 (4.8%)	13 (10.4%)	1	
IIIb ✞	4 (3.2%)	5 (4%)		1
IV	3 (2.4%)	2 (1.6%)		1

✞ One patient with a T4 lesion on CT scan proved to have two synchronous primaries, hence down staged to T2 N0.

Table 4. Clinical and pathological staging and pattern of recurrence in 127 primary NSCLC suitable for VATS resection.

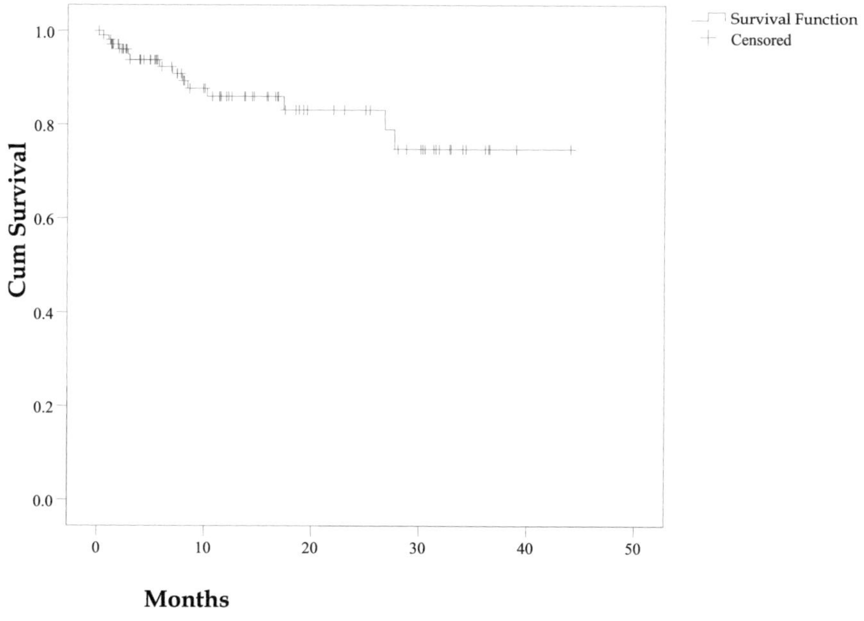

Years	At risk	Events	% survival	SE
0	156	0	100	-
1	92	10	85.0	3.8
2	35	12	82.2	4.2
3	7	16	73.5	7.0

Fig. 11. Kaplan-Meier estimated survival in 156 patients undergoing major VATS resection (all stages).

11. Costing and service commissioning

Cost implications of a surgical procedure are difficult to evaluate [37]. It is difficult to assign a financial value to early return to work, reduced pain and better cosmetic results. Yet we found that VATS lobectomy on average cost £1300 more than an open procedure in terms of operative consumables. On the other hand reduced LOS enable high turnover of beds and improved throughput. The reduced LOS comes at the expense of theatre time, which means fewer cases will get through per operative list.

12. Conclusion

VATS major pulmonary resections are safe and long term results are not compromised. They should be considered first choice for T1-2, N0-1, M0 lung lesions. Aggressive approach to postoperative complications reduced length of hospital stay to a median of 4 days. Air leak remains the most important cause for prolonged hospital stay

13. References

[1] McKenna RJ, Houck W, Fuller CB. Video-assisted thoracic surgery lobectomy: experience with 1,100 cases. Ann Thorac Surg. 2006;81(2):421-5.

[2] Rocco G, Internullo E, Cassivi SD, Van Raemdonck D, Ferguson MK (2008) The variability of practice in minimally invasive thoracic surgery for pulmonary resections. Thorac Surg Clin 18:235–247

[3] Sedrakyan A, van der Meulen J, Lewsey J, Treasure T. Variation in use of video assisted thoracic surgery in the United Kingdom. BMJ. 2004;329(7473):1011-2.

[4] Naruke T: Thoracoscopic surgery for small, non small cell lung cancer. Is video assisted lobectomy an adequate treatment? Data presented at the IVth International Symposium on Thoracoscopy and Video Assisted Thoracic Surgery, Sao-Paulo, May, 1997. Pneumol 1997;23:S17.

[5] McKenna RJ, Wolf RK, Brenner M, Fischel RJ, Wurnig P. Is lobectomy by video-assisted thoracic surgery an adequate cancer operation? Ann Thorac Surg. 1998;66(6):1903-8.

[6] Walker WS: Video assisted thoracic surgery - Pulmonary lobectomy. Semin Laparosc Surg 1996; 4: 233-244.

[7] McKenna RJ, Fischel RJ, Wolf R, Wurnig P. Video-Assisted Thoracic Surgery (VATS) Lobectomy for Bronchogenic Carcinoma. Semin Thorac Cardiovasc Surg 1998;10(4):321-325.

[8] Roviaro GC, Rebuffat C, Varioli F, et al. Videoendoscopic pulmonary lobectomy for cancer. *Surg Laparosc Endosc* 1992;2:244–247.

[9] Kirby TJ, Mack MJ, Landreneau RJ, Rice TW. Initial experience with video-assisted thoracoscopic lobectomy. Ann Thorac Surg 1993:56;1248–1253.

[10] McKenna RJ Jr. Lobectomy by video-assisted thoracic surgery with mediastinal node sampling for lung cancer. J Thorac Cardiovasc Surg. 1994;107(3):879-81.

[11] Walker WS, Carnochan FM, Pugh GC. Thoracoscopic pulmonary lobectomy. Early operative experience and preliminary clinical results. J Thorac Cardiovasc Surg. 1993; 106(6):1111-7.

[12] Coosemans W, Lerut TE, Van Raemdonck DE. Thoracoscopic surgery: the Belgian experience. Ann Thorac Surg. 1993; 56(3):721-30.
[13] Gonzalez D, Paradela M, Garcia J, Dela Torre M. Single-port video-assisted thoracoscopic lobectomy. Interact Cardiovasc Thorac Surg. 2011;12(3):514-5.
[14] D'Amico T A. Robotics in thoracic surgery: Applications and outcomes J Thorac Cardiovasc Surg. 2006;131(1):19-20).
[15] Kirby TJ, Mack MJ, Landreneau RJ, Rice TW. Lobectomy--video-assisted thoracic surgery versus muscle-sparing thoracotomy. A randomized trial. J Thorac Cardiovasc Surg. 1995;109(5):997-1001.
[16] Sugi K, Kaneda Y, Esato K. Video-assisted thoracoscopic lobectomy achieves a satisfactory long-term prognosis in patients with clinical stage IA lung cancer. World J Surg 2000;24:27–31
[17] Craig S.R., Leaver H.A., Yap P.L., Pugh G.C., Walker W.S., Acute phase responses following minimal access and conventional thoracic surgery. Eur J Cardiothorac Surg. 2001;20: 455-463
[18] Walker WS, Codispotilt M, Soon SY, Stamenkovic S, Carnochan F, Pugh G. Long-term outcomes following VATS lobectomy for non-small cell bronchogenic carcinoma. Eur J Cardiothorac Surg 2003;23:397-402.
[19] Pisters KM, Vallières E, Crowley JJ, Franklin WA, Bunn PA , Ginsberg RJ, Putnam JB , Chansky K, Gandara D. Surgery with or without preoperative paclitaxel and carboplatin in early-stage non-small-cell lung cancer: Southwest Oncology Group Trial S9900, an intergroup, randomized, phase III trial. J Clin Oncol. 2010;28:1843-9.
[20] Albain KS, Swann RS, Rusch VW, Turrisi AT 3rd, Shepherd FA, Smith C, Chen Y, Livingston RB, Feins RH, Gandara DR, Fry WA, Darling G, Johnson DH, Green MR, Miller RC, Ley J, Sause WT, Cox JD. Radiotherapy plus chemotherapy with or without surgical resection for stage III non-small-cell lung cancer: a phase III randomised controlled trial. Lancet 2009;374:379-386
[21] Sahai RK, Nwogu CE, Yendamuri S, Tan W, Wilding GE, Demmy TL. Is thoracoscopic pneumonectomy safe? Ann Thorac Surg. 2009;88(4):1086-92.
[22] Nomori H, Ohtsuka T, Horio H, Naruke T, Suemasu K. Thoracoscopic lobectomy for lung cancer with a largely fused fissure. Chest. 2003;123(2):619-22.
[23] Amer K, Khan AZ, Vohra HA. Video-assisted thoracic surgery of major pulmonary resections for lung cancer: the Southampton experience. Eur J Cardiothorac Surg. 2011;39(2):173-9.
[24] Demmy TL, Nwogu CE, Yendamuri S. Thoracoscopic chest wall resection: what is its role? Ann Thorac Surg. . 2010;89(6):S2142-5
[25] Demmy TL, Platis IE, Nwogu C, Yendamuri S. Thoracoscopic extrapleural pneumonectomy for mesothelioma. Ann Thorac Surg. 2011;91(2):616-8
[26] Mahtabifard A, Fuller CB, McKenna RJ Jr. Video-assisted thoracic surgery sleeve lobectomy: a case series. Ann Thorac Surg. 2008;85(2):S729-32.
[27] Walker, W (1999). Video-Assisted Thoracic Surgery. Oxford: Isis Medical Media Ltd. 22.
[28] Kamiyoshihara M, Kakegawa S, Morishita Y. Convenient and improved method to distinguish the intersegmental plane in pulmonary segmentectomy using a butterfly needle. Ann Thorac Surg. 2007;83(5):1913-4.
[29] Solaini L, Prusciano F, Bagioni P, di Francesco F, Solaini L, Poddie DB. Video-assisted thoracic surgery (VATS) of the lung: analysis of intraoperative and postoperative

complications over 15 years and review of the literature. Surg Endosc. 2008;22(2):298-310.
[30] Ueda K, Sudoh M, Jinbo M, Li TS, Suga K, Hamano K. Physiological rehabilitation after video-assisted lung lobectomy for cancer: a prospective study of measuring daily exercise and oxygenation capacity Eur J Cardiothorac Surg. 2006;30(3):533-7.
[31] Walker WS. Video-assisted thoracic surgery (VATS) lobectomy: the Edinburgh experience. Semin Thorac Cardiovasc Surg. 1998;10(4):291-9.
[32] Downey R, McCormack P, LoCicero J. Dissemination of malignant tumors after Video-assisted thoracic surgery. A report of twenty-one cases J Thorac Cardiovasc Surg 1996;111:954-960.
[33] Yan TD, Black D, Bannon PG, McCaughan BC. Systematic review and meta-analysis of randomized and nonrandomized trials on safety and efficacy of video-assisted thoracic surgery lobectomy for early-stage non-small-cell lung cancer. J Clin Oncol. 2009;27(15):2553-62.
[34] Whitson BA, Groth SS, Duval SJ, Swanson SJ, Maddaus MA. Surgery for early-stage non-small cell lung cancer: a systematic review of the video-assisted thoracoscopic surgery versus thoracotomy approaches to lobectomy. Ann Thorac Surg. 2008;86(6):2008-16.
[35] Landreneau RJ, Mack MJ, Hazelrigg SR, Naunheim K, Dowling RD, Ritter P, Magee MJ, Nunchuck S, Keenan RJ, Ferson PF. Prevalence of chronic pain after pulmonary resection by thoracotomy or video-assisted thoracic surgery. J Thorac Cardiovasc Surg I994;107:1079-1086.
[36] Jones RO, Casali G, Walker WS. Does failed video-assisted lobectomy for lung cancer prejudice immediate and long-term outcomes? Ann Thorac Surg. 2008 Jul;86(1):235-9.
[37] Walker WS, Casali G. The VATS lobectomist: analysis of costs and alterations in the traditional surgical working pattern in the modern surgical unit. Thorac Surg Clin. 2008;18(3):281-7.

14

Video-Assisted Thoracic Surgery (VATS) Systematic Mediastinal Nodal Dissection

Khalid Amer
The Cardiovascular & Thoracic Unit, Southampton General Hospital, Southampton, United Kingdom

1. Introduction

VATS lobectomy and other major pulmonary resections (VMPR) are growing in popularity. One of the main criticisms against minimal access in lung cancer surgery is that mediastinal nodes could be difficult to assess. It was shown by different authorities that VATS complete nodal dissection is feasible and does not differ from that performed by an open thoracotomy [1]. Despite conflicting reports, there is an international agreement that nodal dissection does not influence the disease free or the overall survival in lung cancer. However; proper staging of Non Small Cell Lung Cancer (NSCLC) enables standardization of decision on treatment and evaluation of such treatment comparing it to different centres around the world. Recent publications have shown a significant statistical gain in 5 year survival if stage IIa and higher were treated by adjuvant chemotherapy [2, 3]. It is therefore absolutely mandatory to get the staging right in early lung cancer; otherwise patients would be denied a significant chance of cure. In a pressurised service where commissioning is governed by patients waiting times, targets and cost effectiveness, surgeons might feel reluctant to extend the operating time to perform Systematic Nodal Dissection (SND). The risk of improper mediastinal staging in our view is by far greater than extending the duration of the operation. The long-term results of stage migration lead to faulty comparison, and might dictate the wrong management, ending in completely erroneous survival statistics. Oncological randomised controlled trials rely on final histological staging, and therefore it is mandatory to obtain correct staging to avoid erroneous survival statistics in such trials. In our view the only contraindication to SND would be technical difficulty with dissection in the presence of severe adhesions

The way we stage lung cancer has changed over the years. The TNM6 classification [4] is now superseded by the IASLC new TNM7 classification [5]. Fortunately the naming and significance of nodal stations has not changed substantially. Precarinal nodes #3 for a left sided tumour is now considered an N3 stage. Precarinal nodes for a right sided tumour are designated as #4 (there are no #3R), and these are regarded as N2 disease.

2. Definitions

There are different protocols for staging the mediastinum in search of metastasis in N2 nodes. These include:

- Selective node sampling: the surgeon decides which node looked diseased and randomly removes that node (chance node).
- Sentinel nodal sampling: at operation the primary tumour is injected with ^{99}Technitium tracer, and a Geiger counter is used to identify the sentinel hilar nodes which are dissected. If frozen section confirmed absence of metastases, the rest of nodal dissection is omitted (decision node).
- Systematic nodal sampling: one or two nodes sampled from each zonal station (selective).
- Systematic Nodal dissection: at least 2 nodes from each field or station, and at least 3 fields are dissected (total of at least 6 nodes). Must always include subcarinal nodes (universally accepted) [6].
- Lobe-specific nodal sampling: oriented towards the different lymphatic drainage of different lobes e.g. for a right upper lobe tumour, the fields to harvest would be #2-4. Subcarinal lymphadenectomy is not always necessary for tumours of the right upper lobe and left upper trisegmentectomy (selective) [7].
- Extended nodal dissection: by definition means bilateral dissection of nodes (no consensus on extent).

Each of these protocols has points of strengths as well as weaknesses. In general the more the number of harvested nodes, the more likely it is to reveal normal looking nodes with metastatic tumour cells.

- Skip metastases: when stations N2 are involved in the absence of N1 involvement, or N3 involvement in the absence of either N1-N2 nodes. The importance of this phenomenon is not fully understood [8].
- Micrometastases: The prognosis of cancer patients is largely determined by the occurrence of distant metastases. The presence of clinically occult few malignant cells within nodal tissue, bone marrow and pleural fluid, and the clinical relevance of circulating tumour cells are still debatable. The importance of such nodal involvement is not fully understood, as it does not inevitably lead to disease dissemination and disease progression [9, 10].

3. Invasive v non-invasive staging

The tools of staging the mediastinum in NSCLC are either invasive in nature such that histological confirmation of nodal involvement is sought, or non-invasive, whereby an imaging technique is used to infer involvement of nodes by secondary metastasis. Invasive procedures such as mediastinoscopy, mediastinotomy, EBUS-TBNA (Endo Bronchial Ultra Sound - Trans Bronchial Fine Needle Aspirate) and EUS (Endoscopic or trans oesophageal Ultra Sound guided Trucut biopsy or FNA) are still developing. These investigations have limitations in terms of tissue yield, safety profile and cost. At best these are sampling techniques, aimed at sampling specific nodes which have been highlighted by other non-invasive techniques. None of these procedures can claim radical dissection of mediastinal nodes. However, recently VAMLA (Video Assisted Mediastinal Lymph Adenectomy) [11] has claimed bilateral mediastinal clearance of nodes, yet there are still issues with reaching stations #5L & #6L [figure 1] and the distant stations #8 & #9. To enhance the yield of nodes VATS was added to VAMLA to achieve radicality of nodal dissection [12]. On the other hand TEMLA (Transcervical Extended Mediastinal Lymph Adenectomy) was introduced in 2004, which involved a collar incision in the neck, elevation of the sternal manubrium with a special retractor, and claims bilateral dissection of all mediastinal nodes apart from #8 & #9 [13]. The choice of using any of the above mentioned techniques depends on the philosophy of nodal sampling versus radical adenectomy.

Non-invasive preoperative techniques have largely concentrated on CT and PET. Whilst Computed Tomography (CT) can give great anatomical details of the mediastinum and other chest anatomy, it cannot differentiate benign from malignant tissue. Positron Emission Tomography (PET) on the other hand was claimed to make that biological distinction.

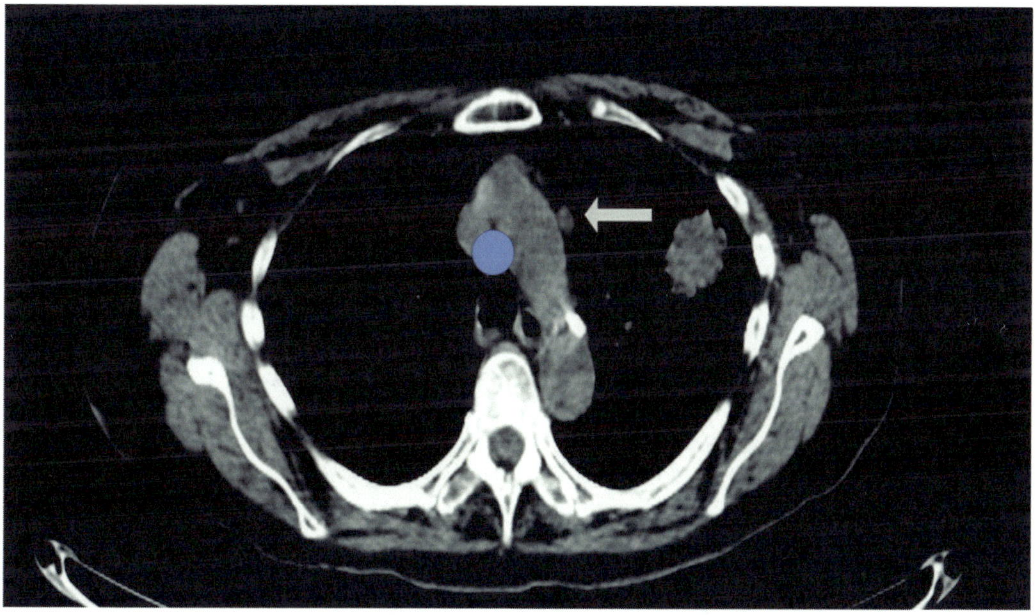

Fig. 1. Station #5L node out of reach of the mediastinoscope (blue circle).

4. The Role of PET

Great hopes were pinned on PET as it seemed to be the most convenient non-invasive staging tool for a fast tract keyhole surgery such as VMPR designed for early lung cancer. PET was expected to identify nodal disease in CT negative and normal looking mediastinum. Recent meta analysis reporting the PET/CT mediastinal staging in patients with NSCLC found the median sensitivity to be 85% (range 67% to 91%) and specificity of 90% (range 82% to 96%) [14]. Gilles et al and Plathow et al summarised the current views about the elevated glucose metabolism in cancers [15,16]. Tumour cells adapt to hypoxia by upregulation of glucose Transporter (GLUTs) and increased activity of Hexokinase. The GLUT is the first energy-independent glucose transporter across the cell membrane down the concentration gradient. Tumours increase their level of energy production by engaging in glycolysis, which is a relatively inefficient way to produce energy compared to aerobic oxidation (2 ATP molecules versus 30 ATPs). The toxic acidic tumour microenvironment results in death of normal tissue while tumour cells evade apoptosis by maintaining normal intracellular pH. It is thought that this process give the tumour cells a competitive advantage for local growth, ultimately leading to invasion of basement membrane and distant metastases. Primary tumours and their nodal secondaries express high GLUT1 upregulation, which in turn is tied to ^{18}F-FDG accumulation in the tumour cell, and hence directly related to SUV_{max} (Maximum Standard Uptake Value). GLUT expression is tied to tumour cell type and differentiation. Squamous cell carcinoma exhibit over expression of GLUT1 whereas adenocarcinoma does not. One of the serious disappointments of PET scanning in lung cancer is the low uptake of carcinoids, adenocarcinoma and bronchioloalveolar carcinomas, in some series up to 40%. This tumour biological behaviour explains why PET is blinded to adenocarcinoma, Bronchiolo-alveolar carcinoma (BAC) and carcinoids tumours. For the same reason the importance of the SUVmax (>3.5) as a surrogate value for malignancy has been played down. Another important snag about the uptake of the FDG metabolite is the mass of active tissue. A node under 1cm in diameter is unlikely to show up as a hot spot on PET even if it was completely replaced by secondary malignant tissue. Al-Sarraf et al found that integrated CT/PET images had reduced sensitivity for non-enlarged <1cm nodes (40%) [17]. Clinicians should be aware of this fact when interpreting the results, and histological confirmation should be sought on CT positive (>1.0cm in its shortest diameter) or PET positive nodes. The international literature seems to suggest that the rate of unexpected (occult) N2 disease in c-N0-1 to be 10%. It is likely that the role of PET will continue to evolve with further clinical studies using other new tracers such as the thymidine analogue 3'-deoxy-3'-[^{18}F]fluorothymidine, which more specifically targets proliferative activity of malignant lesions and can differentiate them from the false-positive inflammatory lesions, as seen with FDG [18]. It should not be forgotten that one of the very useful functions of routinely performed PET in early lung cancer is to exclude obvious metastases to liver, adrenal, bone etc that would have otherwise precluded curative resection [figure 2].

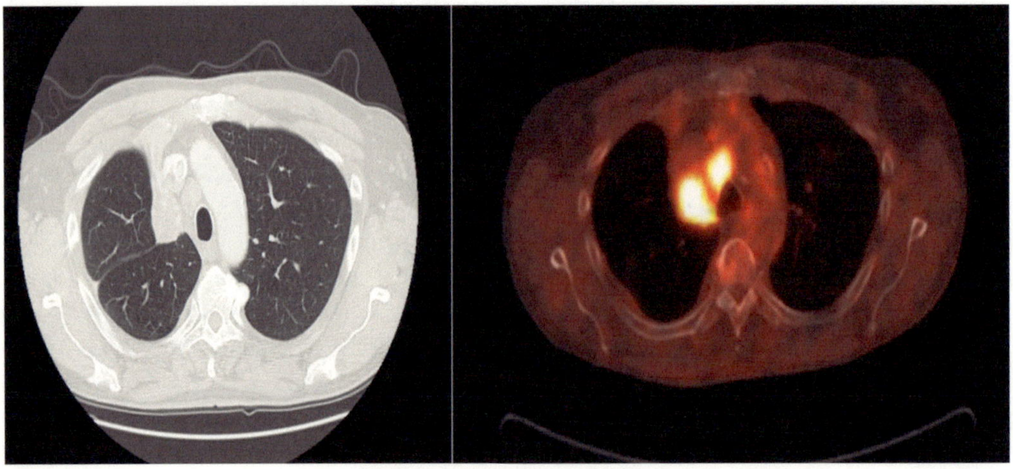

Fig. 2. CT/PET of a patient with right upper lobe lesion. Bronchoscopy obtained squamous cells carcinoma. The high intake of ^{18}FDG seen in precarinal node #4R was sufficient evidence not to proceed with mediastinoscopy. The patient was treated by chemo-Radiotherapy.

5. Preoperative v postoperative staging

The significance of preoperative as opposed to postoperative staging in resectable early lung cancer is tied to what the clinician wants to do with the information. There might be little disagreement about the N1 disease, but controversy surrounds N2 disease. In our opinion For a CT negative and PET negative mediastinum, no further investigation is needed, and patients should proceed to resectional operation + SND. Further multidisciplinary management should be based on SND staging. This is in line with the latest published British Thoracic Society (BTS) guidelines [19]. The dilemma arises when there is histological evidence of single station N2 disease preoperatively. The choices being (1) avoid surgery all together and opt for chemo-radiotherapy (2) induce chemotherapy before surgery, or (3) make a run for surgery while the tumour is operable and follow that by adjuvant chemotherapy / radiotherapy. The first approach is advocated by Albain et al (2009) who showed that lobectomy will add little to Chemo-radiotherapy for patients with stage IIIa (N2) non-small-cell lung cancer, at the expense of higher mortality (evidence level 1b) [20]. The second approach is supported by the S9900 trial follow up published in 2010 which continues to show that the best treatment for N2 resectable lung cancer would be induction chemotherapy followed by surgery (evidence level 1b) [21]. Rocco et al (2010) is supportive of the third approach, concluding that standard treatment of initially resectable stage IIIa NSCLC remains surgery followed by adjuvant chemotherapy (evidence level 2a) [22]. The subject remains controversial, and patients should be involved in decision taking. Surgery is known to give local control and reduce local recurrence, whereas chemotherapy is a systemic treatment designed to reduce disease progression and distant metastases. Currently we rely on CT/PET, mediastinoscopy or EBUS to direct the patient to one form of treatment or prevent unnecessary operation. However, Lim et al conducted a systematic review of all the published meta-analysis of randomised trials in preoperative versus postoperative chemotherapy in patients with resectable lung cancer (evidence level 1a) [23]. They concluded that in patients with resectable lung cancer, there was no difference in overall and disease-free survival between the timing of administration of chemotherapy (postoperative versus preoperative). Clearly this sends a strong message that earnest preoperative investigation of the mediastinum in PET negative resectable early lung cancer might be unnecessary. Myers et al specifically considered the cost effectiveness of routine mediastinoscopy in CT-negative, PET-negative patients with stage I lung cancer [24]. They concluded that routine mediastinoscopy would add an average 0.01 years (3.65 days) of life at a cost of $201,918 per life-year gained. Therefore they do not recommend routine mediastinoscopy in PET-negative patients. Our practice advocates neoadjuvant chemotherapy followed by surgical VMPR-SND followed by adjuvant chemotherapy based on proper SND staging, provided nodal involvement remains single station or single zonal. Multizonal involvement is best served by chemo-radiotherapy, as it is regarded as systemic disease. Surgery alone will not have an impact on the 5 years survival, but might have a palliative effect on local recurrence, and might be considered for instance to control haemoptysis, or continued sepsis precluding the start of other modalities of treatment such as chemotherapy.

6. Where are these mediastinal nodes?

Although nodal mapping has been there for a long time, it seems that there is considerable discordance in nomenclature and designation of nodal stations between Asian and European thoracic surgeons [25]. Historically the Naruke map was the most popular and most followed worldwide until recently [26]. The American Thoracic Society introduced the Mountain-Dressler ATS map in 2007, and finally Rusch et al from the Memorial Sloan-Kettering Cancer Centre introduced the current IASLC nodal map (International Association for the Study of Lung Cancer 2009) to achieve uniformity and to promote analyses of a planned prospective international database [27]. The IASLC map reconciles differences among other used maps, and provides precise anatomic definitions for all lymph node stations. A method of grouping lymph node stations together into "zones" is also proposed for the purposes of future survival analyses [Figure 3]. It goes without saying that surgeons should familiarise themselves with the details of this map to standardise the staging process in any given centre.

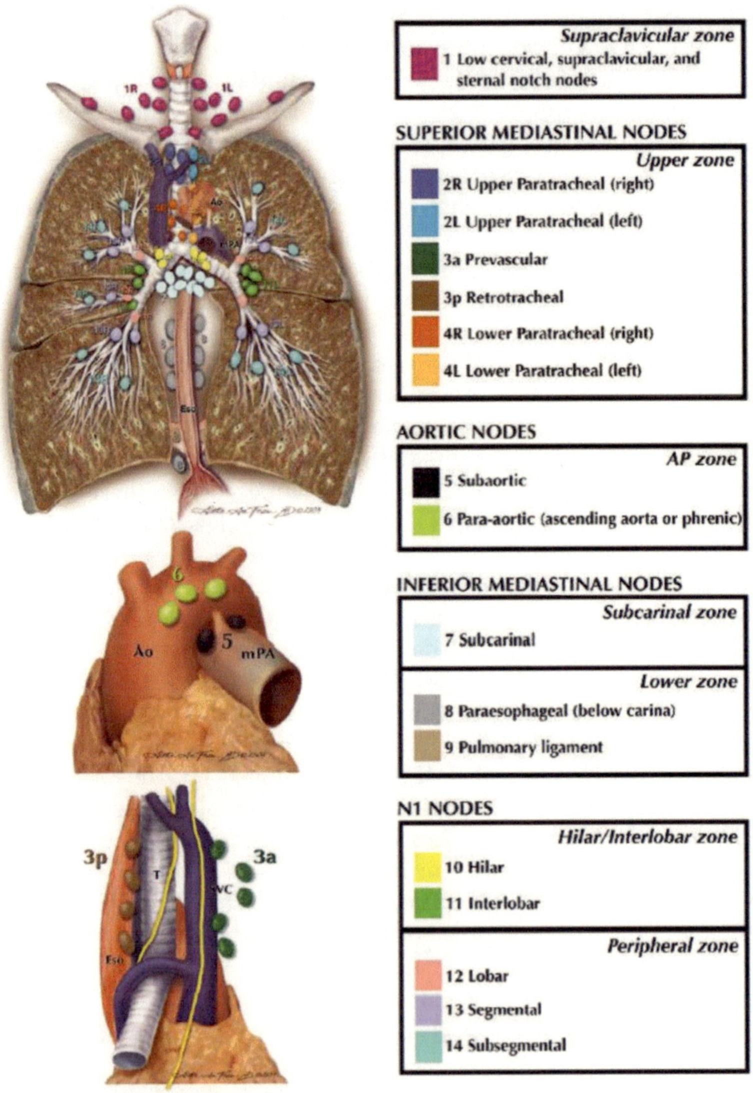

Fig. 3. The IASLC 2009 Nodal map.

7. VATS-SND: Can it be comprehensive?

One of the major criticisms against VATS lung cancer resection is that it is not an oncologically feasible operation, as assessment of the mediastinal nodes is not as complete as open thoracotomy. Comprehensive radical nodal dissection is possible by VATS and should not be different to open thoracotomy, as described by Watanabe et al [1]. The number of harvested nodes is an accepted surrogate to completeness of SND. 99% of patients should have 6 or more nodes harvested from 3 stations as reported in the ACOSOG Z0030 Trial [28]. Racial variations might play a role in the total number of nodes harvested. Video-assisted surgical approach should not adversely affect the yield of lymph node harvest, however; despite extreme care it is sometimes unavoidable to fragment nodes during harvesting [29]. There are few published studies that attest to completeness of VATS-SND, but the most impressive was that of Sagawa et al [30]. After VATS lobectomy-SND, a standard thoracotomy was subsequently opened by a different surgeon to complete systematic nodal dissection and revisit the VATS-SND dissection. The average addition to VATS-SND was 1.2 nodes only. The remnant ("missed" by VATS) lymph nodes and tissues were 2-3%, which seems acceptable for clinical stage I lung cancer. No nodal involvement was observed in the remnant lymph nodes. It would be difficult to obtain clearance for such a study in Europe, but its results are resounding assurance that with practice, VATS SND should be identical to open SND.

8. VATS-SND: How to do it

VMPR is usually considered for early lung cancer T1-2, N0-1 and M0. The decision to include these patients in the VATS series is based on CT/PET studies. The procedure is performed under general anaesthesia, utilising single lung ventilation. 3 ports are fashioned, 2X1cm and a utility port 3-4cm long at the mid-axillary line over the 4th or 5th intercostal space. Nodal harvesting can be performed before, during or after the VATS resection (lobectomy, pneumonectomy, segmentectomy etc) according to published European and international standards [6, 26,28,31].

SND criteria:

- *At least 3 fields nodal dissection*
- *At least 2 nodes from each field*
- *Subcarinal #7 always included*

Southampton "Motto":

- *Every visible node!*
- *"if you see a node, it should be in a pot.."*

We harvest nodes en-block, stations 2-4,7,8,9,10 and 11 on the right, preserving the Azygos vein, and 4,5-6,7,8,9,10, 11 on the left side, preserving the ligamentum arteriosum [32]. We do not harvest #1 bilaterally, or #2 on the left. However, we harvest #3 (precarinal) when indicated on the left chest without dividing the ligamentum arteriosum by retracting the main pulmonary artery up and pushing the carina down[1]. Subcarinal nodes #7 were mandatory for the definition of SND, and if these were not harvested the procedure would have been classified as 'Nodal sampling' and not SND [6]. The procedure extends the operative time by 30 minutes on the right chest and between 45-60 minutes on the left chest. VATS-SND during VMPR requires patience. Whereas en block dissection on the right is straight forward, that on the left is more taxing. Subcarinal #7 on the left is the most time consuming, as the space has to be clearly displayed. We routinely access it from the back of the hilum, starting with SND before resecting the lung. We found great variation in the number and consistency of nodal groups, especially #8 and #9. Nodes could be completely absent, discrete or lumped in a fibro-fatty tissue amenable to block dissection.

Right side:

Planning the port sites is an important part of nodal dissection, and if the ports are set too low the dissection will be a struggle. The anterior utility port should not be lower than the 5th space, and preferably on the 4th space. The posterior port is fashioned over the auscultatory triangle 1-2 finger breadths from the medial border of the scapula. The inferior port is created opposite the highest point in the dome of the diaphragm, in line with the hilar axis [Fig. 4].

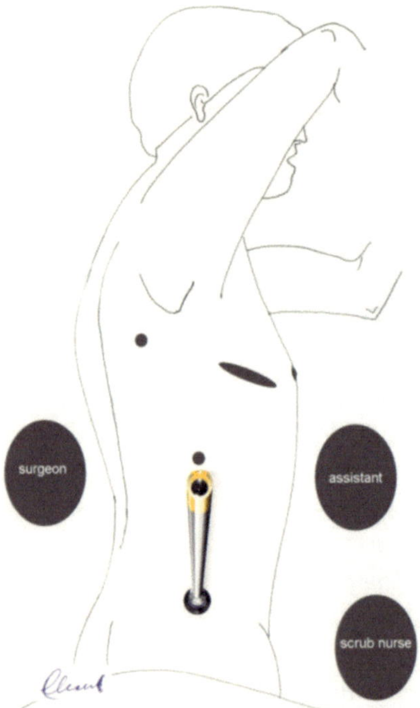

Fig. 4. The camera scope is inserted from the inferior port, and remains there.

[1] Amer K (2011). Routine Systematic Mediastinal Nodal Dissection During VATS Major Pulmonary Resections – The Southampton Technique. Available http://www.ctsnet.org/sections/videosection/videos/vg2011_AmerK_SystematicMediastinal.html. last accessed 01.04.2011

SND is started by releasing the inferior pulmonary ligament, and exposing the inferior pulmonary vein, bringing #9 nodes into light [Fig. 5].

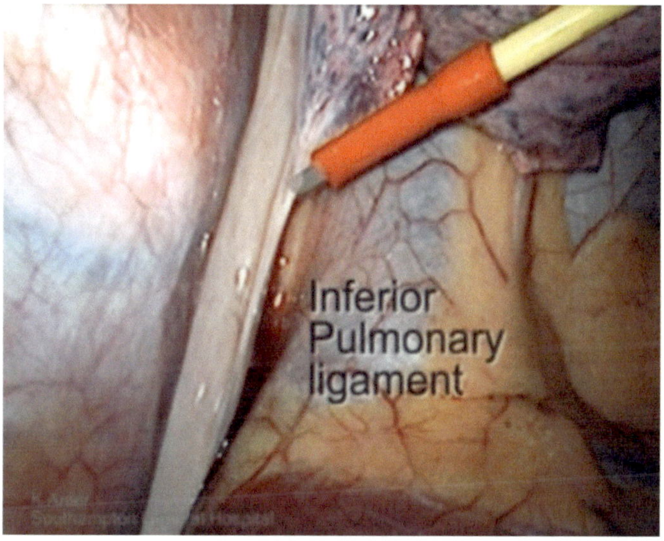

Fig. 5. Releasing the inferior ligament.

The pleural reflection between the SVC and the oesophagus is opened down to the diaphragm, exposing #8 para-oesophageal nodes. The number and consistency of nodes in #8-9 vary greatly. Our method of dissection has evolved into using a malleable diathermy spatula which is insulated albeit for the last 1-2 mm, whilst keeping the energy level at low. Diathermy dissection reduces bleeding and chyle leak, and keeps the operative field neat. Dissection of #8-9 nodes is usually straight forward [Fig. 6-7].

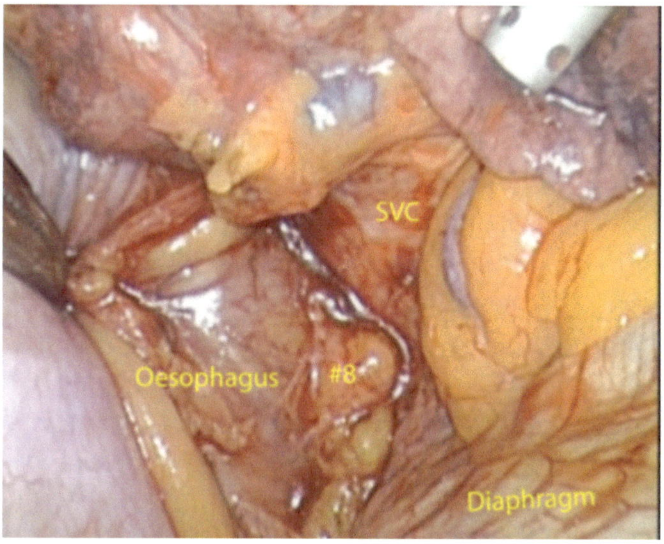

Fig. 6. En-block dissection of #8.

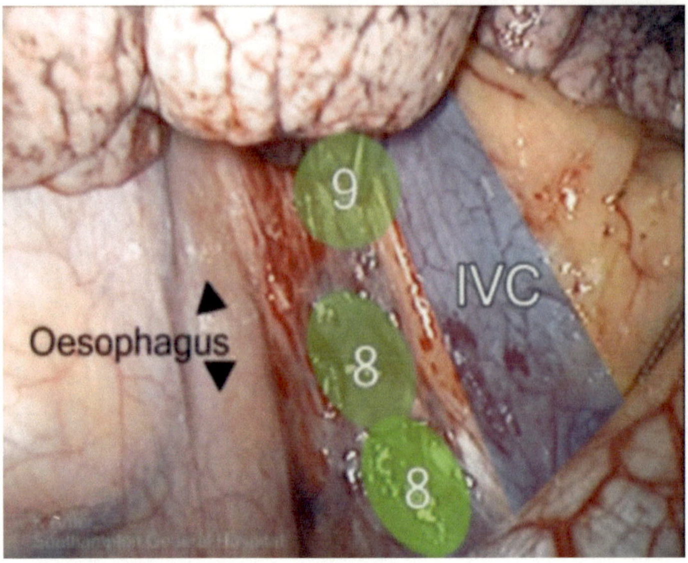

Fig. 7. Schematic location of #8 & #9.

The subcarinal nodes on the right side are found between the right main bronchus and the oesophagus. The lung is retracted anteriorly and the pleural reflection at the back of the hilum is opened from the inferior ligament to the concavity of the Azygos vein, medial to the vagus nerve. All vagal bronchial branches could be cut with impunity [Fig. 8-10].

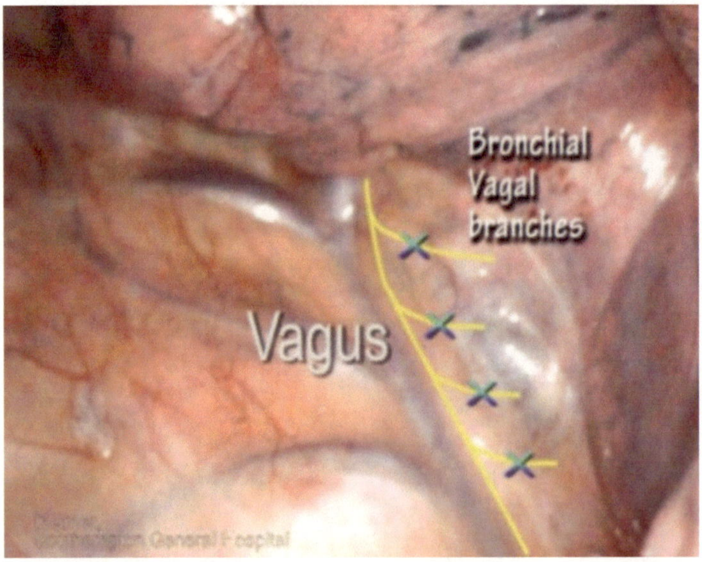

Fig. 8. Vagal bronchial twigs.

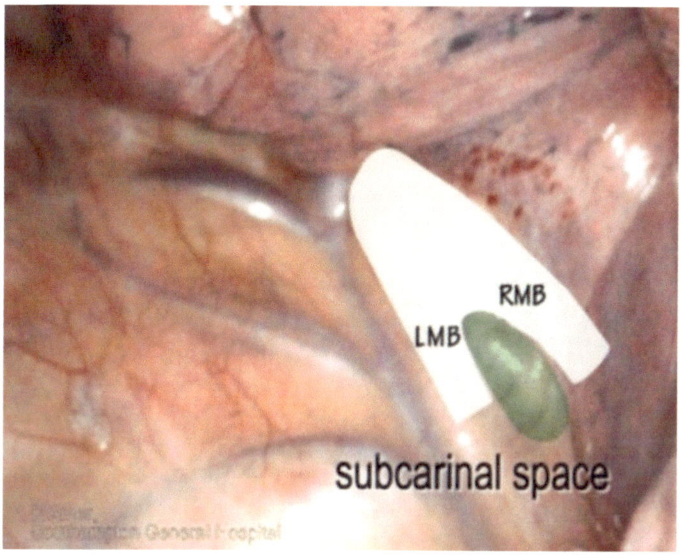

Fig. 9. Schematic location of #7.

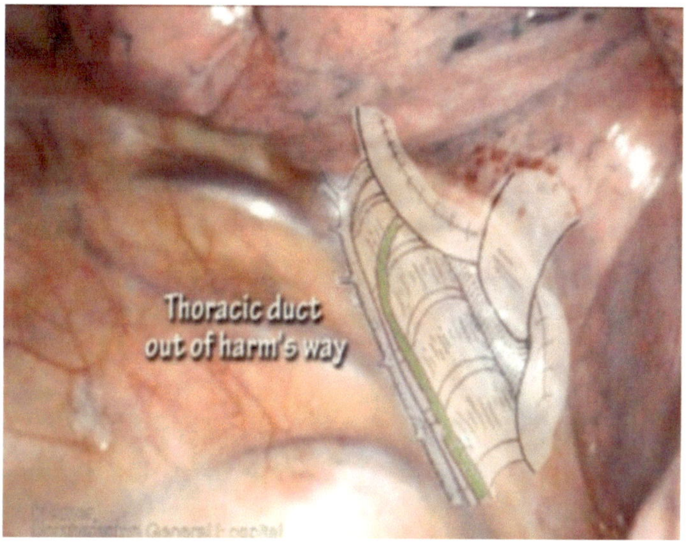

Fig. 10. The thoracic duct surface anatomy.

The right main bronchus is identified and followed proximally until the left main bronchus is seen and identified. The subcarinal nodes are dissected off their blood supply, and for convenience of retrieval a Polythene bag could be used. This is not always necessary. Careful labelling of nodes is to be practiced here as para-oesophageal #8 and para-bronchial #10 nodes could easily be mistaken as #7. Care must be taken not to dig holes in the membranous part of the bronchus or the delicate oesophagus. One should not worry much about thoracic duct injury in this location, as the duct is tucked away from harm's way by the oesophagus [Fig. 10]. At the end of this dissection the right main bronchus, the left main bronchus and the subcarinal space should be well on display [Fig. 11].

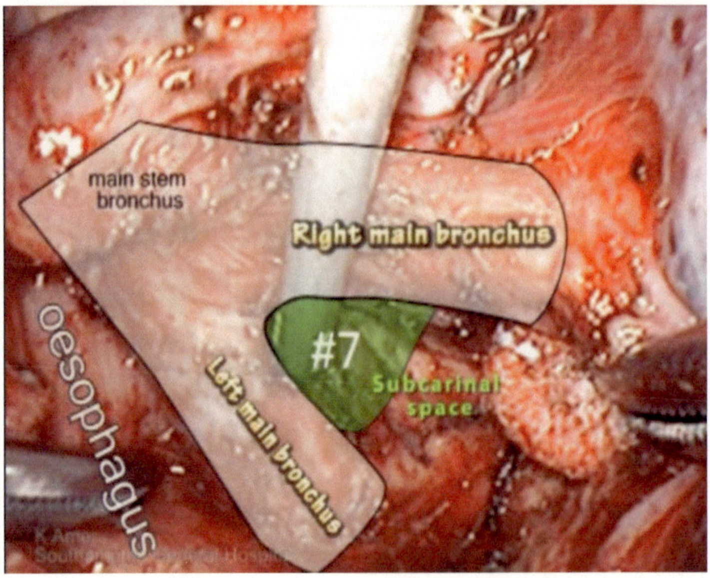

Fig. 11. The right subcarinal space.

Dissection of the parabronchial nodes #2-4 lies within the superior triangle. This triangle is bound by the Vagus and Phrenic nerves, and based on the Azygos vein [Fig. 12].

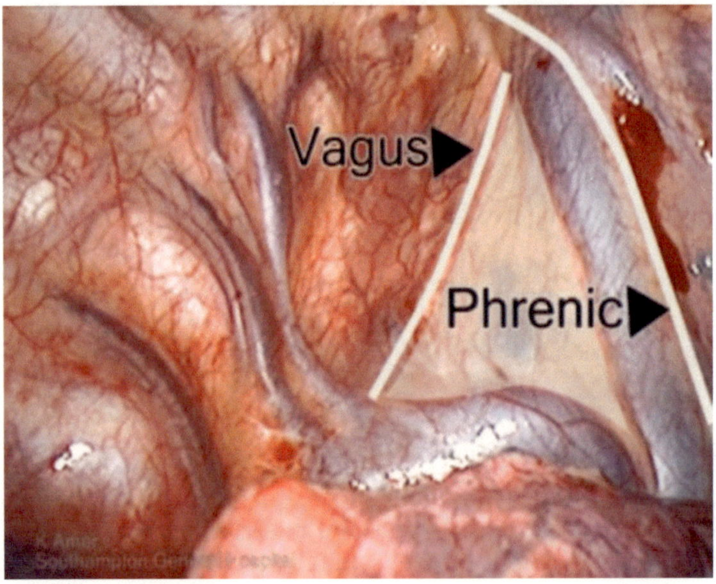

Fig. 12. The right superior triangle.

The pleura is opened like a trap door, just lateral to the SVC and just above the Azygos vein [Fig. 13]. The Vagus nerve sould be found plastered to the inside flap of the pleura. Retraction of the pleura using a Prolene stitch opens the triangle and helps in dissection [Fig. 14].

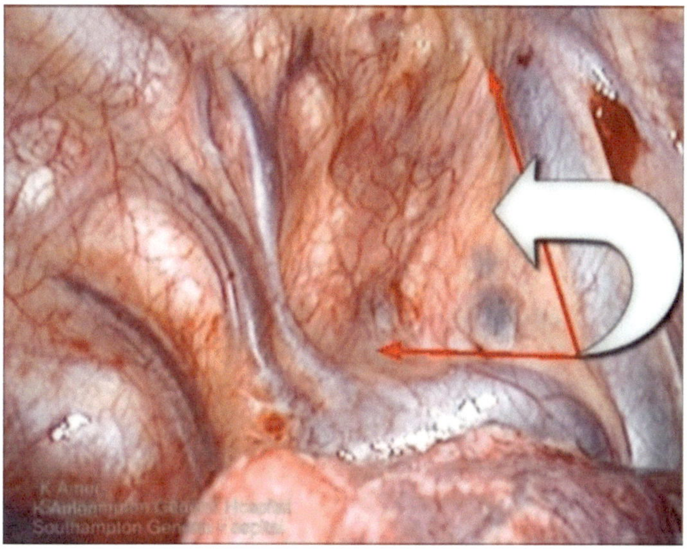

Fig. 13. Trap door to #2-4.

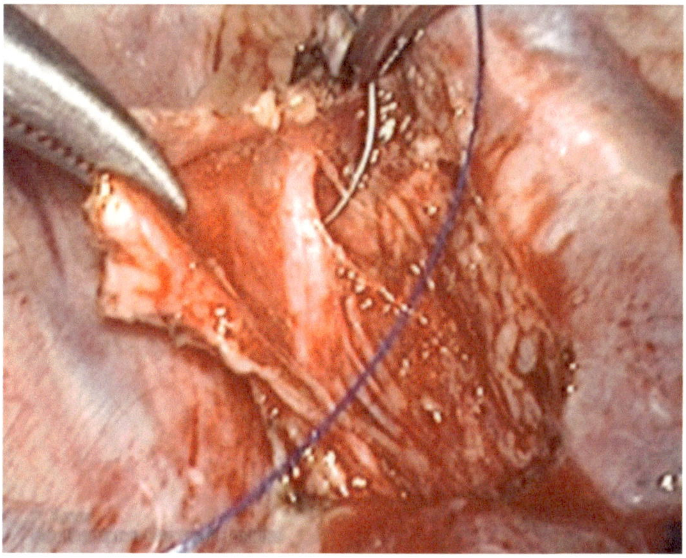

Fig. 14. Retraction of Vagus nerve.

Station #2-4 nodes in the para and pre-tracheal groups exist in a fibro-fatty block that could be dissected en block most of the times. Low energy diathermy is used as before. The dissection is started by pushing the SVC away from the block. One should be aware of the existence of at least one constant vein draining directly from the block to the SVC [Fig. 15]. These veins should be controlled by metal ligaclips or ultrasonic device before proceeding. If they are accidently cut they have the propensity to retract and disappear, making control of the bleeding difficult.

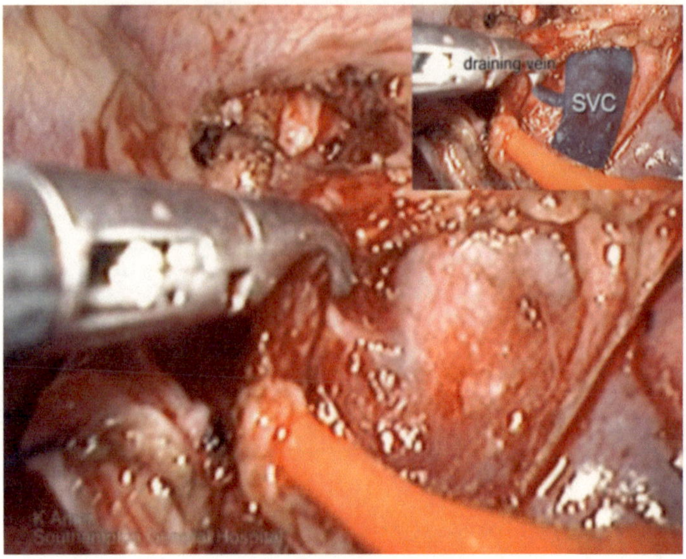

Fig. 15. Direct draining vein from block to SVC.

Further deeper dissection high in the triangle between the SVC and the block identifies the main stem trachea [Fig. 16]. Once the apex of the block is brought down, the dissection becomes easier.

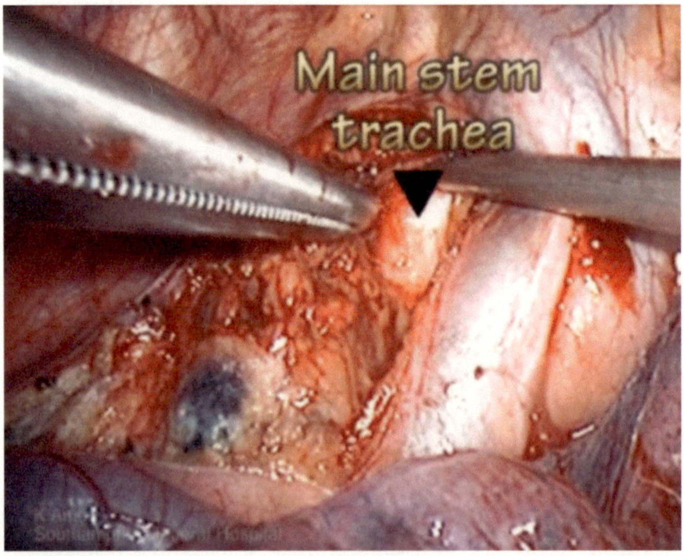

Fig. 16. Identifying the main stem trachea.

Next the lateral part of the block is separated from the vagus nerve. The block is then lifted off the tracheal, and the retrocaval part is freed. Large lymphatic channels could be seen here, and differentiated from nerves by their lobular contour and loss of sheen. Again the block is delivered out of the chest in a Polythene bag for convenience of retrieval only [Fig. 17]. Small discrete nodes are retrieved directly on a surgical instrument.

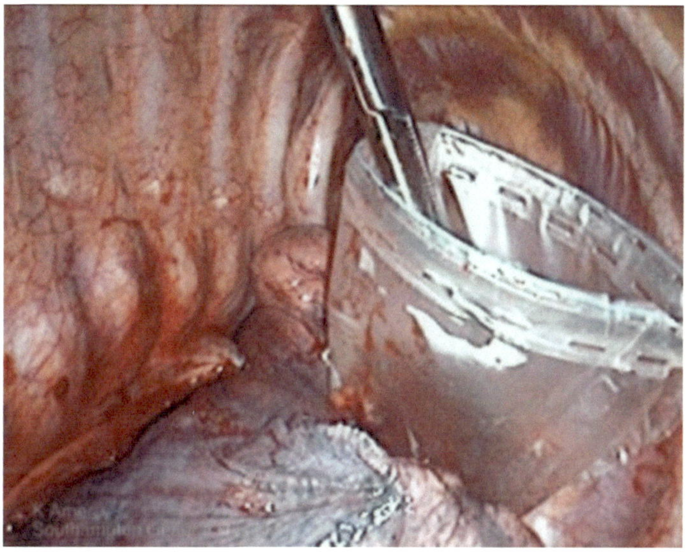

Fig. 17. Retrieval in a Polythene bag of #2-4.

The bed of the superior triangle is made of the arch of the aorta and the right bracheocephalic artery and the main stem trachea [Fig. 18]. The recurrent laryngeal nerve descends into the thoracic inlet parallel to the vagus on the lateral side of the carotid artery. It makes a quick exit out of the chest as it loops around the origin of the right subclavian artery, soon after it enters the thoracic inlet. It continues its course cephalad towards the trachea-oesophageal groove in the neck. This point of looping is approximately 1 cm from the aortic arch, and corresponds to the length of the brachiochephalic trunk [Fig. 18]. It lies at the apex of the superior triangle, and diathermy should be used with extreme caution in this area, especially when the highest #2 nodes are attempted.

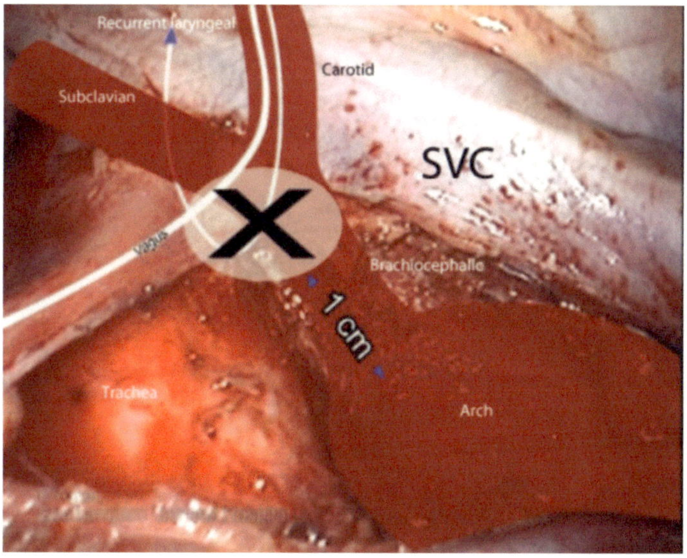

Fig. 18. Location of the right recurrent laryngeal nerve.

Again enthusiasm should be curbed not to cross the median line into the left side, as injury to the thoracic duct could occur. By the end of this dissection the whole length of the trachea should be seen bare of nodes, including a clear retrocaval and retro-azygos spaces [Fig. 19].

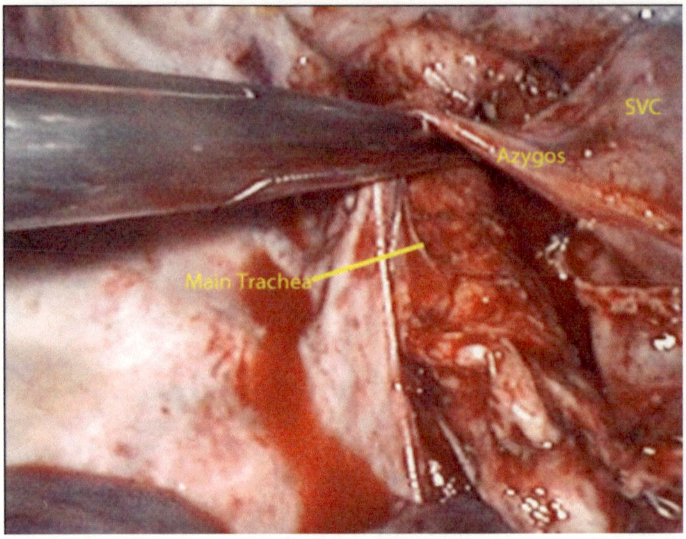

Fig. 19. The view after clearance of #2-4.

Left side:

Dissection is also started here by releasing the inferior pulmonary ligament. This exposes #9 around the inferior vein [Fig. 20]. The pleural reflection between the pericardium and the descending aorta is opened longitudinally from the inferior ligament to the diaphragm. The diaphragm and the pericardium might require retraction using a swab on a stick to expose this area [Fig. 21].

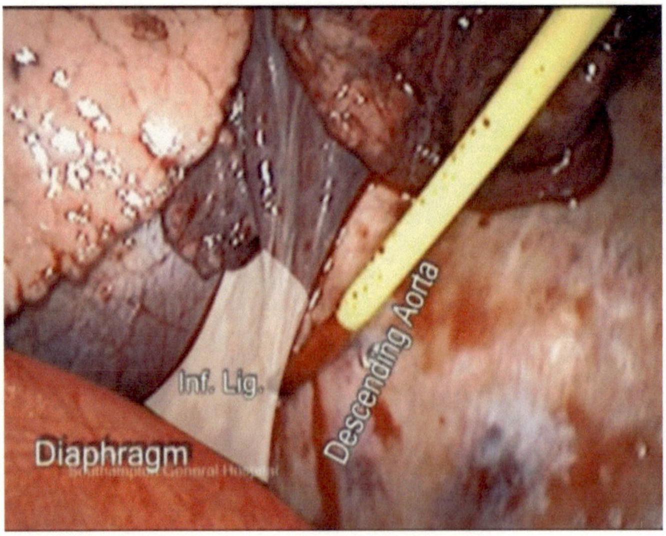

Fig. 20. Exposing left inferior ligament.

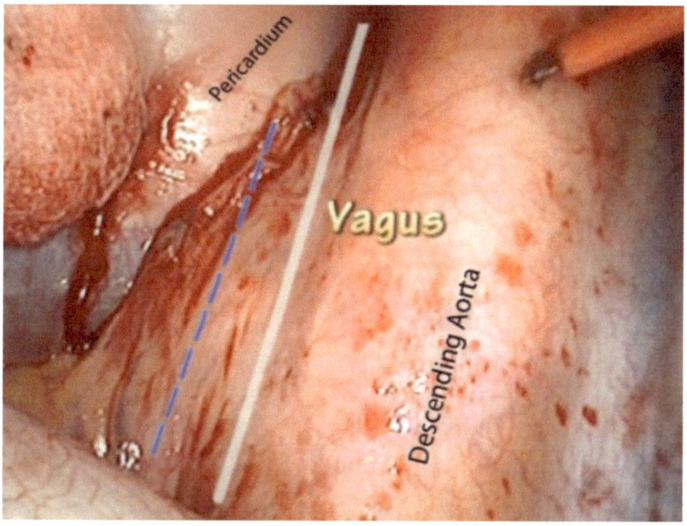

Fig. 21. Pleural landmarks for opening #8 &#9.

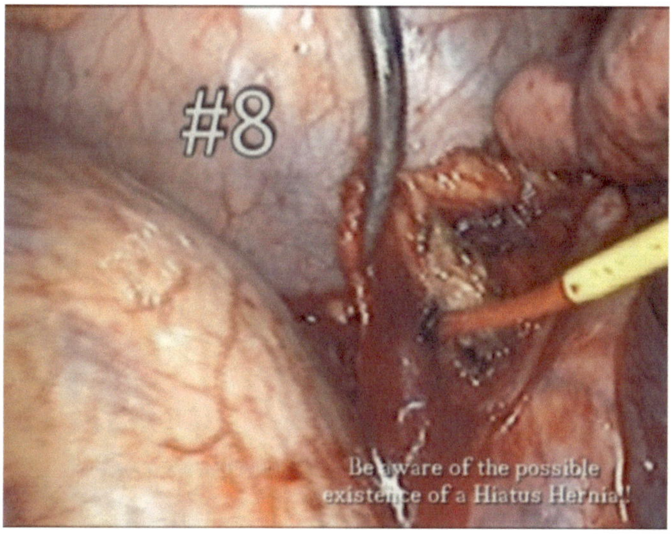

Fig. 22. En-block dissection of left #8.

This exposes #8 nodes which again could be absent, discrete or forming a fibro-fatty block. Care is taken not to injure the vagus, oesophagus, and other organs which are usually not there but could be there, such as a hiatus hernia [Fig. 22].

Dissection of the subcarinal #7 nodes on the left side is time-consuming, and require a prepared plan of action, good suction and detailed mastery of the surrounding anatomy. On retracting the lung anteriorly two nerves and a vein are noted to cross the arch of the aorta. The Phrenic nerve passes anterior to the hilum, whereas the Vagus passes posterior to the hilum. The superior intercostal vein draining the upper 3-4 spaces traverses the upper part of the aorta, crossing the origins of the left subclavian and carotid arteries and drain straight into the innominate vein [Fig. 23].

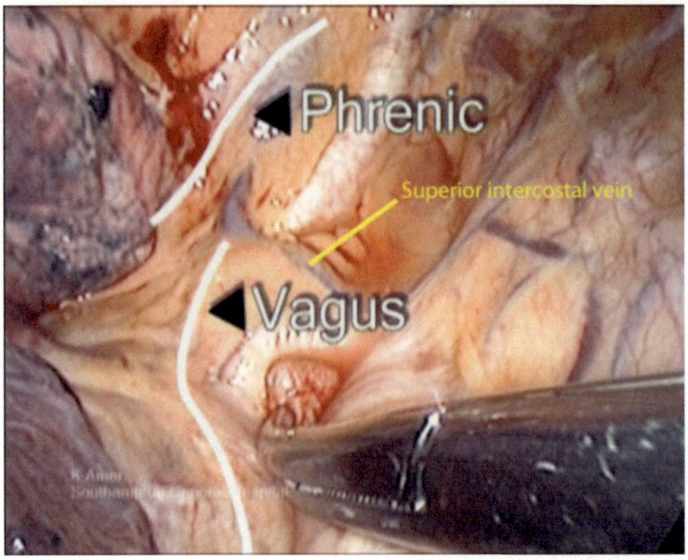

Fig. 23. The hilum watershed between Phrenic and Vagus nerves.

It will be noted that the left recurrent laryngeal nerve descends separate and parallel to the Vagus and hooks around the concavity of the aorta (ligamentum arteriosum) lateral to the vagus. We do not go out of our way to dissect and demonstrate its path, but avoid injury to the recurrent laryngeal by avoiding disturbing the pleura between the arch of aorta and the vagus nerve [Fig. 24]. On the other hand all vagal bronchial branches are cut with impunity [Fig. 25].

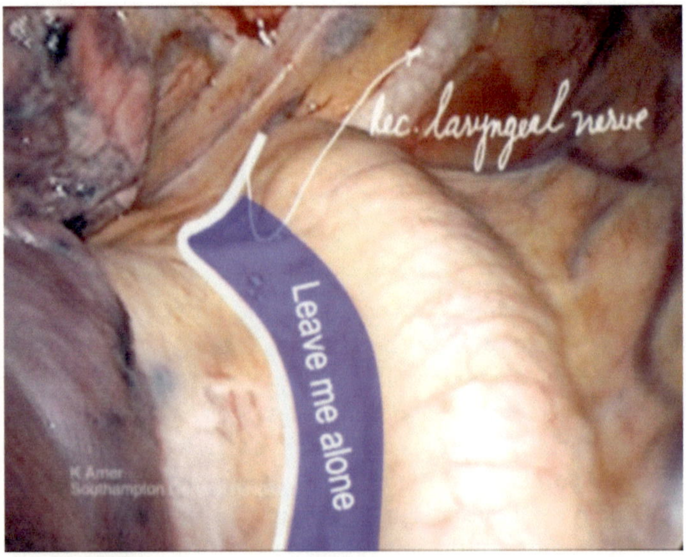

Fig. 24. The no man's land of the recurrent laryngeal nerve.

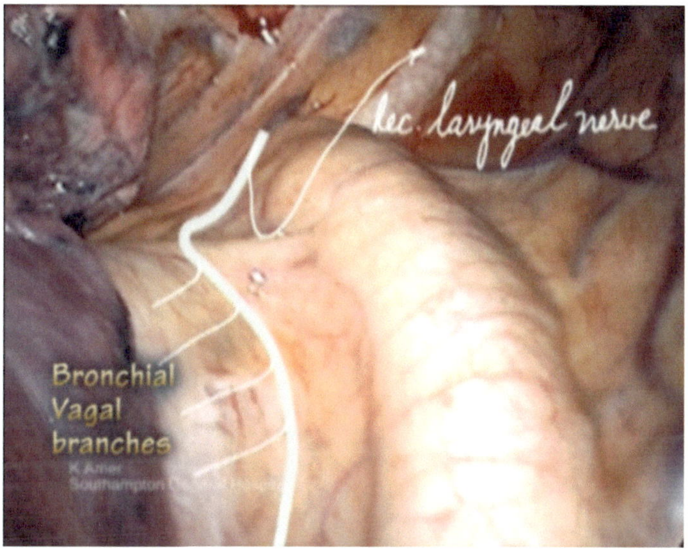

Fig. 25. Left vagal bronchial twigs.

Dissection is started by opening the pleural reflection at the back of the hilum, from the inferior ligament, up to and beyond the aortic arch. Dissection is kept lateral to the vagus, cutting all vagal bronchial branches. One or two bronchial arteries arising directly from the aorta might need to be secured before the space is fully exposed for nodal dissection [Fig. 26].

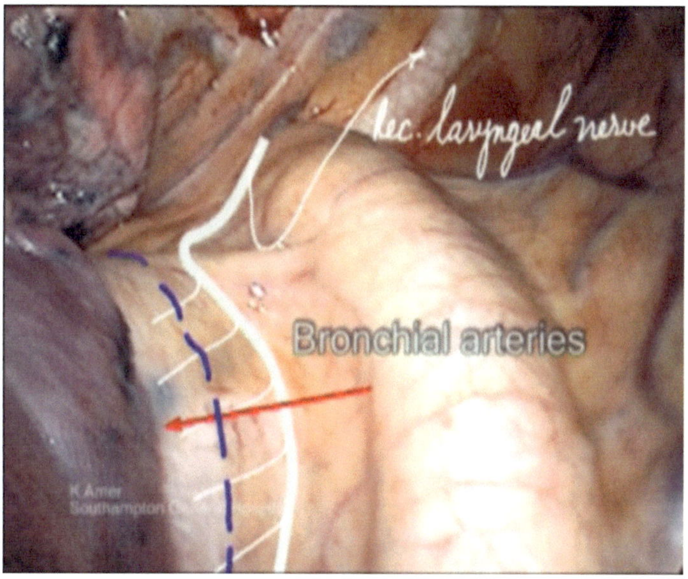

Fig. 26. Vagal bronchial twigs must be cut to access #7.

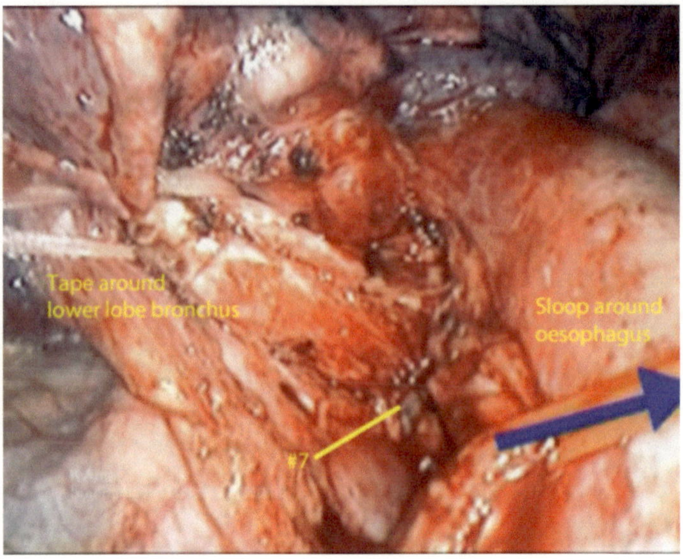

Fig. 27. Exposing the left subcarinal space.

The subcarinal nodes lie in a deep layer, not easily appreciated, deeper than the oesophagus, which is deeper than the aorta. One could make use of strong retraction on the lower lobe bronchus using a tape (has to be sturdy for strong retraction). This will bring the subcarinal space forward into view, and improve vision. A vascular sloop could be used around the oesophagus and *gentle* traction applied to assist in opening the space, but this is not mandatory [Fig. 27].

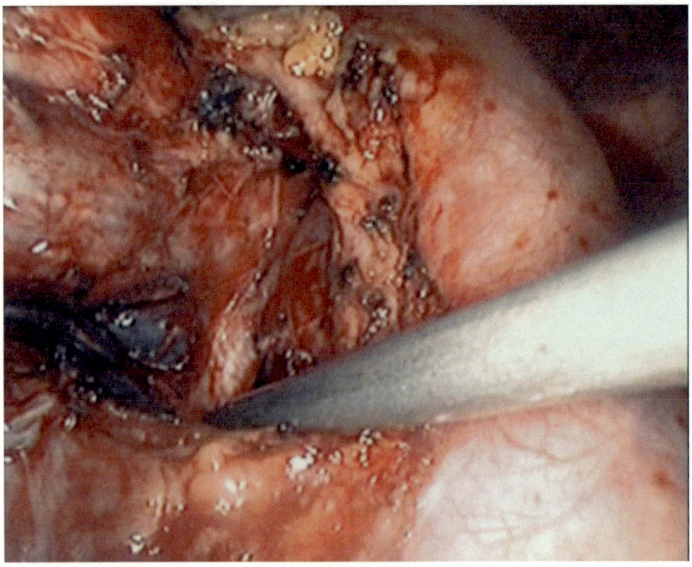

Fig. 28. #7 node.

The principle here is to follow the lower lobe bronchus proximally, as it leads us to the subcarinal space. Pinpoint diathermy dissection of the nodes off their blood supply is performed, taking care not to dig holes in the membranous part of the bronchus. The right main bronchus and the subcarinal space should be well on display by the end of this dissection [Fig. 28-29].

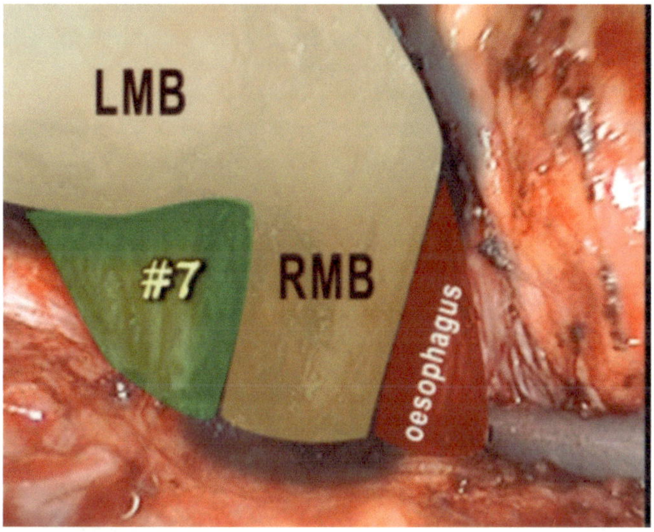

Fig. 29. Anatomy of the subcarinal space.

Nodes that are clearly related to the inferior vein, lower lobe bronchus or the main pulmonary artery are labelled as #10. However; the most lateral of the aorto-pulmonary group are labelled as #4, and these are at a deeper level than #10.

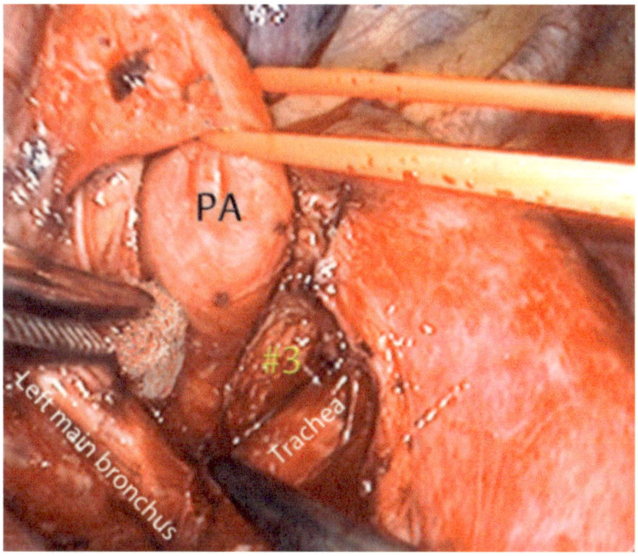

Fig. 30. Exposing pretracheal #3 nodes.

The precarinal #3 nodes could be accessed from the left side if required. The plane of dissection lies below the pulmonary artery, and hence there is no need to dissect and cut the ligamentum arteriosum. The main pulmonary artery is freed from the bronchus and a sloop passed around it. The space under the artery is dissected, and explored by pushing the carina down and the artery up. This manoeuvre exposed the main stem trachea [Fig. 30]. Pretracheal nodes are identified and dissected. Minimal use of diathermy is recommended in this position, as this is the likely position to injure the recurrent laryngeal nerve.

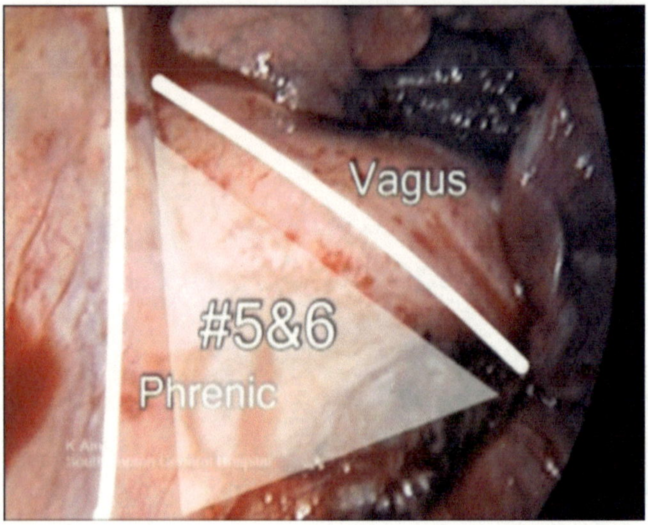

Fig. 31. The left superior triangle.

Dissection of #5 (preaortic) and #6 (sub-aortic and aorto-pulmonary) nodes should be attempted en block. These nodes exist in a triangle similar to the right side, bound by the vagus and Phrenic nerves and the arch of the aorta [Fig. 31]. The fibro-fatty block is lifted off the main pulmonary artery into the aorto-pulmonary space, medial to the vagus nerve. The phrenic nerve is identified and slung using a vascular sloop to avoid harming it. The nodal block is dissected up to the origin of the left subclavian artery, and the block delivered out of the chest.

9. Complications of SND

VATS-SND is safe, and does not add to the morbidity or mortality of the originally planned operation. However there are some complications the surgeon should be aware of:
Major complications:

- Vascular injury; SVC, Aortic arch, Azygos vein etc.
- Bronchial injury; usually the membranous part of major bronchi, especially dissecting around the subcarinal space
- Recurrent laryngeal nerve injury; on the right the danger arises when diathermy is used around the origin of the subclavian artery, and on the left when dissecting #3 (precarinal) at the space between main pulmonary artery and main stem trachea.

- Chyle leak; is rare and usually occurs if dissection involved large lymphatic ducts, mobilisation of oesophagus or in the presence of abnormal anatomical course of the thoracic duct.
- Port-site seedling, which is rare (0.5%) and seems to happen irrespective of whether the nodes were retrieved in a polythene bag or not [32,33].

Minor complications:

- Increased postoperative tube drainage.
- Irritant cough due to diathermy close to the main bronchi.
- Temporary odynophagia (painful swallowing) due to mobilisation of the oesophagus.

10. VATS nodal sampling v dissection

The current evidence suggests that complete mediastinal lymph node dissection is associated with improved survival compared with node sampling in patients with stage I-IIIa NSCLC undergoing resection [34].

11. SND and immune response

It was reported that Systematic lymphadenectomy added to major lung resection performed by open thoracotomy does not increase postoperative humoral immune response in uncomplicated cases [35]. However; there are no studies in the literature that looked into the VMPR-SND and the role of SND in postoperative inflammatory response.

12. Conclusion

VATS Systematic Nodal Dissection during VATS major pulmonary resections is feasible and safe. It should be performed routinely even when nodal involvement is unlikely, as 10% of patients in clinical stage N0-1 will have N2 disease. Multidisciplinary adjuvant treatment of lung cancer should be based on SND staging.

13. References

[1] Watanabe A, Koyanagi T, Ohsawa H, Mawatari T, Nakashima S, Takahashi N, Sato H, Abe T. Systematic node dissection by VATS is not inferior to that through an open thoracotomy: A comparative clinicopathologic retrospective study. Surgery 2005;138:510-517.

[2] Arriagada R, Bergman B, Dunant A, Le Chevalier T, Pignon JP, Vansteenkiste J; Cisplatin-Based Adjuvant Chemotherapy in Patients with Completely Resected Non–Small-Cell Lung Cancer. N Engl J Med. 2004;350:351-60.

[3] Douillard JY, Rosell R, De Lena M, Carpagnano F, Ramlau R, Gonzáles-Larriba JL, Grodzki T, Pereira JR, Le Groumellec A, Lorusso V, Clary C, Torres AJ, Dahabreh J, Souquet PJ, Astudillo J, Fournel P, Artal-Cortes A, Jassem J, Koubkova L, His P, Riggi M, Hurteloup P. Adjuvant vinorelbine plus cisplatin versus observation in patients with completely resected stage IB-IIIA non-small-cell lung cancer (Adjuvant Navelbine International Trialist Association [ANITA]): a randomised controlled trial: Lancet Oncol. 2006;7:719-27.

[4] Union Internationale Contre le Cancer. TNM classification of malignant tumours, Wiley-Liss, New York (1997) 93–7.

[5] Goldstraw P, Crowley J, Chansky K, Giroux DJ, Groome PA, Rami-Porta R, Postmus PE, Rusch V, Sobin L. The IASLC Lung Cancer Staging Project: proposals for the revision of the TNM stage groupings in the forthcoming (seventh) edition of the TNM classification of malignant tumours. J Thorac Oncol 2007;2:706-714.

[6] Lardinois D, De Leyn P, Van Schil P, Rami Porta R, Waller D, Passlick B, Zielinski M, Lerut T, Weder W. ESTS guidelines for intraoperative lymph node staging in non-small cell lung cance. Eur J Cardiothorac Surg 2006;30:787-792.

[7] Asamura H, Nakayama H, Kondo H, Tsuchiya R, Naruke T. Lobe-specific extent of systematic lymph node dissection for non-small cell lung carcinomas according to a retrospective study of metastasis and prognosis. J Thorac Cardiovasc Surg. 1999 Jun;117(6):1102-11.

[8] Misthos P, Sepsas E, Athanassiadi K, Kakaris S, Skottis I. Skip metastases: analysis of their clinical significance and prognosis in the IIIA stage of non-small cell lung cancer Eur J Cardiothorac Surg 2004;25:502-508

[9] Ono T, Minamiya Y, Ito M, Saito H, Motoyama S, Nanjo H, Ogawa J. Sentinel node mapping and micrometastasis in patients with clinical stage IA non-small cell lung cancer. Interact Cardiovasc Thorac Surg. 2009 Oct;9(4):659-61.

[10] Riethdorf S, Wikman H, Pantel K. Review: Biological relevance of disseminated tumor cells in cancer patients. Int J Cancer. 2008 Nov 1;123(9):1991-2006

[11] Witte B, Hürtgen M. Video-assisted mediastinoscopic lymphadenectomy (VAMLA). J Thorac Oncol. 2007 Apr;2(4):367-9.

[12] Witte B, Messerschmidt A, Hillebrand H, Gross S, Wolf M, Kriegel E, Neumeister W, Hürtgen M. Combined videothoracoscopic and videomediastinoscopic approach improves radicality of minimally invasive mediastinal lymphadenectomy for early stage lung carcinoma. Eur J Cardiothorac Surg. 2009 Feb;35(2):343-7. Epub 2008 Dec 16.

[13] Zieliński M. Technical pitfalls of transcervical extended mediastinal lymphadenectomy-how to avoid them and to manage intraoperative complications. Semin Thorac Cardiovasc Surg. 2010 Autumn;22(3):236-43.

[14] Van Tinteren H, Hoekstra OS, Smit EF, van den Bergh JH, Schreurs AJ, Stallaert RA, van Velthoven PC,Comans EF, DiepenhorstFW, VerboomP, van Mourik JC, Postmus PE, Boers M, Teule GJ. Effectiveness of PET in the preoperative assessment of patients with suspected non-small cell lung cancer: The PLUS multicenter randomised trial. Lancet 2002;359:1388-92.

[15] Gillies RJ, Robey I, Gatenby RA. Causes and consequences of increased glucose metabolism of cancers. J Nucl Med. 2008;49:24S-42S.

[16] Plathow C, Weber WA. Tumor cell metabolism imaging. J Nucl Med. 2008;49:43S-63S.

[17] Al-Sarraf N, Gately K, Lucey J, Wilson L, McGovern E, Young V. Lymph node staging by means of positron emission tomography is less accurate in non-small cell lung cancer patients with enlarged lymph nodes: Analysis of 1145 lymph nodes. Lung Cancer 2008;60:62-68

[18] Delphine L. Chen and Farrokh Dehdashti. Advances in Positron Emission Tomographic Imaging of Lung Cancer. J Thorac Cardiovasc Surg. 2004;127:1093-9.

[19] Eric Lim, David Baldwin, Michael Beckles, John Duffy, James Entwisle, Corinne Faivre-Finn, Keith Kerr, Alistair Macfie, Jim McGuigan, Simon Padley, Sanjay Popat, Nicholas Screaton, Michael Snee, David Waller, Chris Warburton, Thida Win.

Guidelines on the radical management of patients with lung cancer. Thorax 2010;65:iii1–iii27
[20] Albain KS, Swann RS, Rusch VW, Turrisi AT 3rd, Shepherd FA, Smith C, Chen Y, Livingston RB, Feins RH, Gandara DR, Fry WA, Darling G, Johnson DH, Green MR, Miller RC, Ley J, Sause WT, Cox JD. Radiotherapy plus chemotherapy with or without surgical resection for stage III non-small-cell lung cancer: a phase III randomised controlled trial. Lancet 2009;374:379-386
[21] Pisters KM, Vallières E, Crowley JJ, Franklin WA, Bunn PA Jr, Ginsberg RJ, Putnam JB Jr, Chansky K, Gandara D. Surgery with or without preoperative paclitaxel and carboplatin in early-stage non-small-cell lung cancer: Southwest Oncology Group Trial S9900, an intergroup, randomized, phase III trial. J Clin Oncol. 2010;28:1843-9.
[22] Rocco G, Perrone F, Rossi A, Gridelli C. Surgical management of non-small cell lung cancer with mediastinal lymphadenopathy. Clinical Oncology 2010;22:325-333
[23] Lim E, Harris G, Patel A, Adachi I, Edmonds L, Song F. Preoperative versus postoperative chemotherapy in patients with resectable non-small cell lung cancer: systematic review and indirect comparison meta-analysis of randomized trials. J Thorac Oncol. 2009;4:1380-8
[24] Meyers BF, Haddad F, Siegel BA, Zoole JB, Battafarano RJ, Veeramachaneni N, Cooper JD and Patterson GA. Cost effectiveness of routine mediastinoscopy in CT and PET-screened patients with stage I lung cancer. J Thorac Cardiovasc Surg 2006;131:822-829.
[25] Watanabe S, Ladas G, Goldstraw P. Inter-observer variability in systematic nodal dissection: comparison of European and Japanese nodal designation. Ann Thorac Surg. 2002 Jan;73(1):245-8
[26] Naruke T, Tsuchiya R, Kondo H, Nakayama Haruhiko, Asamura H. Lymph node sampling in lung cancer: how should it be done? Eur J Cardiothorac Surg 1999;16:17-24.
[27] Rusch VW, Asamura H, Watanabe H, Giroux DJ, Rami-Porta R, Goldstraw P; Members of IASLC Staging Committee.The IASLC lung cancer staging project: a proposal for a new international lymph node map in the forthcoming seventh edition of the TNM classification for lung cancer. J Thorac Oncol. 2009 May;4(5):568-77.
[28] Darling GE, Allen MS, Decker PA, Ballman K, Malthaner RA, Inculet RI, Jones DR, McKenna RJ, Landreneau RJ, Putnam JB Jr. Number of Lymph Nodes Harvested from a Mediastinal Lymphadenectomy: Results of the Randomized, Prospective ACOSOG Z0030 Trial. Chest. 2010 Sep 9. [Epub ahead of print]
[29] Gossot, D (2010). *Atlas of endoscopic Major Pulmonary Resections*. Paris: Springer-Verlag. 22-32.
[30] Sagawa M, Sato M, Sakurada A, Matsumura Y, Endo C, Handa M, Kondo T. A prospective trial of systematic nodal dissection for lung cancer by video-assisted thoracic surgery: can it be perfect? Ann Thorac Surg 2002;73:900-4.
[31] Watanabe A, Koyanagi T, Obama T, Ohsawa H, Mawatari T, Takahashi N, Ichimiya Y. Assessment of node dissection for clinical stage I primary lung cancer by VATS. Eur J Cardiothorac Surg. 2005;27:745-752.
[32] Amer K, Khan AZ, Singh N, Addis B, Jogai S, Harden S, Peebles C, Brown I. Video-assisted thoracic surgery systematic mediastinal nodal dissection and stage migration: impact on clinical pathway. Eur J Cardiothorac Surg. 2011 Apr 13.

[33] McKenna RJ, Houck W, Fuller CB. Video-assisted thoracic surgery lobectomy: experience with 1,100 cases. Ann Thorac Surg. 2006;81(2):421-5.
[34] Scott WJ, Allen MS, Darling G, Meyers B, Decker PA, Putnam JB, McKenna RW, Landrenau RJ, Jones DR, Inculet RI, Malthaner RA. Video-assisted thoracic surgery versus open lobectomy for lung cancer: a secondary analysis of data from the American College of Surgeons Oncology Group Z0030 randomized clinical trial. J Thorac Cardiovasc Surg. 2010 Apr;139(4):976-81
[35] Szczesny TJ, Słotwiński R, Szczygieł B, Stankiewicz A, Zaleska M, Kopacz M, Olesińska-Grodź A. Systematic mediastinal lymphadenectomy does not increase postoperative immune response after major lung resections. Eur J Cardiothorac Surg. 2007 Dec;32(6):868-72. Epub 2007 Oct 17.

15

Pancoast Tumors: Surgical Approaches and Techniques

N. Barbetakis
Consultant Thoracic Surgeon, Thoracic Surgery Department, Theagenio Cancer Hospital, Greece

1. Introduction

1.1 History

Tumors of the superior sulcus represent less than 5% of lung malignancies. The distinctive symptomatology was first described by Edwin Hare in 1838 [1], and it has been nearly 80 years since clinical and radiographic features of this tumor were described by Dr Henry Pancoast, a radiologist, in 1924 [2]. As a radiologist, he noted the difficulty in detecting the tumor on a plain chest radiograph. He initially thought that these tumors arose from epithelial crest cells from the fifth brachial cleft. These tumors have been named Pancoast tumors or Pancoast-Tobias tumors after further descriptions of their features by these authors in 1932 [3, 4]. This was the first time that bronchogenic carcinoma was recognised as the primary cause of this syndrome.

Prior to the 1950s, superior sulcus tumors were uniformly fatal. Chardack and McCallum reported a long-term survival after surgical resection and postoperative irradiation therapy [5]. Paulson, using preoperative irradiation followed by surgical resection, published the first series, which included 18 patients, in 1966 [6]. Shaw and Paulson identified that preoperative irradiation and a well-defined resection were associated with a 5-year survival of 34% [7]. Based upon these studies, preoperative irradiation and an extended posterolateral paravertebral thoracotomy (Shaw Paulson approach) has been the "standard of care" over the last 5 decades. However surgical resection remained limited to tumors invading the ribs only, and any further involvement of vascular or neural structures was still considered to remain a contraindication for an operation. This was changed by Dartevelle who was the first to develop an anterior transcervical approach for the resection of tumors involving subclavian vessels. Later on several other modifications of this technique were reported but with no remarkable improvement on overall survival.

In the last century, the management of the superior sulcus tumor changed from inoperability and incurability to the current regimen of preoperative chemoradiation therapy, with an attempt at complete resection. Interest in trimodality treatment led to the South-West Oncology Group (SWOG) 8805 study of induction chemoradiotherapy (cisplatin, etoposide, 45Gy) followed by surgery that resulted in a complete response rate of 22% and encouraging results [8]. A recent prospective phase II study (SWOG 9416) suggests that preoperative concurrent chemoradiation (cisplatin, etoposide, 45Gy) improves the rate of complete resection, intermediate survival and decreases the rate of local or distal recurrence [9]. The 2-year survival was 55% for all eligible patients and 70% for patients who had a complete resection.

The superior sulcus tumor is a rare tumor posing a unique challenge to thoracic surgeons. The current regimen of preoperative chemoradiation with complete surgical resection leads to reasonable long term survival. Progress is being made in the understanding of the anatomy and biology of this disease. A choice of incisions provides options that have the potential to increase the rate of complete resection. New techniques allow resection of structures that were previously considered unresectable. Future efforts to improve the results will entail not only multidisciplinary approach to en bloc extended resection of adjacent structures but also preoperative therapy (chemotherapy or biologic agents) that yields greater tumor regression, thereby improving complete resection rates that are so critical to long-term survival in this form of non-small cell lung cancer (NSCLC).

2. Definition and surgical anatomy

Pancoast tumor is a cancer of the apex of the lung with no intervening lung tissue between tumor and chest wall. Subsequently, there is involvement of structures of the apical chest wall above the level of the second rib. The chest wall involvement may be limited to invasion of parietal pleura or may extend deeper to involve the periosteum or the bone of the first rib or apical vertebral bodies, or it may include invasion of subclavian vessels, the nerve roots of the brachial plexus or the stellate ganglion. Involvement of the chest wall only at the level of the second rib or lower should not be considered to meet the criteria for Pancoast tumor [10]. An apical tumor involving only the visceral pleura and not the chest wall by clinical staging should not be classified as a Pancoast tumor. However, it seems reasonable to include tumors that are thought to involve chest wall by clinical criteria.

Superior sulcus tumors may occur in the three compartments of the thoracic inlet and symptoms are related to the location. The anterior compartment lies anterior to the insertion of the anterior scalene muscle onto the first rib, the middle compartment extends from there to the posterior border of the middle scalene muscle, whereas the posterior compartment lies behind the middle scalene muscle [11]. Tumors located in the anterior component may invade the subclavian vessels, whereas those in the middle mainly invade the brachial plexus (Figures 1, 2). Posterior Pancoast tumors usually invade the stellate ganglion or vertebral bodies (Figure 3).

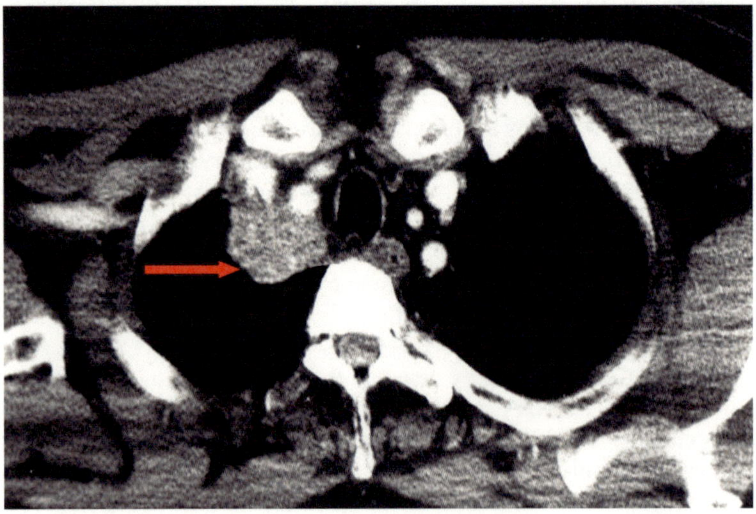

Fig. 1. Pancoast tumor located in the anterior component (anterior Pancoast tumor).

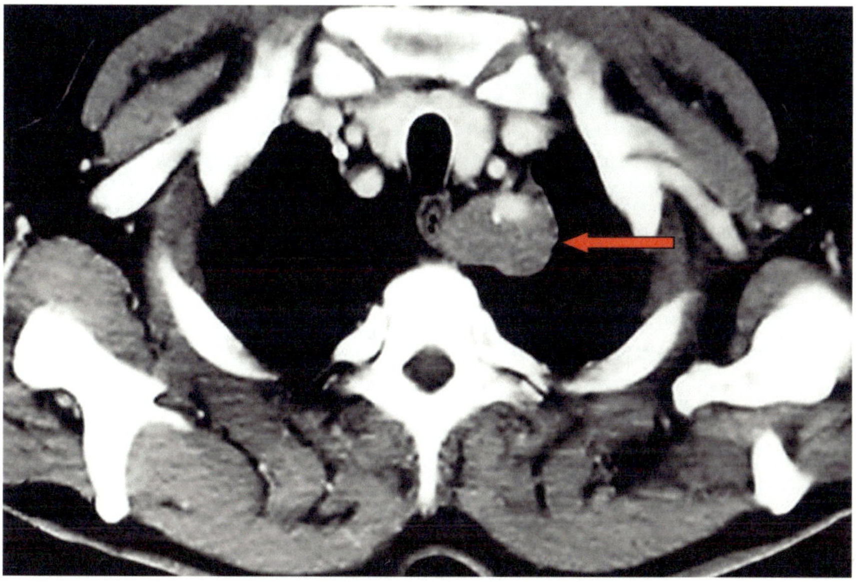

Fig. 2. Pancoast tumor occupying the middle component (median Pancoast tumor).

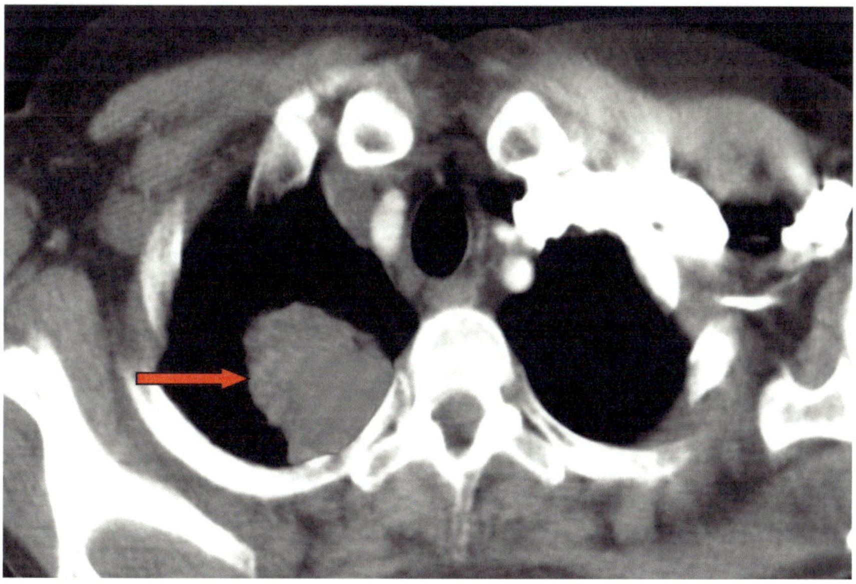

Fig. 3. Pancoast tumor located in the posterior component (posterior Pancoast tumor).

In case of invasion of the brachial plexus, patients often present with intense pain that begins in the shoulder and scapular region and extends down to the ulnar aspect of the arm (T1 dermatome) onto the small and ring fingers (C8 dermatome). Due to increasing pressure on the nerve roots, muscle atrophy of the ulnar aspect of the hand and loss of the triceps reflux can occur. In about 20-30% of patients, tumor invasion of the sympathetic chain and the stellate ganglion causes Horner's syndrome (ipsilateral ptosis, miosis and anhydrosis) [12].

COMPARTMENT	BOUNDARIES	included STRUCTURES	SIGNS AND SYMPTOMS
Anterior	Between sternum and anterior edge of anterior scalene muscle.	Platysma, sternocleidomastoid and omohyoid muscles, jugular and subclavian veins, scalene fat pad.	Pain radiating to the upper anterior chest wall, venous thrombosis.
Middle	Between anterior and posterior border of middle scalene muscle	Anterior and middle scalene muscles, subclavian artery and primary branches, phrenic nerve, trunks of brachial plexus	Pain and parasthesia radiating to the shoulder and upper limb, arterial thrombosis, diaphragmatic paralysis
Posterior	Behind middle scalene muscle	Posterior scalene muscle, posterior scapular artery, posterior aspect of subclavian and vertebral artery, paravertebral sympathetic chain, stellate ganglion, nerve roots of brachial plexus, long thoracic and spinal accessory nerves, neural foramina, vertebral bodies and prevertebral muscles.	Pain in the axilla and in the medial part of the upper arm, Horner's syndrome.

Table 1. Anatomical definition of the thoracic inlet and main clinical features in case of superior sulcus tumor invasion [13].

3. Biological behaviour

Advanced molecular biology techniques have accelerated the understanding of cancer biology. It is well established that the application of such technology has led to the recognition of lung cancer as a molecularly diverse set of tumor types whose only commonality is their origination in the lung [14]. Lung cancer classification is far more complex than the simplistic grouping into small cell and non-small cell variants with a comparable outcome when treated in a similar fashion [15]. Histologic subdivision of lung cancer uses only one of many phenotypic manifestations of the genetic changes that underlie lung cancer development.

Lung cancer development is a result of a stepwise progression of malignant transformation of normal respiratory epithelium. This transformation is driven by the cumulative effect of genetic alterations induced predominantly by inhaled carcinogens from tobacco smoke [16]. The Noguchi classification of lung adenocarcinoma is a pioneering effort to relate tumor histology with clinical and radiologic characteristics. This has resulted in the identification of atypical adenomatous hyperplasia and adenocarcinoma in situ as preinvasive neoplastic lung lesions that serve as precursors to invasive lung adenocarcinoma through a progressive transformation into the type A, B, and C adenocarcinomas with lepidic growth (referring to growth along alveolar structures) characterized by an increasing component of invasive carcinoma but showing excellent survival outcome, and the type D, E, and F solid-type adenocarcinomas with a well-recognized poor prognosis [17]. The most frequently described acquired genetic aberrations within the tumor involve the tumor protein p53 (TP53), KRAS, fragile histidine triad (FHIT), epidermal growth factor receptor (EGFR), cyclin-dependent kinase 2a (CDKN2), LKB1, retinoblastoma (RB), and Myc genes. Larger genomic mishaps such as chromosomal deletions involving the short arms of chromosomes 1, 3, and 9 (del 1p36, del 3p, and del 9p, respectively) are also frequently observed in different lung cancer histologic subtypes and stages. More recently, inversion translocation of the echinoderm microtubule-associated protein-like 4 (EML4) and anaplastic lymphoma kinase (ALK) genes on chromosome 2 (2p21 and 2p23) was shown to characterize a small subset of NSCLC with a characteristic clinical and histologic profile. The discovery of other molecularly defined lung cancer subsets is likely to be hastened by this finding [18].

The treatment options for patients with lung cancer have improved considerably in recent years. Improvements in survival have been noted for patients with every stage of the disease with the integration of new systemic therapy options, improvements to local therapy, and supportive care measures. A number of molecularly targeted agents that modulate a wide array of cell signaling pathways are currently under development. The remarkable success achieved with the use of EGFR tyrosine kinase inhibitors and the ALK inhibitors are the initial steps toward an era of individualized treatment options for patients with NSCLC. Several groups are now involved in screening tumor specimens for dominant oncogenic drivers in individual patients to guide treatment selection. A total of 13 known molecular abnormalities including 8 mutations are evaluated in the tumor specimens. By developing novel clinical trials across institutions to target each of these molecular events, the oncologist is evaluating a variety of individualized treatment approaches for patients with NSCLC. Because these molecular changes are noted in much smaller subsets of patients, such clinical trials are unlikely to complete accrual within a single institution in a reasonable time and therefore require such collaborative efforts to accelerate research.

The tremendous increase in the knowledge of lung cancer biology notwithstanding, a number of important questions remain unanswered. With lung cancer in never-smokers having been recognized as a unique entity, insights into the underlying mechanism and etiological factors will help in the development of novel therapies for this group of patients. The differences in lung cancer biology based on gender are another important area of research that will hopefully lead to the development of gender-driven therapeutic approaches. As newer therapeutic options are developed, participation of patients in clinical trials must be encouraged and supported by health care delivery systems. Currently, fewer than 5% of the patients diagnosed with cancer participate in therapeutic clinical trials [19]

Concerning Pancoast tumors it was traditionally believed that the biology was different from that of other non–small cell lung cancers and in that these tumors had a strong propensity to local invasion and a diminished incidence of spread through lymphatic or hematogenous routes. However, recent data does not support this belief [20]. Additionally the incidence of pathologic N2 disease, is similar to that of other peripheral stage I or II lung tumors and survival is better following a formal lobectomy rather than a wedge resection

alone. The unique feature of Pancoast tumors appears not to lie in the tumor biology but rather in the anatomy of the region in which these tumors occur.
Ipsilateral supraclavicular nodal involvement is classified as N3 disease. However, there is some evidence that such involvement in patients with a Pancoast tumor may not preclude long-term survival. Ipsilateral supraclavicular node involvement in these patients may have a prognostic importance more akin to that of N1 disease [21].

4. Surgical approaches

4.1 Posterior approach

The ideal tumor for the posterolateral approach is situated posteriorly in the superior sulcus and does not invade the anterior structures of the thoracic inlet. It may however invade the vertebral bodies or the brachial plexus. The C8 and T1 nerve roots are most commonly invaded. It is important to assess the patient's neurologic function preoperatively and to inform him properly concerning postoperative neurological morbidity [22].
The patient is placed in the lateral decubitus position. The incision starts anteriorly, allowing exploration of the chest cavity (usually through the fourth/fifth interspace) to assess resectability. The extension of the tumor onto the thoracic chest wall, thoracic inlet, lung, and mediastinum should be assessed. The incision is then extended posteriorly around the tip of the scapula and vertically upward between the spinous processes and posterior edge of the scapula, up to C7 (Figure 4). The division of muscle layers starts from the latissimus dorsi and trapezius to expose and subsequently divide the serratus anterior, rhomboidius major and minor, and levator scapulae muscles. The dorsal scapular nerve and scapular artery branches should be avoided when dividing the rhomboids at their insertion into the medial border of the scapula. These muscles will all be meticulously reapproximated at the end of the case. The chest wall resection is carried out first, in order to release the involved chest wall into the pleural cavity allowing for a safer lobectomy. En bloc resection of the chest wall and lung is preferred to extrapleural dissection without rib sacrifice, which often leads to incomplete resection. In most cases, the first two or three ribs are removed, although more ribs may be resected if required. The resection should guarantee large free margins, resecting 3-4 cm of uninvolved rib anteriorly and one rib and the intercostal muscle below the tumor inferiorly.

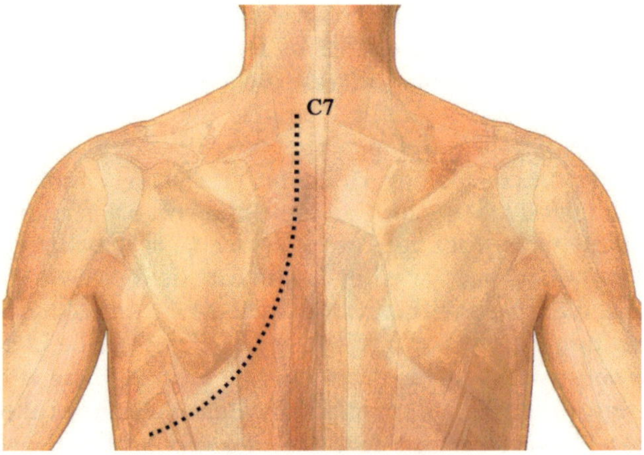

Fig. 4. Posterior approach for Pancoast tumors (Shaw Paulson thoracotomy). The incision extends up to the 7th cervical vertebrae.

First, the anterior and inferior dissection is started along the established resection margins beginning with the healthy rib. The invaded ribs and intercostal muscles are divided using rib shears and electrocautery, in succession from below to above, and the intercostal neurovascular pedicles are ligated. When the first rib is reached, the anterior and middle scalenus insertions to the second and first rib are divided with cautery, exposing the structures of the thoracic inlet crossing above the first rib. It is very important to note the insertions of the anterior and middle scalene on the first rib. Also of note is the phrenic nerve lying on the anterior surface of the anterior scalene. This, as well as the subclavian vein and artery should be identified before dividing the anterior scalene.

The posterior phase of the dissection starts by incising the erector spinae muscle along its anterior border from T1 to T5 and retracting it outward to expose the costotransverse joint. If the tumor involves the parietal pleura only, with no rib or vertebral erosion, the ribs may be disarticulated from the transverse processes, preserving the latter structures. The intercostal nerve and vessel originating from the intervertebral foramen are identified and divided between clips or sutured with 3-0 Prolene. This manoeuvre is repeated for each rib, until the first rib is reached. If the tumor involves the ribs posteriorly, the transverse processes are removed along with the adjacent lateral cortex of the vertebrae using an osteotome.

The lower trunk of the brachial plexus is identified by retracting the first rib downward and can be dissected posteriorly until it splits into the C8 (above the neck of the first rib) and T1 (below the neck of the first rib) nerve roots. Most commonly, the neoplastic invasion is limited to the first thoracic nerve root, which may be divided medial to its entry into the lower trunk and lateral to tumor involvement, keeping the C8 nerve root intact. This is very important in order to avoid the morbidity of loss of function of the intrinsic muscles of the hand [23]. When the tumor involves the C8 nerve, the lower trunk of the brachial plexus should be divided medially, at its origin from the spine. When the T1 nerve root is divided there is usually only a sensory deficit along the medial aspect of the hand.

With a hand inside the chest, the first rib is cut either at its neck if the head is not involved with tumor or beyond the attachment of its tubercle to the transverse process. The chest wall is then released from the apex of the chest en bloc by sequentially dividing the lower portion of the stellate ganglion and first intercostal artery.

Then a formal upper lobectomy with systematic lymph node dissection is the final step. The tumor attached to the chest wall is removed as one specimen. At this time a routine evaluation of the margins is done, obtaining biopsies and placing clips for helping postoperative irradiation.

It is not usually necessary to reconstitute the posterior defect in the chest wall, as it is covered by the scapula. A defect of three or more ribs or over the tip of the scapula should be closed with synthetic mesh. It is well established that meticulous reapproximation and closure with mesh prevents major morbidity in respiratory chest wall motion.

The posterior approach allows excellent exposure of the posterior chest wall including the transverse processes and thoracic nerve roots. It also allows standard exposure of the pulmonary hilum. However, surgical manipulation of the subclavian vessels is very difficult. Furthermore, visualization of the apex is poor making assessment of the appropriate extent of resection problematic.

4.2 Anterior approach

The anterior surgical approach to Pancoast tumors is modified to optimize exposure. Depending on location and size of the tumor there are two basic incisions: 1) a transclavicular incision and 2) a hemi-clamshell incision with supraclavicular extension.

The transclavicular incision (Dartevelle approach) is used with the patient in the supine position with the neck hyperextended and the head turned toward the uninvolved side [24]. The skin is prepared from the mastoid process to the xyphoid process and from the midaxillary line to the contralateral midclavicular line. The cervicotomy uses an L-shaped incision that follows the anterior border of sternocleidomastoid muscle and the inferior border of the clavicle to the deltopectoral groove (Figure 5). In first reports, a standard clavicular resection was included but this was associated with functional disability and suboptimal cosmetic results. An alternative approach involves bisecting the manubrium to preserve the claviculomanubrial junction (Grunenwald approach) (Figure 6) [25].

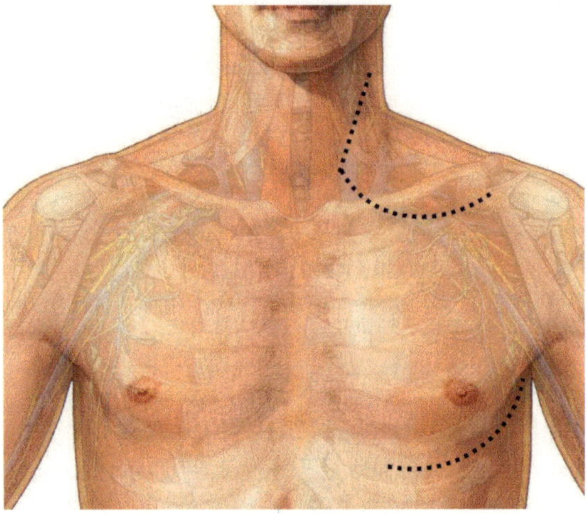

Fig. 5. Anterior transclavicular approach for Pancoast tumors (Dartevelle approach).

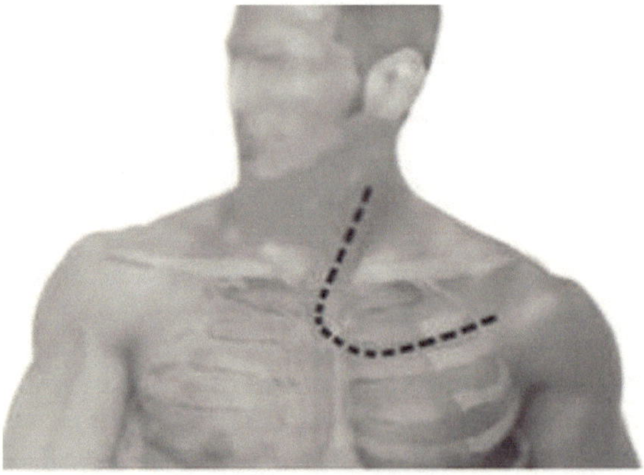

Fig. 6. Anterior approach for Pancoast tumors (Grunenwald approach).

The hemi-clamshell incision is a clavicular-sparing approach [23]. The patient is in full lateral position with slight posterior rotation. The skin is prepared in the same manner as described for the transclavicular approach. In patients requiring a supraclavicular extension, the ipsilateral arm is incorporated in the skin preparation.

The sternocleidomastoid muscle is divided and the medial half of the clavicle is resected. Variations of this approach include simple division of the mid-portion of the clavicle and subsequent reconstruction with plates and screws, or disarticulation of the sternoclavicular joint and lateral retraction of the clavicle.

The sequential steps involve dissection of the jugular veins, dissection of the arteries and exposure of the brachial plexus. Dissection of the jugular veins is important for adequate exposure. Ligation of the internal jugular vein is well tolerated. Especially on the left side, the thoracic duct is ligated with care.

The anterior scalene muscle is divided either at its insertion on the scalene tubercle of the first rib, or as close as it gets to its origin at the transverse processes of C3-C5. The anterior scalene muscle is well defined in 2/3 of patients and may be located behind the subclavian artery or split into two with the artery passing between the bundles [26]. The subclavian artery is mobilized by dividing most of its branches. Care is taken to preserve the vertebral artery and resection of the vessel is done only if it is involved with the tumor. A preoperative Doppler ultrasound is important to detect any extracranial occlusive disease. If the subclavian artery is invaded by the tumor, the affected portion is resected and reconstructed with a PTFE vascular graft. A small dose of heparin is administered during vascular clamping. Following anterior traction of the subclavian artery, the middle scalene muscle comes into good view.

The middle scalene muscle originates from the transverse processes of C2-C7and inserts onto the first rib between the subclavian groove and the posterior tubercle of the transverse process. In tumors invading the middle compartment of the thoracic inlet, the middle scalene muscle may be extensively involved. In these cases resection of the middle scalene muscle requires mobilization along its origin from the lower cervical vertebrae.

At this stage the cords of the brachial plexus are identified laterally. The anterior surface of vertebral bodies C7 and T1 are in view. The sympathetic chain and the stellate ganglion are lying in front of the vertebral bodies of C7 and T1. C8 and T1 nerve roots are visualized and dissected medially up to the lower trunk of the brachial plexus. The C8 nerve component of the plexus is preserved for better functional outcome of the upper limb. For carcinomas affecting the spine a multilevel unilateral laminectomy, nerve root division inside the spinal canal and vertebral body division can be performed by neurosurgeons.

The chest wall resection is performed with progressive resection of the first, second and third ribs. The ribs are resected from the costochondral junction anteriorly to the articulation with the transverse process. To facilitate mobility of the en bloc mass, resection of a short segment of rib (1-2 cm), may create a "mobile" chest wall. Resection of lower ribs is difficult and pulmonary resection by means of a conventional lobectomy is difficult. It may sometimes be necessary to perform a separate posterior thoracotomy to complete the resection and lymph node dissection.

The anterior approach facilitates direct visualization of vascular structures and provides excellent exposure of brachial plexus, sympathetic chain and stellate ganglion. There is freedom for hemi-vertebrectomy for tumors invading anterior parts of the vertebrae. Oncological clearance seems to be optimal due to the fact that the tumor is the last structure to be encountered. Finally the anterior approach seems to offer less morbidity than the posterior one.

A relative disadvantage of the anterior approach is the difficulty in removing the transverse processes and the head of the ribs in order to disarticulate them. The need to perform an additional posterior thoracotomy for the lobectomy and systematic mediastinal lymph node dissection could be seen as a factor that negates the routine use of anterior approach.

4.3 Future perspectives

Although the understanding of the biology and treatment of Pancoast tumors has evolved significantly, it is clear that more progress is needed. When considering that a large randomized trial may not be performed due to the relative rarity of the disease, the present clinical evidence from several phase II studies suggests that induction chemoradiotherapy and surgery be recommended as modern standard of care for Pancoast tumors. However, there are many issues still remaining for debate or are under discussion [27].

1. Recruitment of patients with N2 disease for surgery.
2. Ipsilateral supraclavicular lymph node disease should be considered as N1 disease.
3. The role of high dose preoperative radiotherapy (6000 cGy).
4. The role of prophylactic cranial irradiation.
5. The role of adjuvant postoperative chemotherapy.
6. The role of more aggressive surgery in cases of extensive involvement of the brachial plexus.

5. Acknowledgements

Sincere thanks to:

- Dr Francess Gillespie-Tsilikas (Consultant Anesthesiologist) for her valuable help in language editing.
- Dr Christos Asteriou and Dr Athanassios Kleontas (Residents in Cardiothoracic Surgery) for the photos and figures.
- Dr Christodoulos Tsilikas (Chief Thoracic Surgeon) for his mentoring and endless support.

6. References

[1] Hare ES. Tumor involving certain nerves [Letter]. London Med Gaz 1838;1:16-18.

[2] Pancoast H. Importance of careful roentgen-ray investigation of apical chest tumors. JAMA 1924;83:1407.

[3] Pancoast HK. Superior pulmonary sulcus tumor: tumor characterized by pain, Horner's syndrome, destruction of bone and atrophy of hand muscles. JAMA 1932;99:1391-1396.

[4] Tobias J. Sindrome apico-costo-vertebral doloroso por tumor apexiano: su valor diagnostico en el cancer promitivo pulmonary (Spanish) Rev Med Lat Am 1932;19:1552-1556.

[5] Chardack WM, Mc Callum JD. Pancoast tumor: five-year survival without recurrence or metastases following radical resection and postoperative irradiation. J Thorac Surg 1956;31:532-534.

[6] Paulson DL. The survival rate in superior sulcus tumors treated by presurgical irradiation. JAMA 1966;196:342.

[7] Shaw RR, Paulson DL Kee JL Jr. Treatment of superior sulcus tumor by irradiation followed by resection. Ann Surg 1961;154:29-40.

[8] Albain KS, Rusch VW, Crowley JJ. Concurrent cisplatin/etoposide plus chest radiotherapy followed by surgery for stages IIIA (N2) and IIIB non small cell lung

cancer: mature results of South West Oncology Group phase II study 8805. J Clin Oncol 1995;13:1880-1892.

[9] Rusch VW, Giroux DJ, Kraut MJ. Induction chemoradiation and surgical resection for non-small cell lung carcinomas of the superior sulcus: Initial results of South West Oncology Group Trial 9416 (Intergroup Trial 0160). J Thorac Cardiovasc Surg 2001;121:472-483.

[10] Detterbeck FC. Changes in the treatment of Pancoast tumors. Ann Thorac Surg 2003;75:1990-1997.

[11] Dartevelle P, Macchiarini P. Resection of superior sulcus tumors. In Kaiser LR, Kron IL, Spray TL, eds. Mastery of cardiothoracic surgery. Philadelphia: Lippincott-Raven 1998:257-265.

[12] Komaki R, Putnam JB, Walsh G, Lee JS, Cox JD. The management of superior sulcus tumors. Semin Surg Oncol 2000;18:152-164.

[13] Rea F, Marulli G, Sartori F. Posterolateral (Shaw-Paulson) approach to Pancoast tumor. http://www.ctsnet.org/sections/clinicalresources/thoracic/expert_tech-38.html

[14] Fujii T, Dracheva T, Player A et al. A preliminary transcriptome map of non-small cell lung cancer. Cancer Res 2002;62:3340-3346.

[15] Brambilla E, Travis WD, Colby TW, Corrin B, Shimoshato Y. The new World Health Organization classification of lung tumors. Eur Respir J 2001;18 :1059-1068.

[16] Boyle P. Cancer, cigarette smoking and premature death in Europe: a review including The Recommendations of European Cancer Experts Consensus Meeting. Lung Cancer 1997;17:1-60.

[17] Noguchi M. Stepwise progression of pulmonary adenocarcinoma–clinical and molecular implications. Cancer Metastasis Rev. 2010; 29: 15-21.

[18] Soda M, Choi YL, Enomoto M, et al. Identification of the transforming EML4-ALK fusion gene in non-small-cell lung cancer. Nature. 2007; 448: 561-566.

[19] Ramalingam SS, Owonikoko TK, Khuri FR. Lung cancer: New biological insights and recent therapeutic advances.CA Cancer Journal for Clinicians 2011;61:91-112.

[20] Detterbeck F.C., Jones D.R., Rosenman J.G. Pancoast tumors. In: Detterbeck F.C., Rivera M.P., Socinski M.A., Rosenman J.G., eds. Diagnosis and treatment of lung cancer: an evidence-based guide for the practicing clinician. Philadelphia: WB Saunders, 2001:233-243.

[21] Ginsberg R.J., Martini N., Zaman M., et al. Influence of surgical resection and brachytherapy in the management of superior sulcus tumor. Ann Thorac Surg 1994;57:1440-1445.

[22] Nicastri GD, Swanson JS. Pros and Cons of anterior and posterior approaches to Pancoast tumors: posterolateral superior sulcus tumors resections. Operative Techniques in Thoracic and Cardiovascular Surgery 2006;6:141-153.

[23] Nesbit JC, Wind GG, Rusch VW (Consulting Ed), Walsh GL (Consulting Ed). Superior Sulcus Tumor resection in Nesbit JC, Wind GG (Eds): Thoracic Surgical Oncology: Exposures and Techniques, Philadelphia, Lippincott Williams and Wilkins, 2003.

[24] Dartevelle P, Macchiarini P. Surgical management of superior sulcus tumors. Oncologist 1999;4:398-407.

[25] Grunenwald D, Spaggiari L. Transmanubrial osteomuscular sparing approach for apical chest tumors. Ann Thorac Surg 1997;63:563-566.

[26] Dartevelle P, Mentzer SJ. Anterior approach to superior sulcus tumors. Operative Techniques in Thoracic and Cardiovascular Surgery 2006;6:154-163.

[27] Parissis H, Young V. Treatment of Pancoast tumors from the surgeon's prospective: reappraisal of the anterior-manubrial sternal approach. J Cardiothorac Surg 2010;5:102.

16

Stage I Non-Small Cell Lung Cancer: Recurrence Patterns, Prognostic Factors and Survival

Jung-Jyh Hung and Yu-Chung Wu
Division of Thoracic Surgery, Department of Surgery, Taipei Veterans General Hospital and School of Medicine, National Yang-Ming University, Taipei, Taiwan

1. Introduction

Lung cancer is the leading cause of cancer-related death worldwide. Surgical resection is the treatment of choice for early-stage non-small cell lung cancer (NSCLC).[1,2] Five-year survival in patients with resected stage I NSCLC ranges between 55% and 80%.[3-6] Tumor recurrence is the most common cause of death, and thus the main obstacle for long-term survival after resection.[4-10] The postoperative recurrence rates in stage I NSCLC range between 22% to 38%.[4-8] The incidence of local or regional recurrence in stage I NSCLC after surgical resection has been reported between 7% to 15%,[4-6] while distant metastasis been reported between 14% and 23%.[4-8] Post-recurrence survival in resected stage I NSCLC is poor.[7,10-12]

The fifth edition of the TNM staging system for lung cancer was published in 1997, and stage I NSCLC was subdivided into IA (T1N0M0, tumor size ≤ 3 cm) and IB (T2N0M0, tumor size > 3 cm).[3] In addition to tumor size greater than 3 cm, the T2 descriptor also includes tumors that invade the visceral pleura regardless of size, tumors that involve the main bronchus ≧ 2 cm distal to the carina, and tumors that result in associated atelectasis and obstructive pneumonitis that extends to the hilar region but does not involve the entire lung radiographically.[3] In the sixth edition of the TNM classification (TNM 6)[13] for lung cancer published in 2002, no change was made to the previous edition.[3] The seventh edition of the TNM classification (TNM 7) for lung cancer has been published in 2009.[14,15] The changes to the TNM 6 for lung cancer were based upon the proposals from the International Association for the Study of Lung Cancer (IASLC). In the seventh edition, T1 descriptor has been classified into T1a (≤ 2 cm) and T1b (> 2 to ≤ 3 cm), while size-based T2 descriptor has been classified into T2a (> 3 to ≤ 5 cm), T2b (> 5 to ≤ 7 cm), and T3 (> 7 cm).[16] Stage I NSCLC was subdivided into IA (T1aN0M0, T1bN0M0) and IB (T2aN0M0).17 T2bN0M0 was reclassified as stage IIA.[17]

This review focuses on recurrence patterns of stage I NSCLC after surgical resection, survival after recurrence, and its prognostic factors. Predictors for local recurrence and distant metastasis are analyzed and discussed separately. Recent reports in the literature aiming at recurrence patterns and survival in stage I NSCLC (TNM 7) were also reviewed and included.

2. Prognostic factors for stage I NSCLC

The prognostic factors of stage I NSCLC (TNM 6) have been widely reported in the literature.[4-6,18,19] Martini et al[4] reported that T2 status and sublobar resection were the prognostic factors for poor overall survival in resected stage I NSCLC. Harpole et al[15] reported that presence of symptoms, vascular invasion, visceral pleural invasion and tumor size greater than 3 cm were the factors affecting overall survival in resected stage I NSCLC. Sawyer et al[18] reported that factors predicting poor overall survival included fewer than 15 lymph nodes dissected and tumor size greater than 3 cm. Varlotto et al[19] also reported that lymphadenectomy was associated with improved overall survival and disease-free survival in resected stage I NSCLC. Many other reports also demonstrated the prognostic value of tumor size in stage I NSCLC.[6,20] The number of mediastinal lymph nodes dissected/sampled alternatively represents the quality of lymphadenectomy and affects the survival rate for patients with resected stage I NSCLC.[19,21] Our previous studies[21,22] also showed that number of mediastinal lymph nodes dissected/sampled was a predictor of survival in stage I NSCLC. Cigarette smoking has been shown to be another prognostic factor in patients with NSCLC in the literature.[23-26] Hanagiri et al[23] reported that smoking was a significant postoperative prognostic factor in patients with NSCLC. Bryant et al[24] reported that 5-year survival rate was significantly better for never smokers compared to smokers in stage I NSCLC (TNM 6).

Only few studies reported the prognostic factors of stage I NSCLC (TNM 7).[25-28] In the report by Maeda et al, [27] 5-year overall survival rates for stage IA and IB (TNM 7) were 89.9% and 72.3%, respectively. They also demonstrated that older age, intratumoral vascular invasion, and visceral pleural invasion were poor prognostic factors in stage IB NSCLC.[27] In the report by Maeda et al,[27] 5-year disease-specific survival rates for stage IA and IB NSCLC (TNM 7) were 93.1% and 72.3%, respectively. They also demonstrated that intratumoral vascular invasion and visceral pleural invasion were poor prognostic factors for cancer-specific survival in stage IB NSCLC.[27] Maeda et al[25] reported that overall survival and recurrence-free survival in never smokers were significant better than those of ever smokers in patients with stage I NSCLC (TNM 7). Maeda et al[26] also discovered that a greater smoking extent was associated with the presence of solid components in stage I lung adenocarcinoma, which may have more aggressive biological features resulting in poorer outcomes.

3. Recurrence patterns

For stage I NSCLC (TNM 6), Martini et al[4] reported that the 2- and 5-year recurrence-free rates were 84% and 76%, respectively. Sixty percent of patients developed recurrence within the first 2 years after operation. Sawyer et al[18] reported that 5-year of local recurrence-free and distant metastasis-free rates were 85% and 83%, respectively, in patients with resected stage I NSCLC. In the study by Varlotto et al [29] regarding tumor recurrence in patients with resected NSCLC (including 82% of patients with stage I NSCLC), the 2- and 5-year local recurrence-free rates were 84% and 68%, respectively. The 2- and 5-year distant metastasis-free rates were 87% and 79%, respectively.

Martini et al[4] reported the overall incidence of recurrence in patients with resected stage I NSCLC was 27% (local or regional 7%, systemic 20%). In the study by Harpole et al,[5] the initial location of recurrence of stage I NSCLC after surgical resection was at a distant site in 19%, within the ipsilateral hemithorax in 11% or at both locations in 6% of patients. Distant recurrence rates between 14% to 23% in stage I NSCLC after surgical resection have also been reported in the literature.[6-8] Our studies[11,12] demonstrated that overall incidence of recurrence was 31.0% (distant only in 17.8%, local only in 7.9%, local and distant in 5.3%) in stage I NSCLC after surgical resection. The patterns of local recurrence included local only in 60.2%, local with distant in 15.4%, local before distant in 19.5% and distant before local in 4.9% of patients. Approximately 78% of patients with local recurrence occurred within the first 2 years after operation. We also showed that approximately 84% of patients with distant metastases occurred within the first 2 years after operation. A major proportion of patients (62%) died within one year after distant metastasis.

Most distant metastases appear as multiple foci in multiple organs after treatment of original cancer.[30] Martini et al[4] reported that the most common site of distant metastasis in patients with resected stage I NSCLC was the brain. Yoshino et al[31] demonstrated that pulmonary metastasis was most common in NSCLC patients with recurrence at distant organs, followed by bone metastasis. Our study[12] revealed that bone (32.1%) was the most common site of single organ metastasis in patients with resected stage I NSCLC, followed by the brain (29.2%). We further demonstrated that the patterns of distant metastasis included single and multiple organ metastases in approximately 64% and 36% of patients, respectively.

The recurrence-free rate of stage I NSCLC (TNM 7) has also been reported in the literature.[28,32,33] Maeda et al[32,33] reported that the 5-year recurrence-free rate in patients with stage IA NSCLC (TNM 7) ranges between 84 to 87%. In another article by Maeda et al,[28] they reported that 5-year recurrence-free rate in patients with stage I NSCLC (TNM 7) was 84.2%.

4. Predictors of recurrence

The predictors for recurrence in resected stage I NSCLC (TNM 6) has been well demonstrated in the literature.[4,5,18,29] In the report by Martini et al,[4] the factors having adverse effects on recurrence in resected stage I NSCLC included lesser resection than lobectomy, no lymph node dissection, T2 tumor, and greater tumor size. In the study by Harpole et al,[5] the factors affecting early recurrence in resected stage I NSCLC included presence of symptoms, vascular invasion, visceral pleural invasion, and tumor size greater than 3 cm. Although both Martini et al[4] and Harpole et al[5] performed elegant analysis demonstrating the factors influencing tumor recurrence in resected stage I NSCLC, they did not analyze local recurrence and distant metastasis as separate end-points. Only few studies evaluated the risk factors for local recurrence and distant metastasis separately. Varlotto et al[29] reported that local recurrence in resected NSCLC was associated with lymphatic or vascular invasion, the use of chemotherapy, and diabetes. Distant metastasis in resected NSCLC was significantly higher in patients with non-squamous cell histology, those undergoing pneumonectomy and those with more advanced TNM stage.[29] In the report by Sawyer et al,18 the factors independently predicting local recurrence in resected stage I NSCLC included fewer than 15 lymph nodes dissected and T2 tumor. Tumor size greater than 5 cm and non-squamous histology independently predicted a poor distant metastasis-free rate in resected stage I NSCLC.[18]

The predictors for recurrence in resected stage I NSCLC (TNM 7) has not been widely investigated in the literature. In the reports by Maeda et al,[28,33] they demonstrated that histologic differentiation, intratumoral vascular invasion, and visceral of pleural invasion were significant predictors for recurrence in stage I NSCLC (TNM 7).

5. Postrecurrence survival

In our previous study,[11] the 1- and 2-year post-recurrence survival rates for resected stage I NSCLC patients with local only recurrence were 48.7% and 17.6%, respectively. Tumor size and treatment for initial recurrence were significant predictors for post-recurrence survival in patients with local only recurrence in univariate analyses. The hazard of death was greater in patients with larger tumor size. Treatment for initial recurrence was still significant prognostic indicator in multivariate analysis. Patients underwent re-operation after local recurrence survived longer than those with chemotherapy or/and radiotherapy and those without treatment.

For patients with single organ metastasis, the 1- and 2-year post-recurrence survival rates were 30.2% and 15.1%, respectively.[12] The most common site of single organ metastasis was the bone, followed by the brain. Disease-free interval > 16 months and treatment for distant metastasis (including re-operation, chemotherapy and/or radiotherapy) were significant predictors of better post-recurrence survival in resected stage I NSCLC with single organ metastasis. Post-recurrence survival was not significantly different between single and multiple organ metastases groups of patients. Multiplicity of metastatic organ sites is not a significant prognostic factor in these patients. Yoshino and coworkers[31] reported that the 2-year survival rate of NSCLC patients with postoperative recurrence at distant organs was 15.7 %. Their result is similar to that in our study.

Surgical resection offers a good chance of cure for patients with stage I NSCLC.[3,5,20] However, the outcome of surgical treatment in resected stage I NSCLC after local recurrence have rarely been reported. Walsh et al[34] reported that complete surgical resection or high-dose radiotherapy with curative intent significantly prolonged post-recurrence survival in NSCLC. Sugimura et al[10] demonstrated that whether surgery or combination chemotherapy with radiation significantly improved post-recurrence survival over both no treatment and radiation alone in resected NSCLC after local recurrence. Voltolini et al[35] reported that 5-year survival after re-operation for locally recurrent bronchogenic carcinoma was 15.5%. The 5-year post-recurrence survival in our patients undergoing re-operation after local recurrence was 15%.

Treatment for recurrent NSCLC significantly prolongs overall survival and post-recurrence survival.[10,34] Yoshino et al[31] reported that patients who underwent metastatectomy for recurrence in distant organs had significantly longer survival while those with chemotherapy had marginally prolonged survival. Nakagawa et al[7] reported that treatment for the initial recurrence prolonged survival in stage I NSCLC after recurrence. In our study,[12] treatment for distant metastasis (including surgery and chemotherapy and/or radiotherapy) had a favorable survival in resected stage I NSCLC after distant metastasis than without treatment. There was no significant difference in post-recurrence survival between patients undergoing re-operation and those treated with chemotherapy and/or radiotherapy. However, there were two postoperative deaths due to respiratory failure after pulmonary resection. If the two patients were excluded, patients undergoing re-operation had significantly better post-recurrence survival than those receiving chemotherapy and/or radiotherapy ($P = 0.021$). The differences of therapeutic effects of surgery and chemotherapy and/or radiotherapy need larger series for further investigation.

Disease-free interval has also been shown to be a significant prognostic factor of post-recurrence survival in NSCLC. Longer disease-free interval was associated as with better post-recurrence survival in NSCLC after complete pulmonary resection.[10,34,36] Walsh et al[34] reported that disease-free interval greater than 12 months was a favorable predictor of post-recurrence survival in NSCLC after complete resection. Our study[12] showed that disease-free interval > 16 months was a significant predictor for better post-recurrence survival in patients with stage I NSCLC after distant metastasis.

Although some reports in the literature had tried to figure out the impact of specific distant metastatic organ sites on post-recurrence survival in resected NSCLC, small cohorts or mixtures with local and distant metastasis made it difficult to acquire definite results. Sugimura et al[10] reported that initial recurrence confined to the lung was associated with better post-recurrence survival in resected NSCLC. Yoshino et al[31] demonstrated that intra-pulmonary metastasis was a favorable factor for postrecurrence survival of resected NSCLC, while bone metastasis was a marginally unfavorable factor. Liver metastasis has also been reported as a worse prognostic factor in NSCLC after recurrence.[7,36] In our study, patients with distant metastases confined within the contralateral lung have significantly better post-recurrence survival than those with distant metastases outside the contralateral lung. We further showed that for patients with distant metastases outside the contralateral lung, those with bone metastasis had significantly worse post-recurrence survival.

6. Conclusion

Treatment for initial recurrence is a prognostic predictor for post-recurrence survival in resected stage I NSCLC with local recurrence. Longer disease-free interval and treatment for distant metastasis are indicators for better post-recurrence survival in resected stage I NSCLC with single organ metastasis. Complete surgical resection should be considered in selected candidates with resectable local recurrent disease. Aggressive treatment for distant metastasis in selected patients with longer disease-free interval may prolong the post-recurrence survival.

7. References

[1] Spira A, Ettinger DS. Multidisciplinary management of lung cancer. N Engl J Med. 2004;350:379-392.

[2] Scott WJ, Howington J, Feigenberg S, et al. Treatment of Non-small Cell Lung Cancer Stage I and Stage II: ACCP Evidence-Based Clinical Practice Guidelines (2nd Edition). Chest. 2007;132:234S-242S.

[3] Mountain CF. Revisions in the international system for staging lung cancer. Chest. 1997;111:1710-1717.

[4] Martini N, Bains MS, Burt ME, et al. Incidence of local recurrence and second primary tumors in resected stage I lung cancer. J Thorac Cardiovasc Surg. 1995;109:120-129.

[5] Harpole DH Jr, Herndon JE II, Young WG Jr, et al. Stage I non-small cell lung cancer. Cancer. 1995;76:787-796.

[6] Jones DR, Daniel TM, Denlinger CE, et al. Stage IB nonsmall cell lung cancers: are they all the same? Ann Thorac Surg. 2006;81:1958-1962.

[7] Nakagawa T, Okumura N, Ohata K, et al. Postrecurrence survival in patients with stage I non-small cell lung cancer. Eur J Cardiothorac Surg 2008;34:499-504.

[8] Al-Kattan K, Sepsas E, Fountain SW, et al. Disease recurrence after resection for stage I lung cancer. Eur J Cardiothorac Surg 1997;12:380-384.

[9] Martin J, Ginsberg RJ, Venkatraman ES, et al. Long-term results of combined-modality therapy in resectable non-small-cell lung cancer. J Clin Oncol 2002;20:1989-1995.

[10] Sugimura H, Nichols FC, Yang P, et al. Survival after recurrent nonsmall-cell lung cancer after complete pulmonary resection. Ann Thorac Surg 2007;83:409-418.

[11] Hung JJ, Hsu WH, Hsieh CC, et al. Post-recurrence survival in completely resected stage I non-small cell lung cancer with local recurrence. Thorax. 2009;64:192-196.

[12] Hung JJ, Jeng WJ, Hsu WH, et al. Prognostic factors of post-recurrence survival in completely resected stage I non-small cell lung cancer with distant metastasis. Thorax. 2009;65:241-245.

[13] Sobin L, Wittekind Ch, eds. TNM Classification of Malignant Tumors, Sixth Edition. New York: Wiley-Liss, 2002: 99-103.

[14] American Joint Committee on Cancer. AJCC Cancer Staging Manual. 7th ed. New York: Springer; 2010.

[15] International Union Against Cancer. TNM Classification of Malignant Tumours. 7th ed. Oxford, UK: Wiley-Blackwell; 2009.

[16] Rami-Porta R, Ball D, Crowley J, et al. The IASLC Lung Cancer Staging Project: proposals for the revision of the T descriptors in the forthcoming (seventh) edition of the TNM classification for lung cancer. J Thorac Oncol 2007;2:593-602.

[17] Goldstraw P, Crowley J, Chansky K, et al. The IASLC Lung Cancer Staging Project: proposals for the revision of the TNM stage groupings in the forthcoming (seventh) edition of the TNM Classification of malignant tumours. J Thorac Oncol 2007;2:706-714.

[18] Sawyer TE, Bonner JA, Gould PM, et al. Patients with stage I non-small cell lung carcinoma at postoperative risk for local recurrence, distant metastasis, and death: implications related to the design of clinical trials. Int J Radiat Oncol Biol Phys. 1999;45:315-321.

[19] Varlotto JM, Recht A, Nikolov M, et al. Extent of lymphadenectomy and outcome for patients with stage I nonsmall cell lung cancer. Cancer. 2009;115:851-858.

[20] Nesbitt JC, Putnam JB Jr, Walsh GL, et al. Survival in early-stage non-small cell lung cancer. Ann Thorac Surg 1995;60:466-472.

[21] Hung JJ, Wang CY, Huang MH, et al. Prognostic factors in resected stage I non-small cell lung cancer with a diameter of 3 cm or less: visceral pleural invasion did not

influence overall and disease-free survival. J Thorac Cardiovasc Surg. 2007;134:638-643.

[22] Hung JJ, Jeng WJ, Hsu WH, et al. Prognostic factors in pathological stage IB non-small cell lung cancer greater than 3 cm. Eur Respir J 2010;36:1355-1361.

[23] Hanagiri T, Sugio K, Mizukami M, et al. Significance of smoking as a postoperative prognostic factor in patients with non-small cell lung cancer. J Thorac Oncol 2008;3:1127–1132.

[24] Bryant A, Cerfolio RJ. Differences in epidemiology, histology, and survival between cigarette smokers and never-smokers who develop non-small cell lung cancer. Chest 2007;132:185–192.

[25] Maeda R, Yoshida J, Ishii G, et al. The Prognostic Impact of Cigarette Smoking on Patients with Non-small Cell Lung Cancer. J Thorac Oncol 2011;6:735-742.

[26] Maeda R, Ishii G, Yoshida J, et al. Influence of cigarette smoking on histological subtypes of stage I lung adenocarcinoma. J Thorac Oncol 2011;6:743-750.

[27] Maeda R, Yoshida J, Ishii G, et al. Poor prognostic factors in patients with stage IB non-small cell lung cancer according to the seventh edition TNM classification. Chest 2011;139:855-861.

[28] Maeda R, Yoshida J, Ishii G, et al. Risk factors for tumor recurrence in patients with early-stage (stage I and II) non-small cell lung cancer: Patient selection criteria for adjuvant chemotherapy according to the 7th edition TNM classification. Chest 2011 May 26. [Epub ahead of print]

[29] Varlotto JM, Recht A, Flickinger JC, et al. Factors associated with local and distant recurrence and survival in patients with resected nonsmall cell lung cancer. Cancer 2009;115:1059-1069.

[30] Cady B. Fundamentals of contemporary surgical oncology: biologic principles and the threshold concept govern treatment and outcomes. J Am Coll Surg 2001;192:777-792.

[31] Yoshino I, Yohena T, Kitajima M, et al. Survival of non-small cell lung cancer patients with postoperative recurrence at distant organs. Ann Thorac Cardiovasc Surg 2001;7:204-209.

[32] Maeda R, Yoshida J, Ishii G, et al. Long-term outcome and late recurrence in patients with completely resected stage IA non-small cell lung cancer. J Thorac Oncol 2010;5:1246-1250.

[33] Maeda R, Yoshida J, Ishii G, et al. Long-term survival and risk factors for recurrence in stage I non-small cell lung cancer patients with tumors up to 3 cm in maximum dimension. Chest 2010;138:357-362.

[34] Walsh GL, O'Connor M, Willis KM, et al. Is follow-up of lung cancer patients after resection medically indicated and cost-effective? Ann Thorac Surg 1995;60:1563-1570.

[35] Voltolini L, Paladini P, Luzzi L, et al. Iterative surgical resections for local recurrent and second primary bronchogenic carcinoma. Eur J Cardiothorac Surg 2000;18:529-534.

[36] Williams BA, Sugimura H, Endo C, et al. Predicting postrecurrence survival among completely resected nonsmall-cell lung cancer patients. Ann Thorac Surg 2006;81:1021-1027.

17

Surgical Treatment of Bronchiectasis

Hidir Esme and Sevval Eren
Konya Education and Researc Hospital,
Dicle University, School of Medicine,
Turkey

1. Introduction

Bronchiectasis is pathologically defined as a condition in which there are abnormal and permanent dilatations of proximal bronchi with predominance at the level of the second to the sixth bronchial division. This definition differentiates true bronchiectasis from functional bronchiectasis or pseudobronchiectasis, which is expected to return to normal once control of infection has been achieved (Deslauriers et al., 1998). Bronchiectasis was first described by Laenec in 1819 and, before the antibiotic era, was considered a morbid disease with a high mortality rate from respiratory failure and cor pulmonale (Balkanli et al., 2003). With the development of antibiotics in the 1940s, this entity began to be seen less frequently, but, with the emergence of drug-resistant microorganisms and the increasing frequency of drug-resistant tuberculosis, an increased incidence of postinfectious bronchiectasis is being noted (Miller, 2000). The current increase in tuberculosis rates is directly related to insufficient and irregular medication. Additionally, irregular and inadequate treatment, the cessation of medication shortly after symptom improvement, and a lack of check-ups after treatment are factors accelerating recurrent pulmonary infection in developing countries. As the disease progresses, physical activities become increasingly limited, patients fail to thrive, and ultimately they suffer from social deprivation, intrinsic depression, and respiratory failure (Al-Kattan et al., 2005). Therefore, bronchiectasis is still a major cause of morbidity and mortality in developing countries.

2. Pathophysiology

Reid categorized bronchiectasis as having three main phenotypes: 1) tubular characterized by smooth dilation of the bronchi; 2) varicose in which the bronchi are dilated with multiple indentations; and 3) cystic in which dilated bronchi terminate in blind ending sacs (Reid, 1950). The current major form seen on High resolution computed tomography scanning (HRCT) is the tubular form of bronchiectasis. The most definitive study of the pathology of bronchiectasis was performed by Whitwell (Whitwell, 1952). Whitwell suggested that bronchiectasis should be divided into (1) follicular bronchiectasis, characterized by excessive formation of lymphoid tissue both in the walls of dilated bronchi and in enlarged lymph nodes and thought to be sequelae of whooping cough, measles, or bronchopneumonia, (2) saccular bronchiectasis, characterized by loss of bronchial structures in the sacculi and of alveoli around them, and (3) atelectatic bronchiectasis, in which lung collapse leads to bronchiectasis. Follicular bronchiectasis was the dominant form and this corresponded to tubular bronchiectasis. In his study, he demonstrated marked inflammation of the bronchial wall, principally in the smaller airways. Bronchial dilation was characterized by deficiency/loss of elastin and more advance disease by destruction of muscle and cartilage. There was variable bronchial wall fibrosis, atelectasis and peribronchial pneumonic change (King, 2009).

Follicular bronchiectasis was characterized by the presence of lymphoid follicles in the bronchial wall. The inflammatory process commenced in the small airway. This small airway inflammation caused the release of mediators such as proteases which damaged the large airways causing loss of elastin and other components such as muscle and cartilage which resulted in bronchial dilation. With progression of the disease lymphoid follicles enlarged in size and caused airflow obstruction to the small airways. The final event was spread of the inflammation beyond the airways to cause interstitial pneumonia (King, 2009).

The dominant cell types involved in the inflammatory process in bronchiectasis are neutrophils, lymphocytes, and macrophages. Neutrophils are the most prominent cell type in the bronchial lumen (Loukide et al., 2002; Khair et al., 1996) and release mediators, particularly proteases/elastase which cause bronchial dilation (Khair et al., 1996; Zheng et al., 2000). The infiltrate in the cell wall is predominantly composed of macrophages and lymphocytes (Loukide et al., 2002; Lapa a Silva et al., 1989)

Bronchiectasis can occur as focal or localized disease, or in a diffuse manner. Localized bronchiectasis is usually the result of childhood pneumonia and often has a benign course characterized by recurrent pulmonary infections always in the same anatomic territory. By contrast, diffuse bronchiectasis is often related to immune deficiencies, is bilateral, and may lead to death from respiratory failure (Deslauriers et al., 1998). Karadag et al. found that bronchiectasis most commonly involved the lower lobes. Only one lobe was found to be diseased in 46%, bilobar involvement in 28.1%, and multilobar involvement in 31.9% (Karadag et al., 2005). Karakoc et al. found bronchiectasis affecting the left lower lobe in 30.4%, and multilobar involvement in 56.5% (Karakoc et al., 2001). Dogru et al. found the most common lobe affected by bronchiectasis was the left-lower lobe in the 204 children they evaluated (Dogru et al., 2005). Isolated upper lobe bronchiectasis generally relates to prior tuberculosis, bronchopulmonary aspergillosis, or bronchial obstruction. Overall, one-third of cases of bronchiectasis are unilateral and affect a single lobe, one-third are unilateral but affect more than one lobe, and one-third are bilateral (Figure 1) (Deslauriers et al., 1998).

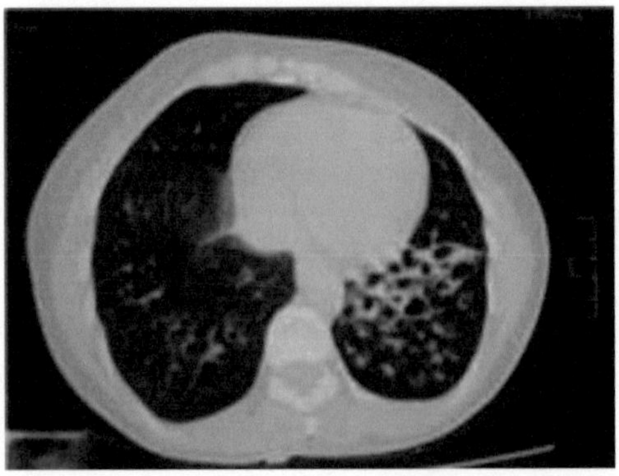

Fig. 1. Chest CT scan showing bilateral cystic bronchiectasis in the lower lobes.

The middle lobe syndrome consists of a small atelectatic lobe, often owing to extrinsic bronchial compression secondary to enlarged peribronchial nodes (Deslauriers et al., 1998). The right middle lobe bronchus is long, often bends sharply at its bifurcation and is of relatively small caliber. A collar of lymph nodes also surrounds the proximal bronchus and any condition that causes a prolonged enlargement of these nodes may lead to obstruction and secondary bronchiectasis. This may also occur in malignancy and in nontuberculous mycobacterial infection (Figure 2) (Bertelsen et al., 1980; Levin, 2002).

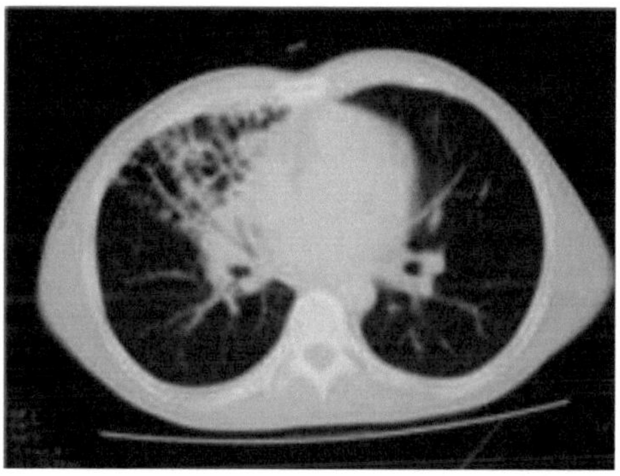

Fig. 2. Chest CT scan showing the bronchiectasis in the right middle lobe

3. Etiology

There have been a large number of factors that have been described as causative for bronchiectasis. A list of etiologic factors in different studies is given in Table 1. Recurrent pulmonary infection during childhood is an important factor in the etiology. Most of patients had recurrent infections in their histories and insufficient medication for pulmonary infection (Prieto et al., 2001; Agasthian et al., 1996; Fujimoto et al., 2001). The insufficient and inadequate use of medications for pulmonary infections and tuberculosis in patients, and the lack of follow-up over time, create a background for lung destruction (Figure 3). Bronchiectasis should not be mistaken with pseudo-bronchiectasis, temporary (up to 6 months) cylindrical dilatation of the bronchi accompanying lung infection in children (Sirmali et al., 2006). In developing countries, tuberculosis is still one of the most important causes of bronchiectasis. Bronchiectasis commonly develops between 1 and 3 months after the initial infection and usually in the same pulmonary region (Karakoc et al., 2001; Haciibrahimoglu et al., 2004).

Deficiencies in immune function, especially in humoral immunity, cause children to be at risk for recurrent sinopulmonary infections, which can lead to the development of bronchiectasis. This includes both primary immunodeficiency and secondary, or acquired, disease states (Boren et al., 2008). Cystic fibrosis is the most common cause of bronchiectasis among Caucasians of North America and Europe. Muco-ciliary clearance is a key defence mechanism against pulmonary infection. Its compromise is important in the development of the vicious cycle of bronchiectasis. The most prominent cilial disorder is primary ciliary dyskinesia which combines upper and lower respiratory tract infection, male infertility and in approximately 50%, situs inversus (King, 2009). Bronchial obstruction from either endobronchial pathology or external compression can also be an acquired factor predisposing to the development of bronchiectasis. Aspirated foreign bodies or gastric contents, slow-growing neoplasms, and mucous impaction can all cause local retention of secretions, secondary infection, and bronchiectasis (Deslauriers et al., 1998).

Etiolgic factor	Balkanli n, %	Eren n; %	Sırmali n, %	Cobanoglu n, %	Giovannetti n, %
Pneumonia	86 (36.1)	22 (15.3)	109 (61.9)	18 (29.0)	10 (22.2)
Childhood infection	63 (26.4)	19 (13.2)	-	7 (11.3)	-
Obstruction due to foreign body	1 (0.4)	4 (2.7)	23 (13)	1 (1.6)	-
Pulmonary sequestration	4 (1.6)	2 (1.4)	-	4 (6.4)	-
Postobstructive pneumonitis	-	34 (23.7)	-	2 (3.2)	-
Measles	-	-	-	4 (6.4)	-
Pertussis	-	-	-	3 (4.8)	4 (8.8)
Tuberculosis	-	22 (15.3)	44 (25)	11 (17.7)	6 (13.3)
Immunodeficiency (IgG, IgA)	-	-	-	1 (1.6)	-
Cystic fibrosis	-	-	-	2 (3.2)	-
Unknown etiology	84 (35.2)	40 (27.9)	-	4 (6.4)	25 (55%)

Table 1. Etiologic factors of bronchiectasis

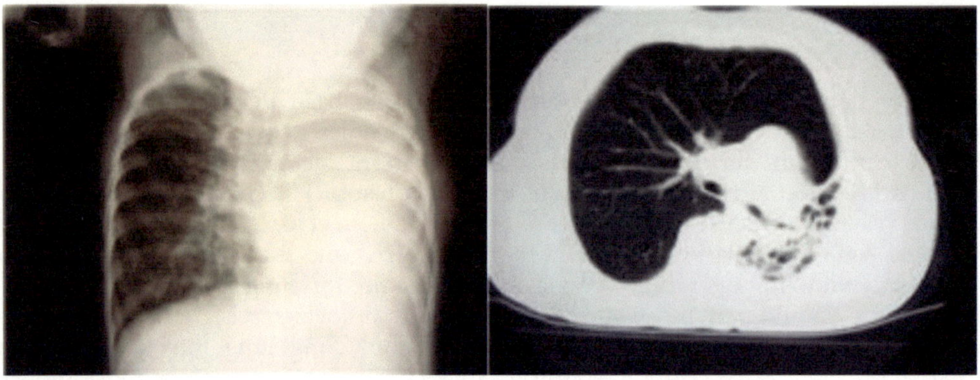

Fig. 3. Standart PA chest radigraph and Chest CT scan of a 4-year-old boy shows a destroyed left lung.

4. Clinical presentation

The clinical presentation of patients with bronchiectasis is variable and depends on the etiology of bronchiectasis and on whether the condition is localized of diffuse. Semptoms of the patients in different studies were presented in Table 2. The primary clinical symptom of bronchiectasis is a recurrent or permanent cough with ample sputum production. The sputum is frequently purulent and is often accompanied by hemoptysis in advanced stages of the disease (Nicotra et al., 1995). In the past, some bronchiectasis has been described as being nonproductive or "dry", although in retrospect these were mostly cases of post-tuberculous bronchiectasis located in the upper lobes (Deslauriers et al., 1998). Severe and life-threatening bleeding may result from erosions of the hypertrophic bronchial arteries or lesions in abnormal anastomoses between the pulmonary and bronchial arterial circulations.

Symptoms may be mild (eg, unproductive cough) or even absent if the disease is restricted to the upper lobes. Patients may also present with symptoms of the underlying disease that has led to the development of bronchiectasis (Zhang et al., 2010). Acute exacerbations of bronchiectasis are defined by symptomatic changes, including increased thick sputum production with change in color, shortness of breath, pleuritic chest pain, and generalized malaise. Chest roentgenograph (CXR) rarely shows new infiltrates, and the patient may lack fever and chills (Boren et al., 2008).

Symptoms	Balkanli n, %	Eren n, %	Zhang n, %	Sirmali n, %	Cobanoglu n, %	Haciibrahimoglu n, %
Productive cough	133 (55.8)	94 (65.7)	671 (85)	167 (94.9)	48 (77.4)	32 (91.4)
Recurrence of pulmonary infection	84 (35.2)	69 (48.2)	-	-	41 (66.1)	33 (94.2)
Fetid sputum	116 (48.7)	72 (50.3)	277 (35)	139 (79)	27 (43.5)	28 (80)
Hemoptysis	39 (12.1)	21 (14.6)	411 (52)	78 (44.3)	7 (11.3)	4 (11.4)
Chest pain	-	12 (8.3)	56 (7.1)	-	7 (11.3)	-
Fatigue	-	-	-	-	17 (27.4)	-
Dyspnea	-	-	-	-	34 (54.8)	-
Growth retardation	-	-	-	34 (19.3)	-	-
Asymptomatic	10 (4.2)	2 (2.0)	25 (3.2)	-	10 (16.1)	-

Table 2. Semptoms of the patients

Physical examination is often nonspecific. Crepitation, wheezing, and coarse expiratory rhonchi may be heard over the lung bases, whereas clinical signs of cor pulmonale and denutrition are uncommon and indicate advanced disease. Routine clinical assessment should include a careful recording of personal and familial history, which may indicate an inherited disorder (Deslauriers et al., 1998).

Pulmonary function testing can help determine the degree of lung damage because of bronchiectasis. Bronchiectasis typically results in obstructive lung function changes as the disease progresses. Typical obstructive changes on lung function testing include a reduced forced vital capacity (FVC), reduced forced expiratory volume in 1 s (FEV1), and reduced FEV1 to FVC ratio. Airway hyperresponsiveness with reversibility after the administration of inhaled bronchodilator should also be evaluated (Boren et al., 2008).

5. Imaging

Diagnosis of bronchiectasis is based on clinical history and imaging. CXR findings that are suggestive but nondiagnostic of bronchiectasis include stranding, cystic lesions, volume loss with crowding of vessels, air-fluid levels and honeycombing, and areas of infiltrates and atelectasis (Agasthian et al., 1996). Computed tomography scanning is currently the best technique to establish the presence, severity, and distribution of bronchiectasis, replacing Lipiodol bronchography, which is considered more invasive and more unpleasant to the patient as well as being occasionally associated with complications such as alveolitis or allergy to the local anesthetic agent or contrast medium. HRCT has replaced this procedure in the diagnosis of bronchiectasis, with only a 2% false negative and a 1% false positive rate (Young et al., 1991). The detailed images demonstrate bronchial dilatation, peribronchial inflammation, and parenchymal disease.

Perfusion isotopic lung scans using 99m Tc albumin particles in microspheres are considered important in the preoperative evaluation of patients with bronchiectasis because they may demonstrate abnormal territories considered normal on CT scans but representing potential areas of bronchial dilatations. This is explained by bronchial artery hyperplasia creating flow reversal through systemic to pulmonary artery shunting, thus causing areas of defective perfusion on the isotopic scan. Bronchial arteriography may be done to document the origin of hemoptysis. Esophageal studies if gastroesophageal reflux is suspected and ultrastructural examination of cilia from biopsy of the nasal respiratory epithelium if ciliary dyskinesia is suspected may be done (Deslauriers et al., 1998).

6. Therapy for bronchiectasis

Treatment options for the management of bronchiectasis include pharmacologic agents such as antibiotics, nonpharmacologic measures such as chest physiotherapy, and surgical procedures involving removal of the affected portion or portions of the lung. In general, treatment goals are to control infections and improve bronchial hygiene. General measures include avoidance of smoking and second-hand smoke, proper nutrition, and ensuring proper immunizations, including yearly influenza vaccinations. Depending on the specific cause of bronchiectasis, additional medical therapies may be warranted. This is especially true in patients with immunoglobulin deficiency, who could benefit from administration of intravenous or subcutaneous immunoglobulin for passive protection (Boren et al., 2008).

The goals of surgical therapy for bronchiectasis are to improve the quality of life for those patients in which medical treatment has failed and to resolve complications such as empyema, severe or recurrent hemoptysis, and lung abscess (Agasthian et al., 1996; Annest et al., 1982). There is a broad consensus concerning the indications for surgical removal. The surgical treatment is based on two physiopathologic hypotheses. First, the resection involves removal of lung tissue with destroyed bronchi that are no longer functional. Second, it permits the removal of a localized area of bronchiectasis, which could otherwise be involved in the infectious contamination of adjacent territories (Mazieres et al., 2003).

Mazierez and colleagues bring some arguments to help in the selection of patients who should be considered for operation (Mazieres et al., 2003). First, respiratory function and performance status must be compatible with the anesthetic risk. Second, the resection should be done quite early in the evolution of the disease because of the risk of contamination of healthy bronchi by an "active" territory and because of the low morbidity when the pulmonary function is good (Etienne et al., 1996). Third, operation is recommended for patients exhibiting disabling bronchiectasis with hemoptysis or a recurring infection that becomes resistant to medical treatment. Fourth, the etiology of bronchiectasis should not be considered in the decision for operation. Some studies showed the benefit of operation in primary ciliary dyskinesia (Simit et al., 1996), Kartagener's syndrome (Figure 4) (Mazieres et al., 2003), and in hypogammaglobulinemia (Cohen et al., 1994). Lastly, the ideal candidate has a nonhomogenous disease. Some territories are more severely involved and constitute real targets. The removal of an active infectious territory may protect the healthy bronchi from infectious contamination. Removal of diseased segments can break the vicious circle as described by Cole and colleagues, and stop the progression of the disease (Cole et al., 1985). In children growth retardation due to bronchiectasis and drop in school attendance secondary to the illness should be included in the indications for surgery as well (Sirmali et al., 2006).

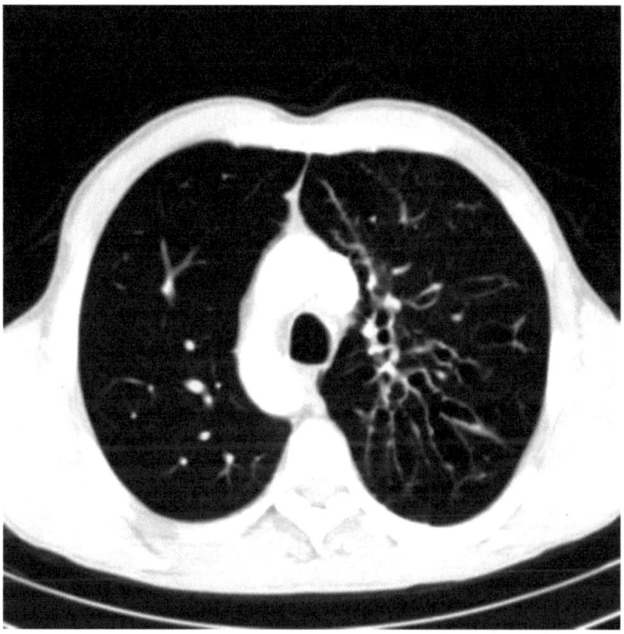

Fig. 4. Computed tomography scan showing the classic image of Kartagener's syndrome caharacterized by dextrocardia and cylindrical bronchiectasis in the right upper lobe (patient's left side).

7. Preoperative preparation

Careful preoperative preparations are of the utmost importance to reduce operation-related morbidity and mortality. The preoperative treatment should include reducing airway obstruction and elimination of microorganisms from the lower respiratory tract, which consists of antimicrobial therapy, postural physiotherapy, bronchodilators, and corticosteroids (Agasthian et al., 1996). Patients should be well prepared during the preoperative period with regard to infection to minimize postoperative complications. Bacterial infections, particularly those involving potentially necrotizing agents such as Staphylococcus aureus, Pseudomonas aeruginosa, Streptococcus pneumonia, and various anaerobes, remain important causes of bronchiectasis, particularly when there is a delay in treatment or other factors that prevent eradication of the infection (Deslauriers et al., 1998). Antimicrobial therapy is particularly true in the setting of mycobacterial disease, such as M. tuberculosis and various environmental mycobacterial species. Patients with focal bronchiectasis and M. avium complex infection typically are started on a three-or four-drug regimen for 2-3 months before surgery based on in vitro susceptibility testing of the isolated organism. The regimen is continued through the hospital stay and for several months thereafter, often to a total of 24 months (Kim et al., 2005).
Preoperative bronchoscopy should be routinely done to rule out benign or malignant cause of obstruction. Preoperative bronchoscopic examinations were performed in 117 (81.8%) of our patients as an adjuvant diagnostic method, to rule out benign or malignant bronchial obstruction, and for localization, collection of samples for microbiology, and bronchial toilet. We consider it essential in the preoperative evaluation and tracheobronchial cleaning of all

patients. In our study, patients in whom bronchoscopy was not performed had a significantly higher rate of postoperative complications (Eren et al., 2007). Patients should be preoperatively monitored until they produced less than 20 mL/day of sputum with little purulence. Operation should be not conducted until bronchofibroscopy showed no engorgement or edema in the tunica mucosa bronchiorum (Zhang et al., 2010).

Most patients with chronic suppurative disease of the lungs are malnourished, often to a considerable degree, as a result of the long-standing catabolic state these patients experience. If malnutrition is present, an aggressive preoperative regimen of nutritional supplementation is advised (Sherwood et al., 2005). Pulmonary function studies should be preoperatively performed in all patients. The patients with bronchiectasis are showed a mixed or obstructive ventilatory pattern. In patients with low FEV1 (<60% of the predicted value) the postoperative complication rate was significantly high. This indicated that surgery should be delayed in cases of severe inflammation until adequate control has been achieved (Eren et al., 2007).

In all patients undergoing pulmonary resection, it is imperative to clearly determine preoperatively the extent of resection to be done because at surgery it may be difficult to judge with great accuracy the segments that are involved.

Balloon tamponade of the bleeding bronchus, which can be performed under emergency conditions is an effective method to manage massive hemoptysis in bronchiectasis patients. Embolization of the bronchial artery is a good alternative, capable of stopping the hemorrhage in 75—90% of the cases (Freitag et al., 1994). On the other hand, once the first episode of hemorrhage is stopped, preoperative assessment should be promptly undertaken because recurrence in the first month after the embolization is frequent and fatal (Fujimoto et al., 2001; Mal et al., 1999). Planning surgical operation in patients with hemoptysis should involve bronchoscopic as well as radiological assessments. Yielding 2% false negative and 1% false positive results, HRCT is a fairly reliable method for the diagnosis of bronchiectasis (Young et al., 1991). In such cases the most appropriate approach is to excise the pathological regions both depicted by HRCT and identified by bronchoscopy.

8. Surgical technique

A left-sided double-lumen endotracheal tube is used to avoid contralateral contamination of secretions. In children under 13 years old, in whom the double-lumen endotracheal tube is not used, bronchoscopy should be performed, and the bronchus of the side ready for resection should be cleaned by aspiration before the introduction of an endotracheal tube. A Fogarty embolectomy catheter may be used as a bronchus blocker in children (Eren et al., 2007). A thoracic epidural catheter is employed when an open approach is planned based on the extent of resection. In patients in whom a thoracoscopic lobectomy or segmentectomy is performed, the epidural is omitted. An arterial line and urinary catheter are placed.

Posterolateral thoracotomy or video-assisted thoracoscopic surgery (VATS) were performed for lung resection. Thoracotomy is performed so as to conserve as much muscle as possible. The resection type is selected according to the affected sides and cardiopulmonary reserve (Balkanli et al., 2003). Excessive bronchial dissection is avoided, and peribronchial tissues are preserved. The bronchial stump may manually be sutured with nonabsorbable materials or closed with a mechanical stapler. The bronchial stump is kept short. Stump covering with mediastinal pleura or tissue is performed. Complete resection is defined as an anatomic resection of all affected segments assessed preoperatively by either HRCT. Two silicon drains are placed into the thoracic cavity before the thorax is closed. All resected specimens are examined histopathologically in order to confirm the diagnosis. At the end of the procedure, the bronchial suture is bronchoscopically checked, and secretions are removed from the airways. Patients are extubated in the operating room. When postoperative mechanical ventilation was necessary, a standard endotracheal tube is substituted for the double-lumen tube (Zhang et al., 20101).

9. Complete resection and preserved segments

Complete and anatomic resection should be done with preservation of as much lung function as possible to avoid cardiorespiratory limitation (Laros et al., 1988). It was reported that the symptoms persisted when incomplete resection was carried out (Campbell & Lilly, 1982). We performed complete resection in 82.5% of our patients and preoperative symptoms resolved completely in 75.9% and improved in 15.7%, i.e. 92.8% benefited from the surgery. In the light of these findings, we suggest that complete resection should be performed for the surgical treatment of bronchiectasis and that incomplete resection should only be used for the palliative treatment of certain life-threatening symptoms. In our study, postoperative complications were observed in 11% of patients that underwent complete resection and in 80% of those that underwent incomplete resection (Eren et al., 2007). When suspicious lung regions are not excised with the aim of sparing as much lung tissue as possible, a second operation that carries a higher morbidity and mortality might be required to remove the residual diseased tissues (Sirmali et al., 2007). Therefore, we suggest that, during intraoperative examinations, if suspected areas that could not be determined by radiological examination are present, these parenchymal areas should be resected to perform complete resection and to decrease relapse rates. Bronchopulmonary development continues during childhood and the space occupied by the resected segments would be filled by the healthy lung segments. Therefore, surgeons should not refrain from wide resection of the lung to achieve complete resection of the diseased area (Sirmali et al., 2007). Incomplete resection should not be preferred in children except for palliative treatment of life threatening complications.

The goal of surgery is to excise all diseased lung areas whenever possible and to preserve as much healthy lung parenchyma as possible. It is known that even 2 or 3 preserved segments can fill the hemithorax (Campbell & Lilly, 1982). As recommended, we suggested to protect the anatomic structure of the superior segment in cases of bronchiectasis of the lower lobe when the superior segment of this lobe was normal (Fujimoto et al., 2001). In such patients, the superior segment had undergone a compensatory increase in volume and the affected basal segments had become small. Thus, the functional value of the superior segment was similar to that of the lower lobe (Yuncu et al., 2006). Patients with an uninvolved apical segment were found to have better spirometric values than those with more extensive disease (Ashour et al., 1996).

10. Resection for multisegmental bilateral bronchiectasis

Surgical treatment is usually offered only when the diseased area is well localized and restricted to one or several segments within the same lobe. Multiple or bilateral bronchiectasis is generally regarded as a contraindication to operation. From the end of the 1970s onward, some thoracic surgeons have suggested that bilateral bronchiectasis is not a contraindication to

resection (George et al., 1979; Fujimoto et al., 2001). Nevertheless, the patients reported in the literature remained quite rare. The therapeutic options in nonfocal bronchiectasis are limited. Most of the time patients are treated with antibiotics and physiotherapy. Recently, progress has been made with the use of new antibiotics and inhalation of tobramycin solution in cases of Pseudomonas aeruginosa colonization (Barker et al., 2000). These therapies allow a good quality of life and symptomatic improvement for several years, but the usual evolution is a progression toward chronic respiratory failure with a poor prognosis and selection of resistant strains (Annest et al., 1982; Keistinen et al., 1997). Transplantation remains indicated for homogenous disease and for patients with advanced disease with seriously compromised pulmonary function and chronic respiratory failure (Hasan et al., 1995). The 3-year survival rate is 75% for patients undergoing double-lung transplantation (Barlow et al., 2000). Some investigators have proposed a radical operation for bilateral bronchiectasis (Kittle et al., 1985; Laros et al., 1988) but others report a higher mortality with pneumonectomy (McGovern et al., 1988). Considering the limited and palliative effect of medical treatment and the risk of transplantation or radical operation, it seems that a limited operation should be offered to some patients with diffuse bronchiectasis.
Mazierez and collegues suggested that surgical indications were offered to patients with multisegmental and severe bronchiectasis if (1) optimal medical treatment and physiotherapy were no longer efficient, (2) bleeding and sputum production were recurrent and abundant, (3) severely damaged territories could be identified, and (4) performance status and pulmonary function were compatible with the anesthetic risk (Mazierez et al., 2003).
Surgery in multiple segments on different lobes is technically more difficult, resulting in higher morbidity and mortality.[21] However, pulmonary resection is indicated early in patients with multisegmentar bronchiectasis, before other portions of the lung become grossly diseased. Our purpose in these patients was to protect as much pulmonary function as possible, with the aim of removing only the affected areas of different lobes. The types of procedures in different studies were presented in Table 3.

Operation type	Balkanli n, %	Eren n; %	Zhang n, %	Sırmali n, %	Haciibrahimoglu n, %	Giovannetti n, %
Pneumonectomy	13 (5.4)	12 (8.3)	90 (11.3)	40 (19.9)	7 (20)	1 (1.7)
Lobectomy	189 (79.4)	82 (55.4)	497 (62.9)	90 (44.7)	17 (48.5)	33 (56.8)
Bilobectomy		7 (4.7)	56 (7.1)	21 (10.4)	2 (5.7)	2 (3.4)
Lobectomy & segmentectomy	31 (13.0)	-	110 (14)	-	5 (14.2)	11 (18.9)
Lobectomy & lingulectomy		-		34 (16.9)	-	
Segmentectomy	10 (4.2)	17 (11.4)	37 (4.7)	16 (7.9)	4 (11.4)	11 (18.9)
Basal segmentectomy	-	16 (10.8)	-	-	-	-
Basal segmentectomy & lingulectomy	-	5 (3.3)	-	-	-	-
Basal segmentectomy & middle lobectomy	-	4 (2.7)	-	-	-	-

Table 3. Type of operation

11. Video-assisted thoracoscopic surgery

VATS for major lung resection has become a more frequent procedure in recent years with promising outcome. VATS represents a new approach; the indications for VATS major resection remain the same as for conventional resection. But not all the patients with bronchiectasis who needed operations were suitable for VATS lobectomy; severe scarring and adhesions on computed tomographic scan should be considered . The severity of adhesions to the chest wall, the hilum, and especially in the fissure, typically seen in inflammatory disease, was the key limiting factor for a safe VATS lobectomy (Weber et al., 2001). Adhesions need to be dissected to explore the relevant anatomy. If there were dense adhesions (such as destroyed lobes mainly after tuberculosis with or without aspergillosis) or enlarged lymph nodes, especially calcified, open operations were required (Zhang et al., 2011).

Bronchiectasis was considered the best lung benign disease suitable for VATS lobectomy (Yim, 2002). The VATS major resection has demonstrated to be a safe procedure when performed by experienced physicians. Postoperative pain after VATS is uncommon as compared with open surgery. Other documented advantages include better preservation of pulmonary function in the early postoperative period, earlier return to full activities, and better quality of life after recovery. One major advantage of VATS resection is that it allows recruitment of older and sicker patients with multiple comorbidities who would otherwise not be candidates for resection through a conventional thoracotomy approach (Farjah et al., 2009; Gonzales-Aragoneses et al., 2009). In study of Zhang and collegeus, the patients with VATS had a shorter length of stay in the hospital, fewer complications, and less pain in the postoperative period than those with thoracotomies (Zhang et al., 2011).

12. Postoperative complication

Bronchiectasis is an inflammatory disease of the lungs and the risk of developing postoperative empyema is higher than in other cases. Empyema, on the other hand, is a risk factor for bronchopleural fistula (Sirmali et al., 2006). Therefore, we suggest reinforcement of the bronchial stump in all patients. Bronchopleural fistula can be observed in as many as 9.1% of the cases (Fujimoto et al., 2001). Fujimoto and colleagues argued that the bronchial stump should be reinforced when the inflammation in the lung of bronchiectasis patients could not be effectively controlled (Fujimoto et al., 2001). We, however, suggest reinforcement the bronchial stump in all cases. Additionally, to avoid empyema, we recommend postoperative bacterial culture of thoracic effusion if the remaining lung shows signs of persisting inflammation. Sputum retention is common because patients with this disease might have problems with ciliary motion and postoperative expectoration, which would be easily disrupted (Fujimoto et al., 2001). In our series, respiratory physiotherapy was re-initiated on the first post-operative day, and continued for 2 weeks after discharge. We used bronchoscopy for sputum aspiration during the early postoperative period if physiotherapy was not effective. Virtually all patients had specific or large-spectrum intravenous antibiotic therapy for 1 week (Eren et al., 2007).

In bronchopleural fistula, drainage of the infected space is a key initial step to limit damage to the remaining lung. Bronchopleural fistula noted very early after the initial resection may be treated with primary reclosure and rebuttressing of the stump; later bronchopleural fistula usually require rib resection and creation of an Eloesser flap, followed by bronchopleural fistula closure and subsequent Clagett procedure, for successful treatment (Sugarbaker et al., 2009). The presence of a significant intrathoracic "space" appears to be more common after major lung resection for infectious lung disease such as bronchiectasis compared with other indications for surgery. The use of transposed muscle such as latissimus dorsi minimizes the potential complications in this setting, including postresection empyema or prolonged air leak (Sugarbaker et al., 2009). The rate of complications in the current literature varies between 9.4% and 24.6%. Mortality ranges from 0% to 8.3% in the literature (Fujimoto et al., 2001). Postoperative complications in different studies were presented in Table 4.

Complication	Balkanli n, %	Eren n, %	Zhang n, %	Sırmali n, %	Cobanoglu n, %	Haciibrahimoglu n, %	Giovannetti n, %
Postoperative Pneumonia	-	3 (2.0)	24 (3)	3 (1.7)	-	3 (8.8)	2 (4.4)
Atelectasis	7 (2.9)	11 (7.6)	16 (2)	8 (4.5)	4 (6.4)	-	
Prolonged air-leak	6 (2.5)	7 (4.8)	21 (2.7)	3 (1.7)	2 (3.2)	1 (2.9)	1 (2.2)
Residual air-space	-	-	-	-	-	-	1 (2.2)
Sputum retention	-	-	-	-	-	-	1 (2.2)
Bronchial infection	-	-	-	-	-	-	1(2.2)
Bronchopleural fistula	2 (0.8)	-	3 (0.4)	-	2 (3.2)	-	-
Postoperative hemorrhage	4 (1.6)	2 (1.3)	9 (1.1)	2 (1.1)	1 (1.6)	-	-
Empyema	2 (0.8)	5 (3.4)	5 (0.6)	5 (2.8)	2 (3.2)	2 (5.8)	-
Severe supraventricular arrhythmias	-	3 (2.0)	32 (4)	-	1 (1.6)	-	-
Respiratory insufficiency	-	2 (1.3)	10 (1.3)	-	-	-	-
Total	21 (8.8)	33 (23)	128 (16.2)	-	-	6 (17.6)	6 (13.2)

Table 4. Postoperative complications

13. Conclusion

Bronchiectasis is pathologically defined as a condition in which there are abnormal and permanent dilatations of proximal bronchi. Bronchiectasis can occur as focal or localized disease, or in a diffuse manner. Overall, one-third of cases of bronchiectasis are unilateral and affect a single lobe, one-third are unilateral but affect more than one lobe, and one-third are bilateral. Recurrent pulmonary infection during childhood is an important factor in the etiology. In developing countries, tuberculosis is still one of the most important causes of bronchiectasis. Bronchial obstruction from either endobronchial pathology or external compression can also be an acquired factor predisposing to the development of bronchiectasis.

Treatment options for the management of bronchiectasis include pharmacologic agents such as antibiotics, nonpharmacologic measures such as chest physiotherapy, and surgical procedures involving removal of the affected portion or portions of the lung. The goals of surgical therapy for bronchiectasis are to improve the quality of life for those patients in which medical treatment has failed and to resolve complications such as empyema, severe or recurrent hemoptysis, and lung abscess. The preoperative treatment should include reducing airway obstruction and elimination of microorganisms from the lower respiratory tract, which consists of antimicrobial therapy, postural physiotherapy, bronchodilators, and corticosteroids. Preoperative bronchoscopy should be routinely done to rule out benign or malignant cause of obstruction.

Complete and anatomic resection should be done with preservation of as much lung function as possible to avoid cardiorespiratory limitation. It was reported that the symptoms persisted when incomplete resection was carried out. When suspicious lung regions are not excised with the aim of sparing as much lung tissue as possible, a second operation that carries a higher morbidity and mortality might be required to remove the residual diseased tissues. Therefore, we suggest that, during intraoperative examinations, if suspected areas that could not be determined by radiological examination are present, these parenchymal areas should be resected to perform complete resection and to decrease relapse rates.
Surgery in multiple segments on different lobes is technically more difficult, resulting in higher morbidity and mortality. However, pulmonary resection is indicated early in patients with multisegmentar bronchiectasis, before other portions of the lung become grossly diseased. Our purpose in these patients was to protect as much pulmonary function as possible, with the aim of removing only the affected areas of different lobes. VATS represents a new approach; the indications for VATS major resection remain the same as for conventional resection. But not all the patients with bronchiectasis who needed operations were suitable for VATS lobectomy; severe scarring and adhesions on computed tomographic scan should be considered. When necessary, surgical treatment of bronchiectasis can be performed with acceptable morbidity and low mortality.

14. References

Agasthian, T.; Deschamps, C., Trastek, VF., Allen, MS. & Pairolero, PC. (1996). Surgical management of bronchiectasis. *Ann Thorac Surg*, Vol.62, No.4 , pp. 976-978

Al-Kattan, KM.; Essa, MA., Hajjar, WM., Ashour, MH., Saleh, WN. & Rafay, MA. (2005). Surgical results for bronchiectasis based on hemodynamic (functional and morphologic) classification *J Thorac Cardiovasc Surg* , Vol.130, No.5, pp. 1385-1390

Annest, LS.; Kratz, JM. & Crawford, FA Jr. (1982). Current results of treatment of bronchiectasis. *J Thorac Cardiovasc Surg*, Vol.83, No.4, pp. 546-550

Ashour, M.; Al-Kattan, KM., Jain, SK., Al-Majed, S., Al-Kassimi, F., Mobaireek, A., Al-Hajjaj, M. & Al-Zear, A. (1996). Surgery for unilateral bronchiectasis: results and prognostic factors. *Tuber Lung Dis*, Vol.77, No.2, pp. 168-72

Balkanli, K.; Genc, O., Dakak, M., Gurkok, S., Gozubuyuk, A., Caylak, H. & Yucel, O. (2003). Surgical management of bronchiectasis: analysis and short-term results in 238 patients. *Eur J Cardiothorac Surg*, Vol.24, No.5, pp. 699-702

Barker, AF.; Couch, L., Fiel, SB., Gotfried, MH., Ilowite, J., Meyer, KC., O'Donnell, A., Sahn, SA., Smith, LJ., Stewart, JO., Abuan, T., Tully, H., Van, Dalfsen J., Wells, CD. & Quan, J. (2000). Tobramycin solution for inhalation reduces sputum Pseudomonas aeruginoa density in bronchiectasis. *Am J Respir Crit Care Med* , Vol.162, No.2 Pt 1, pp. 481–485

Barlow, CW.; Robbins, RC., Moon, MR., Akindipe, O., Theodore, J. & Reitz, BA. (2000). Heart-lung versus double-lung transplantation for suppurative lung disease. *J Thorac Cardiovas Surg*,Vol.119, No.3, pp. 466–476

Bertelsen, S.; Struve-Christensen, E., Aasted, A. & Sparup, J. (1980). Isolated middle lobe atelectasis: aetiology, pathogenesis, and treatment of the so-called middle lobe syndrome. *Thorax*, Vol.35, No.6, pp. 449–452

Campbell, DN. & Lilly, JR. (1982). The changing spectrum of pulmonary operations in infants and children. *J Thorac Cardiovasc Surg*, Vol.83, No5. , pp. 680-685.

Cobanoglu, U.; Yalcinkaya, İ., Er, M., Isik, AF., Sayir, F. & Mergan, D. (2011). Surgery for bronchiectasis: The effect of morphological types to prognosis. *Ann Thorac Med, Vol.*6, No.1, pp. 25–32

Cohen, AJ.; Roifman, C., Brendan, J., Mullen, M., Reid, B., Weisbrod, G. & Downey, GP. (1994). Localised pulmonary resection for bronchiectasis in hypogammaglobulinaemic patients. *Thorax,* Vol.49, No.5, pp. 509–510

Cole, PJ.; Roberts, DE., Higgs, E. & Prior, C. (1985). Colonising microbial load a cardinal concept in the pathogenesis and treatment of progressive bronchiectasis due to "vicious circle" host mediated damage. *Thorax*, Vol.40, pp. 227

Deslauries, J.; Goulet, S. & Francois, B. (1998). Surgical treatment of bronchiectasis and broncholithiasis. In: *Advanced therapy in thoracic surgery,* Franco, LF., Putnam, JB, (ed.), pp. 300–309, ON: Decker, Hamilton

Dogru, D.; Nik-Ain, A., Kiper, N., Gocmen, A., Ozcelik, U., Yalcin, E. & Aslan, AT. (2005). Bronchiectasis: the consequence of late diagnosis in chronic respiratory symptoms. *J Trop Pediatr,* Vol.51, No.6; pp. 362–365

Eller, J.; Lapa, e Silva JR., Poulter, LW., Lode H. & Cole, PJ. (1994). Cells and cytokines in chronic bronchial infection. *Ann N Y Acad Sci*, Vol.725, pp. 331–345

Eren, S.; Esme, H. & Avci, A. (2007). Risk factors affecting outcome and morbidity in the surgical management of bronchiectasis. *J Thorac Cardiovasc Surg*, Vol.134, No.2, pp. 392-398

Boren, EJ.; Teuber, SS. & Gershwin, ME. (2008). A Review of Non-Cystic Fibrosis Pediatric Bronchiectasis. *Clinic Rev Allerg Immunol*, Vol.34, pp. 260–273

Etienne, T.; Spiliopoulos, A. & Megevand, R. (1993). Bronchiectasis: indication and timing for surgery. *Ann Chir*, Vol.47, No.8, pp. 729–735

Farjah, F.; Wood, DE., Mulligan, MS., Krishnadasan, B., Heagerty, PJ., Symons, RG. & Flum, DR. (2009). Safety and efficacy of video-assisted versus conventional lung resection for lung cancer. *J Thorac Cardiovasc Surg,* Vol.137, No.6, pp. 1415–1421

Freitag, L.; Tekolf, E., Stamatis, G., Montag, M. & Greschuchna, D. (1994). Three years experience with a new balloon catheter for the management of haemoptysis. *Eur Respir J*, Vol.7, No.11, pp. 2033—2037

Fujimoto, T.; Hillejan, L. & Stamatis, G. (2001). Current strategy for surgical management of bronchiectasis. *Ann Thorac Surg,* Vol.72, No.5, pp. 1711-1715

George, SA.; Leonardi, HK. & Overholt, RH. (1979). Bilateral pulmonary resection for bronchiectasis: a 40-year experience. *Ann Thorac Surg*, Vol.28, No.1, pp. 48–53

Giovannetti, R.; Alifano, M., Stefani, A., Legras, A., Grigoroiu, M., Collet, JY., Magdelenat, P. & Regnard, JF. (2008). Surgical treatment of bronchiectasis: early and long-term results Interactive. *CardioVascular and Thoracic Surgery*, Vol.7,No.4 ,pp. 609–612

Gonzalez-Aragoneses, F,; Moreno-Mata, N., Simon-Adiego, C., Peñalver-Pascual, R., Gonzalez-Casaurran, G. & Perea, LA. (2009). Lung cancer surgery in the elderly. *Crit Rev Oncol Hematol*, Vol.71, No.3, pp. 266 -271

Haciibrahimoglu, G.; Fazlioglu, M., Olcmen, A., Gurses, A. & Bedirhan, MA. (2004). Surgical management of childhood bronchiectasis due to infectious disease. *J Thorac Cardiovasc Surg*, Vol.127, No.5, pp. 1361-1365

Hasan, A.; Corris, PA., Healy, M., Wrightson, N., Gascoigne, AD., Waller, DA., Wilson, I., Hilton, CJ., Gould, FK. & Forty, J. (1995). Bilateral sequential lung transplantation for end-stage septic lung disease. *Thorax*, Vol.50, No.5, pp. 565–566

Karadag, B.; Karakoc, F., Ersu, R., Kut, A., Bakac, S. & Dagli, E. (2005). Non-cystic fibrosis bronchiectasis in children: a persisting problem in developing countries. *Respiration*, Vol.72, No.3, pp. 233–238

Karakoc, GB.; Yilmaz, M., Altintas, DU. & Kendirli, SG. (2001). Bronchiectasis: still a problem. *Pediatr Pulmonol*, Vol.32, pp. 175–178

Keistinen, T.; Saynajakangas, O., Tuuponen, T. & Kivela, SL. (1997). Bronchiectasis: an orphan disease with a poorly understood prognosis. *Eur Respir J*, Vol.10, No.12, pp. 2784–2787

Khair, OA.; Davies, RJ. & Devalia, JL. (1996). Bacterial-induced release of inflammatory mediators by bronchial epithelial cells. *Eur Respir J*, Vol.9, pp. 1913–1922

Kim, JS.; Tanaka, N., Newell, JD., Degroote, MA., Fulton, K., Huitt, G. & Lynch, DA. (2005). Nontuberculous mycobacterial infection: CT scan findings, genotype, and treatment responsiveness. *Chest* Vol.128, No.6, pp. 3863–3869

King, PT. (2009). The pathophysiology of bronchiectasis. *International Journal of COPD*, Vol.4, pp. 411–419

Kittle, CF.; Faber, LP., Jensik, RJ. & Warren, WH. (1985). Pulmonary resection in patients after pneumonectomy. *Ann Thorac Surg*, Vol.40, pp 294–299

Lapa e Silva, JR.; Guerreiro, D., Noble, B., Poulter, LW. & Cole, PJ. (1989). Immunopathology of experimental bronchiectasis. *Am J Respir Cell Mol Biol*, Vol.1, pp. 297–304

Laros, CD.; Van den Bosch, JM., Westermann, CJ., Bergstein, PG., Vanderschueren, RG. & Knaepen, PJ. (1988). Resection of more than 10 lung segments. A 30-year survey of 30 bronchiectatic patients. *J Thorac Cardiovasc Surg*, Vol.95, pp. 119-123

Levin, DL. (2002). Radiology of pulmonary Mycobacterium avium-intracellulare complex. *Clin Chest Med*, Vol.23, pp. 603–612

Loukides, S.; Bouros, D., Papatheodorou, G., Lachanis, S., Panagou, P. & Siafakas, NM. (2002). Exhaled H2O2 in steady-state bronchiectasis: relationship with cellular composition in induced sputum, spirometry, and extent and severity of disease. *Chest*, Vol.121, pp. 81–87

Mal, H.; Rulon, I., Mellot, F., Brugiere, O., Sleiman, C., Menu, Y. & Fournier, M. (1999). Immediate and long-term results of bronchial artery embolization for life-threatening hemoptysis. *Chest*, Vol.115, pp. 996—1001

Mazie`res, J.; Murris, M., Didier, A., Giron, J., Dahan, M., Berjaud, J. & Le´ophonte, P. (2003). Limited Operation for Severe Multisegmental Bilateral Bronchiectasis *Ann Thorac Surg*, Vol.75, pp.382–387

McGovern, EM.; Trastek, VF., Pairolero, PC. & Payne, WS. (1988). Completion pneumonectomy: indications, complications and results. *Ann Thorac Surg*, Vol.46, pp. 141–146

Miller, JI. (2000). Bacterial infections of the lungs and bronchial compressive disorders. In: Shields TW, editor. *General thoracic surgery*. 5th ed. Pp. 1048-1051, Lippincott Williams & Wilkins, Philadelphia

Nicotra, MB.; Rivera, M., Dale, AM., Shepherd, R. & Carter, R. (1995). Clinical, pathophysiologic, and microbiologic characterization of bronchiectasis in an aging cohort. *Chest*, Vol.108, pp. 955- 961

Prieto, D.; Bernardo, J., Matos, MJ., Eugenio, L. & Antunes, M. (2001). Surgery for bronchiectasis. *Eur J Cardiothorac Surg*, Vol.20, pp. 19-23

Reid, L. (1950). Reduction in bronchial subdivisions in bronchiectasis. *Thorax*, Vol.5, pp. 223–247

Sherwood, JT.; Mitchell, JD. & Pomerantz, M. (2005). Completion pneumonectomy for chronic mycobacterial disease. *J Thorac Cardiovasc Surg*, Vol.129, pp. 1258–1265

Sirmali, M.; Karasu, S., Turut, H., Gezer, S., Kaya, S., Tastepe, I. & Karaoğlanoğlu, N. (2006). Surgical management of bronchiectasis in childhood. *Eur J Cardiothorac Surg*, Vol.31, No.1, pp. 120-123

Smit, HJ.; Schreurs, AJ., Van den Bosch, JM. & Westermann, CJ. (1996). Is resection of bronchiectasis beneficial in patients with primary ciliary dyskinesia? *Chest*, Vol.109, pp. 1541–1544

Sugarbaker DJ.; Bueno R, Krasna MJ, Mentzer ZJ & Zellos L. (2009). *Adult Chest Surgery*, The McGraw-Hill Companies, ISBN 978-0-07-145912-9, China

Weber, A.; Stammberger, U., Inci, I., Schmid, RA., Dutly, A. & Weder, W. (2001). Thoracoscopic lobectomy for benign disease–a single centre study on 64 cases. *Eur J Cardiothorac Surg*, Vol.20, pp. 443– 844

Whitwell, F. (1952). A study of the pathology and pathogenesis of bronchiectasis. *Thorax*, Vol.7, pp. 213–219

Yim, AP. (2002). VATS major pulmonary resection revisited– controversies, techniques, and results. *Ann Thorac Surg*, Vol.74, pp. 615–623

Young, K.; Aspestrand, F. & Kolbenstvedt, A. (1991). High resolution CT and bronchography in the assessment of bronchiectasis. *Acta Radiol*, Vol.32, pp. 439-441

Yuncu, G.; Ceylan, KC., Sevinc, S., Ucvet, A., Kaya, SO., Kiter, G., Unsal, S. & Ozsinan, F. (2006). Functional results of surgical treatment of bronchiectasis in a developing country. *Arch Bronconeumol*, Vol.42, No.4, pp. 183-188

Zhang, P.; Zhang, P., Jiang, S., Jiang, G., Zhou, X., Ding, J. & Gao, W. (2011). Video-Assisted Thoracic Surgery for Bronchiectasis. *Ann Thorac Surg*, Vol.91, pp. 239–243

Zheng, L.; Tipoe, G., Lam, WK., Leung, RY., Ho, JC., Shum, IH., Ooi, GC., Ip, MS. & Tsang, KW. (2000). Up-regulation of circulating adhesion molecules in bronchiectasis. *Eur Respir J*, Vol.16, No.4, pp. 691–696

18

Role of Thoracomyoplasty Procedures in Modern Surgery for Intrathoracic Suppurations

Petre Vlah-Horea Botianu and Alexandru Mihail Botianu
Surgical Clinic 4, University of Medicine and Pharmacy from Targu-Mures, Romania

1. Introduction

Both thoracoplasty and muscle transposition are rarely performed procedures in modern thoracic surgery (Deslauriers et al., 2002). Their importance comes from the fact that these procedures are usually indicated in desperate cases, with failed medical treatments and who cannot be cured through standard procedures such as resection or decortication. For these patients, thoracomyoplasty operations are often the last chance for cure and sometimes even life-saving procedures (Botianu et al., 2010a).

2. Modern indications of thoracomyoplasty procedures

In our days, most of the intrathoracic suppurations can be managed without surgery, through antibiotics and minor procedures such as thoracocenthesis or tube-thoracostomy (Davies et al., 2011). Overall, about 10-15% of patients with intrathoracic suppurations still require some form of major surgical treatment. Out of them, most can be managed through less invasive and mutilating procedures (Pardos-Gea et al., 2011, Zahid et al., 2011), which make thoracomyoplasty a quite rarely indicated procedure:

- for pleural empyema: in cases not amenable to decortication - usually chronic cases with no cleavage plane and subjacent lesions in the parenchyma limiting the re-expansion of the lung;
- for pulmonary lesions (abscesses, tuberculosis, aspergilloma etc.): in cases not amenable to lung resection - usually a combination of poor biological and cardio-pulmonary status (including pulmonary hypertension), contralateral disease, fixed and adherent lesions with major technical difficulties.

Tuberculosis (TB) requires a special attention. Although TB infection by itself is not an indication for such procedures, many cases with chronic disease present with features making them candidates for thoracomyoplasty procedures. In our experience, almost half of the patients requiring thoracomyoplasty operations had different forms of TB lesions (Botianu P. et al., 2010a).

Bronchial fistula is frequently solved with the use of muscle flaps, alone or in combination with thoracoplasty. Simple closure by suturing through an inflamed tissue has very few chances of success, making reinforcement with a viable flap almost mandatory in most cases. In many cases, the muscle flaps are used as a plug to close the bronchial defect, without direct suture of the edges of the fistula (Hollaus et al., 1999, Zaheer et al., 2009).

Postoperative empyema is also an indication for thoracomyoplasty procedures in selected cases (Garcia-Yuste et al., 1998, Regnard et al., 2000). A particular technical aspect is that the previous thoracotomy reduces the availability of the neighbourhood flaps. The need to have some flaps available in case of postoperative complications is the main argument for the use of muscle-sparing thoracotomies (Nosotti et al., 2010).
Intrathoracic muscle transposition (without thoracoplasty) has also some other indications such as reinforcement of high-risk sutures (Abolhoda et al., 2009, Thingnam et al., 2011), repair of esophageal and tracheal defects (Kotzampassakis et al., 2009, Meyer et al., 2004), pericardial and diaphragmatic reconstruction (Kobayashi et al., 2009), dynamic cardiomyoplasty for end-stage heart failure (Chachques et al., 2008), salvage of infected vascular prosthesis (Mitra et al., 2005) etc.

3. Thoracoplasty

3.1 Historical background

The term "thoracoplasty" was introduced by Estlander (1879) who performed resection of multiple fragments of ribs ("resectio costorum multiplex") to achieve obliteration of an underlying empyema (Estlander, 1879). The operation became popular mainly as a method of lung collapse to achieve healing of tuberculosis before the introduction of modern TB chemotherapy. In fact, thoracoplasty procedures dominated chest surgery before the 1950's and played an essential role in the development of thoracic surgery as a distinct specialty. After 1950-60's, the interest for this procedure decreased due to the introduction of medical treatment (antibiotics and specific TB drugs) and development of other less mutilating and more effective surgical procedures (Deslauriers et al., 2002, Horrigan & Snow, 1990).

3.2 Terminology

Thoracoplasty is a procedure that targets the resolution of a cavity (pleural or pulmonary) by collapsing the chest wall through rib resection and/or plombage; according to the way this collapse is achieved, there are different terms which are used to describe the procedure:

- **in one or more stages** - according to the number of operative steps used. In the past many authors preferred to perform the thoracoplasty in more steps, with resection of 2-3 ribs in each step, in order to lower the magnitude of the operative aggression and to reduce mortality (Alexander 1936). This was a reasonable attitude in the early years of thoracic surgery, when a lot of things that are today standard were not available (general anesthesia, oro-tracheal intubation, blood transfusion, antibiotics, electrocautery etc). Besides the need for more procedures, a specific disadvantage is the cavity movement phenomenon, in which the cavity just moves in one direction without any resolution; at the end, the patient will have some ribs resected and the same cavity in another position (Archibald 1926). In our days, most of these procedures are done in a single step.
- **extra-pleural or intra-pleural** - according to the intact preservation or opening of the parietal pleural. In the past, opening of the pleural space during thoracoplasty was considered as a major accident (fear for wound contamination, pneumothorax etc.) (Archibald 1926). In our days, in most cases the pleura is opened deliberately to achieve a direct access to the pleural and/or pulmonary lesion.

- **sub-periostal or extra-periostal** - according to the plane used for rib resection, with or without preservation of the periosteum. In our days, in most cases the ribs are resected using a subperiostal plane. Leaving the periosteum intact allows some form of bone regeneration which helps the long-time stabilization of the chest wall (Alexander 1936).

Many authors use the term "classic" thoracoplasty, with different meanings depending on time and geographical location. For example, in Europe, in the 1910-20's, "classic" thoracoplasty referred to the procedures described by Estlander and Schede, which were then replaced by the procedures described by Andre Maurer and Sauerbruch; the later became also "classic" for the American surgeons who trained in Europe. In the USA, after 1930, the technique described by Alexander became the standard thoracoplasty performed for lung collapse in order to heal lung TB. In the 1950's, the osteoplastic techniques and plombage with different materials became popular, being then almost abandoned.

In our days, most thoracoplasties are done in a single operative step, intrapleural and using a subperiosteal plane for rib resection (Hopkins et al., 1985).

3.3 Main types of thoracoplasty

Over the time, more than 100 thoracoplasty procedures were described, many of them being in fact minor modifications or combinations of previously described techniques; such a big number of techniques is by itself an indication for the dificulties encountered in this kind of surgery. We present a brief description of the most important techniques, all of them being very popular at a certain moment of the development of thoracic surgery.

The Schede thoracoplasty is a very "radical" procedure developed for empyema and involving the resection of ribs, intercostal spaces and parietal pleura overlying the empyema cavity. The wound was left opened and the visceral pleura from the empyema cavity was placed in direct contact with healthy tissues represented by extracostal chest wall muscles and subcutaneous tissue (Schede 1890). For small empyema cavities it may be a reasonable procedure but for big cavities the procedure is a very mutilant one. With different modifications, it is still used today for highly selected cases of empyema (Stobernack et al., 1997, Botianu 2005, 2008).

The Sauerbruch thoracoplasty (paravertebral) was indicated for empyema cavities that extended more in the vertical axis than in the horizontal one and involved a 4-6 cm length resection of the posterior part of the ribs. The main disadvantages were the risk of respiratory failure due to the paradoxical movements of the chest wall and the secondary scoliosis.

The Andre Maurer thoracoplasty (descendant) involves complete excision of the first 2 ribs and partial removal of the ribs 3-5, leaving intact only the anterior part of them; it was performed extrapleurally, in one or more steps according to the patient's biological status.

The Alexander thoracoplasty was designed for treatment of lung TB and involved a subperiosteal and extrapleural removal of the first 8-9 ribs; for a better collapse the removal of the first rib and the transverse vertebral apophyses was considered to be mandatory. For a better tolerance of the procedure, it was performed in 3 steps at 3 weeks intervals. With this strategy and a good selection of the patients, Alexander achieved an important improvement of the results, with a 10% mortality and 90% rate of healing in survivors (Alexander 1936).

The Archibald thoracoplasty involved resection of the first 3 ribs and introduction of the pectoral muscles in the extrapleural space to maintain the collapse of the lung; a particular aspect is the ingenious separate mobilization of the two flaps: the pectoralis major was mobilized based on the branches from the internal mammary vessels and the pectoralis minor was mobilized based on the thoraco-acromial pedicle (Entin 1995).

Extrapleural plombage (plombage thoracoplasty) achieves lung collapse with the use of different materials that are introduced inside the chest using an extrafascial or extraperiosteal plane (fig. 1). The main advantages of the plombage thoracoplasties are the absence of chest wall mutilation and the fact that the procedure is easy, quick and well-tolerated, even by patients with poor biological status; the procedure was quite popular in the 1950-60's, with immediate good results (Wilson et al., 1956). The main disadvantage is the high risk of complications related to the introduction inside the chest of a foreign material, including overinfection, migration and erosion of major vessels, which may frequently require the removal of the plombage material (Massard et al., 1997).

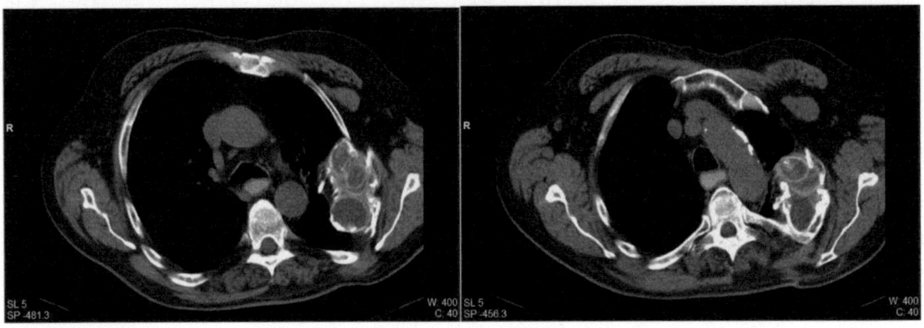

Fig. 1. CT aspect of an 81 years-old patient who underwent a plombage thoracoplasty 46 years ago for left upper lobe tuberculosis. The patient presented no TB recurrence and no chest complaints.

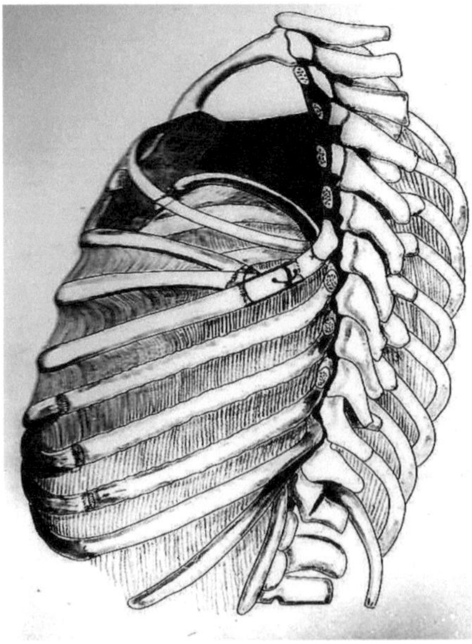

Fig. 2. Osteoplastic thoracoplasty developed by Naftali (1964) for apical TB lesions. Note the rib grafts placed in a paramediastinal position which induce also a transversal collapse.

The osteoplastic thoracoplasty was popularized by Holst and Björk in the 1950's and aimed to create a new roof for the chest cavity. The posterior parts of the upper ribs were resected in a growing length, from superior towards inferior and their new posterior ends were sutured to the first rib that was left intact. This resulted in a smaller thoracic cage with a stable wall that prevented the reexpansion of the lung above the new roof (Holst 1952, Bjork 1954, Krasnov et al., 1989). Besides lung TB, these procedures were also frequently performed for the prophylaxis or treatment of pleural space problems after upper lobectomies. In our unit, Naftali Zoltan has developed and used in the 1960's an original technique of osteoplastic thoracoplasty (fig. 2) which involved also the use of rib grafts placed in a paramediastinal position, achieving a collapse not only in the vertical plane, but also in the transversal one - from medial towards lateral (Naftali, 1964).
Apycolisis was introduced by Semb (1937) and involved the division of the adhesions between the pleural dome at the apex and the soft tissues from the base of the neck. This manoeuver, which was used by many surgeons during thoracoplasties for apical TB lesions, allowed a more complete collapse of the lung apex.
Resection of the first rib was mandatory in many of the classic thoracoplasties, being considered the key to achieve an adequate collapse in the vertical plane. However, it's resection is associated with severe adverse effects such as scoliosis, asymmetry and functional impairment of the shoulder and upper extremity. For these reasons, we believe that it's preservation is nowadays manatory; if there is a space below the first rib it can be easily filled with local flaps (Botianu P. et al., 2010a, c, Deslauriers et al., 2002).

3.4 Modern thoracoplasty – The Andrews procedure and it's modifications

In our time, thoracoplasty is almost always performed for pleural or pleuro-pulmonary cavities, with opening of the pleura and subperiostal rib resection. Most surgeons use the Andrews thoracoplasty, with or without various modifications (Cornet et al., 1965, Icard et al., 1999). The technique was first described as a solution for postpneumonectomy empyema / thoracomediastinal plication (Andrews 1961) and then used for other types of empyema (Andrews 1965).
The original technique involved:

- thoracotomy;
- subperiostal rib resection, limited to the portion of the chest wall located above the empyema cavity;
- wide opening of the suppurated pleural cavity with careful removal of the pus and detrituses;
- closure of the bronchial fistula (if present);
- removal of the parietal pleura;
- obliteration of the cavity by fixation of the remaining periosto-intercostal plane to the visceral/mediastinal pleura; this is achieved by mattressing using separate "U" stitches;
- drainage of the subscapulary space and closure of the wound.

The main original idea of this technique was to open the infected pleural cavity, clean it and obliterate it, with primary wound closure.
In our unit, we have tried to improve the results of the Andrews thoracoplasty by several modifications which resulted in a personal procedure (Botianu A.M., 1996 - licence no. 100297/1989/RO) which was used with good results in the last 25 years. The main steps of the procedure are:

- postero-lateral incision and opening of the empyema cavity (fig. 3a);
- wide debridement and toilet of the cavity; if bronchial fistulas are present, they are temporary closed using small gauzes to avoid bronchial inundation.
- subperiosteal removal of ribs overlying the empyema cavity (fig. 3b);
- the remaining chest wall (consisting of parietal pleura, periosteum and intercostal spaces) is sectioned using several cranio-caudal and transversal incisions, which are placed according to how we plan to use the resulting intercostal flaps. The transversal incisions are made through the bed of the resected ribs to avoid damage to the intercostal vessels. The parietal pleura is carefully cleaned but without attempting a complete excision. The resulting pleuro-periosto-intercostal flaps must remain well vascularised and are used for:
    - closure-reinforcement of the bronchial fistulas, using always atraumatic needles and late resorbable suture materials;
    - plombage of the cul-de-sacs and dead angles (such as below the first rib or paravertebral), diminishing the extent of the rib resection;
    - plombage of intrapulmonary cavities (fig. 3c);

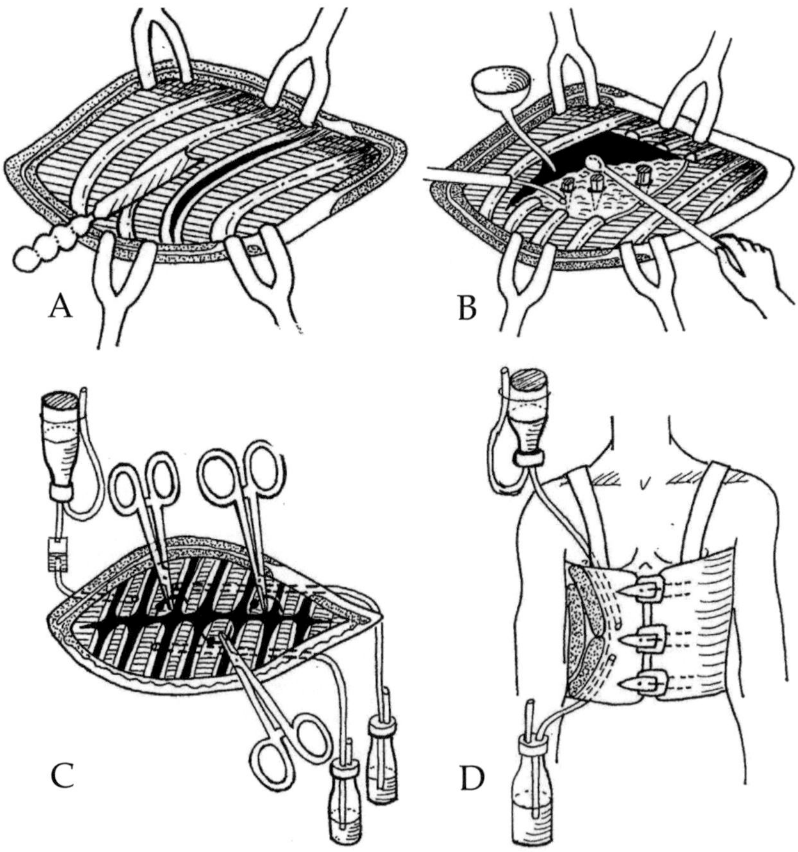

Fig. 3. Main steps of the thoracopleuroplasty procedure used in Surgical Clinic 4, University of Medicine and Pharmacy from Targu-Mures, Romania (Botianu A.M., 1996 /licence no. 100297/1989/RO).

- installation of a closed-circuit irrigation-aspiration system which consists of 1-2 usual drains which are placed in a declive position and are connected to a standard chest drainage system and a separate smaller drain placed in the upper part of the cavity and connected to a standard perfusion set (fig. 3d). This system allows postoperative elimination of pus and secretions, as well as lavages with different antibiotic and antiseptic solutions; in case of postoperative bleeding, local hemostatics may also be introduced in the cavity. Before having CT and US highly available, we also used this system to introduce contrast inside the chest to follow the resolution of the lesion.
- we have completely abandoned the matressing described by Andrews by suturing with "U" stitches the remaining chest wall to the visceral or mediastinal pleura. We consider that this manoeuver is not only time-consuming but has several disadvantages such as the danger to damage the underlying lung or mediastinal structures, ischemia of the remaining pleuro-periosto-intercostal plane and an overall fixation of the chest wall in a non-physiologic position.
- suturing of the remaining planes (skin, subcutaneous fat and chest wall muscles) in a single layer with separate stitches;

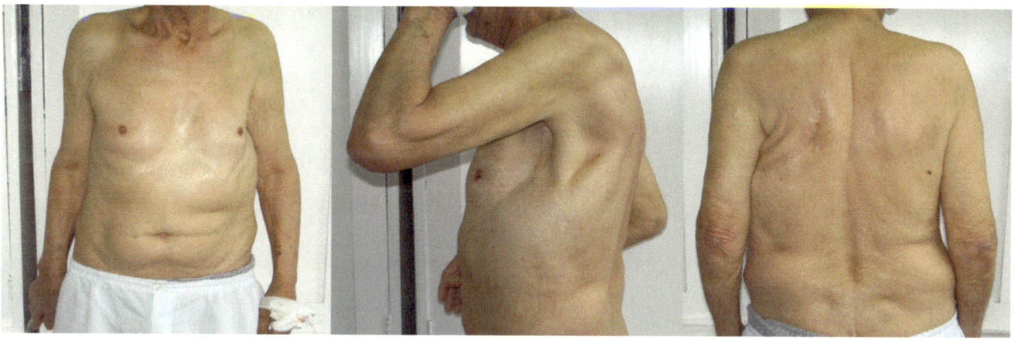

Fig. 4. Postoperative aspect at 10 years after a thoracomediastinal plication for a left post-pneumonectomy empyema, performed according to the technique described previously. The cosmetic result is acceptable, with no soliosis and no major chest difformity.

- temporary fixation of the chest wall using compressive bandage and an external contention (fig. 3d); this allows a definitive fixation of the new chest wall in a more natural position, after the cavity is obliterated and the patient starts to breathe normally (fig. 4).

4. Intrathoracic muscle transposition

4.1 Historical background

The idea to bring muscle flaps inside the chest is not a new one, as it was described at the beginning of the 20th century by surgeons like Abrashanoff (1911), Robinson (1915) or Archibald (1921). However, these techniques did not become very popular, mainly due to the fear of infection (large dissections without the possibility to use antibiotics) and absence of precise anatomical knowledge (Arnold & Pairolero, 1989).

In the 1960-70's, plastic and reconstructive surgeons developed the techniques for extensive mobilization of muscle and musculo-cutaneous flaps, based on precise anatomic knowledge.

The use of muscle flaps in thoracic surgery was popularized in the 1990's mainly through the work of the Mayo Rochester team of surgeons, with an excellent cooperation between thoracic and plastic surgeons (Arnold & Pairolero, 1989, Pairolero et al., 1990).

4.2 Basic principles

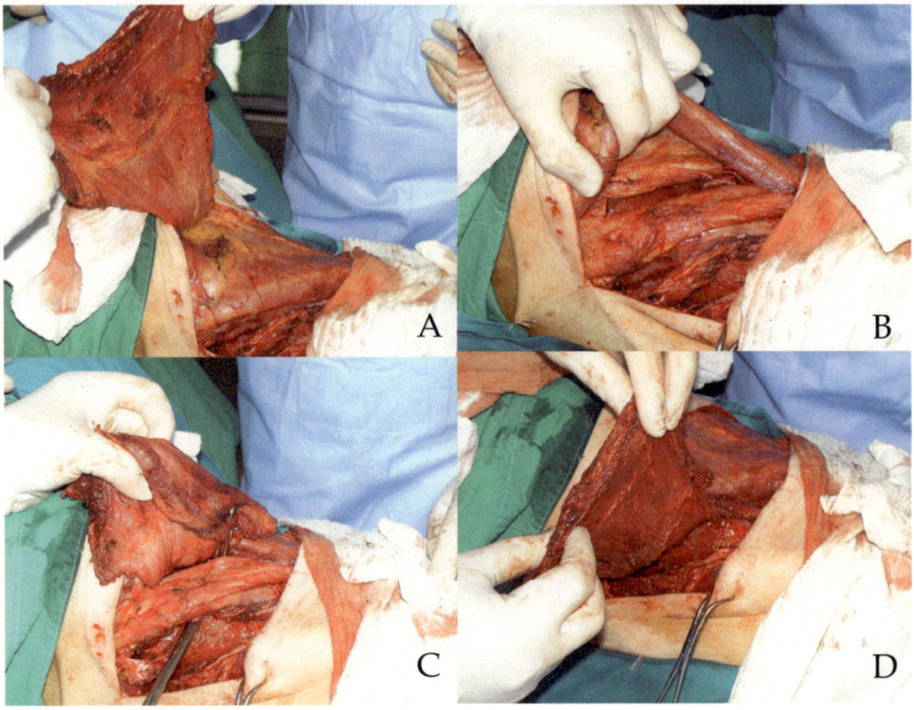

Fig. 5. Intrathoracic transposition of a latissimus dorsi flap. A: The flap raised from the chest wall with preservation of the thoraco-dorsal vessels B: Aspect of the small opening ("second thoracotomy") C: introduction of the flap inside the chest D: final aspect of the flap after intrathoracic transposition.

The basic idea is that muscle flaps bring a well vascularized tissue able to fight actively against infection and promote angiogenesis and healing. These characteristics were proven by the experience of plastic and reconstructive surgeons, who have used them with good results in a great variety of defects – including chronic infections, traumatic lesions or irradiated wounds (Mathes et al., 1977). In order to maintain the aforementioned qualities, the entire muscle flap should remain viable at the end of the procedure and in the postoperative period. A correct mobilization requires precise anatomic knowledge about vascularization and cleavage planes and an accurate dissection with preservation of the vascular pedicles - both arterial and venous (Mathes & Nahai, 1979). As a general rule, in most cases of intrathoracic transposition the flaps do not require such an extensive mobilization as it is needed in plastic surgery procedures.

The surgeon who performs intrathoracic muscle transposition must be familiar with the anatomy of the local flaps, in terms of cleavage planes, relationships with other structures and blood supply, as well as with the dimensions of the flap and its limits of mobilization.

Most muscles have several vascular sources, not all of them allowing a complete mobilization of the flap. Anatomical variations may also play an important role. The nutritive pedicle must be carefully prepared using a combination of blunt and sharp dissection, avoiding any damage since this is equivalent to the loss of the flap (McCraw & Arnold, 1987).

At the end of the mobilization, the viability of the entire flap must be carefully evaluated. In case of ischemic changes, the affected portion of the flap must be resected; from our experience, severe ischemia of extended portions of the flap is very rare if the mobilization is correctly performed. Any severe ischemia leads to flap necrosis with subsequent recurrence of the intrathoracic suppuration and failure of the surgical procedure.

Introduction of the flap inside the thorax requires usually a second window created through a limited rib resection (less than 10 cm length, no more than one rib). When introducing the flap inside the chest, care must be taken to avoid any compression, kinking or twisting of the vascular pedicle in order to avoid thrombosis and loss of the flap. The muscle must reach the defect without any tension and without torsion. Haemostasis must be carefully checked, since postoperative bleeding from the flap will lead to hemothorax. The wound is usually closed, with separate chest and subcutaneous drainage to avoid the postoperative development of seroma in the space resulted from muscle flap dissection (fig. 5).

Mobilization of any flap and it's transposition in a different position involves a certain degree of functional morbidity. For most of the flaps used for intrathoracic transposition, these functional sequelae are minor, since there are some other muscles with synergic action that compensate their absence. When put in balance, these functional sequelae are minor compared to the gravity of the situation of the patients that require thoracomyoplasty procedures. However, these aspects must be discussed with the patient before the procedure and a signed informed consent should be obtained (Pairolero & Arnold, 1989, Arnold & Pairolero, 1989).

4.3 Surgical anatomy and techniques of mobilization of the most important flaps

The techniques of muscle flap mobilization were described in detail by the plastic surgeons (Mathes & Nahai, 1979, McCraw & Arnold, 1987), and are based on very precise anatomical knowledges concerning the blood supply (Mathes & Nahai, 1981).

The latissimus dorsi flap is probably the most used flap in thoracic surgery. It may be prepared using a skin incision running parallel with the anterior border of the muscle or through a standard postero-lateral skin incision. The standard latissimus dorsi flap involves detachment of the muscle from the iliac crest and sacrum and mobilization from the chest wall keeping intact the main blood supply represented by the thoraco-dorsal vessels, which run parallel with the anterior margin on the deep side of the muscle. If necessary, the insertion tendon and the vascular branch for the serratus anterior may be sectioned in order to increase the length. The flap is quite easy to prepare since there are distinct cleavage planes and the nutrient blood vessels are large enough and with very few anatomical variants; it has a large volume and a long arch of rotation, which allows it to reach almost every part of the thorax (Abolhoda et al., 2008, Seify et al., 2007).

The reversed latissimus dorsi flap is much rarely used. It involves sectioning of the flap in the upper part and mobilization based on the secondary blood supply represented by some perforator branches from the last intercostal and first lumbar vessels; these branches are small and have an extremely variable anatomy, which make this mobilization more limited and difficult compared to the standard one. However, it may be used with good results in certain circumstances, the main indication being repair or filling of defects located in the supradiaphragmatic area (Botianu P et al., 2010b).

Due to the synergic activity of other muscles, mobilization of the latissimus dorsi is not associated with serious functional impairment, having no impact on daily activities.

The serratus anterior flap has two main sources of blood supply: the thoracic lateral artery (originating from the axillary artery) and a branch originating from the thoraco-dorsal artery. Since the two vessels have an almost parallel traject, we prefer to preserve both of them if the entire muscle is mobilized; the veins run parallel to the arteries, draining in the axillary vein. The muscle can be easily dissected from the surrounding structures and detached from the chest wall and the scapula. It reaches easily the hilum and is excellent for defects located in the upper half of the thorax. Another advantage is that almost the entire muscle remains intact after the standard postero-lateral thoracotomy, making it suitable for postoperative complications. A specific complication described in the literature is the winged scapula ("scapula allata"), which is very unpleasant for the patient and difficult to treat (Arnold et al., 1984). If several prophylactic measures are taken, this complication is very rare. In our personal experience with over 70 serratus anterior flaps, we had no case of true winged scapula, only some cases of minor asymmetry (Botianu P et al., 2010c).

If necessary, the serratus anterior and the latissimus dorsi can be mobilized together using the common thoraco-dorsal vascular pedicle.

The pectoralis flap may also be mobilized in more ways. The most used is the mobilization of the pectoralis major, with or without the pectoralis minor muscle, by detachment from the chest wall and subcutis using the thoracoacromial vessels for blood supply. For an increased mobilization, it is necessary to section the insertion tendon on the humerus. Another common way of mobilization is based on the perforator branches that arise from the internal thoracic and anterior intercostal vessels in the parasternal region. The pectoralis flap is usefull for defects located in the apical region (Kalweit et al., 1994, Nomori et al., 2001), although it's mobilization is difficult through a standard thoracotomy incision; it is also frequently used to prevent and treat infectious complications after median sternotomy (Gao et al., 2010).

The rectus abdominis flap can be mobilized based on the superior epigastric vessels, which continue the internal thoracic ones. The second pedicle, represented by the inferior epigastric vessels, can also support the entire flap but does not allow it's mobilization inside the chest and therefore cannot be used for intrathoracic transposition. Usually, a paramedian vertical incision is made in the abdominal wall and the anterior rectus sheath is opened, allowing exposure of the muscle. The rectus abdominis is raised from the posterior sheath and the inferior epigastric vessels are ligated. A special care must be taken when the flap is turned towards the chest in order to avoid damaging of the vascular pedicle. Specific complications for this flap are represented by the abdominal wall problems, with the risk of developing an incisional hernia. It is preferred by some authors for the treatment of sterno-mediastinal infections following sternotomy (Oh et al., 2004) but it is also usefull for different infections located in the inferior part of the thorax (Ojika et al., 1995).

Intercostal flaps are very easy to prepare during thoracomyoplasty procedures (Sarkar et al., 1985). These flaps usually contain the intercostal spaces (including the muscles), the parietal pleura and the periosteum remaining after the rib resection. The arterial blood supply is represented by the posterior intercostal arteries arising from the thoracic aorta and the anterior intercostal arteries arising from the internal thoracic artery; the veins have a parallel traject and drain into the azygos veins, respectively the internal thoracic veins. There is a very rich network connecting the anterior and the posterior intercostal vessels, as well as the vessels from adjacent intercostal spaces and neighbourhood muscles. According to the location of the defect, both the anterior and the posterior intercostal vessels may be used as blood supply for the flaps. When creating the intercostal flaps, the incision should be always made through the bed of the resected ribs in order to minimize the risk of damaging the main intercostal vessels. We found these intercostal flaps particularly usefull for bronchial fistula closure and filling of some dead angles and cul-de-sacs (Botianu P et al., 2010a, c).

The omentum flap - although it is not a muscle, it should be included here since it is preferred in many instances with the same purposes and principles as the muscle flaps (Petrov et al., 1999). The main vessels are represented by the left gastro-epiploic artery (originating from the splenic artery) and the right gastro-epiploic artery (originating from the gastro-duodenal artery). These two arteries create the gastro-epiploic arcade which runs along the great curvature of the stomach and gives small branches for the stomach and the so-called epiploic arteries for the omentum. The veins run parallel with the arteries, creating similar arcades. These epiploic vessels have a descendant traject and form a second arcade along the inferior edge of the omentum (Barkow's arcade). There are many ways to mobilize the omentum based on the vessels and arcades described. However, the anatomy of the omental vascularization is extremely variable and it should be carefully evaluated before planning the flap and making any incision (Kirikuta, 1980). Specific complications are related to the risk of incisional hernia and development of adhesions with intestinal obstruction. The omentum flap is preferred by some authors for sterno-mediastinal infections (Hountis et al., 2009), closure of large bronchial fistulas - especially after pneumonectomy (Chichevatov & Gorshenev, 2005) and reinforcement of high-risk sutures (D'Andrilli et al., 2009). Recent publications have shown good results with the laparoscopic mobilization, which makes the omental flap more attractive (van Wingerden et al., 2010).

Other rarely used flaps have been reported in case-reports or small series, with more or less good results: trapezius, subscapularis, infraspinatus, external oblique, teres major etc. Such flaps should be taken into consideration especially when other standard flaps are not available or have failed (Fuchs et al., 2010, Schreiner et al., 2010).

5. Thoracomyoplasty – combining thoracoplasty and muscle flaps

The idea of this kind of procedures is to combine thoracoplasty with intrathoracic muscle transposition in an attempt to achieve safe obliteration of the diseased intrathoracic space. Since for suppurated defects complete filling is mandatory for safe primary wound closure, combining thoracoplasty and muscle transposition acts as a compromise between:

- an extended thoracoplasty (rib resection) with major chest wall mutilation;
- the use of multiple muscle flaps, with added donor-site morbidity and postoperative functional deficits.

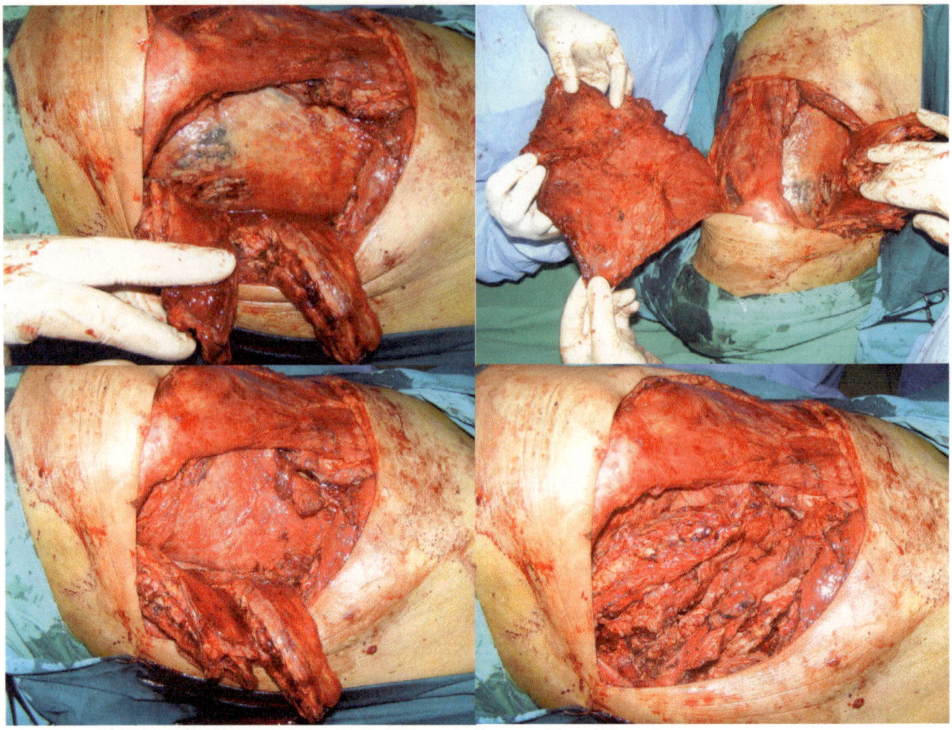

Fig. 6. Intraoperative aspects of a complex space-filling procedure / thoracomyoplasty: a limited 5-ribs thoracoplasty, transposition of the latissimus dorsi based on the thoracodorsal vessels and 2 intercostal flaps with posterior vascularization.

There is no standardized technique of thoracomyoplasty. Both rib resection and muscle transposition should be performed trying to reduce the chest wall mutilation and functional morbidity to minimum, but without compromising the definitive obliteration of the cavity (fig. 6).

The local anatomy should be carefully evaluated when planning the procedure:

- location and dimensions of the cavity, which can be easily assessed on preoperative CT scans;
- presence of bronchial fistula, whose safe closure is mandatory. The presence of a bronchial fistula may be suggested preoperatively by the clinical course; bronchoscopy and CT may detect some large and centrally located fistula but the exact position of the smaller ones can be evaluated only intraoperative.
- available flaps - in many cases, the neighbourhood muscles may be compromised by previous procedures; typical examples are postero-lateral thoracotomy which divides the latissimus dorsi, upper digestive surgery which compromises the omentum, subcostal laparotomy or myocardial revascularization with the internal mammary artery which compromise the rectus abdominis flap.

The terminology used for this kind of procedures is not very clear. The term "thoracoplasty" should be reserved for cases not associating any muscle flap mobilization. Some authors talk about myoplasty, muscle flaps or intrathoracic muscle transposition, which can quite rarely solve alone a large suppurated cavity without associating any rib resection. As well as other authors, we find the terms "thoracomyoplasty" and "complex space-filling procedures" are the most appropriate to describe this kind of procedures (Botianu P et al., 2010a, García-Yuste et al., 1998, Naumov et al., 1991, Riquet 2010).

6. Personal experience and results from the literature

During the last 8 years we have performed thoracomyoplasty procedures in 102 patients, with almost one half of them having different TB lesions. The procedure was adapted to the local anatomy of the lesion, with an average of 5 resected ribs/patient and 1.9 flaps/patient. Our recently published analysis of the first 76 patients showed an acceptable mortality (5%) and rate of recurrence requiring an open-window procedure (5%); other minor local complications included a few skin necrosis and persistent small thoracic fistulae solved under local anesthesia with no need for a major reoperation.

Postoperative hospitalization ranged between 4 and 180 days, with an average of 40 ± 5 days; all the patients with hospitalizations longer than 60 days presented recurrence of the infection requiring on open-window procedure. At the moment of discharge, all the patients had healed wounds with no need for any other surgical care. TB patients were referred to our pneumology colleagues to continue the specific chemotherapy.

Five patients presented a mild impairment of the shoulder function, but without interfering with the daily activities; 4 patients presented a minor asymmetry of the two shoulders and scapulas but we had no case of true winged scapula and no major functional disturbance secondary to the extrathoracic muscle flap mobilization. None of our patients presented severe scoliosis or a major chest deformity. At 3 months follow-up, 91% (66 patients) of the survivors returned to an almost normal life compared with their preoperative status.

A comparative evaluation showed no statistically significant difference between the pre- and post-operative values of the the functional respiratory tests (VC preoperative - mean 1050 ml/62% of predicted vs postoperative - mean 1100 ml/63% of predicted, FEV1 preoperative - mean 850 ml/61% of predicted vs postoperative - mean 890 ml/62% of predicted, Wilcoxon signed-rank test, $p>0.05$). The main explanation is that the parenchyma underlying the thoracomyoplasty is more or less diseased, therefore with a lower contribution to the respiration; also, closure of the bronchial fistula improves the respiratory function (Botianu P et al., 2010a).

Other authors have also recently published important series with quite similar results, with mortality, morbidity and hospitalization falling within an acceptable range of values. These data recommend the use of thoracomyoplasty procedures to solve difficult cases of intrathoracic suppurations (García-Yuste et al., 1998, Icard et al., 1999, Jadczuk 1998, Krassas et al., 2010, Regnard et al., 2000, Stefani et al., 2011).

7. Future challenges

During the recent years, a few new ideas emerged:

- the use of free-transfers, which increases the number and volume of the flaps available for filling of the infected spaces (Walsh et al., 2011). However, they involve a multidisciplinary approach and complicated procedures; the microsurgical anastomoses of the vessels require experience and special technical skills, are time-consuming and involve a specific morbidity.

- the use of less-invasive procedures for flap mobilization, using special retractors, light sources, instruments and dissection techniques borrowed from endoscopic surgery. Proponents consider that with the use of these techniques the mobilization of the muscle flaps may be performed using shorter skin incisions and less donor-site morbidity, making them more acceptable (Blidisel et al., 2008).

A major problem is the difficulty to study these procedures according to the modern principles of evidenced-based medicine. These procedures are rarely performed and address to a small number of desperate cases, not comparable to those submitted to the standard treatment consisting of lung resection and/or pleural decortication. The rarity of these procedures and the great heterogenicity of the patients (in terms of local anatomy, etiology and biological status) makes any kind of randomised trial or fair comparison impossible (Botianu P. et al., 2010a, b).

The most important challenge remains probably training, since many surgeons are not familiar with the techniques of thoracoplasty or muscle flaps mobilization; most young surgeons have neither performed, nor seen such procedures. Specific training and/or a good cooperation with a plastic and reconstructive surgery colleague is mandatory.

8. Conclusions

Both thoracoplasty and muscle transposition remain in the armamentarium of modern thoracic surgery (Riquet 2010). Due to the recrudescence of TB and other infectious diseases of the chest, it is possible that the number of patients requiring this kind of surgery will increase in the near future. We believe that sooner or later any thoracic surgeon will meet a patient requiring such a procedure. Thoracomyoplasty may solve a complicated case with good immediate and long-term outcome. In such situations, training, careful evaluation and an accurate surgical technique are essential to achieve good results (Botianu P. et al., 2010a, Krassas et al., 2010, Stefani et al., 2011).

9. References

Abolhoda A,; Bui T.D.; Milliken J.C. & Wirth G.A. (2009) *Pedicled latissimus dorsi muscle flap: routine use in high-risk thoracic surgery,* Tex Heart Inst J; 36(4):298-302

Abolhoda A.; Wirth G.A.; Bui T.D. & Milliken J.C. (2008) *Harvest technique for pedicled transposition of latissimus dorsi muscle: an old trade revisited,* Eur J Cardiothorac Surg; 33(5):928-30

Abrashanoff G. (1911) *Plastische Methode der Schliessung von Fistelgangen, welche von inneren Organen kommen,* Zentralbl Chir; 38:186-7

Alexander J. (1936) *Some advances in the technic of thoracoplasty,* Ann Surg; 104(4):545-51

Andrews NC. (1961) *Thoracomediastinal plication: a surgical technique for chronic empyema,* J Thorac Cardiovasc Surg; 41:809-16

Andrews NC. (1965) *The surgical treatment of chronic empyema,* Dis Chest; 47:533-8

Archibald E. (1926) *On extra-pleural thoracoplasty,* Can Med Assoc J;16(4)433-5

Arnold P.G. & Pairolero P.C. (1989) *Intrathoracic muscle flaps: a 10-year experience in the management of life-threatening infections,* Plast Reconstr Surg; 84(1):92-8

Arnold P.G.; Pairolero P.C. & Waldorf J.C. (1984) *The serratus anterior muscle: intrathoracic and extrathoracic utilization,* Plast Reconstr Surg; 73(2):240-8

Bjork V.O. (1954) *Thoracoplasty, a new osteo plastic technique,* J Thorac Surg; 28(2):194-211

Blidisel A.; Maciuceanu B.; Jiga L.; Papurica M. & Ionac M. (2008) *Endoscopy-assisted harvesting and free latissimus dorsi muscle flap transfer in reconstructive microsurgery,* Chirurgia (Bucur); 103(1):67-72

Botianu A.M. (1996) *Procedeu de toracopleuroplastie pentru tratamentul chirurgical al empiemului toracic cu sau fara fistula bronsica/Personal procedure of thoracopleuroplasty for the treatment of the thoracic empyema, with or without bronchial fistula,* Jurnalul de Chirurgie toracică/Journal of Thoracic Surgery; 1:3:251-260

Botianu P. V.-H. (2005) *Re-evaluation of the Schede thoracoplasty,* Jurnalul de Chirurgie Toracica - Journal of Thoracic Surgery; 7(1):71-78

Botianu P.V.-H.; Butiurca A.; Dobrica A.; Damian V.; Ionica S.; Lupu C. & Stoica S. (2008) *Schede procedure and muscular plombage for a multirelapsed TB empyema with pleuro-cutaneous fistula,* Revista de Medicina şi Farmacie-Orvosi es Gyogyszereszeti Szemle (Acta Medica Marisiensis); 54(S3): 69-72

Botianu P.V.-H.; Botianu A.M.; Bacarea V. & Dobrica A.C. (2010) *Thoracodorsal versus reversed mobilisation of the latissimus dorsi muscle for intrathoracic transposition,* Eur J Cardiothorac Surg; 38(4):461-5

Botianu P.V.-H.; Botianu A.M.; Dobrica A.C. & Bacarea V. (2010) *Intrathoracic transposition of the serratus anterior muscle flap--personal experience with 65 consecutive patients,* Eur J Cardiothorac Surg; 38(6):669-73

Botianu P.V.-H.; Dobrica A.C.; Butiurca A. & Botianu A.M. (2010) *Complex space-filling procedures for intrathoracic infections - personal experience with 76 consecutive cases,* Eur J Cardiothorac Surg; 37(2):478-81

Chachques J.C.; Jegaden O.J.; Bors V.; Mesana T.; Latremouille C.; Grandjean P.A.; Fabiani J.N. & Carpentier A. (2008) *Heart transplantation following cardiomyoplasty: a biological bridge,* Eur J Cardiothorac Surg; 33(4):685-90

Chichevatov D. & Gorshenev A. (2005) *Omentoplasty in treatment of early bronchopleural fistulas after pneumonectomy,* Asian Cardiovasc Thorac Ann; 13(3):211-6

Cornet E.; Dupon H.; Coiffard P. & Rembeaux A. (1965) *Thoracopleuroplasties for empyema according to Andrews' method (18 cases),* Ann Chir Thorac Cardiovasc; 4(4):509-15

D'Andrilli A.; Ibrahim M.; Andreetti C.; Ciccone A.M.; Venuta F. & Rendina E.A. (2009) *Transdiaphragmatic harvesting of the omentum through thoracotomy for bronchial stump reinforcement,* Ann Thorac Surg; 88(1):212-5

Davies H.E.; Rosenstengel A. & Lee Y.G. (2011) *The diminishing role of surgery in pleural disease,* Curr Opin Pulm; 17(4):247-54

Deslauriers J.; Jacques L.F. & Grégoire J. (2002) *Role of Eloesser flap and thoracoplasty in the third millennium,* Chest Surg Clin N Am; 12(3):605-23

Entin MA. (1995) *Romance and tragedy of tuberculosis: Edward Archibald's contribution to the surgical treatment of pulmonary tuberculosis,* The Canadian Journal of Plastic Surgery; 3(4):213-6

Estlander J.A. (1879) *Résection des côtes dans l'empyème chronique,* Rev Med Chir (Paris); 3:157-70

Fuchs P.; Schreiner W.; Wolter T.P.; Autschbach R.; Sirbu H. & Pallua N. (2011) *A four-muscle-flap for thoracomyoplasty in patients with sacrificed thoracodorsal vessels,* J Plast Reconstr Aesthet Surg; 64(3):335-8

Gao J.; Wang Y.L.; Lu S.Q.; Cai A.B., Yang Z.F., Han Z.Y., Li J.J., Wen Y.M., Geng F.Y. & Wang W.Z. (2010) *Management of sternal osteomyelitis and mediastinal infection following median sternotomy,* Chin Med J (Engl); 123(20):2803-6

García-Yuste M.; Ramos G.; Duque J.L.; Heras F.; Castanedo M.; Cerezal L.J. & Matilla J.M. (1998) *Open-window thoracostomy and thoracomyoplasty to manage chronic pleural empyema,* Ann Thorac Surg; 65(3):818-22

Hollaus P.H.; Huber M.; Lax F.; Wurnig P.N.; Böhm G. & Pridun N.S. (1999) *Closure of bronchopleural fistula after pneumonectomy with a pedicled intercostal muscle flap,* Eur J Cardiothorac Surg; 16(2):181-6

Holst J. (1952) *Technique of so-called dome thoracoplasty; preliminary report,* Nord Med; 19:48(38):1290-3

Hopkins R.A.; Ungerleider R.M.; Staub E.W. & Young W.G. Jr. (1985) *The modern use of thoracoplasty,* Ann Thorac Surg; 40(2):181-7

Horrigan T.P. & Snow N.J. (1990) *Thoracoplasty: current application to the infected pleural space,* Ann Thorac Surg; 50(5):695-9

Hountis P.; Dedeilias P. & Bolos K. (2009) *The role of omental transposition for the management of postoperative mediastinitis: a case series,* Cases J; 23;2(1):142

Icard P.; Le Rochais J.P.; Rabut B.; Cazaban S.; Martel B. & Evrard C. (1999) *Andrews thoracoplasty as a treatment of post-pneumonectomy empyema: experience in 23 cases,* Ann Thorac Surg; 68(4):1159-63

Jadczuk E. (1998) *Posptneumonectomy empyema,* Eur J Cardiothorac Surg; 14(2):123-6

Kalweit G.; Feindt P.; Huwer H.; Volkmer I. & Gams E. (1994) *The pectoral muscle flaps in the treatment of bronchial stump fistula following pneumonectomy,* Eur J Cardiothorac Surg; 8(7):358-62

Kirikuta I. (1980) *Use of the omentum in plastic surgery,* Ed. Medicala/Medical Publishing House, Bucuresti

Kobayashi H.; Nomori H.; Mori T.; Shibata H.; Yoshimoto K. & Ohba Y. (2009) *Extrapleural pneumonectomy with reconstruction of diaphragm and pericardium using autologous materials,* Ann Thorac Surg 2009; 87(5):1630-2

Kotzampassakis N.; Christodoulou M.; Krueger T.; Demartines N.; Vuillemier H.; Cheng C.; Dorta G. & Ris H.B. (2009) *Esophageal leaks repaired by a muscle onlay approach in the presence of mediastinal sepsis,* Ann Thorac Surg; 88(3):966-72

Krasnov V.A.; Kozhevnikov N.N.; Gorbunov G.M. & Andrenko A.A. (1989) *Long-term results of the use of osteoplastic thoracoplasty in the treatment of destructive tuberculosis of the lungs in patients with antisocial behavior,* Probl Tuberk; (1):41-4

Krassas A.; Grima R.; Bagan P.; Badia A.; Arame A.; Barthes F.P. & Riquet M. (2010) *Current indications and results for thoracoplasty and intrathoracic muscle transposition,* Eur J Cardiothorac Surg; 37(5):1215-20

Massard G.; Thomas P.; Barsotti P.; Riera P.; Giudicelli R.; Reboud E.; Morand G.; Fuentes P.A. & Wihlm J.M. (1997) *Long-term complications of extraperiosteal plombage,* Ann Thorac Surg; 64(1):220-4

Mathes S.J. & Nahai F. (1981) *Classification of the vascular anatomy of muscles: experimental and clinical correlation,* Plast Reconstr Surg; 67(2):177-87

Mathes S.J. & Nahai S. (1979) *Clinical atlas of muscle and musculocutaneous flaps,* CV Mosby Co, St. Louis

Mathes S.J.; Vasconez L.O. & Jurkiewicz M.J. (1977) *Extensions and further applications of muscle flap transposition,* Plast Reconstr Surg; 60:6-13

McCraw J.B. & Arnold P.G. (1987) *McCraw and Arnold's Atlas of Muscle and Musculocutaneous Flaps,* Hampton Press, Norfolk, VA

Meyer A.J.; Krueger T.; Lepori D.; Dusmet M.; Aubert J.D.; Pasche P. & Ris H.B. (2004) *Closure of large intrathoracic airway defects using extrathoracic muscle flaps,* Ann Thorac Surg; 77(2):397-404

Mitra A.; Spears J.; Perrotta V.; McClurkin J. & Mitra A. (2005) *Salvage of infected prosthetic grafts of the great vessels via muscle flap reconstruction,* Chest; 128(2):1040-3

Naftali Z. (1964) *Toracoplastia osteoplastica cu transplant paramediastinal de coastă in tratamentul tuberculozei cavernoase (Osteoplastic thoracoplasty with paramediastinal transplantation of rib grafts in the treatment of cavernous tuberculosis),* PhD Thesis

Naumov V.N.; Shaikhaev A.I. & Testov V.V. (1991) *Thoracomyoplastic operations in the surgery of tuberculosis of the lungs,* Grud Serdechnososudistaia Khir; (7):46-8

Nomori H.; Horio H.; Hasegawa T. & Suemasu K. (2001) *Intrathoracic transposition of a pectoralis major and pectoralis minor muscle flap for empyema in patients previously subjected to posterolateral thoracotomy,* Surg Today; 31(4):295-9

Nosotti M.; Baisi A.; Mendogni P.; Palleschi A.; Tosi D. & Rosso L. (2010) *Muscle sparing versus posterolateral thoracotomy for pulmonary lobectomy: randomised controlled trial,* Interact Cardiovasc Thorac Surg; 11(4):415-9

Oh A.K.; Lechtman A.N.; Whetzel T.P. & Stevenson T.R. (2004) *The infected median sternotomy wound: management with the rectus abdominis musculocutaneous flap,* Ann Plast Surg; 52(4):367-70

Ojika T.; Mukoyama N.; Suzuki M.; Senda Y. & Namiki Y. (1995) *Two cases of empyema treated with rectus abdominis myocutaneous flap and muscle flap,* Kyobu Geka; 48(5):394-6

Pairolero P.C. & Arnold P.G. (1989) *Intrathoracic transfer of flaps for fistulas, exposed prosthetic devices, and reinforcement of suture lines,* Surg Clin North Am; 69(5):1047-59

Pairolero P.C.; Arnold P.G.; Trastek V.F.; Meland N.B. & Kay P.P. (1990) *Postpneumonectomy empyema. The role of intrathoracic muscle transposition.* J Thorac Cardiovasc Surg; 99(6):958-66

Pardos-Gea J.; Maza Ú.; Pérez-López J. & San José Laporte A. (2011) *Home intravenous antibiotic therapy of empyema and lung abscess: safety and efficacy,* Enferm Infecc Microbiol Clin; 29(3):237-9

Petrov D.; Dzhambazov V.; Minchev T.; Plochev M.; Goranov E.; Krupev M. & Petkov R. (1999) *Omentoplasty in surgical management of postpulmonectomy pleural empyema,* Khirurgiia (Sofiia); 55(6):13-5

Regnard J.F.; Alifano M.; Puyo P.; Fares E.; Magdeleinat P. & Levasseur P. (2000) *Open window thoracostomy followed by intrathoracic flap transposition in the treatment of empyema complicating pulmonary resection,* J Thorac Cardiovasc Surg; 120(2):270-5

Riquet M. (2010) *Thoracomyoplasty (Editorial comment),* Eur J Cardiothorac Surg; 37(2):482

Sarkar S.K.; Sharma T.N.; Singh H.; Singh A.; Purohit S.D. & Sharma V.K. (1985) *Thoracoplasty with intercostal myoplasty for closure of an empyema cavity and bronchopleural fistula,* Int Surg; 70(3):219-21

Schede M. (1890) *Die behandlung der empyeme,* Verh Long Innere Med Wiesbaden; 9:41-141

Schreiner W.; Fuchs P.; Autschbach R.; Pallua N. & Sirbu H. (2010) *Modified technique for thoracomyoplasty after posterolateral thoracotomy,* Thorac Cardiovasc Surg; 58(2):98-101

Seify H.; Mansour K.; Miller J.; Douglas T.; Burke R.; Losken A.; Culbertson J.; Jones G.; Nahai F. & Hester T.R. (2007) *Single-stage muscle flap reconstruction of the postpneumonectomy empyema space: the Emory experience,* Plast Reconstr Surg; 120(7):1886-91

Semb C. (1937) *Thoracoplasty with extrafascial apicolysis,* Br Med J; 2(4004):650-6

Stefani A.; Jouni R.; Alifano M.; Bobbio A.; Strano S.; Magdeleinat P. & Regnard J.F. (2011) *Thoracoplasty in the current practice of thoracic surgery: a single-institution 10-years experience,* Ann Thorac Surg; 91(1):263-8

Stobernack A.; Achatzy R. & Engelmann C. (1997) *Delayed complications after extrapleural pneumonolysis for lung tuberculosis,* Chirurg; 68(9):921-7

Thingnam S.K.; Mohite P.N.; Raju G.; Ranade S.D. & Saklani R. (2011) *Triple reinforcement of bronchial stump,* Thorac Cardiovasc Surg; 59(3):169-71

van Wingerden J.J.; Coret M.E.; van Nieuwenhoven C.A.; Totté E.R. (2010) *The laparoscopically harvested omental flap for deep sternal wound infection,* Eur J Cardiothorac Surg 2010; 37(1):87-92

Walsh M.D.; Bruno A.D.; Onaitis M.W.; Erdmann D.; Wolfe W.G.; Toloza E.M. & Levin L.S. (2011) *The role of intrathoracic free flaps for chronic empyema,* Ann Thorac Surg; 91(3):865-8

Wilson N.J.; Armada 0.; Vindzberg V. & O'Brien WB (1956) *Extraperiosteal plombage thoracoplasty: operative technique and results with 161 cases with unilateral surgical problems,* J Thorac Surg; 32:797-813

Zaheer S.; Allen M.S.; Cassivi S.D.; Nichols F.C. 3rd; Johnson C.H.; Deschamps C. & Pairolero P.C. (2006) *Postpneumonectomy empyema: results after the Clagett procedure,* Ann Thorac Surg; 82(1):279-86

Zahid I.; Nagendran M.; Routledge T. & Scarci M. (2011) *Comparison of video-assisted thoracoscopic surgery and open surgery in the management of primary empyema,* Curr Opin Pulm Med; 17(4):255-9

19

Lung Volume Reduction Surgery

James D. Maloney, Nicole K. Strieter and Joshua L. Hermsen
University of Wisconsin School of Medicine and Public Health,
William S. Middleton Memorial VA,
USA

1. Introduction

Lung volume reduction surgery (LVRS) was first reported by Drs Brantigan and Mueller from the University of Maryland in 1957. (1) Since that time it has enjoyed both fame and infamy but has never experienced widespread acceptance. Although subjective and often quantitative improvements in breathing were documented, early results were plagued by high mortality. Since those early reports the selection process for patients undergoing LVRS has been refined and has resulted in a safe and effective procedure. Regardless of selection criteria, however, numbers of LVR cases remain small. This is in contrast to the burgeoning population of patients with emphysema.

Chronic Obstructive Pulmonary Disease (COPD) is a major cause of morbidity and mortality in the United States. COPD includes both chronic bronchitis and emphysema as these conditions often coexist. It is estimated that 12.1 million adults aged 18 and over have a diagnosis of COPD. As many as 24 million U.S. adults have some evidence of impaired lung function This suggests that the disease in under diagnosed. (2,3) COPD is currently the fourth leading cause of death in the United States, and is projected to be the third most common by 2020. The disease no longer predominates in men. The number of women dying from the disease has surpassed the number seen in men. (2) As we move outside the United States to areas still seeing a rise in tobacco consumption millions more are affected. Chronic bronchitis and emphysema dramatically increase healthcare costs. COPD leads to high resource utilization, including frequent clinician office visits, hospitalizations due to acute exacerbations, and chronic therapy. (3) According to the National Heart Lung and Blood Institute, the national projected annual cost for COPD in 2010 was $49.9 billion. This includes $29.5 billion in direct health care expenditures, $8.0 billion in indirect morbidity costs and $12.4 billion in indirect mortality costs. (2,3)

The primary cause of COPD is smoking. COPD is under-diagnosed, with only 15 to 20 percent of smokers confirmed as having the disease although the majority develop some degree of airflow obstruction (4,6). Inhalation of tobacco smoke causes destruction of lung tissue that occurs in several ways. Tobacco exposure directly disrupts clearance of mucous secretions by injuring and destroying the cilia in turn increases mucus production from mucosal irritation leads to infection and injury. Chronic inflammation from direct irritation and subclinical infection results in elevated levels of inflammatory mediators. With continued exposure, there is loss of proteins and destruction of normal parenchymal architecture with decreased elasticity and alveolar destruction.(7)

2. Emphysema

DEFINITION —The Global Initiative for Chronic Obstructive Lung Disease (GOLD) — a report produced by the National Heart, Lung, and Blood Institute (NHLBI) and the World Health Organization (WHO) — defines COPD as follows (8):
"COPD is characterized by airflow limitation that is not fully reversible. The airflow limitation is usually progressive and associated with an abnormal inflammatory response of the lungs to noxious particles or gases."
There are commonly three distinct forms of COPD: chronic bronchitis, asthma and emphysema (9). Chronic bronchitis is characterized by chronic productive cough for three months in each of two successive years. This requires exclusion of other causes of chronic cough (9, 10). Asthma is "a chronic inflammatory disorder of the airways in which many cells and cellular elements play a role. The chronic inflammation is associated with airway responsiveness that leads to recurrent episodes of wheezing, breathlessness, chest tightness, and coughing. Asthma manifests airflow obstruction that is reversible, spontaneously or with treatment". (11) Asthma is not dependent on the noxious stimuli of smoking and does not have the same effect on survival that is seen in other forms of COPD. Emphysema is abnormal, permanent enlargement of the airspaces that are distal to the terminal bronchioles. (12)Emphysema is normally accompanied by moderate or severe airflow obstruction and destruction of alveolar walls without evidence of fibrosis. Emphysema causes dyspnea through airflow limitation, hyperinflation, and loss of gas exchanging surfaces in the lungs (13). In contrast to asthma, chronic bronchitis and emphysema typically manifest in the sixth decade of life and have a higher mortality to prevalence ratio. Emphysema is separated into radiographic definitions of centrilobular, panacinar and distal acinar(14) . In centrilobular emphysema the areas of disease are located near the center of the secondary pulmonary lobule. Arterial deficiency in the upper lobes accompanies this, but the distal acinus is unaffected. *Panacinar* emphysema affects the entire respiratory acinus, from respiratory bronchiole to alveoli. It occurs more commonly in the lower lobes, especially basal segments, and anterior margins of the lungs. Similar to centrilobular disease, affected areas demonstrate arterial defficiency. Most candidates for LVRS will have centrilobular emphysema.
COPD can be categorized as mild, moderate, severe and very severe, based primarily on forced expiratory volume in 1 second (FEV1).(8) In cases of very severe COPD, classification is impacted by pulmonary hypertension and pCO2. (table 1) Most candidates for LVRS will be classified as very severe based on GOLD criteria.

• Stage 1: Mild
FEV1 ≥ 80% predicted
• Stage 2: Moderate
80> FEV1 ≥ 50%
• Stage 3: Severe
50 > FEV1 ≥30% predicted
• Stage 4: Very Severe
FEV1 < 30% or
FEV1 < *50%* + chronic respiratory failure
(PaO_2 < 60mmHg, $PaCO_2$ > 50mmHg, cor pulmonale)

Table 1. Gold executive summary for staging of emphysema.
Klaus FR, et al. Global Strategy for the Diagnosis, Management, and Prevention of Chronic Obstructive Pulmonary Disease: GOLD Executive Summary. Am L Respir Crit Care Med. Vol 176. Pp 532-55, 2007.

3. Lung Volume Reduction Surgery (LVRS)

Lung volume reduction attempts to correct loss of elastic recoil by reducing the volume of the most damaged lung segments and allowing the remaining less damaged tissues to expand within the chest. By eliminating parts of emphysematous lung with the longest expiratory time and removing dead space, dynamic air trapping is reduced and exercise capacity can be increased. The operating length of respiratory muscles is also normalized improving both inspiratory and expiratory effort. (14) Surgical removal of diseased lung restores the normal dimensions of both the chest wall and the diaphragm and augments the force exerted by the diaphragm. In addition it addresses dead space and ventilation/perfusion mismatch. The underlying mechanisms of improvement have not been fully elucidated. Increased elastic recoil, reduction in dynamic hyperinflation, and augmented force exerted by the diaphragm (15,16) have been suggested to explain the improvement in (FEV_1). There are quantitative increases in FVC, FEV_1, RV, and RV/TLC after LVRS in appropriately chosen candidates. These results support the hypothesis that the improvement in airflow rates resulted from a decrease in static hyperinflation and an increase in elastic recoil, resulting in greater radial traction on peripheral airways.(16) In short, respiratory mechanics are improved with LVRS.

Cremona and colleagues studied pulmonary gas exchange in COPD patients and recorded a very wide range of physiologic abnormality pre-operatively. (17) Post-LVRS Pa_{O2} increases were related to improvement in ventilation/perfusion mismatch, mainly due to a reduction in hyperinflation and dead space. There was no direct contribution from changes in lung mechanical properties. In contrast, the changes in Pa_{CO2} were accounted for by improvement in lung mechanical properties and not V/Q mismatch. (17) This corroborate data provided by Criner et al that also showed a downward shift in PaCo2 post LVRS in upper lobe predominant patients.(18)

Dr Joel Cooper reinvigorated the concept of lung volume reduction surgery as a successful therapy for emphysema. (19) It was in 1996 after publication of his results in the JCTVS that the volume of LVRS cases performed in the United States ballooned. Unfortunately the thoracic surgical community was not able to duplicate his results. Morbidity and mortality were excessive, and the cost to medicare and other third party payers extravagant. The outcomes were not consistent with Dr Cooper's published data. CMS took notice and quickly ceased reimbursement for the procedure. This discrepancy ultimately led to the NETT a study that was in part initiated to determine medicare reimbursement.

4. NETT (national emphysema treatment trial) review

The NETT was and continues to be the most influential trial of surgical lung volume reduction despite the fact that it was closed for accrual almost 10 years ago. To this day, it continues to be exhaustively reviewed and analyzed. This study determined not only the patient population should undergo LVRS for maximum benefit and the population who were high risk of mortality, but also criteria to circumscribe the number of centers able to offer the therapy. The NETT was a randomized, controlled, multicenter, long-term trial that examined the effects of LVRS. The primary endpoints were survival and maximum exercise performance and secondary endpoints were post surgical lung function, patient symptoms and quality of life all compared to medical therapy alone.(20) The initial data was published in 2003 and reported the effects of LVRS on survival and maximum exercise capacity.

Median follow-up was 2.4 years in its primary iteration.(21) In 2006, NETT investigators reported updated analyses with a median follow-up of 4.3 years.(22) Over 1200 patients were randomized in the trial giving it sufficient statistical power. 608 patients were randomized to the surgery arm, 70% were by median sternotomy, the remainder by VATS. Quantitative improvement was seen in the LVRS group as compared to the medically managed patients. Exercise capacity, a primary endpoint, improved following LVRS after 6, 12 and 24 months compared to medically treated patients. In comparison to medically treated patients, LVRS patients performed better in 6 minute walk distance (6MWD), percent predicted forced expiratory volume in one-second (FEV1), the severity of dyspnea, and quality of life assessments. (21) Though overall mortality was not statistically different, 90 day mortality for the surgery arm was approaching 8%, far higher than the medical arm (1.3 %). Upon further review, it was determined that there was a subgroup who posed prohibitive surgical risk. This subgroup, defined by FEV1 < 20 % predicted and either a diffusing capacity for carbon monoxide (DLCO) < 20% predicted or homogeneous emphysema represented prohibitive risks with a 30-day mortality of 16% (23). Identification of this subgroup helped to delineate the pulmonary function testing criteria appropriate for LVRS and led to categorizing non-high risk patients into four distinct groups for analysis.
The basis for grouping non high risk patients was the craniocaudal distribution of emphysema on chest CT (upper lobe predominance) and post rehabilitation exercise test maximum wattage (low or high exercise).

4.1 NETT Subgroup analysis

1. Upper lobe predominant low exercise capacity

This group demonstrated the most benefit from LVRS. Patients with upper lobe predominant emphysema and low exercise capacity had a lower risk of death with LVRS than medical therapy. This LVRS group was more likely to achieve > 10 W improvement in maximum exercise wattage at 24 months, and > an 8 point improvement in St. George's Respiratory Questionnaire (SGRQ) score at 24 months.

2. Upper lobe predominant high exercise capacity

Patients with upper lobe predominant emphysema and high exercise tolerance, LVRS had no effect on survival even in extended follow up. Following LVRS, however, patients were more likely to have > 10 W improvement in maximum exercise wattage at 24 months and significant improvement in SGRQ as compared to medical therapy.

3. Non-upper lobe predominant low exercise capacity

Patients with non-upper lobe predominant disease and low exercise capacity, LVRS had no effect on the risk of death or maximum exercise capacity at 24 months. However, LVRS patients were more likely to have significant improvement in SGRQ at 24 months.

4. Non-upper lobe predominant high exercise capacity

Patients with non-upper lobe predominant emphysema and high exercise at baseline, LVRS increased the risk for death and had no beneficial impact on maximum exercise capacity at 24 months or SGRQ.

4.2 Patient outcomes

The above groupings were instrumental in determining appropriate patients for LVRS. In the non-high risk population the 30-day mortality was 2.2% with LVRS and 0.2% with medical treatment ($p< 0.001$). 90-day mortality rate was 5.2% with LVRS and 1.5% with medical treatment (21). LVRS did not demonstrate short term survival benefit over medical treatment. LVRS showed significant and sustained increases in exercise capacity and 6 minute walk distance, reduction in dyspnea, and improvements in disease-specific and general quality of life measurements.(24) In patients with upper lobe predominant emphysema and low exercise capacity, total mortality rate was 0.11 deaths per person-year with LVRS and 0.13 with medical treatment, respectively. In upper lobe predominant, low exercise tolerance patients, LVRS increased survival, and improved exercise capacity and quality of life compared to medical therapy. (22)

Postoperative morbidity was not a primary endpoint in the NETT but is important in assessing the success of a procedure. 58.7% of the patients had at least one complication within 30 days of surgery. Major pulmonary and cardiovascular morbidity occurred in approximately 30% and 20% respectively during the NETT. Cardiac arryhtmia occurred in almost 25%. 18% developed pneumonia, 21% were re-intubated and 8% underwent tracheostomy.(24,25) Despite significant morbidity, quality of life measures were improved with LVRS over medical therapy. Outcomes related to mortality and morbidity continue to improve. Ginsburg et al recently published their series of 49 patients undergoing LVRS selected using the criteria defined by the NETT. Both BODE index and FEV1 showed statistically significant improvement, and operative mortality (90 day) was zero, with acceptable morbidity. (26) Boley and colleagues published a recent series with morbidity and mortality lower than that documented in the NETT. (27) Despite improved mortality, predicting response in LVRS patients continues to be difficult. Imfeld and colleagues demonstrated that post-operative BODE index accurately predicts survival, however preoperative values do not.(28) (see table 2) Similarly there is no perfect instrument to determine an expected increase in FEV1 or 6 minute walk that will positively influence BODE index and subsequently survival.

Variable	Points on BODE Index			
	0	1	2	3
FEV_1 (% of predicted)†	≥65	50–64	36–49	≤35
Distance walked in 6 min (m)	≥350	250–349	150–249	≤149
MMRC dyspnea scale‡	0–1	2	3	4
Body-mass index§	>21	≤21		

Table 2. Variables for BODE index a predictor of survival in COPD patients

5. Indications for LVRS

Criteria for LVRS in our institution is based on the NETT inclusion and exclusion criteria with some limited changes. We have not set firm age limitations in our patient exclusion criteria for LVRS but review them on a case by case basis in patients over 65 years of age. With few exceptions, in patients with FEV1 > 35% predicted, we have chosen to manage medically barring substantial symptoms in a patient with severe bullous disease and significant segmental or lobar compression.

History and physical exam consistent with emphysema
Imaging with evidence of heterogeneous emphysema
Pre-rehabilitation postbronchodilator TLC ≥ 100% predicted
Pre-rehabilitation postbronchodilator RV ≥ 150% predicted
FEV1 % predicted 20-35 %
Pre-rehabilitation room air, resting $PaCO_2$ ≤ 60 mm Hg (≤ 55 mm Hg in Denver)
Pre-rehabilitation room air, resting PaO_2 ≥ 45 mm Hg (≥ 30 mm Hg in Denver)
Body-mass index ≤ 32 (males) or ≤ 35 (females)
Nonsmoker for 6 months prior to initial review with negative urine cotinines
Completion pulmonary rehabilitation program (prior to surgery)

Table 3. Inclusion Criteria for LVRS at UWHC.

CT scan evidence of diffuse emphysema judged unsuitable for LVRS
Previous LVRS
Previous sternotomy (relative) or lobectomy
Significant untreated coronary disease
CHF and ejection fraction < 45%
Pulmonary hypertension: mean≥ 40 mm Hg or peak systolic >50 mm
History of recurrent infections with daily sputum production judged clinically significant
Daily use of > 20 mg of prednisone or its equivalent
Evidence of systemic disease or neoplasia that may compromise survival
Inability to complete screening, baseline data or pulmonary rehabilitation

Table 4. Exclusion Criteria for UWHC.

Questions remain regarding two patient groups, Alpha 1 antitrypsin and homogeneous emphysema. There is data to suggest benefit from LVRS in both patient populations. (29,30) The overall benefit has been less pronounced than patients with heterogeneous upper lobe predominant emphysema patients. Patients have been shown to have a slightly reduced survival without transplant when compared with upper lobe predominant group. (29) Our institution has not as yet recommended LVRS in homogeneous disease. Similarly, we recommend transplantation primarily for Alpha-1-antitrypsin, though LVRS is considered as a bridge to transplant in specific individuals.

6. Pre-operative evaluation

PreOperative assessment for LVRS should parallel evaluation for lung transplantation. The goals are similar: the patient should be physiologically capable of tolerating the procedure, there are no non-pulmonary conditions which exist that would limit the expected benefit of the procedure, and the pulmonary status is such that the patient's quality of life or overall health is positively impacted by the surgery. Referral is often through the auspices of lung transplantation at our institution. The advent of the lung allocation score has changed the lung transplant recipient profile substantially. Therefore, all patients referred with COPD/emphysema are additionally reviewed for LVRS.

Pulmonary evaluation begins with pulmonary function testing and 6 minute walk as an assessment of exercise tolerance. Clear indications for transplantation evaluation include FEV1 or DLCO ≤ 20% predicted. In patients with FEV1 ≥ 35% symptoms appear reasonably controlled with medical management alone and observation is typically recommended in our institution. Patients at higher risk of acute exacerbations post -operatively such as those with significant chronic bronchitic, asthmatic, or bronchiectatic components, may not be optimal surgical candidates. If COPD exacerbation occurs we generally delay surgery 1 month and confirm that steroid dosage is down to a level less than or equal to 10 mg /day. Computed Tomography scanning is performed with a graded degree of emphysema (1-4) in the upper, middle and lower lung fields. A change in score of 2 or more is considered significant and suggests heterogeneous disease.(14,31) We have found the lung perfusion scan to be immensely helpful in determining appropriate candidates and anecdotally in predicting response from surgery. The geometric mean of the perfusion score is quantitative and not dependent on the interpreting radiologist. CT scan quality may affect interpretation though this is less influential with improved technology and dissemination into the community.

The importance of perfusion scanning in determining appropriate patient selection has become evident. Recent analysis of the existing NETT data emphasized the importance of perfusion scintigraphy in the evaluation of potential LVRS patients. Low upper lobe perfusion was defined as less than 20% of blood flow to the upper third of the lungs. (24) We believe that this should be lateralized to 10% of perfusion per lung. In patients with upper lobe predominance and low exercise capacity who were confirmed as having low upper zone perfusion by scintigaraphy there was lower mortality with LVRS vs. medical therapy ($p=0.008$) Similarly, in upper lobe predominant emphysema and high exercise, patients with confirmed low upper lobe zone perfusion had lower mortality with LVRS ($p=0.02$). (24) Though perfusion scintigraphy this appears to be a predictor of mortality we cannot definitively state that it is a predictor of change in FEV1.

It is important to underscore the multidisciplinary nature of LVRS evaluation. In addition to meeting screening criteria and confirming an absence of comorbidity that would increase the risk of complication or mortality, patients should be medically optimized. This is crucial during pulmonary rehabilitation for the individuals to get the best response possible from this surgery. Minor modifications in COPD medications may be important such as discontinuing inhaled corticosteroid as this may be a risk factor for prolonged airleak.(32) Some have advocated preoperative initiation of B blockade or even amiodarone due to the high (approaching 25% incidence) of arrhythmia. We routinely administer prophylactic beta blockade B blockers in the immediate postoperative period in patients who are at high risk, but have not yet moved to more aggressive amiodarone regimen.

6.1 Technical considerations

Our institutional bias is to perform LVRS with bilateral thoracoscopy. We use lateral positioning, starting on the side that has greater perfusion, then repositioning for the contralateral side. The more severely affected lung is more likely to have significant air leak post resection. This may create ventilatory difficulty intraoperatively during single lung ventilation. A double lumen tube is preferred for lung isolation, though Arndt bronchial blockers have been used successfully. A three Port exposure is normally adequate. We recommend placing ports at the seventh intercostal space anterior axillary line, the fourth intercostal space anteriorly, and just inferior to the scapula. (figure 2) The amount of lung resected is based on surgeon discretion, estimating the residual pleural volume appropriate for the patient and the severity of the disease. Typically this means resection of approximately 40-50% of the left upper lobe volume and 50-60% of the right upper lobe volume. Resection is performed with a linear cutter stapling device and buttressing material. Surgeon preference dictates choice of both stapler and buttress material and there is no data suggesting significantly improved outcome with a specific model. (25,26) We do not routinely use sealant in our procedures, but perform an extended pleural tent extending from the 4th intercostal port site anteriorly around the apex and down to the hilum medially and posteriorly. Straight chest tubes are placed anteriorly and posteriorly extending to the height of the tent, not the apex of the bony thorax.

Surgical approach does not appear to significantly alter outcomes. In the NETT 90 day mortality and all cause mortality did not show significant differences. Mean operative time was less with median sternotomy (MS). Transfusion requirements were equivalent. There was a higher incidence of intraoperative complication in the VATS group related to a higher occurrence of hypoxemia. (24,27) A recent study by Boley and colleagues showed equivalent early outcomes with VATS and MS. Pain scores, narcotic requirement and incentive spirometry scores were similar (27). The NETT did show some differences. At 30 days post LVRS a higher percentage of VATS patients were living independently than MS patients, 80% vs 70% respectively. (22) Surprisingly, though functional outcomes were equivalent at 1 and 2 years, LVRS related cost and total medical costs were higher for MS patients than VATS patients. (24) My personal and institutional preference for VATS stems from the following. A more effective pleural tent can be created with VATS than median sternotomy. Second is my concern that sternal precautions limits early return to preoperative lifestyle. A VATS LVRS patient can be back to driving 2 weeks after discharge which I would not allow in MS patients.

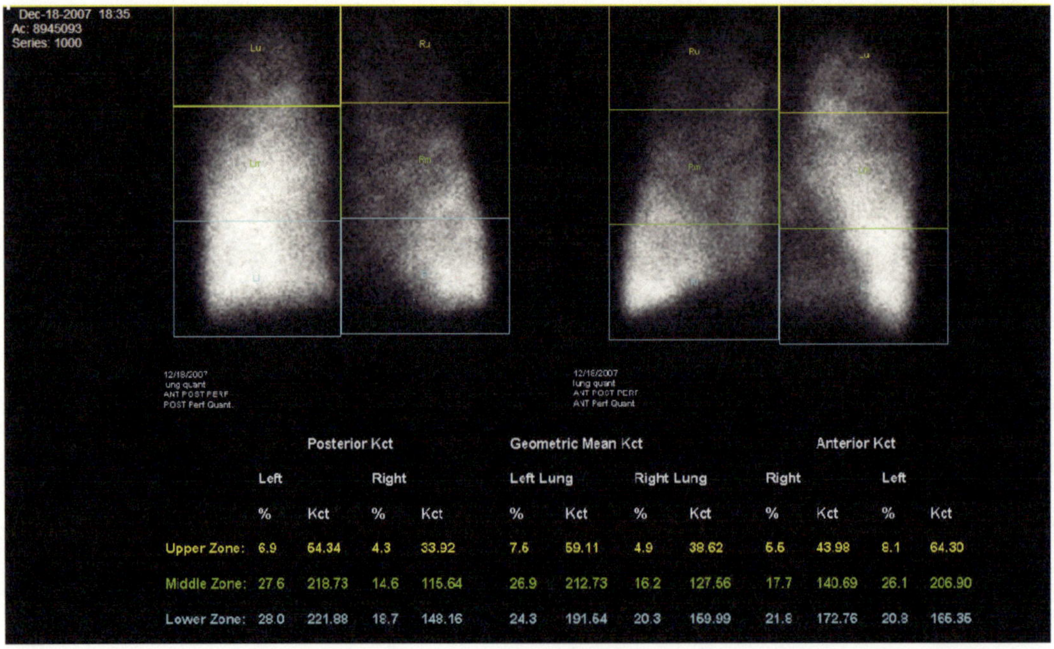

Fig. 1. Perfusion scan demonstrating favorable upper lobe distribution of emphysema.

Unilateral LVRS in patients with anatomic or other contraindications to bilateral therapy has been reported. Meyers et al showed that FEV1 was increased 32% at 12months and 28% at 3 years.(33) Exercise capacity and QOL measures were also improved. The increase in FEV1 however, was not maintained at 5 years. (33) This reflects our experience in unilateral LVRS and patients undergoing incidental LVR effects during upper lobectomy for lung malignancy.

6.2 Peri-operative care

Perioperative care for LVRS patients in our institution is provided in an adaptable acuity care unit for cardiothoracic surgical patients. All beds within the Unit are ICU capable and require only an electronic order to change patient status. Not all patients require ICU care, however it is easily and immediately available when required. In our recent series 25% of patients required ICU care. One patient remained intubated overnight after a combined robotic off pump coronary artery bypass and LVRS. Three patients required reintubation. In all three patients, we moved quickly to tracheostomy and all were off ventilator support at the time of discharge. Average days in the ICU is 2, reflecting the few patients who have been reintubated and required tracheostomy. Overall median LOS was 7 days in our series. We have had no 30 or 90 day mortality. Mean preoperative FEV1 was 26% predicted and mean FEV1 increase was 44% over baseline. The extent of quantifiable respiratory functional improvement is variable, as demonstrated in Table 2

Pain control postoperatively is quite different from our thoracic oncology patients due to the frequent need for prolonged chest drainage and the bilateral nature of the procedure. We use a combination of epidural and oral narcotic analgesics. We try to avoid ketoralac and other NSAIDs in the early postoperative period. An aggressive respiratory therapy protocol is used for pulmonary toilet. With this approach we have reduced our need for bronchoscopy for secretion clearance. In patients where unilateral or staged LVRS is performed we employ a protocol similar to that for lobectomy. Paravertebral blocks for preemptive pain control and patient controlled or oral narcotic analgesia are utilized. Chest tubes are maintained to water seal unless subcutaneous emphysema or increasing pneumothorax develops. Air leaks are currently the most common reason for longer LOS. Examining the NETT data, following LVRS 90% of patients had air leak at some point within 30 days of surgery. (22) Median air leak duration was 7 days, but 12% had air leaks > 30 days. As expected air leak was longer in patients with lower FEV1. Post operative complications were greater in patients with a prolonged air leak and the post-operative stay was longer. With new ways of managing air leaks as an outpatient there is less effect on LOS. Easily maintained, miniature, waterless pleural drainage systems have allowed safe discharge with weekly outpatient clinic visits. These drainage systems allow extra time healing and give patients more mobility post discharge.

6.3 LVRS as alternative to lung transplant

Comparisons of LVRS to lung transplant have been reported. However, it is currently not a fair comparison as patients who undergo LVRS would not generate a LAS high enough to be considered for lung transplantation. A retrospective series compared functional outcomes (pulmonary function tests, arterial blood gas analysis, six-minute walk distance) in 33 patients who underwent LVRS versus 39 patients who had single lung transplantation and 27 patients who had bilateral sequential lung transplantation (34). The patients were evaluated before the operation and at 3, 6, and 12 months after surgery. In the LVRS group mean FEV1 improved by 79% and 82% at 6 and 9 months, respectively. Improvement in PFTS was far more dramatic in the transplant population. Mean FEV1 increases were over 200% in the single lung transplant group and approaching 500% in the bilateral lung transplant group. 6 MW showed similar differences in response(34). While lung transplant demonstrated far superior function at 12 months than LVRS, improvements in survival for COPD patients from lung transplant have been difficult to identify though it appears from recently published reports that adjusted mortality is improved with lung transplant in COPD patients with a high LAS.(35) Overall survival after lung transplantation at one and 3 years is currently 84% and 70% respectively.(36) This is juxtaposed to the results of LVRS. Longterm follow-up of NETT data published in 2006 demonstrated improved survival in the upper lobe predominant, low exercise capacity cohort.(22) In another recent series three year survival was 95%. (26)

Organ availability is currently the major limitation in lung transplantation. Organ allocation has therefore been a matter of much controversy. The lung transplant population has had a remarkable shift in the last 5 years due to the Lung Allocation Score. Components of the score are listed in table 6 (37). Of Note FEV1 is not present within the scoring system though it appears to have an effect on mortality and is represented in the Bode Index. In 2000, 43% of lung transplants done within the US were for COPD and 14.6%for IPF. In 2008 that ratio had shifted to 28.6% and 33.5% for COPD and IPF, respectively (36). Shortly after initiation of the LAS, we reviewed patients undergoing evaluation for lung transplantation at the William S. Middleton Memorial VA Hospital to determine the need for a dedicated LVRS program. 162 patients were referred from 2002 to 2007. 69 patients were listed and 93 deferred. 60% of the deferred group (56 patients) had COPD. 29% met screening criteria for LVRS. (Maloney, unpublished abstract). We compared the functional status and overall severity of disease as measured by an estimated Lung Allocation Score (LAS) between the 29 patients who met criteria for LVRS and patients undergoing lung transplant during that time period. In addition to demographic differences there was a significant difference in LAS. (table 7) The mean age was older in the LVRS group but the value was not statistically significant.

LVRS has been used as a bridge to transplant. As with any re-operative technique there is increased complexity related to postoperative scarring and adhesion. Dissection of the hilum with phrenic nerve injury or praxia is the foremost concern. In one prospective study, LVRS prior to lung transplantation improved symptoms and lung function enough to delay lung transplantation for a median of 33 months. A second series stated LVRS could potentially delay lung transplant for up to five years.(39) Patients undergoing LVRS prior to transplant had a similar response to surgical intervention as patients not being considered for transplantation, with the exception of lower lung field predominance which had a shorter duration of improvement. (39,40)

Patient 1				
	PreOP	%	Post OP	%
FVC	1.76	59	2.53	84
FEV1	0.51	23	0.77	35
Patient 2				
	PreOP	%	Post OP	%
FVC	1.53	51	2.61	81
FEV1	0.47	21	1.09	40

Table 5. Representative Patient data demonstrating the variability of response to LVRS.

Lung Diagnosis
Date of birth
Functional Status
Assisted Ventilation
Height and Weight
Diabetes
Supplemental Oxygen
Percent predicted FVC
Six minute walk distance
Serum creatinine
PA pressures (especially systolic & mean)
Pulmonary capillary wedge mean
PCO2

Table 6. Data elements used in determining the LAS.

LVRS	Transplant	
Age 61	Age 54	NS
LAS (estimated) 31.9	LAS 43.9	P=0.0154
	FEV1 16.4 ± 3.7	

Table 7. Comparison of potential LVRS patients to transplant recipients after adopting LAS as means for recipient selection.

1. Anatomic lobar resection of the most hyperinflated lobe is performed through an axillary muscle sparing thoracotomy.
2. The medial anterior mediastinal parietal pleura is incised in a craniocaudal fashion, ideally from the apex to the diaphragm.
3. Using primarily blunt, manually assisted dissection, generous pleural flaps are developed.
4. Ideally these flaps are dissected back to the edge of remaining lung (anterior flap) and to the medial hilum (posterior flap)
5. The pleural flaps are trimmed (if needed), overlapped (in whichever orientation seems most appropriate), and tacked in place with 3-0 braided, absorbable suture.

Table 8. Mediastinal Pexy Technique for native lung hypertrophy after Single lung transplant

7. LVRS post lung transplant

Although the optimal approach to end-stage COPD is argued, the International Society for Heart and Lung Transplantation Registry demonstrates that single lung transplant for COPD has been the most common lung transplantation procedure performed.(40) When single lung transplant is performed, there is risk of developing native lung hyperinflation. A percentage of these patients have decreased function resulting from graft compression by the native lung, which can compromise oxygenation, pulmonary function tests and exercise capacity. While the physiology of the transplanted lung becomes restrictive, the overall pulmonary function picture is one of obstruction dominated by the native lung. Chest CT scans can facilitate diagnosis in these patients, with demonstration of increasing native lung expansion at the cost of allograft volume. It is critical to identify chronic rejection or bronciolitis obliterans syndrome prior to native LVRS as mortality in this setting is prohibitive. Bronchoscpy with biopsy, lung scintigraphy, PFTs and CT imaging are helpful but clinical suspicion of confounding causes of functional decline can be difficult to rule out. Native side LVRS (nLVRS) was first described in such patients in the 1990's although it remains an uncommon procedure. (41) Both anatomic and non-anatomic resection has been described for this purpose. The largest series, comprised of 8 pts, was reported by Reece et al in 2008. (42) This experience and others show that while nLVRS can reliably relieve graft compression and improve lung function/patient symptomatology, it is high risk with considerable morbidity and mortality. It is important to note that the patterns of disease amenable to LVRS as determined by the National Emphysema Treatment Trial do not necessarily apply to the post-transplant patient given that the main problem is compression of the functional transplant lung graft. Much of the morbidity following nLVRS is owed to prolonged air leak and infectious complication in the native lung. We have developed a technique of mediastinal pexy that fixes the mediastinum towards, and minimizes pleural space on the volume reduced side.

2004	2010
27 transplants total	37 transplants total
12/27 COPD = 44.4%	8/37 COPD = 21.6 %
7/27 IPF = 25.9%	15/37 IPF = 40.5%

Table 9. UW distribution of Lung transplants by disease

7.1 Technique

1. Anatomic lobar resection of the most hyperinflated lobe is performed through an axillary muscle sparing thoracotomy.
2. The medial anterior mediastinal parietal pleura is incised in a craniocaudal fashion, ideally from the apex to the diaphragm.
3. Using primarily blunt, manually assisted dissection, generous pleural flaps are developed.
4. Ideally these flaps are dissected back to the edge of remaining lung (anterior flap) and to the medial hilum (posterior flap)
5. The pleural flaps are trimmed (if needed), overlapped (in whichever orientation seems most appropriate), and tacked in place with 3-0 braided, absorbable suture.

The 20% mortality rate in the largest series of this technique underscores the high-risk nature of this procedure. Both patient mortalities in Reece's series ultimately died of infectious respiratory complications, one in the setting of bronchial stump leak and the other was ultimately diagnosed with bronchiolitis obliterans at autopsy. The average ICU LOS was 13d and average hospital LOS was 21 days. Their functional results were excellent with 87.5% of patients having significant and sustained pulmonary function and symptom improvement. Other authors have reported smaller experiences with 1-yr survival rates of 50% or less. (41,42) We propose that the mediastinal pexy technique allows for both minimization and fixation of pleural space on the volume reduced side greater than can be achieved with standard pleural tenting and/or physiologic shifting following volume reduction. Our experience is small but encouraging. ICU length of stay is less than previously reported and there seems to be at least a trend towards decreased chest tube duration. Other authors have reported use of endobronchial valves acutely for native lung hyperinflation (43).

8. Endobronchial treatments for LVRS

Bronchoscopic techniques for volume reduction of emphysematous lung are inherently attractive because of decreased periprocedural mortality and morbidity. Currently available data on efficacy of bronchoscopic lung volume reduction are not conclusive. Patients appear to derive a subjective benefit in relief of dyspnea, however improvements in spirometry or exercise tolerance have not been demonstrated. Endobronchial technique for LVR include; one-way endobronchial valves implanted into the airway, self-activating coils, targeted destruction and remodeling of emphysematous tissue and bypass tract airway stenting. Of the multiple forms of bronchoscopic therapy we will concentrate on endobrochial valves which have the most data, and touch briefly on other options.

8.1 Endobronchial valves

Endobronchial valves are designed to exclude the most emphysematous regions from ventilation and reduce air trapping. Valves allow expiration, but prevent any distal flow during inspiration (44). There are two distinct endobronchial valve designs; duckbill (zephyr) and umbrella-shaped (spiration) valves. The VENT trial was a prospective multicenter randomized trial comparing endobronchial valve therapy to medical management.(44,45) Post procedure (6 month) FEV1 increased 4.3% over baseline and an increase in 6MW of 2.5%. Though both were statistically significant it is hard to determine the clinical value of these increases. In patients with complete fissures, the increase in FEV1 was 17%. Patients showed subjective improvements based on St. George Respiratory Questionnaire (SGRQ). Major complications occurred in 6% demonstrating safety. Acute COPD exacerbations however were increased substantially over the medically managed group. The Spiration IBV valve did not demonstrate increased FEV1 or quantitative functional assessment. Subjective improvements were seen in some patients. Morbidity and mortality also were low demonstrating feasibility and safety of the device. (44) Lobar atelectasis appears to be evidence of clinically favorable response to valve placement. Less than 25% of reported cases achieved this effect. (45,46) Of note neither device is approved in the US for volume reduction in emphysema. The spiration IBV valve is approved for persistent air leaks and there is good documentation of its efficacy in that arena.(47)
The greatest limitation in effective endobronchial LVR is crossventilation. Incomplete fissures between lobes of the lung and collateral ventilation accounts for this finding. However, the greatest benefits appear to be found in patients who actually do develop such target lobe atelectasis because of favorable changes in chest wall dimensions. (22,48) If valves are to be used in the future, bronchoscopic LVR trials may need to incorporate assessment techniques to preferentially select patients with high collateral ventilation resistance as they are more likely to obtain greater benefit. Other means of bronchoscopic LVR are not as affected by cross ventilation and may have greater long term value.

8.2 Biological lung volume reduction

Biological agents aim to reduce lung volume by sealing off the most emphysematous areas. The rapidly polymerizing sealant is designed to work at the alveolar level rather than in the airways. The mechanism of action involves resorption atelectasis from airway occlusion, subsequent airspace inflammation, and then remodeling resulting in contraction of lung parenchyma. This therapy should not be affected by collateral ventilation as it works on an alveolar level.

The sealant, a mixture of fibrinogen suspension and thrombin solution, is instilled into targeted areas determined by preoperative imaging. Serious adverse events were limited and no fatalities documented. Improvement was identified in FEV_1 (38% to 44%); 6-minute walk (27%), and in SGRQ (32% to 46%). Concern has been expressed regarding the longevity of the treatment as smaller dose therapy did not appear to maintain results even with short term follow up. (49)

8.3 LVRC

Lung volume reduction coils (LVRS) are wire implants placed into the parenchyma bronchoscopically. The coil once deployed, acts to contract the tissue leading to a volume reduction effect. This concept is not affected by the influence of cross ventilation, so may have an advantage over endobronchial valves. A small series has been reported that demonstrated safety and additional trials are necessary to confirm efficacy. (50)

9. Cost-effectiveness of LVRS

As discussed previously the costs of caring for patients with COPD are staggering and increase as the severity of emphysema worsens regardless of therapy used to palliate the disease. However, it is a small portion of patients with emphysema and even smaller percentage that are candidates for LVRS. A review of the NETT data showed that costs for LVRS was higher than best medical care and this was confirmed in a different healthcare system in a Canadian trial. (51,52) The mean total costs per person ($98,952 vs. $62,560, $p<0.001$) and per-person medical costs ($80,818 vs. $43,689, $p<0.001$) at three years.(49,51) Cost effectiveness for LVRS improves over time as care for a medically managed patient increases in expense. There is a significant difference in costs for the four groups defined by the NETT. The cost-effectiveness of LVRS vs. medical therapy was $140,000 per quality-adjusted life-year (QALY) gained at 5 years, and was projected to be $54,000 per QALY gained at 10 years. In the subgroup with upper lobe–predominant emphysema and low baseline exercise capacity, which showed the greatest overall benefits after LVRS, the cost per quality-adjusted life year gained was $98,000 at 3 years and $21,000 at 10 years.(53) Bronchoscopic LVR is less costly initially, but without a significant change in BODE score that decrease in amount per QALY seen in surgical LVRS over time may not occur. The financial impact of endobronchial therapy is not trivial as workup, implants, and surveillance are costly, and potentially without the quantifiable improvement of surgical therapy. As healthcare dollars become less available we must make sure that emerging therapies are measured against the gold standard of surgical LVRS instead of being driven by market forces. At the same time we must continue to improve morbidity and mortality in LVRS which will limit costs related to adverse events.

10. Summary

LVRS along with supplemental oxygen and smoking cessation is only one of few therapies that can improve survival in selected patients with severe emphysema. Despite the impressive conclusions demonstrated by the NETT data and more recent trials that show substantial benefit, relatively few patients undergo LVRS relative to the prevalence of emphysema.(24) In 2009 118 medicare patients underwent the procedure based on STS data. This number is down from approximately 250 patients in 2004, shortly after the initial NETT data was published. At that time in 2004 there were 42 approved centers. This number has decreased as participation in the NETT no longer results in automatic center approval. Only CMS certified centers and transplant centers now may be reimbursed through medicare for the procedure. In addition, some of the LVRS literature has stigmatized the surgery, suggesting that the risk is prohibitive. Many pulmonologists remain unaware of the benefits of LVRS and the consistently improving procedure related morbidity, mortality and LOS. Also as non-surgical options consistently achieve below expected results and remain investigational, the pulmonary community loses interest. One appropriate ongoing concern is the cost of therapy to the healthcare system as funds become increasingly limited. This will minimize cost and improve the QALY in comparison to best medical treatment. Education of the community pulmonologist and availability of information to patients will limit referrals to patients who are likely to benefit from surgery. This too will minimize costs in patient evaluation. Another is that LVRS functional and quantitative PFTS results show substantial variation between patients. Ongoing assessment of more recent LVRS series will be crucial in determining predictive capabilties of preoperative testing and minimizing morbidity and streamlining care and hospital stay.

11. References

[1] Brantigan OC, Mueller E, Kress MB. A surgical approach to pulmonary emphysema. Am Rev Respir Dis 1959; 80:194.

[2] National Heart Lung and Blood Institute. Morbidity and Mortality: 2009 Chart Book on Cardiovascular, Lung and Blood Diseases.

[3] Centers for Disease Control and Prevention. National Center for Health Statistics. National Health & Nutrition Examination Survey, 1988-1994.

[4] Rennard SI, Vestbo J. COPD: the dangerous underestimate of 15%. Lancet 2006; 367:1216.

[5] Buist AS, McBurnie MA, Vollmer WM, et al. International variation in the prevalence of COPD (the BOLD Study): a population-based prevalence study. Lancet 2007; 370:741.

[6] Petty, RL, Nett, LM. COPD: Prevention in the primary care setting, The National Lung Health Education Program, 2001. p.341.

[7] Bridges RB, Wyatt RJ, Rehm SR. Effects of smoking on inflammatory mediators and their relationship to pulmonary dysfunction Eur J Respir Dis Suppl. 1986;146:145-52.

[8] Global strategy for the diagnosis, management, and prevention of chronic obstructive pulmonary disease: Executive summary 2006. Global Initiative for Chronic Obstructive Lung Disease (GOLD). http://www.goldcopd.org (Accessed on December 14, 2009).

[9] Standards for the diagnosis and care of patients with chronic obstructive pulmonary disease. American Thoracic Society. Am J Respir Crit Care Med 1995; 152:S77.

[10] BTS guidelines for the management of chronic obstructive pulmonary disease. The COPD Guidelines Group of the Standards of Care Committee of the BTS. Thorax 1997; 52 Suppl 5:S1.

[11] GINA report, global strategy for asthma management and prevention 2006. Global Initiative for Asthma (GINA) http://www.ginasthma.com (Accessed on August 31, 2007).

[12] Hogg JC. Pathophysiology of airflow limitation in chronic obstructive pulmonary disease. Lancet 2004; 364:709.

[13] Obstructive lung disease. Med Clin North Am 1990; 74:547.

[14] Radiology paper

[15] Travaline j, Sudarshan S, Obrien G, Kuzma AM, Furukawa S. Effect of lung volume reduction surgery on diaphragm strength. Am J Respir Crit Care Med 157: 1578–1585, 1998.

[16] Martinez FJ, deOca MM, Whyte RI, Stetz J, Gay SE, Celli BR. Lung-volume reduction improves dyspnea, dynamic hyperinflation, and respiratory muscle function. Am J Respir Crit Care Med 155: 1984–1990, 1997.

[17] Cremona G, Barbara J, Melgosa T, Appendini L, Roca J, Casaio C. Mechanisms of gas exchange response to lung volume reduction surgery in severe emphysema. J Appl Physiol. 2011 Apr;110(4):1036-45. Epub 2011 Jan 13

[18]

[19] J.D. Cooper, A.G. Patterson, S.R. Sundaresan, E.P. Trulock, R.D. Yusen, M.S. Pohl and S.S. Lefrak, Results of 150 consecutive bilateral lung volume reduction procedures in patients with severe emphysema, J Thorac Cardiovasc Surg 112 (1996), pp. 1319–1330.

[20] NETT Research Group. Rationale and design of the national emphysema treatment trial,A prospective randomized trial of lung volume reduction surgery. Chest. 1999;116:1750

[21] A. Fishman, F. Martinez, K. Naunheim et al., "A randomized trial comparing lung-volume-reduction surgery with medical therapy for severe emphysema," The New England Journal of Medicine, vol. 348, no. 21, pp. 2059–2073, 2003.

[22] Naunheim KS, Wood DE, Mohsenifar Z, et al. Long-term follow-up of patients receiving lung-volume-reduction surgery versus medical therapy for severe emphysema by the National Emphysema Treatment Trial Research Group. Ann Thorac Surg 2006; 82:431.

[23] National Emphysema Treatment Trial Research Group. Patients at high risk of death after lung-volume-reduction surgery. N Engl J Med 2001; 345:1075.

[24] Criner GJ, Cordova F, Sternberg AL, Martinez FJ. The NETT: Part II- Lessons learned about lung volume reduction surgery. Am J Respir Crit Care Med. 2011 Jun 30. [Epub ahead of print]

[25] M. M. DeCamp, R. J. McKenna, C. C. Deschamps, and M. J. Krasna, "Lung volume reduction surgery: technique, operative mortality, and morbidity," Proceedings of the American Thoracic Society, vol. 5, no. 4, pp. 442–446, 2008

[26] Ginsburg ME, Thomashow BM, Yip CK, DiMango AM, Maxfield RA, Bartels MN, Jellen P, Bulman WA, Lederer D, Brogan FL, Gorenstein LA, Sonett JR. Lung volume reduction surgery using the NETT selection criteria. Ann Thorac Surg. 2011 May;91(5):1556-60; discussion 1561. Epub 2011 Apr 2

[27] Boley TM, Reid A, Manning BT, Markwell SJ, Vassileva CM, Hazelrigg SR.Sternotomy or bilateral thoracospy: pain and post-operative complicationsafter lung-volume reduction surgery. Eur J Cardiothorac Surg. 2011 May 19. [Epub ahead of print]

[28] Imfeld S, Bloch KE, Weder W, Russi EW. The BODE index after lung volume reduction surgery correlates with survival. Chest 2006; 129:873.

[29] Weder W, Tutic M, Bloch KE. Lung volume reduction surgery in nonheterogeneous emphysema. Thorac Surg Clin. 2009 May;19(2):193-9.

[30] Donahue JM, Cassivi SD. Lung volume reduction surgery for patients with alpha-1 antitrypsin deficiency emphysema. Thorac Surg Clin. 2009 May;19(2):201-8.

[31] Washko GR, Hoffman E, Reilly JJ. Radiographic evaluation of the potential lung volume reduction surgery candidate. Proc Am Thorac Soc 2008; 5:421.

[32] DeCamp MM Jr, Lipson D, Krasna M, Minai OA, McKenna RJ Jr, Thomashow BM The evaluation and preparation of the patient for lung volume reduction surgery. Proc Am Thorac Soc. 2008 May 1;5(4):427-31

[33] Meyers BF, Sultan PK, Guthrie TJ, et al. Outcomes after unilateral lung volume reduction. Ann Thorac Surg 2008; 86:204.

[34] Gaissert HA, Trulock EP, Cooper JD, et al. Comparison of early functional results after volume reduction or lung transplantation for chronic obstructive pulmonary disease. J Thorac Cardiovasc Surg 1996; 111:296.

[35] OPTN/SRTR database annual report 2009

[36] Chest. 2007 Nov;132(5):1646-51

[37] Tutic M, Lardinois D, Imfeld S, et al. Lung-volume reduction surgery as an alternative or bridging procedure to lung transplantation. Ann Thorac Surg 2006; 82:208.

[38] Meyers BF, Yusen RD, Guthrie TJ, et al. Outcome of bilateral lung volume reduction in patients with emphysema potentially eligible for lung transplantation. J Thorac Cardiovasc Surg 2001; 122:10.

[39] Nathan SD, Edwards LB, Barnett SD, et al. Outcomes of COPD lung transplant recipients after lung volume reduction surgery. Chest 2004; 126:1569.

[40] E.P. Trulock, L.B. Edwards, D.O. Taylor, M.M. Boucek, B.M. Keck and M.I. Hertz et al., Registry of the International Society for Heart and Lung Transplantation: twenty-third official adult lung and heart-lung transplantation report—2006, J Heart Lung Transplant 25 (2006), pp. 880–892.

[41] Fitton, B.T. Bethea, M.C. Borja, D.D. Yuh, S.C. Yang and J.B. Orens et al., Pulmonary resection following lung transplantation, Ann Thorac Surg 76 (2003), pp. 1680–1685.

[42] Reece TB, Mitchell JD, Zamora MR, Fullerton DA, Cleveland JC, Pomerantz M, Lyu DM, Grover FL, Weyant MJ. Native lung volume reduction surgery relieves functional graft compression after single-lung transplantation for chronic obstructive pulmonary disease. J Thorac Cardiovasc Surg. 2008 Apr;135(4):931-7.

[43] Crespo MM, Johnson BA, McCurry KR, Landreneau RJ, Sciurba FC. Use of endobronchial valves for native lung hyperinflation associated with respiratory

failure in a single-lung transplant recipient for emphysema. Chest. 2007 Jan;131(1):214-6.
[44] I. Y. P. Wan, T. P. Toma, D. M. Geddes et al., "Bronchoscopic lung volume reduction for end-stage emphysema: report on the first 98 patients," Chest, vol. 129, no. 3, pp. 518–526, 2006.
[45] F. C. Sciurba, A. Ernst, F. J.F. Herth et al., "A randomized study of endobronchial valves for advanced emphysema," The New England Journal of Medicine, vol. 363, no. 13, pp. 1233–1244, 2010.
[46] S. C. Springmeyer, C. T. Bolliger, T. K. Waddell, X. Gonzalez, and D. E. Wood, "Treatment of heterogeneous emphysema using the spiration IBV valves," Thoracic Surgery Clinics, vol. 19, no. 2, pp. 247–253, 2009.
[47] J. M. Travaline, R. J. McKenna, T. De Giacomo et al., "Treatment of persistent pulmonary air leaks using endobronchial valves," Chest, vol. 136, no. 2, pp. 355–360, 2009.
[48] E. J. Cetti, A. J. Moore, and D. M. Geddes, "Collateral ventilation," Thorax, vol. 61, no. 5, pp. 371–373, 2006.
[49] Berger RL, Decamp MM, Criner GJ, Celli BR Lung volume reduction therapies for advanced emphysema: an update. Chest. 2010 Aug;138(2):407-17.
[50] F. J. Herth, R. Eberhard, D. Gompelmann, D. -J. Slebos, and A. Ernst, "Bronchoscopic lung volume reduction with a dedicated coil: a clinical pilot study," Therapeutic Advances in Respiratory Disease, vol. 4, no. 4, pp. 225–231, 2010.
[51] Ramsey SD, Berry K, Etzioni R, et al. Cost effectiveness of lung-volume-reduction surgery for patients with severe emphysema. N Engl J Med 2003; 348:2092.
[52] Miller JD, Malthaner RA, Goldsmith CH, et al. A randomized clinical trial of lung volume reduction surgery versus best medical care for patients with advanced emphysema: a two-year study from Canada. Ann Thorac Surg 2006; 81:314.
[53] Ramsey SD, Shroyer AL, Sullivan SD, Wood DE. Updated evaluation of the cost-effectiveness of lung volume reduction surgery. Chest 2007; 131:823.

20

Endoscopic Lung Volume Reduction for Emphysema

Paulo F. Guerreiro Cardoso
Department of Cardio-Pneumology, Division of Thoracic Surgery,
Heart Institute (InCor)-Hospital das Clínicas,
Faculdade de Medicina, Universidade de São Paulo,
Brazil

1. Introduction

In advanced stages of emphysema there is a sequence of events that start with hyperinflation, followed by a reduction in diaphragmatic mobility, an increase in resting pleural pressures that intensifies expiratory muscle recruitment and reduces elastic recoil of the lungs.

During exercise, the limitation to expiratory flow prolongs the expiratory phase causing dynamic hyperinflation and ultimately reducing exercise tolerance. Such factors altogether will predispose to respiratory infections, will cause body mass consumption, muscular deconditioning and weight loss. This ominous cycle of events in the emphysema patient impacts negatively and progressively on the quality of life. The patient experiences breathlessness during ordinary activities and even at rest. At this stage of the disease process, palliation becomes a more relevant goal than increased longevity (Berger, Decamp et al. 2010).

The medical treatment of this condition includes bronchodilators, costicosteroids, oxygen and the management of exacerbations and infections. The pulmonary rehabilitation programs, when added to the medical management has been shown to reduce dyspnea, improve quality of life, reduce the frequency of hospital admitions but it does not impact on survival (ATS 1999).

The current options for the surgical treatment are surgical ablation of bulous disease (bullectomy), lung volume reduction surgery (LVRS) and lung transplantation. Despite its unequivocal benefits in selected patients, all such procedures carry a considerable morbidity and mortality.

The LVRS was initially proposed by Brantigan in the 1950's, but mortality was a major issue in the early years (Brantigan, Mueller et al. 1959). In the 1990's, Cooper et al published the first successful, series of pacientes submitted to LVRS (Cooper, Patterson et al. 1996). This was followed by randomized studies that demonstrated functional benefits and acceptable mortality in patients with low exercise capacity and upper lobe predominant heterogeneous disease (Ciccone, Meyers et al. 2003). Despite the promising results of LVRS, mortality has remained high and duration of the benefits remained a controversial issue as shown in the National Emphysema Treatment Trial (NETT) (Fishman, Martinez et al. 2003). The application of LVRS for homogeneous emphysema has added to the controversy (Weder,

Tutic et al. 2009). A recent reassessment of the NETT results revealed that only 45% of the LVRS were actually performed in upper lobe predominant heterogeneous emphysema, and more that one half of the patients were lost to follow up at 5 years, both in the medical and the surgical arms of the trial (Sanchez 2009).
The loss of enthusiasm in LVRS was followed by the development of several endoscopic methods and devices for lung volume reduction. There have been several experimental and clinical studies on such devices based on the asumption that a bronchoscopic procedure is less invasive and a safer alternative for achieving LVR. Furthermore, a non-surgical procedure will probably extend the current indications for LVR, resulting in a broader access to a larger number of patients with emphysema (Herth, Gompelmann et al. 2010).
This chapter focuses on the description of the current methods and devices for bronchoscopic lung volume reduction for emphysema and the results of the clinical trials.

2. Principles of bronchoscopic lung volume reduction (BLVR)

Some procedures have shared the same principle of LVRS in which, by reducing the hyperinflated lung size, there is an improvement in elastic recoil of the emphysematous lungs and consequently in the breathing mechanics (Ingenito, Wood et al. 2008).
The one-way valves promote size reduction as a result of selective atelectasis mostly when the devices are applied in the upper lobes. However, this relies upon poor collateral ventilation in order to function properly and to provide sizeable volume reduction (Gompelmann, Eberhardt et al. 2010). A complete fissure is a feature that ensures that there is little or no connection with the ajacent lobe, and therefore less collateral ventilation.
Biologic lung volume reduction (BioLVR) uses polymers administered endobronchially to produce a similar effect. It causes selective occlusion of segmental areas where it is instilled, and blocks collateral ventilation because of the inflammatory reaction it causes across the area treated and permeates deeply into the alveoli. Such properties makes BioLVR amenable to be used for either homogeneous or heterogeneous emphysema.
The production of local fibrosis has also been attempted using endobronchial thermal vapor ablation. The principle here is a definitive volume reduction, only achieved at the cost of an inflammatory response and subsequent local scarring that is not reversible (Snell, Hopkins et al. 2009).
The emphysema with predominantly homogeneous destruction calls for different measures. The principle is opposed to what is found in heterogeneous emphysema. Collateral ventilation is usually abundant in homogeneous emphysema, and the procedure must take advantage of it. The production of extra-anatomic passages communicating the distal bronchi with the lung parenchyma is known as airway bypass. This was originally proposed as communications or "spiracles" between the lung and the chest wall (Macklem 1978; Moore, Cetti et al. 2010). Recently, this procedure was then modified to accomodate such passages within the bronchi, thus enabling it to be performed bronchoscopically (Choong, Macklem et al. 2008). This procedure will reduce hyperinflation and provide a diaphragmatic remodelling that will ultimately improve ventilatory mechanics.

3. Devices and results

The devices developed for endoscopic treatment of heterogeneous emphysema can be divided into 3 categories: Blocking devices (e.g. one-way valves); Reversible non-blocking or removable (e.g. *coils*); Non-reversible or non-blocking definitive (e.g. vapor thermoablation, endobronchial polymers, airway bypass).

3.1 Blocking devices

3.1.1 One-way valves

These devices have been validated for clinical use in some countries. The Zephyr® (Pulmonx, Redwood City-CA, EUA) (FIGURE 1) is a model that can be placed bronchoscopically.

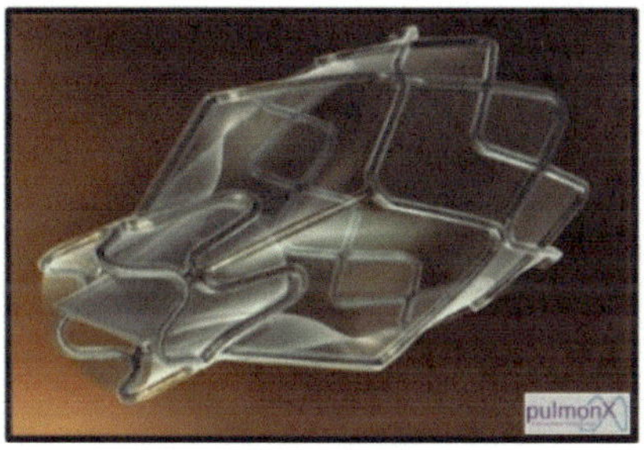

Fig. 1. The Zephyr® one-way valve (Pulmonx, Redwood City-CA, USA)

The success of the procedure is related to presence of complete fissures, high heterogeneity and the presence of atelectasis of the treated lobe. The manufaturer has recently introduced a device for measuring collateral flow which is composed of a catheter with a baloon tip and a flow transducer Chartis™, Pulmonx, Redwood City-CA, EUA) (Figure 2).

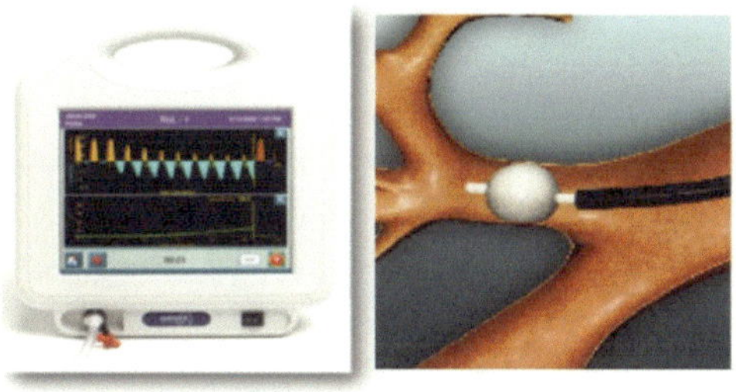

Fig. 2. The console and catheter for the measurement of collateral ventilation (Chartis® system; Pulmonx, Redwood City-CA, USA).

Once the target area is identified radiologically, the catheter is passed through the working channel of the bronchoscope, advanced into the lobar bronchus, the baloon tip is inflated in place occluding the bronchus. The collateral ventilation is then measured on site by the flow transducer connected to the tip of the catheter (Aljuri and Freitag 2009). This allows the examiner to choose the area with the least collateral ventilation for installing the valves. A study with 25 patients using this method of measuring collateral flow showed that in 90% of the cases the resistance measurements correlated with the post-implantation atelectasis visualized on a chest X-ray (Gompelmann, Eberhardt et al. 2010).

The clinical studies carried out so far have been done in a heterogeneous population of emphysema patients and this has impacted the results negatively. A safety and efficacy non-randomized study showed that 90 days post-implant of one-way valves has revealed a 4,9% decrease in residual volume (RV) and a 10% increase in FEV1. There were 8% serious adverse events and 1% mortality (Wan, Toma et al. 2006).

To date, the largest randomized study with one-way valves was the **VENT** study (**V**alve for **E**mphysema PalliatioN **T**rial). There were 321 patients included accross 31 centers in the United States and 23 centers in Europe. Major inclusion criteria were: FEV1 between 15-45%; RV ≥ 150% and total lung capacity (TLC) ≥ 100% predicted. All patients underwent a full pulmonary rehabilitation program before and after the procedure. A 2:1 randomization (treatment with valves : control with best medical care) resulted in 214 patients receiving valves and the results have been published recently (Sciurba, Ernst et al.). At 6 months there was a small but significant improvement in FEV1 of 4,3% with a mean difference between treatment versus control group of 6,8% ($p<0.005$). There was a 2,5% increase in exercise tolerance on the 6-minute walk test (6MWT) in the treatment group, versus a decrease of -3,4% in the control group (mean difference of 5,8% $p=0.04$). There were small improvements in dyspnea, a reduction in suplemmental O_2 requirements (-12L/day), and better quality of life (-3,4 points in the St. George Respiratory Questionnaire).
The high heterogeneity (> 15% between lobes by CT) subset analysis at 6 months post-procedure showed that enhanced effects on FEV1 improvements of 10,7% ($p=0,004$) and of 12,4% in the 6MWT ($p=0,002$).
The presence of complete fissure also yielded improvements in FEV1 difference between treatment and control at 6 months (16,2%; $p<0,001$) and at 12 months (17,9%; $p<0,001$). The results at 6 months are summarized in (Figure 3). Major adverse events occurring within 90 days after placement of the one-way valves were mostly COPD exacerbations requiring hospitalization (7,9% in the treated group versus 1,1% in controls;$p=0,03$). Pneumothorax occurred in 4.2% of patients in the treated group early post-procedure follow-up and it was similar between groups in the late follow-up (valves=1%; control=2,4%). All but one resolved spontaneously (Hopkinson, Toma et al. 2005) (de Oliveira, Macedo-Neto et al. 2006).

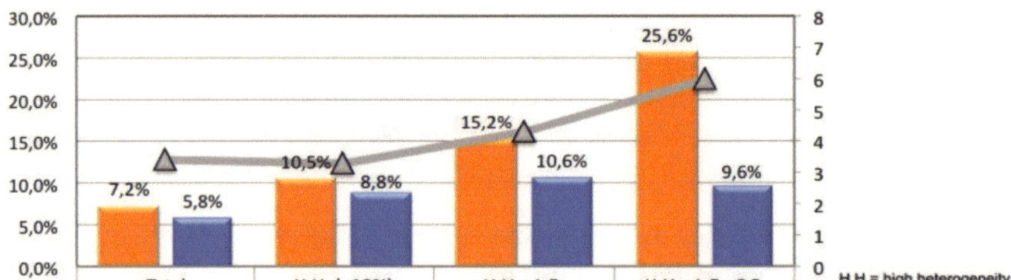

	Total	H.H. (>10%)	H.H.+ L.E.	H.H.+ L.E.+C.F.
FEV1 % Change	7,2%	10,5%	15,2%	25,6%
6MWT % Change	5,8%	8,8%	10,6%	9,6%
SGRQ Delta (abs)	3,4	3,28	4,29	5,96

FEV1 % Change   6MWT % Change   SGRQ Delta (abs)

Compiled from Sciurba et al. New Engl J Med 2010;363:1233

Fig. 3. Overall % changes (left axis) in FEV1 (orange), 6 MWT (purple) and the delta in the points (right axis) of the Saint George Respiratory Questionnaire (SGRQ) triangle (gray) are shown. The subset of high heterogeneity above 10% increased in about 30% the differences from baseline. When high heterogeneity was added to lobar exclusion, the functional parameters have doubled the differences and, in the subset that congregates high heterogeneity with lobar exclusion and low collateral flow, FEV1 jumped to 25%, 6 MWT to 10% and the delta in SGRQ went up to 6 points.

Hopkinson et al (Hopkinson, Toma et al. 2005) demonstrated that in a series of 19 patients patients treated with one-way valves who developed persisting lobar atelectasis at 1 month after the procedure, showed an improved survival at 6 years of follow-up.
One-way valves have been employed for BLVR as a bridge to lung transplantation in severe COPD patients. There is one report on 4 patients undergoing Zephyr® valve placement (average on 3,5 valves/patient), that showed no procedure related morbidity or mortality. BLVR was able to reduce RV and improve the 6MWT mMRC score. Three out of the four patients were transplanted successfully between 6-7 months, and one patient died 13 months after valve placement still on the transplant waiting list. The authors concluded that in a selected group of COPD patients awaiting lung transplantation, BLVR with one-valves can improve functional status and help patients awaiting lung transplantation for severe emphysema (Venuta, Diso et al. 2011).
Another valve device with a different design has been developed and tested (IBV®, Olympus Co., Spiration, Redmond-WA, EUA) (FIGURE 4). It has the ability of obstructing the airflow selectively in the segments where it is placed and, by the same token, allows secretions to exit the segment. One study with 30 patients showed improvements in quality of life, however without significant differences in pulmonary function (Wood, McKenna et al. 2007). This study has used outcome measures similar to LVRS. An expansion of this study has been published recently and included 91 patients with severe obstruction, hyperinflation and upper lobe predominant emphysema (Sterman, Mehta et al. 2010). A total of 609 bronchial valves placed bilaterally into the upper lobes. There were no procedure-related deaths. Thirty-day morbidity and mortality were 5.5 and 1.1%, respectively and pneumothorax was the most frequent serious device-related complication. There were no significant differences at 1,3,6 and 12 months in pulmonary function, exercise tolerance and gas exchange. There was a significant health-related quality of life improvement (-8.2+/-16.2) change at 6 months and it was associated with a decreased volume in the treated lobes without visible atelectasis.
In another recent study, the IBV® valves were tested and validated for clinical use in persistent air leaks (Wood, Cerfolio et al. 2010).

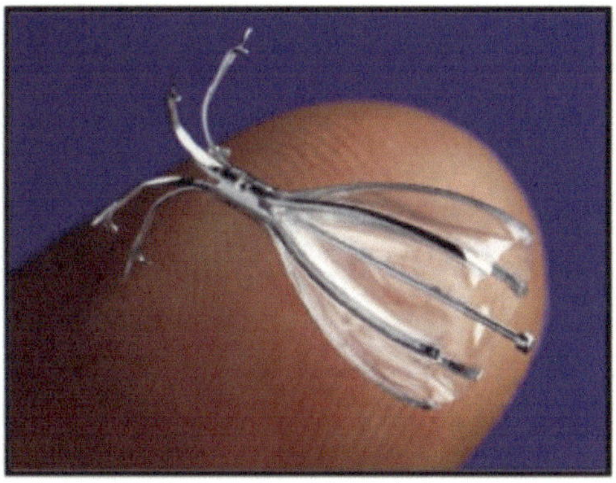

Fig. 4. The IBV® one-way valve (Spiration-Olympus, Redmond-WA, USA)

The studies using one-way valves concluded that this procedures have a good safety profile with low mortality and can be effective in selected subgroups of patients.

3.2 Removable non-blocking devices
3.2.1 Coils

This device is made out of a single nitinol wire with a memory (RePneu® Lung Volume Reduction Coil, PneumRx Inc., Mountain View, CA-EUA) (FIGURE 5). It is placed in a straight position within an introducer sheath that fits in the working channel of the flexible bronchoscope. Once the target segmental bronchus is reached, the device is deployed and its memory causes it to curve around its own axis, forcing the bronchus along with the adjacent lung parenchyma. Volume reduction is achieved when several of such devices are placed within the same lobe.

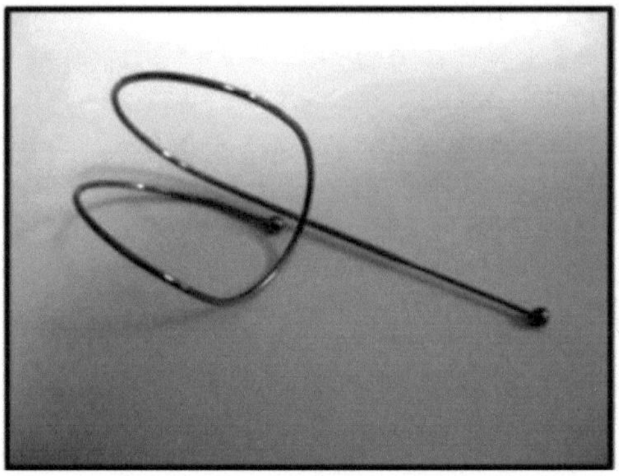

Fig. 5. Endobronchial nitinol coil utilized for BLVR (RePneu® Lung Volume Reduction Coil, PneumRx Inc, Mountain View, CA-USA)

The device a used in a preliminary safety trial on 11 patients, in whom 21 procedures were required to place the coils (average of 4.9 ± 0.6 coils per procedure), lasting 45 minutes each in average. After a follow-up of 7-11 months, efficacy was superior in patients with heterogeneous emphysema (Herth, Eberhardt et al. 2009; Herth, Eberhard et al. 2010).

3.3 Definitive (non-removeable) non-blocking devices
3.3.1 Bronchial thermal vapor ablation (BTVA)

This is a new technology that uses hot water vapor administered via a flexible bronchoscope by means of a baloon occlusion catheter (BTVA-*bronchial thermal vapor ablation*; Uptake Medical Corporation, Seattle-WA, EUA) (FIGURE 6). The system was designed to deliver a precise amount of vapor per gram of lung tissue. The early experimental studies carried out in animal models concluded that an amount of 5cal/gram of lung tissue was sufficient to cause a thermal lesion with subsequent fibrotic scarring and lung volume reduction. A preliminary clinical study on 11 patients with severe heterogeneous emphysema showed no significant improvements in FEV1 or RV at 6 months. However, gas transfer improved, the Medical Research Council Dyspnea Score (mMRC) improved 0,5 points from baseline, and the St. George Respiratory Questionnaire Score improved from 64,4 at baseline to 49,1 (Snell, Hopkins et al. 2009). The complication most frequently found with this procedure was bacterial pneumonia and COPD exacerbation. This technology is still under clinical testing, and new studies with higher amounts of vapor are under way.

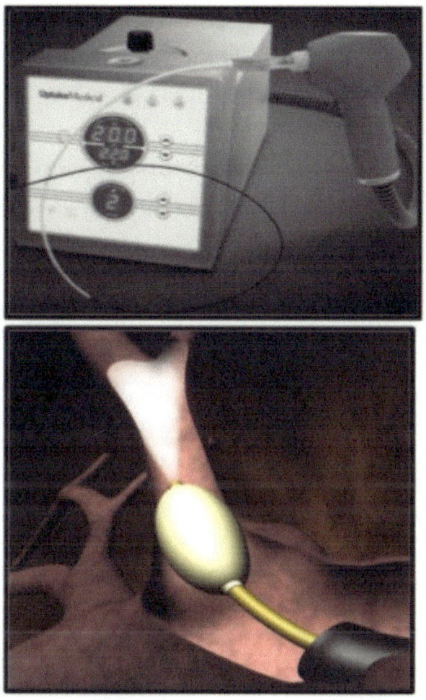

Fig. 6. Vapor generator (top) and catheter (bottom) used for bronchial thermal vapor ablation (BTVA-Uptake Medical Corporation, Seattle-WA, EUA).

3.3.2 Biological lung volume reduction (BioLVR) with polymers

This procedure consists of achieving lung volume reduction after obstruction with biodegradeable polymers instilled endobronchially under flexible bronchoscopy. This substance is a polymer mixed with fibrin and thrombin (*Aeriseal®*, Aeris Therapeutics Woburn-MA, EUA). Once it is delivered via a catheter into the segmental bronchi, its components polymerize resulting in a gel that blocks the bronchi. This substance progresses into the alveoli causing a local inflammatory reaction that causes scarring formation which will ultimately perpetuate the lung volume reduction (Ingenito and Tsai 2007).

The BioLVR has been applied to upper lobe predominant emphysema, both homogeneous and heterogeneous. Experimental data has shown that, by reaching deep into the alveoli, the polymer promotes blockage of the collateral ventilation. A clinical study on patients with homogeneous emphysema has been concluded recently (Reilly, Washko et al. 2007; Refaely, Dransfield et al. 2010). Among the 25 patients that underwent BioLVR, 17 received a dose of 10ml per treated site and 8 received 20ml. The higher dose group had the best results at 6 months. FEV1 reduced 8%, the mMRC dyspnea score reduced by 0,4 points and the St.George's Respiratory Questionnaire reduced by 4.9%. The authors concluded that in homogeneous emphysema the higher dose and the number of segmental bronchi treated were related to a better functional result (Murgu and Colt 2010).

The largest series published on BioLVR included 50 patients with upper lobe predominant emphysema. The FEV1 increased 15.6% at 6 months relative to pre-treatment values ($p=0.002$). On the other hand, subjects receiving higher doses of the polymer experienced more serious adverse events (8%), including pneumonia, pulmonary thromboembolism ad aspiration (Criner, Pinto-Plata et al. 2009).

3.3.3 Airway bypass

As mentioned earlier in this chapter, this procedure was designed to take advantage of the collateral ventilation that occurs naturally and is greatly enhanced in homogeneous emphysema.

This procedure evolved from the earlier concept of extra-anatomical communications between the lung parenchyma and the skin created by Macklem (Macklem 1978), to the production of fenestrations between the segmental bronchi and the adjacent lung proposed by Macklem and Cooper (Macklem, Cardoso et al. 2006).

The procedure consists of the production of orifices in the wall of the distal segmental and subsegmental bronchi (fenestrations), which are kept open with small self-expandable metal stents covered with a thin layer of medical silicone (Choong, Haddad et al. 2005).

The airway bypass procedure uses a proprietary system (Exhale Emphysema Treatment System™, Broncus Technologies Inc., Mountain View, CA-EUA) that includes: a doppler probe, catheter and a processor used for the location of extraluminal vessels through the bronchial wall; a needle-baloon dilator and a baloon catheter that expands the stents and the drug eluting stents loaded with paclitaxel. All devices described above were designed to pass through the 2mm or larger working channel of a flexible bronchoscope (FIGURE 7).

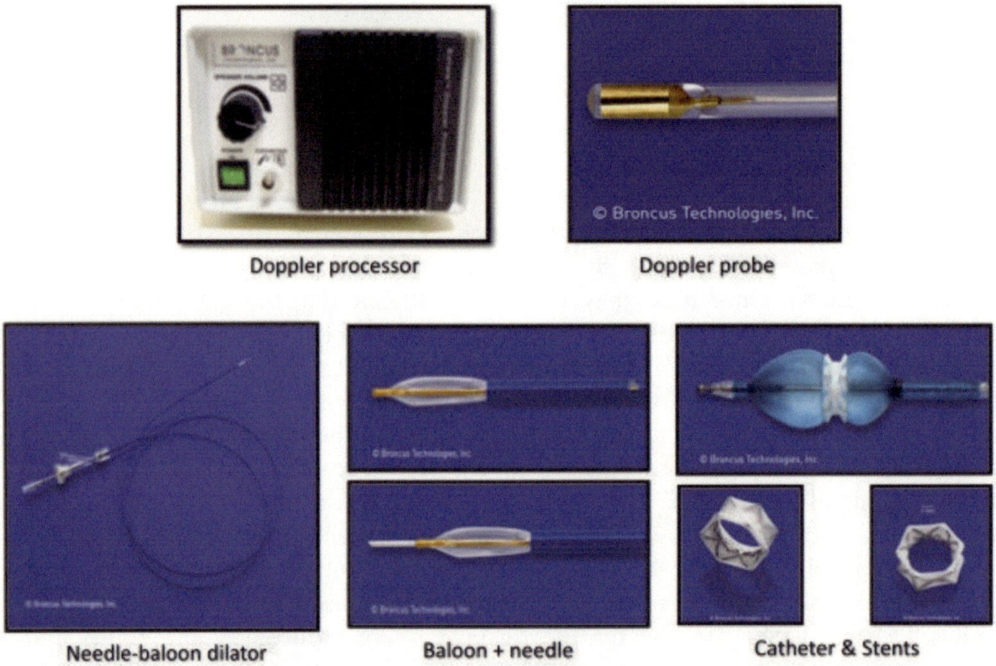

Fig. 7. The Exhale Emphysema Treatment System™, Broncus technologies Inc., Mountain View, CA-USA) used for the airway bypass procedure: doppler processor and probe (top row); needle-baloon dilator and a baloon catheter that expands the stents and the drug eluting stents loaded with paclitaxel (bottom row).

The proof of concept was achieved in a preliminary study on 12 explanted emphysematous lungs extracted from recipients of lung transplants. The lungs were placed in an airtight negative pressure ventilation chamber and connected to a pneumotachometer. Passages were created in the distal bronchi using a radiofrequency probe and stents were placed to hold the passage open. The creation of the passages resulted in an increase in the cumulative expiratory volumes in a direct proportion to the number of passages created (Lausberg, Chino et al. 2003). Further studies in the same model concluded that airway bypass was able to improve mechanics of breathing in severely emphysematous lungs, therefore supporting that it can improve ventilatory function in patients by reducing gas trapping and flow resistance (Choong, Macklem et al. 2008).

This was followed by a feasibility and safety study in humans prior to lobectomy and lung transplantation using radiofrequency generators to create the passages communicating the distal bronchi with the emphysematous lung parenchyma (Rendina, De Giacomo et al. 2003). The next step was to prolong the patency of the stents. This was achieved experimentally with the use of mitomycin-C in the stents (Choong, Haddad et al. 2005) and later by the development of drug eluting stents loaded with paclitaxel (Choong, Phan et al. 2006).

Prior to the procedure itself, the preferred sites for stent placement were identified on the chest CT scans based on the areas of most emphysematous destruction within the lung parenchyma (FIGURE 8). Efforts were made to place a minimum of three stents in each lung bilaterally. The middle lobe was not treated.

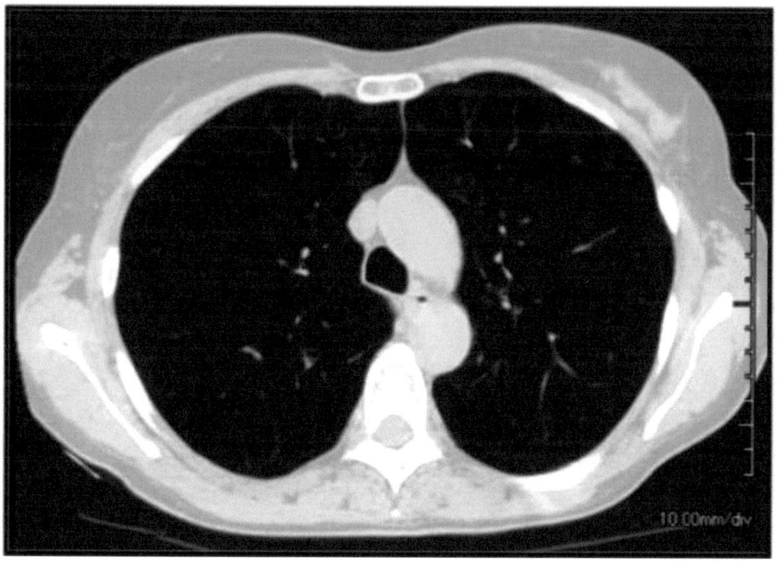

Fig. 8. CT scan showing homogeneous destruction by emphysema in a potentially suitable candidate for the airway bypass procedure.

The creation of each stented passage requires the following steps: 1) identification of a blood vessel-free location with a Doppler probe at the level of segmental bronchi; 2) fenestration of the bronchial wall by means of the needle-baloon dilator; 3) re-scanning the fenestration and its adjacent area with the the doppler probe to ascertain that no vessels were in the vicinity of the puncture site; 4) passage of the stent loaded catheter and deployment of the paclitaxel-eluting stent into the hole by expanding the hidrostatic baloon with a comercially available inflation syringe (FIGURES 9, 10).

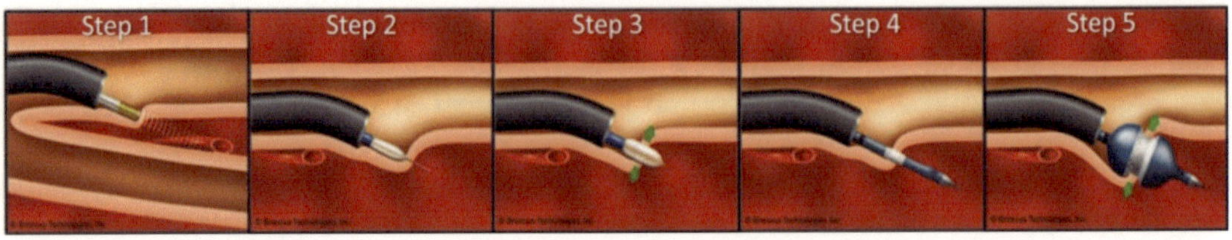

Fig. 9. Steps of the airway bypass procedure: 1- flexible bronchoscope is advanced into the distal airway, the area is scanned by the doppler probe; 2- the needle is passed, the airway pierced; 3- the passage is dilated with the baloon, and scanned again with the doppler probe to ascertain the absence of blood vessels in the vicinity of the passage; 4- the stent is then positioned into the passage; 5- the stent is deployed using a special baloon coupled to the catheter.

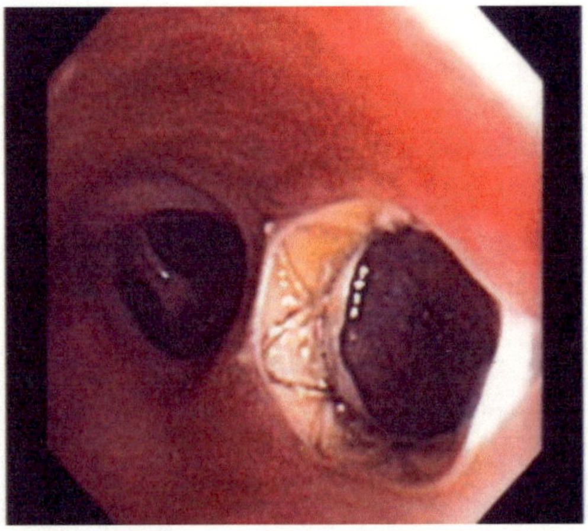

Fig. 10. Paclitaxel eluting stent (right) placed adjacent to a segmental bronchus (left).

The initial feasibility studies were followed by the first clinical studies to evaluate efficacy and safety (Macklem, Cardoso et al. 2006; Cardoso, Snell et al. 2007). A multicentric study included 35 patients with a RV ≥ 220%, FEV1 ≤ 40% and mMRC ≥ 2. Two hundred and sixty four stents were implanted, with an average of 8 stents per patient. There was 1 death secondary to bleeding in this series (mortality of 2,6%). This event triggered an extensive safety revision that resulted in several recommendations made, including re-scanning puncture sites, and the placement of a stand-by bronchial blocker into the airway during the procedure. At 1 month after the procedure there were significant differences in all functional parameters, however such changes got smaller and were restricted to rv ($p=0,04$) and mmrc ($p=0.02$) at 6 months. The subset of patients with RV/TLC ≥ 0.67 sustained the best benefits with significant changes in RV (-14,1% ; $p=0,02$) and mMRC (-0,5% ; $p=0,03$). The most frequent serious adverse events were COPD exacerbation (32%) and respiratory infection (27%), most of them have occurred in the first monthy after procedure. One additional death occurred due to bowel obstruction in the late follow up, which was considered as unrelated to the procedure.

These results led to the design of the *E*xhale *A*irway *S*tents for *E*mphysema (*EASE* Trial) (Shah, Slebos et al. 2011). This was a multicenter phase III trial of airway bypass with paclitaxel-eluting stents. The EASE trial was the first double-blind, randomised, sham-

controlled study on bronchoscopic lung volume reduction in severe homogeneous emphysema.
The EASE Trial used a 2:1 (treatment:sham) randomization. Double-blinding was maintained by dividing the investigators into two teams (blinded Team A with access to pre and post-procedure assessments ; and blinded Team B that performed only the bronchoscopic procedures without further patient contact). All patients underwent a full 6-10 week program of pulmonary rehabilitation prior to the procedure and 8 weeks after the procedure. Follow-up visits were scheduled for 1, 3, 6 and 12 months emphysema (Shah, Slebos et al. 2011).
The 6-month efficacy endpoints required both an improvement greater than 12% in FVC, and a more than 1 point decrease in mMRC over baseline. This trial enrolled 315 patients at 38 centers with homogeneous emphysema and severe hyperinflation (RV ≥ 180% predicted; RV/TLC ≥ 0.65). There were 208 patients randomised for airway bypass and 107 for sham bronchoscopy.
The results of the EASE trial were submitted for publication recently (Shah, Slebos et al. 2011). The airway bypass group received a mean of 4.7±1.4 stents per patient. The 6-month co-primary endpoint was 14.4%for AB vs 11.2% for SC. On day 1, RV decreased significantly in the airway bypass group (change of 379mL from baseline ; *p=0,006*), and this was associated with increases in FEV_1 and FVC. At months 1, 3, 6 and 12 the changes were no longer significant between the groups on FVC, FEV1, mMRC. The functional assessment by Saint George Respiratory Questionnaire was better in the airway bypass group at 1 month, but this coincided with the post-procedural rehabilitation program. The 6MWT showed no significant differences after the first month of follow-up between the groups.
Composite safety endpoints at 6 months were 14,4% in the airway bypass group and 11,2% in the sham controls (*p=1,0*). There was one death after the airway bypass procedure due to a ruptured abdominal aortic aneurysm. Overall mortality at 12 months was similar between airway bypass and sham controls (6,7% and 6,5% respectively).
Further CT analysis showed that there were lobar volume decreases after stent placement at day 1. However, at month 6 the RV increased coincidently with stent loss by expectoration or stent occlusion. Such findings have suggested that the loss of stents or its occlusion were the limiting factors for achieving long term benefit. Further studies must be redesigned with special attention to the functional endpoints and focus on new imaging methods.
Targeting trapped air regions with more accurate mapping in COPD patients is another issue that has to be addressed. Better monitoring for loss of effect and sequential interventions to prolong effect durability with the current technology are therefore required.
In summary, despite the early promising results in the first clinical trial with the airway bypass procedure, the paclitaxel eluting stents used in the EASE trial showed only short term good results. The trial exposed both the need for technical improvements in the stents and for preventing its early occlusion. This will then prolong effect durability if this technology is to be pursued in the future.
The common denominator in all procedures and the few trials on BLVR is the lack of common endpoints and the need for new assessment methods that are both non-invasive and accurate.

4. New methods for the assessment in BLVR

The assessment methods used in BLVR today are essentially the same used a decade ago for LVRS and during the NETT trial.

As BLVR has evolved, this has led the centers to enroll patients with worse pulmonary function and poor performance requiring a more thorough evaluation. On the other hand, all major trials on BLVR did not share the same endpoints, making interpretation of results not only difficult, but sometimes confusing.

All procedures proposed for BLVR so far are based on lung deflation. Surprisingly, none of the methods currently employed have the ability to provide dynamic information as the procedure is being carried out along with the pattern of lung deflation.

Based on the facts abovementioned, new methods for patient selection and post-treatment evaluation must be studied to correct this idiosyncrasy. Such new methods shall be ideally less invasive, able to provide meaningful information and add on to the current evaluation strategy (PFTs, performance testing, Chest CT scan, etc).

4.1 Chest CT scan imaging analysis

Advanced helical scanners have enabled much better imaging management. This has been particularly useful for the detection of target areas in emphysema and airway navigation for bronchoscopy planning. The ability to quantify emphysema based on the CT scan is also a powerful tool for post-treatment assessment.

There are commercially available softwares able to provide an accurate volumetry of each lobe. This is accomplished by mapping the emphysematous areas using the -910 and -950 Hounsfield unit cut-offs and applying the information to complex algorithms. The software will calculate many parameters such as air and tissue volumes. It will generate histograms with the less dense (and more emphysematous) areas, comparing them between the lobes and giving numerical information about heterogeneity. This has become a key for the success of certain procedures such as BLVR with one-way valves (Coxson, Nasute Fauerbach et al. 2008). The software can generate multiplannar images of the airway and its relation to the emphysematous areas, in addition to schematic depictions of the target emphysematous areas with accurate volume calculations (Figure 11). This is particularly useful for obtaining post-procedure static volumetry and to determine heterogeneity between lobes.

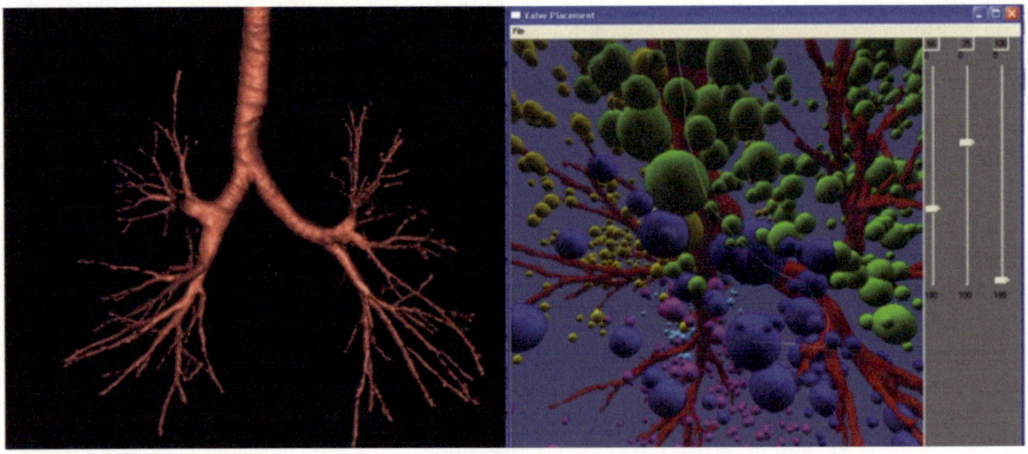

Fig. 11. Images of the airway (left) and a schematic depiction of the emphysematous lobes and its distribution (right) to facilitate navigation and device placement (Apollo®-Vida Diagnostics, Iowa-USA).

The problem limiting repeat CT scans for post-treatment assessment is the cumulative radiation dose. Standard-dose CT for follow-up of BLVR is limited by the risk of administration of a radiation dose of 8-12 mSv for each CT examination. Low-dose CT, in which the radiation dose is six to ten fold less than in conventional CT, has been used for the evaluation of emphysema patients (Gierada, Pilgram et al. 2007). This technique was recently used for the evaluation of the feasibility of thin-section low-dose CT in the radiologic monitoring of patients after placement of bronchial stents for airway bypass (Grgic, Wilkens et al. 2008).

4.2 Electrical impedance tomography (EIT)

EIT uses the injection of high frequency and low amplitude electrical currents through 16 or 32 electrodes placed around the chest to obtain images of a cross section of the lungs. These currents travel through the thorax following pathways that vary according to chest wall shape and thoracic distribution of impeditivities. The resulting electric potentials on the surface of the chest wall are measured and used to obtain the electric impedance distribution within the thorax using a reconstruction algorithm (Figure 12). The output image of such algorithms is usually a 32 by 32 or a 64 by 64 array from which each element corresponds to a pixel on the image and contains the change in impedance in relation to a reference frame, expressed as a percentage (Costa, Lima et al. 2009). This method has been extensively investigated in the intensive care setting for patients undergoing mechanical ventilation.

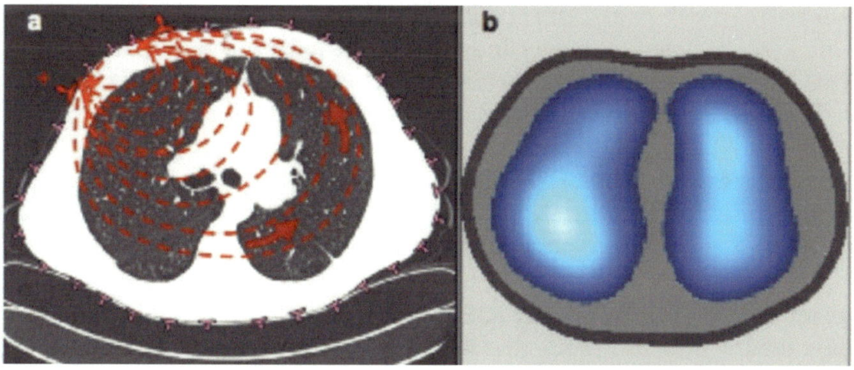

Fig. 12. Electrical impedance tomography (EIT): a) the 32 electrode belt around the chest and the electrical current between 2 electrodes; b) image generated by the software representing the average variation of impedance.

EIT combines two interesting features: it is not invasive and can be performed at the bedside. It has been proven useful for PEEP titration, to optimize ventilation strategies by detecting the imbalances in regional lung ventilation, as well as to detect pneumothorax and small pleural effusions (Victorino, Borges et al. 2004; Costa, Lima et al. 2009). More recently there have been studies showing that EIT can assess lung perfusion through intravenous injection of hypertonic saline, which is a contrast agent for EIT images because of its extremely low impeditivity (Tanaka, Ortega et al. 2008).

The characteristics of EIT makes it a potentially useful tool for the assessment of BLVR. It combines the ability of quantifying lung deflation, to show the redistribution of ventilation during and after the procedure and, by the same token, to detect pneumothorax..

Furthermore, this is the only procedure that can be done at the bedside. We have recently embarked on an experimental study of the patterns on lung deflation after BLVR to detect its feasibility prior to its clinical application.

4.3 Diaphragmatic mobility by ultrasound (US)

One of the hallmarks of advanced COPD is diaphragmatic flattening and dysfunction, both caused by chronic hyperinflation. This causes muscular deconditioning of the diaphragm, that contributes to dyspnea and low exercise tolerance. It is therefore expected that the improvements in diaphragmatic mobility should follow the improvements in breathing mechanics after BLVR in severe COPD patients. Surprisingly, insofar this has not been studied in BLVR protocols.

The US measurement of craniocaudal displacement of the left intrahepatic branches of the portal vein was described as an indirect assessment of right hemidiaphragmatic mobility (Toledo, Kodaira et al. 2003). Paulin et al (Paulin, Yamaguti et al. 2007) created a classification of diaphragmatic dysfunction based on the degree of its mobility. They showed that COPD patients with less than 33.9mm of diaphragm mobility as measured by US had greater dyspnea upon exertion and covered shorter 6MWT distances if compared to patients with more than 34mm of diaphragmatic mobility. Based on this assumption, Yamaguti et al (Yamaguti, Paulin et al. 2009) published an interesting study on the risk of death on COPD individuals with and without diaphragmatic dysfunction based on US evaluation of mobility. They concluded that COPD patients with lower diaphragm mobility had a higher risk of death than COPD patients without diaphragmatic dysfunction and that quality of life was unrelated to the decline in diaphragmatic function in their studies COPD subjects. This has yielded to another major study currently under way at the University of Sao Paulo, Brazil to specifically assess the "Evaluation of ins and expiratory muscles in respiratory diseases".

The US for the measurement of diaphragmatic mobility is also non-invasive and its reproducibility and reliability in COPD patients has been demonstrated. Its use for the assessment of BLVR shall be contemplated in future studies.

4.4 Opto-electronic plethismography (OEP) method

OEP is a new noninvasive technique that is highly accurate method for measuring the total chest wall volume variations, allowing partitioning of the complex shape of the chest wall into basically three different functional compartments (upper chest, thoraco-abdominal and abdominal). It measures breathing patterns and, if combined with pressure measurements, can be used to study statics, dynamics and energetics of the respiratory system (Aliverti, Dellaca et al. 2001). It uses non-invasive video imaging capturing the movement of skin markers while the patient breathes spontaneously. Studies on severe COPD patients using OPE have shown that dynamic hyperinflation is not the only mechanism limiting exercise performance. The measurement of chest wall volumes by OPE can identify the different patterns of respiratory muscle activation during exercise (Aliverti, Stevenson et al. 2004). Another important feature of OPE is its ability to evaluate coordination. One of the semiologic features of COPD is the paradoxical ventilation. This is also known as the Hoover's sign, in which the flattened diaphragm contracts inwards instead of downwards, thereby pulling the inferior ribs inwards with its movement. In normal subjects the expansion of both rib cage and abdomen happen synchronously and in phase. In COPD a

less effective diaphragm alters this mechanism. Lower ribcage paradox at rest is associated with early-onset hyperinflation of the chest wall and predominant dyspnea at exercise. When paradox is absent, the sense of leg effort has been shown to be a more important symptom limiting exercise. On the other hand, COPD patients with an asynchronous abdominal rib cage breathing pattern showed more dynamic hyperinflation and dyspnea as the exercise limiting factor (Aliverti, Quaranta et al. 2009).
Given this is a non-invasive method of measuring both breathing, coordination and chest wall volumes, it makes OPE an excellent tool for screening and evaluating patients for BLVR. We are currently using OPE to measure coordination and lung volume integration in the assessment of COPD patients in our bronchoscopic lung volume reduction program.

5. Conclusion

Bronchoscopic lung volume reduction is an emerging non-surgical alternative for palliation in severe emphysema patients. Despite all the efforts and resources spent into trials and device development, BLVR remains mostly investigational. With the exception of the one-way valves that have been approved for use in Europe and Latin America, all other devices are still under scrutiny. A number of new devices have been proposed and only a few have shown modest benefits if compared to surgical lung volume reduction. Nevertheless, most of the devices have shown a good safety profile and their effectiveness depends greatly on the technology used and on subject selection. The need for development of new methods for evaluation and follow-up following BLVR is another issue that must be addressed in conjunction to the creation of a more uniform data aquisition and interpretation accross the clinical trials.

6. References

Aliverti, A., R. Dellaca, et al. (2001). "Optoelectronic plethysmography: a new tool in respiratory medicine." Recenti Prog Med 92(11): 644-647.
Aliverti, A., M. Quaranta, et al. (2009). "Paradoxical movement of the lower ribcage at rest and during exercise in COPD patients." Eur Respir J 33(1): 49-60.
Aliverti, A., N. Stevenson, et al. (2004). "Regional chest wall volumes during exercise in chronic obstructive pulmonary disease." Thorax 59(3): 210-216.
Aljuri, N. and L. Freitag (2009). "Validation and pilot clinical study of a new bronchoscopic method to measure collateral ventilation before endobronchial lung volume reduction." J Appl Physiol 106(3): 774-783.
ATS (1999). "Pulmonary rehabilitation-1999. American Thoracic Society." Am J Respir Crit Care Med 159(5 Pt 1): 1666-1682.
Berger, R. L., M. M. Decamp, et al. (2010). "Lung volume reduction therapies for advanced emphysema: an update." Chest 138(2): 407-417.
Brantigan, O. C., E. Mueller, et al. (1959). "A surgical approach to pulmonary emphysema." Am Rev Respir Dis 80(1, Part 2): 194-206.
Cardoso, P. F., G. I. Snell, et al. (2007). "Clinical application of airway bypass with paclitaxel-eluting stents: early results." J Thorac Cardiovasc Surg 134(4): 974-981.
Choong, C. K., F. J. Haddad, et al. (2005). "Feasibility and safety of airway bypass stent placement and influence of topical mitomycin C on stent patency." J Thorac Cardiovasc Surg 129(3): 632-638.

Choong, C. K., P. T. Macklem, et al. (2008). "Airway bypass improves the mechanical properties of explanted emphysematous lungs." Am J Respir Crit Care Med 178(9): 902-905.

Choong, C. K., L. Phan, et al. (2006). "Prolongation of patency of airway bypass stents with use of drug-eluting stents." J Thorac Cardiovasc Surg 131(1): 60-64.

Ciccone, A. M., B. F. Meyers, et al. (2003). "Long-term outcome of bilateral lung volume reduction in 250 consecutive patients with emphysema." J Thorac Cardiovasc Surg 125(3): 513-525.

Cooper, J. D., G. A. Patterson, et al. (1996). "Results of 150 consecutive bilateral lung volume reduction procedures in patients with severe emphysema." J Thorac Cardiovasc Surg 112(5): 1319-1329; discussion 1329-1330.

Costa, E. L., R. G. Lima, et al. (2009). "Electrical impedance tomography." Curr Opin Crit Care 15(1): 18-24.

Coxson, H. O., P. V. Nasute Fauerbach, et al. (2008). "Computed tomography assessment of lung volume changes after bronchial valve treatment." Eur Respir J 32(6): 1443-1450.

Criner, G. J., V. Pinto-Plata, et al. (2009). "Biologic lung volume reduction in advanced upper lobe emphysema: phase 2 results." Am J Respir Crit Care Med 179(9): 791-798.

de Oliveira, H. G., A. V. Macedo-Neto, et al. (2006). "Transbronchoscopic pulmonary emphysema treatment: 1-month to 24-month endoscopic follow-up." Chest 130(1): 190-199.

Fishman, A., F. Martinez, et al. (2003). "A randomized trial comparing lung-volume-reduction surgery with medical therapy for severe emphysema." N Engl J Med 348(21): 2059-2073.

Gierada, D. S., T. K. Pilgram, et al. (2007). "Comparison of standard- and low-radiation-dose CT for quantification of emphysema." AJR. American journal of roentgenology 188(1): 42-47.

Gompelmann, D., R. Eberhardt, et al. (2010). "Predicting atelectasis by assessment of collateral ventilation prior to endobronchial lung volume reduction: a feasibility study." Respiration 80(5): 419-425.

Grgic, A., H. Wilkens, et al. (2008). "Low-dose MDCT for surveillance of patients with severe homogeneous emphysema after bronchoscopic airway bypass." AJR. American journal of roentgenology 191(3): W112-119.

Herth, F., R. Eberhardt, et al. (2009). "Pilot Study of an Improved Lung Volume Reduction Coil for the Treatment of Emphysema." Am J Respir Crit Care Med 179: A6160.

Herth, F. J., R. Eberhard, et al. (2010). "Bronchoscopic lung volume reduction with a dedicated coil: a clinical pilot study." Ther Adv Respir Dis 4(4): 225-231.

Herth, F. J., D. Gompelmann, et al. (2010). "Endoscopic lung volume reduction." Respiration 79(1): 5-13.

Hopkinson, N. S., T. P. Toma, et al. (2005). "Effect of bronchoscopic lung volume reduction on dynamic hyperinflation and exercise in emphysema." Am J Respir Crit Care Med 171(5): 453-460.

Ingenito, E. P. and L. W. Tsai (2007). "Evolving endoscopic approaches for treatment of emphysema." Semin Thorac Cardiovasc Surg 19(2): 181-189.

Ingenito, E. P., D. E. Wood, et al. (2008). "Bronchoscopic lung volume reduction in severe emphysema." Proc Am Thorac Soc 5(4): 454-460.

Lausberg, H. F., K. Chino, et al. (2003). "Bronchial fenestration improves expiratory flow in emphysematous human lungs." Ann Thorac Surg 75(2): 393-397; discussion 398.

Macklem, P., Cardoso P., et al. (2006). Airway Bypass: A New Treatment for Emphysema. Annual Meeting of the American Thoracic Society, San Diego-CA.

Macklem, P. T. (1978). "Collateral ventilation." N Engl J Med 298(1): 49-50.

Moore, A. J., E. Cetti, et al. (2010). "Unilateral extrapulmonary airway bypass in advanced emphysema." Ann Thorac Surg 89(3): 899-906.

Murgu, S. D. and H. G. Colt (2010). "Interventional bronchoscopy from bench to bedside: new techniques for central and peripheral airway obstruction." Clin Chest Med 31(1): 101-115, Table of Contents.

Paulin, E., W. P. Yamaguti, et al. (2007). "Influence of diaphragmatic mobility on exercise tolerance and dyspnea in patients with COPD." Respir Med 101(10): 2113-2118.

Refaely, Y., M. Dransfield, et al. (2010). "Biologic lung volume reduction therapy for advanced homogeneous emphysema." Eur Respir J 36(1): 20-27.

Reilly, J., G. Washko, et al. (2007). "Biological lung volume reduction: a new bronchoscopic therapy for advanced emphysema." Chest 131(4): 1108-1113.

Rendina, E. A., T. De Giacomo, et al. (2003). "Feasibility and safety of the airway bypass procedure for patients with emphysema." J Thorac Cardiovasc Surg 125(6): 1294-1299.

Sanchez, P. (2009). "NETT trial: a reassessment." AATS meeting-Abstracts.

Sciurba, F. C., A. Ernst, et al. (2010). "A randomized study of endobronchial valves for advanced emphysema." N Engl J Med 363(13): 1233-1244.

Shah, P., D. Slebos, et al. (2011). "Bronchoscopic lung volume reduction with Exhale Airway Stents for Emphysema (EASE): A Randomised, Sham Controlled Multicenter Trial." Lancet 378: 997-1005.

Shah, P. L., D. J. Slebos, et al. (2011). "Design of the exhale airway Stents for emphysema (EASE) trial: an endoscopic procedure for reducing hyperinflation." BMC Pulm Med 11(1): 1.

Snell, G. I., P. Hopkins, et al. (2009). "A feasibility and safety study of bronchoscopic thermal vapor ablation: a novel emphysema therapy." Ann Thorac Surg 88(6): 1993-1998.

Sterman, D. H., A. C. Mehta, et al. (2010). "A multicenter pilot study of a bronchial valve for the treatment of severe emphysema." Respiration 79(3): 222-233.

Tanaka, H., N. R. Ortega, et al. (2008). "Fuzzy modeling of electrical impedance tomography images of the lungs." Clinics 63(3): 363-370.

Toledo, N. S., S. K. Kodaira, et al. (2003). "Right hemidiaphragmatic mobility: assessment with US measurement of craniocaudal displacement of left branches of portal vein." Radiology 228(2): 389-394.

Venuta, F., D. Diso, et al. (2011). "Bronchoscopic lung volume reduction as a bridge to lung transplantation in patients with chronic obstructive pulmonary disease." Eur J Cardio-Thorac Surg 39(3): 364-367.

Victorino, J. A., J. B. Borges, et al. (2004). "Imbalances in regional lung ventilation: a validation study on electrical impedance tomography." Am J Respir Crit Care Med 169(7): 791-800.

Wan, I. Y., T. P. Toma, et al. (2006). "Bronchoscopic lung volume reduction for end-stage emphysema: report on the first 98 patients." Chest 129(3): 518-526.

Weder, W., M. Tutic, et al. (2009). "Persistent benefit from lung volume reduction surgery in patients with homogeneous emphysema." Ann Thorac Surg 87(1): 229-236; discussion 236-227.

Wood, D. E., R. J. Cerfolio, et al. (2010). "Bronchoscopic management of prolonged air leak." Clin Chest Med 31(1): 127-133, Table of Contents.

Wood, D. E., R. J. McKenna, Jr., et al. (2007). "A multicenter trial of an intrabronchial valve for treatment of severe emphysema." J Thorac Cardiovasc Surg 133(1): 65-73.

Yamaguti, W. P., E. Paulin, et al. (2009). "Diaphragmatic dysfunction and mortality in patients with COPD." J Bras Pneumol 35(12): 1174-1181.

21

Mediastinal Parathyroidectomy: Preoperative Management of Hyperparathyroidism

Dariusz Sagan[1*], Jerzy S. Tarach[2], Andrzej Nowakowski[2], Maria Klatka[3], Elżbieta Czekajska-Chehab[4], Andrzej Drop[4], Beata Chrapko[5] and Janusz Klatka[6]
[1]*Department of Thoracic Surgery,*
[2]*Department of Endocrinology,*
[3]*Department of Paediatric Endocrinology and Neurology,*
[4]*1st Department of Radiology,*
[5]*Department of Nuclear Medicine,*
[6]*Department of Otolaryngology and Laryngeal Oncology,*
Medical University of Lublin,
Poland

1. Introduction

1.1 Anatomy and embryology of parathyroid glands

The normal parathyroid gland is oval or spherical in shape, has a distinct yellowish color, and averages 2x3x7 mm. The total mean weight of four normal parathyroids is about 150 mg. Majority of the population have four parathyroid glands typically located at the posterior capsule of the thyroid gland (Fig. 1; Fig.2), however in nearly 15% of individuals more than four glands are present. Phylogenetically, the parathyroid glands appear in amphibia, and arise from pharyngeal pouches III and IV. They may be arrested in the development as high as

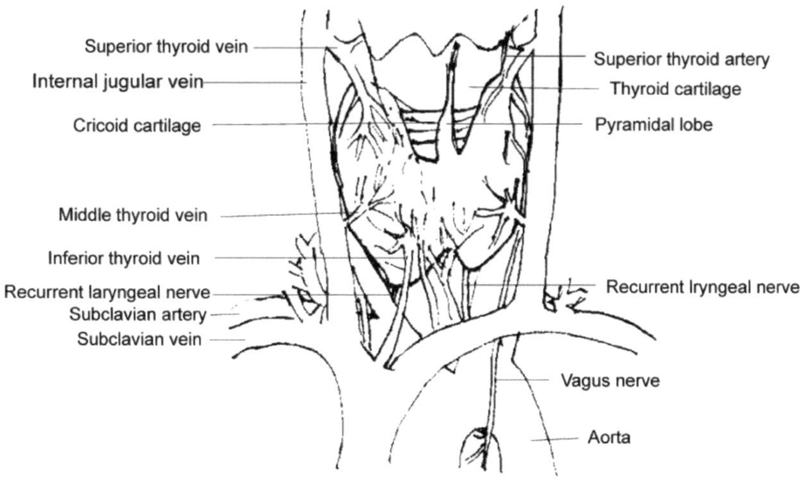

Fig. 1. Thyroid & parathyroid anatomy

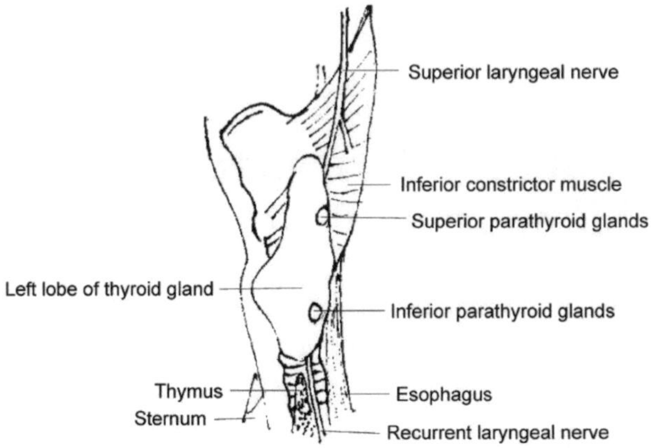

Fig. 2. Parathyroid glands anatomy. Left side view

at the level of the hyoid bone on the way of their descent to their typical location. Occasionally, parathyroids may be incorporated into the thyroid gland or thymus (intrathyroidal or mediastinal location). Lower (inferior) parathyroid glands (parathyroid III) may be found in the anterior mediastinum, while the upper (superior) parathyroids (parathyroid IV) usually remain in close association with the upper portion of the lateral thyroid lobes but may descend caudally along the esophagus into the posterior mediastinum (Fig. 3).

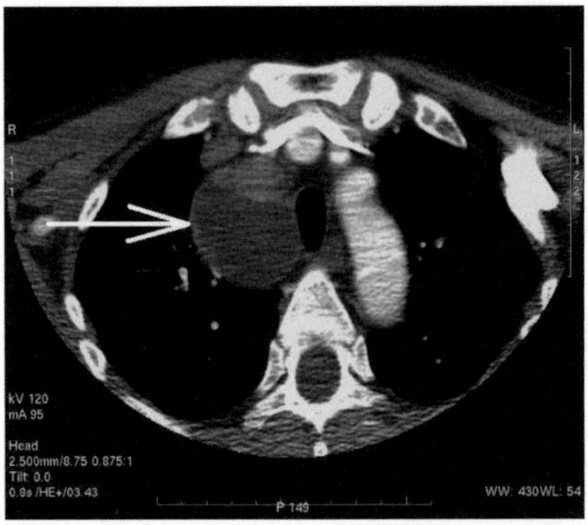

Fig. 3. Computed tomography scan showing a large mediastinal parathyroid adenoma (indicated with an arrow)

The parathyroid glands may lie in front of or behind the internal jugular vein and common carotid artery. Parathyroids are usually supplied by a branch of the inferior thyroid artery but may be supplied by the superior thyroid or, rarely, the thyroid ima arteries. The vessels can be seen entering a hilum-like structure, a feature that may be practically utilized to differentiate parathyroid glands from fat.

2. Physiology

Parathyroid glands secrete parathyroid hormone (PTH), which together with vitamin D, and calcitonin plays a vital role in precise regulation of calcium and phosphorus metabolism in bone, kidney, and gut. PTH and calcitonin work in concert to regulate plasma levels of ionized calcium. Fall in the ionized calcium level stimulates the parathyroids to secrete more PTH, and inhibits the parafollicular cells within the thyroid to produce less calcitonin. The rise in PTH and fall in calcitonin stimulate increased resorption of calcium in the renal tubules and from bones, thus more calcium enters the blood, and ionized calcium levels normalize. PTH in the blood stream is heterogeneous and consists of the intact hormone, the amino terminal (N-terminal) fragment and the carboxyl terminal (C-terminal) fragment. C-terminal fragment is biologically inert, whereas N-terminal fragment maintains hormonal activity, however substantially lower than the intact hormone. Currently available diagnostic tests are capable of intact hormone level determination, which is important for reliability of the measurement in particular for intraoperative use.

3. Primary hyperparathyroidism

Primary hyperparathyroidism is a disease characterized by autonomous overproduction of PTH resulting in hypercalcemia. In majority of cases it is caused by a single parathyroid adenoma (80-85%), and less frequently by hyperplasia (10%), multiple adenomas (6%), or carcinoma (1%). Currently, primary hyperparathyroidism occurs in 0.1-0.3% of the general population and in unselected patients is considered the most common cause of hypercalcemia. It is almost three times more common in women than in men, with peak incidence between the third and fifth decades.

Excess production of PTH results in mobilization of calcium from bone and inhibition of the renal reabsorption of phosphate, leading to hypercalcemia and hypophosphatemia. Besides, it causes a wasting of calcium and phosphorus, which eventually may result in osseous mineral loss and osteoporosis. Other conditions which may be associated with hyperparathyroidism include nephrocalcinosis, nephrolithiasis, osteitis fibrosa cystica, pancreatitis, peptic ulcer, hypertension, and gout. Diagnosis of any of these diseases should evoke suspicion for hyperparathyroidism and the patient should be referred for more precise tests.

Hyperparathyroidism is occasionally associated with multiple endocrine neoplasia (MEN) type 1, or type 2. MEN type 1 is characterized by tumors of the parathyroid, pituitary, and pancreas (hyperparathyroidism, pituitary tumors, and islet cell pancreatic tumors) that may lead to gastrinoma (Zollinger-Ellison syndrome), glucagonoma, insulinoma (hypoglycemia), somatostatinoma, lipoma and pancreatic polypeptide tumors (PPomas). Adrenocortical tumors, carcinoid tumors, and multiple lipomas have also been reported in these patients. MEN type 2 is divided into 2 subtypes: MEN 2a and MEN 2b. MEN 2a is characterized by hyperparathyroidism associated with pheochromocytoma and thyroid medullary carcinoma. Hyperparathyroidism is rare in MEN 2b patients who often have multiple neuromas and a marfanoid habitus.

Parathyroid adenomas may range in weight from 65 mg to over 35 g, but occasionally the weight of these tumors may exceed 35g. Usually the size of the tumor parallels the degree of hypercalcemia (the larger the tumor, the more severe hypercalcemia). Microscopic examination of parathyroid adenomas shows chief cell, water cell, or, rarely, oxyphil cell type.

Primary parathyroid hyperplasia may be another cause of hyperparathyroidism. This condition involves all of the parathyroid glands, which vary considerably in size but are usually larger than normal. Microscopic examination may reveal two types: chief cell hyperplasia and water-clear cell hyperplasia. Parathyroid carcinoma is rare but usually leads to severe hypercalcemia, and should be suspected at operation when the parathyroid gland is hard, has a whitish or irregular capsule, or shows signs of invasiveness. Rupture of the parathyroid tumor or breaching of the tumor capsule during rough dissection may result in seeding hyperactive tissue. This, and less frequently multiple embryologic rests may lead to a rare condition called parathyromatosis characterized by persistent hypercalcemia.

4. Signs and symptoms

Clinical signs and symptoms of hyperparathyroidism range from barely recognizable by patients, like muscle fatigablility, weakness, psychiatric disturbances, constipations, polydipsja and polyuria to severely impairing normal activities, like bone and muscle pains, nephrolithiasis, nephrocalcinosis, hypertension, peptic ulcer, pancreatitis or gout. Osteitis fibrosa cystica with bone pains and deformities, which was a prevailing symptom in patients with hyperparathyroidism a few decades ago, now became less frequent because majority of cases are detected early in the course of the disease. Also the incidence of renal complications decreased markedly and many patients are diagnosed by routine screening while still asymptomatic.

5. Laboratory tests

Serum calcium, parathyroid hormone and phosphates level are the principal laboratory tests used for the diagnosis of hyperparathyroidism. Elevated serum calcium and low phosphates are highly suggestive of hyperparathyroidism, however in about 50% of patients serum phosphates level is normal. Measurement of serum intact parathyroid hormone (PTH) concentration is the key test in diagnostic workout for patients with hypercalcemia, because the PTH level is low or nil in all cases except for those caused by primary hyperparathyroidism and familial hypocalciuric hypercalcemia, where PTH is markedly elevated.

Complementary laboratory tests include chlorides, protein electrophoretic pattern, alkaline phosphatase, creatinine, uric acid and urea nitrogen, urinary calcium, blood hematocrite and pH, serum magnesium and ESR. Sometimes, when previous tests are equivocal, measurement of nephrogenous cAMP, 1,25-hydroxy vitamin D levels and tubular resorption of phosphates may be helpful. Serum chloride concentration is elevated in nearly half of patients with hyperparathyroidism and may be a useful diagnostic clue. It's due to direct influence of PTH on the proximal renal tubule decreasing the resorption of bicarbonate, which leads to increased resorption of chloride. Other causes of hypercalcemia do not give rise in chloride concentration.

6. Secondary hyperparathyroidism

Secondary hyperparathyroidism (sHPT) is a condition characterized by excess secretion of parathyroid hormone stimulated by external factors, mainly hypocalcemia. Chronic renal failure is the most common cause of secondary hyperparathyroidism, as it results in hypocalcemia due to impaired conversion of vitamin D into active form, and excessive loss of calcium with urine. Sporadically sHPT may be caused by malabsorption, like chronic pancreatitis, small bowel disease or malabsorbtion-dependent bariatric surgery. Prolonged stimulation of parathyroid tissue by hypocalcemia results in enlargement of parathyroids in the form of their hyperplasia and less frequently parathyroid adenoma.

7. Tertiary hyperparathyroidism

Tertiary hyperparathyroidism (tHPT) is a condition of autonomic excessive secretion of parathyroid hormone developing from secondary parathyroidism, that maintains despite restoration of renal function. It is caused by development of autonomous (unregulated) parathyroid function following a prolonged period of persistent parathyroid stimulation. It is no longer responsive to treatment by medication and requires surgical removal of three and a half parathyroid glands.

8. Indications for surgical treatment

Parathyroidectomy is currently recognized as the treatment of choice for patients with primary hyperparathyroidism. For virtually all these patients surgical resection of hyperactive parathyroid tissue is curative. It provides both metabolic improvement and symptoms relief. Medical observation is contraindicated. Furthermore, parathyroidectomy is recommended as early as possible in the course of the disease because once systemic complications such as renal dysfunction or hypertension develop, they tend to progress despite elimination of the underlying hyperparathyroidism.

9. Preoperative imaging techniques

Various techniques are currently available for parathyroid glands imaging. Noninvasive studies include ultrasonography, scintigraphy, computed tomography (CT) scanning, and magnetic resonance imaging (MRI). Scintigraphy with use of the radiopharmaceuticals technetium ^{99m}Tc sestamibi or technetium ^{99m}Tc tetrofosmin is widely recommended as the preferred imaging technique for parathyroids. Parathyroid selective arteriography or selective parathyroid venous sampling have been used occasionally as invasive techniques in select cases.

9.1 Ultrasonography

Parathyroid ultrasonography is currently the most easily accessible and a relatively inexpensive non-invasive test that is routinely used for the assessment of the thyroid and parathyroid glands. It is utilized for preoperative investigation in patients with hyperparathyroidism not only to localize and visualize enlarged parathyroids, but also to rule out thyroid nodules that may need to be evaluated prior to parathyroid surgery. For best results a high-frequency (7.5- or 10-MHz) linear ultrasound transducer should be available. The patient should be supine with the neck moderately hyperextended. It is recommended to start the evaluation from the carotid bifurcation superiorly and proceed down to the sternal notch inferiorly and to the carotid artery laterally.

Normal parathyroids are barely visualized with ultrasonography. Parathyroid adenomas appear on gray-scale images as hypoechoic or anechoic, discrete, oval masses. They are located posterior to the lobe of the thyroid gland and anterior to the longus colli muscles. Usually, the common carotid artery confines the parathyroid-bearing region laterally. An

echogenic line separating the thyroid tissue from the enlarged parathyroid gland can be often visualized. Cystic changes, lobulations, increased echogenicity due to fatty deposition, and occasional calcifications are more frequent in larger adenomas.
Parathyroid adenomas, in particular lesions larger than 1 cm in diameter, tend to be hypervascular, and therefore color Doppler ultrasonography is useful in localizing these enlarged glands. Besides, Doppler ultrasound can easily disclose the extrathyroidal vessel supplying parathyroid and this finding may constitute a road map to the otherwise inconspicuous gland.
Ultrasonography is efficient in diagnosing cervical parathyroid lesions with reported sensitivity up to 80% and specificity up to 90%, but fails to detect majority of parathyroid adenomas located in the mediastinum. Additionally, intrathyroidal lesions cannot be differentiated as a parathyroid adenoma or thyroid nodule based on imaging only, and a biopsy is required.

9.2 ^{99m}Tc sestamibi imaging

Nuclear imaging with use of ^{99m}Technetium (^{99m}Tc) sestamibi is currently approved as a standard technique for preoperative imaging of parathyroid glands. ^{99m}Tc sestamibi is a complex of the radioisotope technetium-^{99m}Tc with the ligand methoxyisobutylisonitrile (MIBI). ^{99m}Tc sestamibi, first applied as a myocardial perfusion agent, for parathyroids assessment is combined with either sodium iodide I^{123} or ^{99m}Tc pertechnetate in a procedure called subtraction scintigraphy. It is based on a fenomenon that ^{99m}Tc sestamibi is accumulated by both thyroid and abnormal parathyroids, whereas sodium iodide I^{123} and ^{99m}Tc pertechnetate are taken up by only thyroid tissue. To visualize parathyroids and differentiate them from thyroid tissue the sodium iodide I^{123} or ^{99m}Tc -pertechnetate image is subtracted from the ^{99m}Tc-sestamibi image.
Another, more recent imaging modality is the dual-phase technique with ^{99m}Tc sestamibi as the sole imaging agent. Both thyroid tissue and abnormal parathyroid tissue incorporate ^{99m}Tc sestamibi from circulating blood rapidly after intravenous administration. The test is based on the differential washout of ^{99m}Tc sestamibi from thyroid compared with abnormal parathyroids. The rate of washout from hyperactive parathyroid tissue, such as parathyroid adenoma, is much slower than that of normal thyroid tissue. Routine protocol includes intravenous administration of 20mCi of ^{99m}Tc Sestamibi and sequencial acquisition of early and delayed images of the neck and upper mediastinum. The early image, obtained 10-15 minutes after the injection, is called the thyroid phase as ^{99m}Tc sestamibi is rapidly taken up in the thyroid gland at this time. 1.5-3 hours after the injection the delayed image called the parathyroid phase is recorded. At this phase, ^{99m}Tc sestamibi has been washed out from thyroid but remains accumulated in the hyperactive parathyroid tissue, and this allows for localization of abnormal parathyroid glands. Planar images may be complemented with lateral or oblique acquisitions, or even SPECT images when appropriate equipment is applied. Sensitivity of the ^{99m}Tc sestamibi dual phase protocol has been reported to achieve 70-100%. Small or pedunculated, mobile adenomas may, however, be missed at this test.
^{99m}Tc sestamibi may also be used in minimally invasive parathyroid surgery, as an intraoperative adjunct facilitating localization of hyperactive parathyroid adenoma and confirming curative resection. The radionuclide is injected 1.5 to 3 hours prior to surgery, and a hand-held gamma probe is used to guide the incision, localize the abnormal gland and confirm identity of the resected parathyroid tissue ex-vivo. This technique called

intraoperative nuclear mapping proved to be successful, and is a standard procedure in a number of centers.

^{99m}Tc tetrofosmin is another radiopharmaceutical agent recently introduced into parathyroid imaging. It has a slightly different mechanism of accumulation in tissues, but imaging characteristics similar to those of ^{99m}Tc sestamibi. Also imaging protocols are similar with intravenous injections of 20-25 mCi of radionuclide prior to early (10-30 minutes) and delayed (1.5-3 hours) acquisition images.

9.3 Computed tomography (CT) scanning

Assessment of parathyroid glands with use of a typical CT protocol involves the acquisition of contiguous axial 2- to 3-mm images ranging from the hyoid bone down to the carina. Nonenhanced images of parathyroid adenomas have an attenuation similar to that of muscle. Substantial degree of enhancement is usually shown in parathyroid adenomas after administration of contrast material, as these lesions tend to be hypervascular structures. Typically, parathyroid adenomas present at CT as enlarged, enhancing, soft-tissue masses in the expected location of the parathyroids. The sensitivity of CT in detecting parathyroid adenomas attains 90%. However, the use of ionizing radiation and required intravenous administration of contrast material accompanied by associated risks are considered remarkable disadvantages of this imaging technique. Besides, thyroid nodule, tortuous vessel, or laterally displaced esophagus may be misidentified as a false-positive finding, whereas small or ectopic lesion, poor visualization of neck structures or distorted neck anatomy due to prior surgery may lead to false-negative result.

9.4 Magnetic resonance imaging

MRI is occasionally used for parathyroid imaging. A typical MRI protocol for the assessment of parathyroids involves axial images of the neck and mediastinum. Images are acquired using T1-weighted spin-echo sequences (short recovery time [TR], short echo time [TE]) followed by T2-weighted spin-echo sequences (long TR, long TE). Parathyroid adenomas are seen on MRI images as soft-tissue masses, whereas normal parathyroids are usually not detected. Parathyroid adenomas commonly have low-to-medium signal intensity on T1-weighted images and high signal intensity on T2-weighted images. After gadolinium contrast administration, abnormal parathyroid glands show strong enhancement on T1-weighted images, comparable to conventional T2-weighted imaging.

9.5 Parathyroid arteriography and venous sampling

Parathyroid arteriography and parathyroid venous sampling are invasive tests burdened by a remarkable risk of embolic stroke and spinal cord injury, and therefore should be considered only when the findings of noninvasive imaging modalities are nondiagnostic. Parathyroid adenomas, like many endocrine tumors, tend to be hypervascular and have a characteristic appearance on angiograms. They appear as round or oval lesions with smooth margins and dense vascular blush. Localization of parathyroid adenoma may be visualized with use of digital subtraction angiography (DSA) and/or conventional arteriography. Thyrocervical trunks and common carotid arteries should be subject to selective arteriography in typical cases. Ectopic mediastinal or thymic glands may be better identified by examination of internal thoracic arteries.

Selective venous sampling with parathyroid hormone measurement may be performed to determine the general location of hypersecreting parathyroid tissue. Right and left thymic veins, inferior thyroid veins, and vertebral veins have been reported to be sampled in this regimen. A 2-fold gradient in PTH concentration in the sampled vein as referenced to that of the peripheral vein confirms the location of hyperactive parathyroid tissue. Similar technique may also be used intraoperatively to confirm curative resection of parathyroid adenoma.

10. Preoperative anesthetic management

Since renal function is likely to be impaired in hyperparathyroidism, prior to surgical treatment hypercalcemic patients require thorough rehydration. In some of these patients urinary catheterization and central venous pressure monitoring may be indicated. After rehydration, loop diuretics may be administered to decrease renal calcium reabsorption and promote urinary excretion, which in result will alleviate hypercalcaemia. Excessive diuresis may in turn lead to increased maintenance fluid requirements. Corticosteroids, bisphosphonates, calcium chelators such as trisodium edentate, calcitonin, or even dialysis are occasionally indicated in severe cases. Hypertension, if present, should be controlled with fast-acting antihypertensive medication. In patients with end-stage renal failure, perioperative invasive central venous pressure monitoring may be helpful for thorough monitoring of circulatory system. Occasionally, tumors of other organs may secrete PTH, for example, bronchial or tracheal carcinomas. This condition is called pseudohyperparathyroidism and should be brought to attention preoperatively to avoid intreaoperative ventilatory problems in theses rare cases when the lesion occludes bronchial or tracheal lumen.

11. References

[1] Fernández-Fernández FJ, Sesma P. Primary hyperparathyroidism. N Engl J Med. 2012 Mar 1;366(9):860; author reply 860-1.

[2] Afzal A, Gauhar TM, Butt WT, Khawaja AA, Azim KM. Management of hyperparathyroidism: a five year surgical experience. J Pak Med Assoc. 2011 Dec;61(12):1194-8.

[3] Wang CC, Hsu YJ, Wu CC, Yang SS, Chen GS, Lin SH, Chu P. Serum fetuin-A levels increased following parathyroidectomy in uremic hyperparathyroidism. Clin Nephrol. 2012 Feb;77(2):89-96. doi: 10.10.5414/CN106757.

[4] Emilion E, Emilion R. Estimation of the 25(OH) vitamin D threshold below which secondary hyperparathyroidism may occur among African migrant women in Paris. Int J Vitam Nutr Res. 2011 Jul;81(4):218-24.

[5] Francucci CM, Ceccoli L, Caudarella R, Rilli S, Vescini F, Boscaro M. Asymptomatic primary hyperparathyroidism: surgical and medical management. J Endocrinol Invest. 2011 Jul;34(7 Suppl):50-4.

[6] Nuti R, Merlotti D, Gennari L. Vitamin D deficiency and primary hyperparathyroidism. J Endocrinol Invest. 2011 Jul;34(7 Suppl):45-9. Review.

[7] Pepe J, Cipriani C, Pilotto R, De Lucia F, Castro C, Lenge L, Russo S, Guarnieri V, Scillitani A, Carnevale V, D'Erasmo E, Romagnoli E, Minisola S. Sporadic and

hereditary primary hyperparathyroidism. J Endocrinol Invest. 2011 Jul;34(7 Suppl):40-4. Review.

[8] Cetani F, Pardi E, Borsari S, Marcocci C. Molecular pathogenesis of primary hyperparathyroidism. J Endocrinol Invest. 2011 Jul;34(7 Suppl):35-9. Review.

[9] Francucci CM, Ghigo E, Boscaro M. Primary hyperparathyroidism and skeleton. Foreword. J Endocrinol Invest. 2011 Jul;34(7 Suppl):1-2.

[10] Ardito G, Revelli L, Giustozzi E, Giordano A. Radioguided parathyroidectomy in forearm graft for recurrent hyperparathyroidism. Br J Radiol. 2012 Jan;85(1009):e1-3.

[11] Peiris AN, Youssef D, Grant WB. Secondary hyperparathyroidism: benign bystander or culpable contributor to adverse health outcomes? South Med J. 2012 Jan;105(1):36-42. Review.

[12] Marcocci C, Cetani F. Clinical practice. Primary hyperparathyroidism. N Engl J Med. 2011 Dec 22;365(25):2389-97.

[13] Piedra M, García-Unzueta MT, Berja A, Paule B, Lavín BA, Valero C, Riancho JA, Amado JA. "Single nucleotide polymorphisms of the OPG/RANKL system genes in primary hyperparathyroidism and their relationship with bone mineral density". BMC Med Genet. 2011 Dec 20;12:168.

[14] Duh QY. The Bayes theorem wins: comment on "Impact of localization studies and clinical scenario in patients with hyperparathyroidism being evaluated for reoperative neck surgery". Arch Surg. 2011 Dec;146(12):1403.

[15] Shin JJ, Milas M, Mitchell J, Berber E, Ross L, Siperstein A. Impact of localization studies and clinical scenario in patients with hyperparathyroidism being evaluated for reoperative neck surgery. Arch Surg. 2011 Dec;146(12):1397-403.

[16] Sorensen MD, Duh QY, Grogan RH, Tran TC, Stoller ML. Urinary parameters as predictors of primary hyperparathyroidism in patients with nephrolithiasis. J Urol. 2012 Feb;187(2):516-21. Epub 2011 Dec 15.

[17] Shlapack MA, Rizvi AA. Normocalcemic primary hyperparathyroidism-characteristics and clinical significance of an emerging entity. Am J Med Sci. 2012 Feb;343(2):163-6. Review.

[18] Bhadada SK, Bhansali A, Shah VN, Rao DS. Changes in serum leptin and adiponectin concentrations and insulin resistance after curative parathyroidectomy in moderate to severe primary hyperparathyroidism. Singapore Med J. 2011 Dec;52(12):890-3.

[19] Wang TS, Cheung K, Farrokhyar F, Roman SA, Sosa JA. Would scan, but which scan? A cost-utility analysis to optimize preoperative imaging for primary hyperparathyroidism. Surgery. 2011 Dec;150(6):1286-94.

[20] Perrier ND, Evans DB. Population-level predictors of persistent hyperparathyroidism. Surgery. 2011 Dec;150(6):1120-1.

[21] Yeh MW, Wiseman JE, Chu SD, Ituarte PH, Liu IL, Young KL, Kang SJ, Harari A, Haigh PI. Population-level predictors of persistent hyperparathyroidism. Surgery. 2011 Dec;150(6):1113-9.

[22] Wallace LB, Parikh RT, Ross LV, Mazzaglia PJ, Foley C, Shin JJ, Mitchell JC, Berber E, Siperstein AE, Milas M. The phenotype of primary hyperparathyroidism with normal parathyroid hormone levels: how low can parathyroid hormone go? Surgery. 2011 Dec;150(6):1102-12.

[23] Press D, Politz D, Lopez J, Norman J. The effect of vitamin D levels on postoperative calcium requirements, symptomatic hypocalcemia, and parathormone levels following parathyroidectomy for primary hyperparathyroidism. Surgery. 2011 Dec;150(6):1061-8.

[24] Mshelia DS, Hatutale AN, Mokgoro NP, Nchabaleng ME, Buscombe JR, Sathekge MM. Correlation between serum calcium levels and dual-phase (99m)Tc-sestamibi parathyroid scintigraphy in primary hyperparathyroidism. Clin Physiol Funct Imaging. 2012 Jan;32(1):19-24. doi: 10.1111/j.1475-097X.2011.01048.x. Epub 2011 Aug 24.

[25] Lumachi F, Camozzi V, Luisetto G, Zanella S, Basso SM. Arterial blood pressure, serum calcium and PTH in elderly men with parathyroid tumors and primary hyperparathyroidism. Anticancer Res. 2011 Nov;31(11):3969-72.

[26] El-Shafey EM, Alsahow AE, Alsaran K, Sabry AA, Atia M. Cinacalcet hydrochloride therapy for secondary hyperparathyroidism in hemodialysis patients. Ther Apher Dial. 2011 Dec;15(6):547-55. doi: 10.1111/j.1744-9987.2011.00994.x.

[27] Cheungpasitporn W, Suksaranjit P, Chanprasert S. Acute kidney injury from bilateral ureteral calcium stones in the setting of primary hyperparathyroidism. Am J Emerg Med. 2012 Feb;30(2):383-4. Epub 2011 Nov 17.

[28] Schmidt MC, Kahraman D, Neumaier B, Ortmann M, Stippel D. Tc-99m-MIBI-negative parathyroid adenoma in primary hyperparathyroidism detected by C-11-methionine PET/CT after previous thyroid surgery. Clin Nucl Med. 2011 Dec;36(12):1153-5.

[29] Sanadgol H, Bayani M, Mohammadi M, Bayani B, Mashhadi MA. Effect of vitamin C on parathyroid hormone in hemodialysis patients with mild to moderate secondary hyperparathyroidism. Iran J Kidney Dis. 2011 Nov;5(6):410-5.

[30] Carneiro-Pla D, Solorzano C. A summary of the new phenomenon of normocalcemic hyperparathyroidism and appropriate management. Curr Opin Oncol. 2012 Jan;24(1):42-5.

[31] Suwan N. Secondary hyperparathyroidism and risk factors in patients undergoing peritoneal dialysis in a tertiary hospital. J Med Assoc Thai. 2011 Sep;94 Suppl 4:S101-5.

[32] Iwata S, Walker MD, Di Tullio MR, Hyodo E, Jin Z, Liu R, Sacco RL, Homma S, Silverberg SJ. Aortic valve calcification in mild primary hyperparathyroidism. J Clin Endocrinol Metab. 2012 Jan;97(1):132-7. Epub 2011 Oct 26.

[33] Amin AL, Wang TS, Wade TJ, Quiroz FA, Hellman RS, Evans DB, Yen TW. Nonlocalizing imaging studies for hyperparathyroidism: where to explore first? J Am Coll Surg. 2011 Dec;213(6):793-9. Epub 2011 Oct 19.

[34] Pilz S, Kienreich K, Drechsler C, Ritz E, Fahrleitner-Pammer A, Gaksch M, Meinitzer A, März W, Pieber TR, Tomaschitz A. Hyperparathyroidism in patients with primary aldosteronism: cross-sectional and interventional data from the GECOH study. J Clin Endocrinol Metab. 2012 Jan;97(1):E75-9. Epub 2011 Oct 19.

[35] Jabiev AA, Lew JI, Garb JL, Sanchez YM, Solorzano CC. Primary hyperparathyroidism in the underinsured: a study of 493 patients. Surgery. 2012 Mar;151(3):471-6. Epub 2011 Oct 13.

[36] Wilson SD, Doffek KM, Wang TS, Krzywda EA, Evans DB, Yen TW. Primary hyperparathyroidism with a history of head and neck irradiation: the consequences of associated thyroid tumors. Surgery. 2011 Oct;150(4):869-77.
[37] Lu KC, Wu CC, Ma WY, Chen CC, Wu HC, Chu P. Decreased blood lead levels after calcitriol treatment in hemodialysis patients with secondary hyperparathyroidism. Bone. 2011 Dec;49(6):1306-10. Epub 2011 Oct 1.
[38] Witteveen JE, van Lierop AH, Papapoulos SE, Hamdy NA. Increased circulating levels of FGF23: an adaptive response in primary hyperparathyroidism? Eur J Endocrinol. 2012 Jan;166(1):55-60. Epub 2011 Oct 7.
[39] Udelsman R. Approach to the patient with persistent or recurrent primary hyperparathyroidism. J Clin Endocrinol Metab. 2011 Oct;96(10):2950-8.
[40] Bollerslev J, Marcocci C, Sosa M, Nordenström J, Bouillon R, Mosekilde L. Current evidence for recommendation of surgery, medical treatment and vitamin D repletion in mild primary hyperparathyroidism. Eur J Endocrinol. 2011 Dec;165(6):851-64. Epub 2011 Sep 29.
[41] Adachi M, Miyoshi T, Shiraishi N, Shimada H, Sakaguchi S, Tomita K, Kitamura K. A study of maintenance therapy after intravenous maxacalcitol for secondary hyperparathyroidism. Clin Nephrol. 2011 Oct;76(4):266-72.
[42] Ishimura E, Okuno S, Tsuboniwa N, Ichii M, Yamakawa K, Yamakawa T, Shoji S, Nishizawa Y, Inaba M. Effect of cinacalcet on bone mineral density of the radius in hemodialysis patients with secondary hyperparathyroidism. Clin Nephrol. 2011 Oct;76(4):259-65.
[43] Shapey IM, Jaunoo SS, Hanson C, Jaunoo SR, Thrush S, Munro A. Primary hyperparathyroidism: how many cases are being missed? Ann R Coll Surg Engl. 2011 May;93(4):294-6.
[44] Pyram R, Mahajan G, Gliwa A. Primary hyperparathyroidism: Skeletal and non-skeletal effects, diagnosis and management. Maturitas. 2011 Nov;70(3):246-55. Epub 2011 Sep 23.
[45] Jithpratuck W, Garrett LH, Peiris AN. Treating vitamin D insufficiency in primary hyperparathyroidism: a cautionary tale. Tenn Med. 2011 Aug;104(7):47-9.
[46] Espiritu RP, Kearns AE, Vickers KS, Grant C, Ryu E, Wermers RA. Depression in primary hyperparathyroidism: prevalence and benefit of surgery. J Clin Endocrinol Metab. 2011 Nov;96(11):E1737-45. Epub 2011 Sep 14.
[47] Boucher BJ. Re Yu et al. The natural history of treated and untreated primary hyperparathyroidism: the Parathyroid Epidemiology and Audit Research Study. Q J Med 2011; 104:513-521. QJM. 2011 Dec;104(12):1107-8. Epub 2011 Sep 10.
[48] Sorensen MD, Duh QY, Grogan RH, Tran TC, Stoller ML. Differences in metabolic urinary abnormalities in stone forming and nonstone forming patients with primary hyperparathyroidism. Surgery. 2012 Mar;151(3):477-83. Epub 2011 Sep 3.
[49] Frazão JM, Messa P, Mellotte GJ, Geiger H, Hagen EC, Quarles LD, Kerr PG, Baños A, Dehmel B, Urena P. Cinacalcet reduces plasma intact parathyroid hormone, serum phosphate and calcium levels in patients with secondary hyperparathyroidism irrespective of its severity. Clin Nephrol. 2011 Sep;76(3):233-43.
[50] Stephani J, Akinli AS, von Figura G, Barth TF, Weber T, Hartmann B, Adler G, von Boyen GB. Acute Pancreatitis in a patient with hypercalcemia due to tertiary hyperparathyroidism. Z Gastroenterol. 2011 Sep;49(9):1263-6. Epub 2011 Sep 1.

[51] Kovesdy CP, Lu JL, Malakauskas SM, Andress DL, Kalantar-Zadeh K, Ahmadzadeh S. Paricalcitol versus ergocalciferol for secondary hyperparathyroidism in CKD stages 3 and 4: a randomized controlled trial. Am J Kidney Dis. 2012 Jan;59(1):58-66. Epub 2011 Aug 31.

[52] Hoi WH, Leow MK, Sule A, Lee HY, Mmed TA, Tay JC. Hyperparathyroidism due to eutopic PTH secretion from an ectopic intrathymic parathyroid cyst. Ann Thorac Cardiovasc Surg. 2011 Oct 25;17(5):511-3. Epub 2011 Jul 13.

[53] Zitt E, Woess E, Mayer G, Lhotta K. Effect of cinacalcet on renal electrolyte handling and systemic arterial blood pressure in kidney transplant patients with persistent hyperparathyroidism. Transplantation. 2011 Oct 27;92(8):883-9.

[54] Macfarlane DP, Yu N, Donnan PT, Leese GP. Should 'mild primary hyperparathyroidism' be reclassified as 'insidious': is it time to reconsider? Clin Endocrinol (Oxf). 2011 Dec;75(6):730-7. doi: 10.1111/j.1365-2265.2011.04201.x.

[55] Lucchi L, Carboni C, Stipo L, Malaguti V, Ferrari F, Graziani R, Arletti S, Graziosi C. Early initiation of cinacalcet for the treatment of secondary hyperparathyroidism in hemodialysis patients: a three-year clinical experience. Artif Organs. 2011 Dec;35(12):1186-93. doi: 10.1111/j.1525-1594.2011.01270.x. Epub 2011 Aug 17.

[56] Plosker GL. Cinacalcet: a pharmacoeconomic review of its use in secondary hyperparathyroidism in end-stage renal disease. Pharmacoeconomics. 2011 Sep;29(9):807-21. doi: 10.2165/11207220-000000000-00000.

[57] Akizawa T, Kido R, Fukagawa M, Onishi Y, Yamaguchi T, Hasegawa T, Fukuhara S, Kurokawa K. Decreases in PTH in Japanese hemodialysis patients with secondary hyperparathyroidism: associations with changing practice patterns. Clin J Am Soc Nephrol. 2011 Sep;6(9):2280-8. Epub 2011 Aug 11.

[58] Hansen D, Rasmussen K, Danielsen H, Meyer-Hofmann H, Bacevicius E, Lauridsen TG, Madsen JK, Tougaard BG, Marckmann P, Thye-Roenn P, Nielsen JE, Kreiner S, Brandi L. No difference between alfacalcidol and paricalcitol in the treatment of secondary hyperparathyroidism in hemodialysis patients: a randomized crossover trial. Kidney Int. 2011 Oct;80(8):841-50. doi: 10.1038/ki.2011.226. Epub 2011 Aug 10.

[59] Kırış A, Erem C, Kırış G, Nuhoğlu I, Karaman K, Civan N, Örem C, Durmuş I, Kutlu M. The assessment of left ventricular systolic asynchrony in patients with primary hyperparathyroidism. Echocardiography. 2011 Oct;28(9):955-60. doi: 10.1111/j.1540-8175.2011.01468.x. Epub 2011 Aug 9.

[60] Maniero C, Fassina A, Guzzardo V, Lenzini L, Amadori G, Pelizzo MR, Gomez-Sanchez C, Rossi GP. Primary hyperparathyroidism with concurrent primary aldosteronism. Hypertension. 2011 Sep;58(3):341-6. Epub 2011 Aug 8.

[61] Islam MZ, Viljakainen HT, Kärkkäinen MU, Saarnio E, Laitinen K, Lamberg-Allardt C. Prevalence of vitamin D deficiency and secondary hyperparathyroidism during winter in pre-menopausal Bangladeshi and Somali immigrant and ethnic Finnish women: associations with forearm bone mineral density. Br J Nutr. 2012 Jan;107(2):277-83. Epub 2011 Aug 9.

[62] Padmanabhan H. Outpatient management of primary hyperparathyroidism. Am J Med. 2011 Oct;124(10):911-4. Epub 2011 Aug 3.

[63] Rudofsky G, Tsioga M, Reismann P, Leowardi C, Kopf S, Grafe IA, Nawroth PP, Isermann B. Transient hyperthyroidism after surgery for secondary hyperparathyroidism: a common problem. Eur J Med Res. 2011 Aug 8;16(8):375-80.

[64] Jain SK, Roy SP, Nagi ON. Alendronate induced femur fracture complicated with secondary hyperparathyroidism. Mymensingh Med J. 2011 Jul;20(3):501-6.
[65] Park JH, Kang SW, Jeong JJ, Nam KH, Chang HS, Chung WY, Park CS. Surgical treatment of tertiary hyperparathyroidism after renal transplantation: a 31-year experience in a single institution. Endocr J. 2011 Oct 29;58(10):827-33. Epub 2011 Jul 30.
[66] Isaksen T, Nielsen CS, Christensen SE, Nissen PH, Heickendorff L, Mosekilde L. Forearm bone mineral density in familial hypocalciuric hypercalcemia and primary hyperparathyroidism: a comparative study. Calcif Tissue Int. 2011 Oct;89(4):285-94. doi: 10.1007/s00223-011-9517-x. Epub 2011 Jul 22.
[67] Lieberman SM, Vouyiouklis M, Elangovan S, Morris LG. Image of the month. Tertiary hyperparathyroidism after parathyroidectomy with autotransplantation. Arch Surg. 2011 Jul;146(7):879-80.
[68] Bellavia M, Gioviale MC, Damiano G, Palumbo VD, Cacciabaudo F, Altomare R Buscemi G, Lo Monte AI. Is secondary hyperparathyroidism-related myelofibrosis a negative prognostic factor for kidney transplant outcome? Med Hypotheses. 2011 Oct;77(4):557-9. Epub 2011 Jul 16.
[69] Agorastos A, Weinas A, Agorastos AD, Wiedemann K. Psychosis-induced vitamin D deficiency with secondary hyperparathyroidism and osteoporotic fractures. Gen Hosp Psychiatry. 2011 Nov-Dec;33(6):641.e3-5. Epub 2011 Jul 16.
[70] Nagar S, Reid D, Czako P, Long G, Shanley C. Outcomes analysis of intraoperative adjuncts during minimally invasive parathyroidectomy for primary hyperparathyroidism. Am J Surg. 2012 Feb;203(2):177-81. Epub 2011 Jul 14.
[71] De Rosa A, Rinaldi C, Tucci T, Pappatà S, Rossi F, Morra VB, Faggiano A, Colao A, De Michele G. Co-existence of primary hyperparathyroidism and Parkinson's disease in three patients: an incidental finding? Parkinsonism Relat Disord. 2011 Dec;17(10):771-3. Epub 2011 Jul 5.
[72] Bargren AE, Repplinger D, Chen H, Sippel RS. Can biochemical abnormalities predict symptomatology in patients with primary hyperparathyroidism? J Am Coll Surg. 2011 Sep;213(3):410-4. Epub 2011 Jul 1.
[73] Meola M, Petrucci I, Colombini E, Barsotti G. Use of ultrasound to assess the response to therapy for secondary hyperparathyroidism. Am J Kidney Dis. 2011 Sep;58(3):485-91. Epub 2011 Jun 29.
[74] Schreinemakers JM, Pieterman CR, Scholten A, Vriens MR, Valk GD, Rinkes IH. The optimal surgical treatment for primary hyperparathyroidism in MEN1 patients: a systematic review. World J Surg. 2011 Sep;35(9):1993-2005.
[75] Alhefdhi A, Pinchot SN, Davis R, Sippel RS, Chen H. The necessity and reliability of intraoperative parathyroid hormone (PTH) testing in patients with mild hyperparathyroidism and PTH levels in the normal range. World J Surg. 2011 Sep;35(9):2006-9.
[76] Ikegami S, Kamimura M, Uchiyama S, Kato H. Women with insufficient 25-hydroxyvitamin D without secondary hyperparathyroidism have altered bone turnover and greater incidence of vertebral fractures. J Orthop Sci. 2011 Sep;16(5):573-80. Epub 2011 Jun 29.

[77] van Ginhoven TM, Morks AN, Schepers T, de Graaf PW, Smit PC. Surgeon-performed ultrasound as preoperative localization study in patients with primary hyperparathyroidism. Eur Surg Res. 2011;47(2):70-4. Epub 2011 Jun 23.

[78] Christensen MH, Dankel SN, Nordbø Y, Varhaug JE, Almås B, Lien EA, Mellgren G. Primary hyperparathyroidism influences the expression of inflammatory and metabolic genes in adipose tissue. PLoS One. 2011;6(6):e20481. Epub 2011 Jun 17.

[79] Stubbs JR, Wetmore JB. Does it matter how parathyroid hormone levels are suppressed in secondary hyperparathyroidism? Semin Dial. 2011 May-Jun;24(3):298-306. doi: 10.1111/j.1525-139X.2011.00935.x.

[80] Fujii T, Yamaguchi S, Yajima R, Tsutsumi S, Uchida N, Asao T, Oriuch N, Kuwano H. Use of a handheld, semiconductor (cadmium zinc telluride)-based gamma camera in navigation surgery for primary hyperparathyroidism. Am Surg. 2011 Jun;77(6):690-3.

[81] Kaji H, Imanishi Y, Sugimoto T, Seino S. Comparisons of serum sclerostin levels among patients with postmenopausal osteoporosis, primary hyperparathyroidism and osteomalacia. Exp Clin Endocrinol Diabetes. 2011 Jul;119(7):440-4. doi: 10.1055/s-0031-1275661. Epub 2011 Jun 10.

[82] Frank-Raue K, Haag C, Schulze E, Keuser R, Raue F, Dralle H, Lorenz K. CDC73-related hereditary hyperparathyroidism: five new mutations and the clinical spectrum. Eur J Endocrinol. 2011 Sep;165(3):477-83. Epub 2011 Jun 7.

[83] Rejnmark L, Vestergaard P, Mosekilde L. Nephrolithiasis and renal calcifications in primary hyperparathyroidism. J Clin Endocrinol Metab. 2011 Aug;96(8):2377-85. Epub 2011 Jun 6.

[84] Schillaci G, Pucci G, Pirro M, Monacelli M, Scarponi AM, Manfredelli MR, Rondelli F, Avenia N, Mannarino E. Large-artery stiffness: a reversible marker of cardiovascular risk in primary hyperparathyroidism. Atherosclerosis. 2011 Sep;218(1):96-101. Epub 2011 May 18.

[85] Mannstadt M, Holick E, Zhao W, Jüppner H. Mutational analysis of GCMB, a parathyroid-specific transcription factor, in parathyroid adenoma of primary hyperparathyroidism. J Endocrinol. 2011 Aug;210(2):165-71. Epub 2011 Jun 3.

22

Pulmonary Transplantation and Ischemia-Reperfusion Injury

Ashish K. Sharma, Matthew L. Stone,
Christine L. Lau and Victor E. Laubach
University of Virginia Health System, Charlottesville, VA, USA

1. Introduction

Lung transplantation provides a curative hope for many with end-stage pulmonary disease. Since the first attempt at human lung transplantation in 1963, scientific and surgical advancements have supported improved survival and quality of life for lung transplant recipients (Hardy, et al., 1963). Significant contributions in cardiopulmonary bypass, pharmacologic immunosuppression, and donor-recipient risk stratification have increased the success and associated clinical adoption of this treatment strategy. Continued research efforts in novel methods for organ preservation, donor graft selection, and recipient risk stratification support a promising future for lung transplantation.

Improvements in surgical technique and perioperative care over the past two decades have led to a 30-fold increase in the number of lung transplant recipients worldwide to 2,769 patients in 2008 (Christie, et al., 2010). Since 1994, bilateral lung transplantation has supplanted single lung transplantation as the primary strategy for organ replacement to now account for 71% of lung transplants performed worldwide (Christie, et al., 2010). In 2010, the primary indications for lung transplantation included chronic obstructive pulmonary disease (35.5%), idiopathic pulmonary fibrosis (22.1%), and cystic fibrosis (16.0%) (Christie, et al., 2010). Despite this promising evolution and the increasing number of indications for lung transplantation, long-term survival has shown minimal improvement. Lung transplant outcomes remain the poorest of any solid organ transplant, with international survival estimates demonstrating a 21% one-year and 50% five-year mortality (Christie, et al., 2010).

Lung ischemia-reperfusion (IR) injury following transplantation imposes a significant threat to graft and recipient survival (Diamond & Christie, 2010). IR injury is the main cause of primary graft failure and significantly increases the risk for acute rejection and long-term graft dysfunction (de Perrot, et al., 2003). Multivariate analysis of long-term graft function has implicated IR injury as an independent predictor for bronchiolitis obliterans syndrome (BOS), the most common cause of long-term morbidity and mortality after lung transplantation (Fiser, et al., 2002). IR-induced lung injury is characterized by nonspecific alveolar damage, lung edema, and hypoxemia occurring within 72 hours after lung transplantation (de Perrot, et al., 2003). The estimated incidence of IR injury is 41% following lung transplantation with an associated 30-day mortality of 40%, compared to 7% for patients with no IR injury (Granton, 2006). Clinical studies have demonstrated increased in-hospital mortality and morbidity associated with IR injury resulting in prolonged ventilation, postoperative systolic pulmonary hypertension, longer intensive care unit stay, and increased cost of hospitalization (Cottini, et al., 2006; King, et al., 2000).

Currently no clinical therapies are available to prevent IR injury. The standard method used to help minimize IR injury for lung transplantation incorporates a universal cold crystalloid flush of the donor organ prior to explantation. Cold storage on ice during the preservation period limits metabolic activity, vasospasm, and thrombosis (Puri & Patterson, 2008). Reimplantation into the recipient restores warm perfusion to the allograft, initiating a characteristic inflammatory cascade leading to IR injury. Hypothermic organ storage is associated with oxidative stress, sodium pump inactivation, intracellular calcium overload, iron release, and cell death that induce cell surface expression patterns and proinflammatory mediators for leukocyte activation during the reperfusion period (de Perrot, et al., 2003). This inherent response mechanism implicates IR injury as a primary determinant of both immediate and long-term graft survival.

Quality of the donor allograft and nature of recipient pathophysiology are primary determinants for the severity of IR injury, with a defined spectrum from mild pulmonary infiltration to the most severe acute respiratory distress syndrome (King, et al., 2000). A significant research commitment in lung transplantation is focused on organ selection and preservation to limit the deleterious effects of IR injury. Currently a disparaging 10-30% of donor lungs are approved for transplantation based on predictive criteria incorporating donor history, arterial blood gas assessment, chest x-ray and bronchoscopic findings, and physical examination upon lung retrieval. Inherent limitations are present in the subjective assessment of the donor allograft, as evidenced in comparable outcomes with extended donor criteria with marginal donor organs (Sundaresan, et al., 1995). This finding supports continued research commitment to risk stratification and predictive modeling for IR injury in donor lung selection.

Allograft selection and donor pool expansion are primary aims for current lung transplantation research. Traditional organ procurements for lung transplantation involve donation following brain death, excluding donations after cardiac death as a result of the inherent extended period of ischemia. Study of systemic markers for inflammation in brain dead donors has established interleukin-8 as a predictive cytokine marker for primary graft failure after reperfusion (Fisher, et al., 2001). This foundational research exemplifies the potential role for systemic markers of inflammation in the predictive modeling of graft survival.

A recent study on lung donation after controlled cardiac death has demonstrated comparable early- and medium-term outcomes in contrast to donation after brain death (de Vleeschauwer, et al., 2011). These promising results introduce a potential for donor pool expansion in coordination with lung rehabilitation strategies prior to recipient lung implantation. A multicenter study has demonstrated a close relationship between graft ischemic time and both early gas exchange and long-term survival following single and double lung transplantation. The coordinated aim to increase the donor pool with donation after cardiac death and the principle strategy to minimize periods of warm and cold ischemia have inspired novel *ex-vivo* perfusion methods for the donor lung prior to recipient implantation (Cypel, et al., 2011a). An international commitment to technologic advancement and scientific understanding promises to support improved outcomes and needed expansion of the donor pool for future generations.

The focus of this chapter is to define the principle immunologic and inflammatory mediators of IR injury, providing a mechanistic understanding for the multi-factorial pathogenesis of this clinical condition. Novel treatment strategies and current clinical methods for donor allograft treatment are reviewed as a foundational discussion for future research initiatives in the prevention of IR injury.

2. Cellular mediators of lung IR injury

A major complication after lung transplantation is IR injury. After the ischemic insult, reperfusion of the lungs is critical to maintain organ viability; however, reperfusion can also cause a wide variety of complex pathophysiological changes to the lung leading to inflammation and injury. IR causes a multi-faceted cascade of signal transduction events involving a milieu of pro-inflammatory cytokines and chemokines and the generation of reactive oxygen species (ROS) by a myriad of cells in the lung. The crosstalk between these cells via a plethora of molecules leads to the initiation and amplification of a signaling cascade that ultimately culminates in pulmonary injury and dysfunction. Many studies have now established that cells of the innate immune system (bone marrow-derived cells such as T cells, macrophages, dendritic cells and neutrophils) play an important role in lung IR injury. In addition, resident pulmonary cells, such as alveolar epithelial cells and endothelial cells, are also critical mediators of lung IR injury. These cell populations will be discussed below.

2.1 Neutrophils

One of the effector cells responsible for causing lung inflammation and injury are known to be neutrophils. Lung injury can be manifested by the multi-faceted role of infiltrating neutrophils to the site of injury, which adhere to and cross the endothelium upon activation. Although neutrophils play an important role in perpetuating lung IR injury, the role of neutrophils in the early phase is less predominant. Studies from Deeb and colleagues have shown that during the first few hours of IR injury, it is the neutrophil-independent events that play a major role and that neutrophil-dependent events exert their effects after several hours of reperfusion (Deeb, et al., 1990). Other studies have confirmed this biphasic cellular response and have suggested that T cells and macrophages have a more prominent role in the early phase of IR injury while neutrophils play a late, effector role in the execution of lung IR injury (Eppinger, et al., 1995; Fiser, et al., 2001). The infiltration and activation of neutrophils causes lung injury via release of oxygen free radicals and disruption of capillary-epithelial barrier which leads to increased microvascular permeability and pulmonary edema causing irreversible tissue damage.

2.2 Macrophages and dendritic cells

The role of antigen presenting cells such as macrophages and dendritic cells has been implicated in lung IR injury. Several studies suggest that lung IR injury is biphasic, with distinct acute macrophage-mediated injury followed later by neutrophil-dependent injury (Eppinger, et al., 1995, 1997; Fiser, et al., 2001a, 2001b). Abundant evidence suggests that alveolar macrophages in the donor lung are quickly activated by IR to subsequently release pro-inflammatory chemokines and cytokines, and it has been demonstrated that depletion of alveolar macrophages attenuates lung IR injury (Naidu, et al., 2003; Zhao, et al., 2006). This acute pulmonary damage is followed by a cascade of events leading to activation of the recipient inflammatory system against the already damaged vascular endothelium and airway epithelium. A number of studies have strengthened a position for alveolar macrophages and TNF-α in acute IR injury (Eppinger, et al., 1997; Maxey, et al., 2004; Zhao, et al., 2006). One possible mechanism for decreased injury after suppression of macrophage function involves the attenuation of TNF-α or IFN-γ in respiratory burst activity and other inflammatory functions of macrophages (Arenzana-Seisdedos, et al., 1985; Eden & Turino, 1986; Issekutz & Issekutz, 1993; Mayer, et al., 1993; Phillips, et al., 1990). These studies indicate that IR injury is in part initiated by activated macrophages whereas delayed injury is mediated by activated neutrophils.

Recent studies have implicated a contributory role for dendritic cells in organ injury after transplantation including lung IR injury (He, et al., 2007; Saemann, et al., 2009). The cross-talk between antigen presenting cells like macrophages or dendritic cells and T lymphocytes has been postulated to play an important role in the initiation of lung IR injury. A detailed role for dendritic cells in lung IR injury, however, remains to be defined.

2.3 T lymphocytes

Involvement of T cells in IR injury until recently has not been considered; however, it has been demonstrated that T cells can be activated by antigen-independent mechanisms including oxygen radicals and cytokines such as TNF-α, IFN-γ, IL-23, IL-6, and RANTES (Bacon, et al., 1995). It is well known that the lung harbors a substantial reservoir of lymphocytes, and various subsets of T cells such as CD4+ T cells, CD8+ T cells, iNKT cells and γδT cells, have been implicated in lung IR injury. Yang *et al.* have recently demonstrated a key role for CD4+ T cells in an *in vivo* hilar clamp model of lung IR injury (Yang, et al., 2009). In the microcirculation, T cells may amplify inflammation by simultaneously binding to endothelial cells, macrophages, platelets and neutrophils. Several studies describe lung, renal and hepatic protection from IR injury in either null mice or T cell-depleted mice (Le Moine, et al., 2000; Rabb, et al., 2000; Sharma, et al., 2008; Zwacka, et al., 1997). These studies demonstrate significantly reduced neutrophil recruitment and inflammation in T cell-deficient mice after IR injury and suggest a role for T cells in the amplification of innate inflammatory signals. Clavien *et al.* described the activation of T cells by ROS during rat liver IR (Clavien, et al., 1993), and it appears that CD4+ T cells, but not CD8+ T cells, play a key role in the initiation of lung IR injury in mice (Sharma, et al., 2008). It has also been shown that acute lymphocyte-mediated lung IR injury involves CD40-CD40L signaling mechanisms (Moore, et al., 2002). CD4+ T cells play an important role in the initiation of immune responses by providing help to other cells and by taking on a variety of effector functions during immune reactions. CD4+ T cell priming results in the differentiation of various T cell subsets distinguished by the production of particular cytokines and effector functions.

Classically, CD4+ effector cells were viewed in the context of the Th1-Th2 cell paradigm, but other subsets have recently emerged including IL-17-producing T cells (Th17 cells), T cells with regulatory function (Treg cells) and invariant natural killer T (iNKT) cells (Larosa & Orange, 2008). There is also evidence that IL-23, IL-6, and TGF-β are proximal regulators of

IL-17 production by Th17 cells (Kolls & Linden, 2004) and iNKT cells (Rachitskaya, et al., 2008). iNKT cells are typically CD4+ T cells that share receptor structure with conventional T and NK cells and are characterized by their ability to rapidly produce immunoregulatory cytokines such as IL-4 and/or IFN-γ. NKT cells also constitutively express IL-23R and RORγt which can be rapidly activated during a variety of infections and inflammatory responses, and are recruited to produce IL-17 under emergency conditions. In the setting of renal IR, iNKT cell activation mediates neutrophil infiltration, IFN-γ production, and renal IR injury (Li, et al., 2007). Accumulating evidence suggest that Th17 cells are highly pro-inflammatory in that IL-17 is a key cytokine for the recruitment, activation and migration of neutrophils (Kolls & Linden, 2004), and Th17 cell-produced IL-17 is implicated in the pathogenesis of autoimmunity in various animal models (Bettelli, et al., 2007). However, the acute time frame of IL-17 production in lung IR injury is not consistent with a role for Th17 cells, which are not normally present in the lung and which require differentiation from naïve CD4+ T cells. Recent studies have revealed a critical role for the IL-23/IL-17 axis in various models of inflammation including IR injury (Edgerton, et al., 2008; Hanschen, et al., 2008; Wu, et al., 2007; Yen, et al., 2006). A critical role for iNKT cells and their rapid production of IL-17A in lung IR injury and neutrophil infiltration has been recently demonstrated using a mouse lung IR model (Sharma, et al., 2011). These studies support the concept that T lymphocytes can and do mediate IR injury.

2.4 Alveolar epithelial cells

The role of alveolar type II epithelial cells in lung IR injury has been described in recent studies (Sharma, et al., 2007). Alveolar type II epithelial cells contribute to lung IR injury via release of pro-inflammatory cytokines and chemokines. For example, it is well known that KC mediates lung injury by promoting infiltration of neutrophils. The crosstalk between macrophages and type II epithelial cells also contributes to the exacerbation of lung injury after IR. Sharma *et al.* showed that TNF-α production by alveolar macrophages mediates alveolar type II epithelial cell activation and KC production in an *in vitro* hypoxia-reoxygenation model (Sharma, et al., 2007). Recent studies also implicate alveolar type I cell-released mediators such as soluble receptor for advanced glycation end products (sRAGE) as a potential biomarker and indicator of lung injury after lung transplantation (Calfee, et al., 2007). This new marker may be useful given the recent discovery of the role of alveolar type I cells in alveolar fluid clearance (Johnson, et al., 2006). However, the exact role of alveolar type I cells in lung transplant biology remains less understood.

2.5 Endothelial cells

Increased endothelial permeability has been postulated to be the primary cause of IR-induced pulmonary edema (Hidalgo, et al., 1996). In a syngeneic rat lung transplantation model, it has been reported that the destruction of endothelial cell barrier promotes pulmonary edema and lymphocyte migration and that sphingosine 1-phosphate, a G protein coupled receptor agonist, reduces endothelial cell permeability and protects lung function and injury after IR (Okazaki, et al., 2007). Lung endothelial cells also mediate lung injury by contributing to oxidative stress (Balyasnikova, et al., 2005; Shuvaev & Muzykantov, 2011). Free radical production in endothelial cells via NADPH oxidase- or xanthine oxidase-dependent pathways results in elevated lung oxidant burden during reperfusion (Al-Mehdi, et al., 1998). However, other cells such as leukocytes also contribute to free radical-mediated lung damage during IR injury (Shimoyama, et al., 2005). The prevention of the disruption of endothelial cell barrier is crucial for attenuation of lung injury after IR.

3. Reactive oxygen species (ROS) in lung IR injury

Lung IR injury is a complex pathological phenomenon encompassing various cellular, biochemical and molecular mechanisms. One of the key signaling pathways involving multiple cell types includes oxidative stress due to the generation of reactive oxygen species (ROS). Several groups have demonstrated that inhibition of enzymes involved in ROS generation can dramatically reduce the pro-inflammatory profile after IR.

3.1 ROS generation

A burst of ROS production occurs immediately upon reperfusion of hypoxic cells including leukocytes, epithelial cells and endothelial cells. The antioxidant defense capabilities of the lung are unable to cope with this ROS burst leading to altered cellular metabolic functions and redox signaling. Oxidative stress due to ROS generation causes pro-inflammatory cytokine release and enhanced transcription of numerous genes resulting in inflammation, cell injury, and neutrophil recruitment and activation in the lung after IR. Reperfusion of ischemic tissue results in generation of ROS such as superoxide ($\bullet O_2^-$), hydrogen peroxide (H_2O_2), and the hydroxyl radical (•OH), which leads to oxidative damage to lung tissue (Al-Mehdi, et al., 1994; Al-Mehdi, et al., 1997; Ayene, et al., 1992; Eckenhoff, et al., 1992; Fisher, et al., 1991; Zhao, et al., 1997). This oxidative burst begins to directly increase the adherence of neutrophils to the endothelium (McIntyre, et al., 1995). The release of ROS not only induces cellular lipid membrane peroxidation and the production of inflammatory cytokines, but also plays a role in regulating the activity of several antioxidant enzymes (e.g. glutathione peroxidase, catalase and superoxide dismutase) as well as key transcription factors such as NF-κB and activator protein-1 (AP-1) (Cho, et al., 2006; Morimoto, 1993; Schreck, et al., 1992). Fisher *et al.* demonstrated oxygen-dependent lipid peroxidation during rat lung ischemia (Fisher, et al., 1991). Two key mechanisms of ROS generation in the lung include the NADPH oxidase system and activated xanthine oxidase, as discussed further below.

3.2 NADPH oxidase

Recent studies have demonstrated a key role of the NADPH-oxidase enzyme complex in ROS generation after IR (Goyal, et al., 2004; Jackson, et al., 2004; van der Vliet, 2008; Yang, et al., 2008; Yao, et al., 2007). NADPH oxidase, which is present in epithelial cells, endothelial cells, macrophages, T cells and neutrophils, among others, utilizes NADPH as a substrate to generate superoxide from molecular oxygen. Superoxide is usually rapidly converted to hydrogen peroxide (H_2O_2) or can react with nitric oxide (NO•) to generate peroxynitrite ($ONOO^-$). Thus NADPH oxidase activity is a major source of ROS in the lung after IR. The upregulation of NADPH oxidase-generated ROS can contribute to IR injury through important redox signaling pathways such as the activation of MAP kinases, NF-κB and AP-1, which stimulates the production of proinflammatory cytokines. Pharmacological antagonism of NADPH oxidase by apocynin has been shown to protect against lung IR injury (Pearse & Dodd, 1999; Zhu, et al., 2008).

3.3 Xanthine and xanthine oxidase

Xanthine oxidase-dependent superoxide generation after IR is also a possible mechanism of lung injury (Kennedy, et al., 1989; Lynch, et al., 1988). Under ischemic conditions, xanthine dehydrogenase is converted to xanthine oxidase, which in turn converts hypoxanthine to xanthine and then further catalyzes the oxidation of xanthine to uric acid. In lung endothelium and alveolar type II epithelial cells, this conversion changes the normal degradation of hypoxanthine to uric acid into a source of oxygen radicals. The xanthine oxidase-generated free radicals damage endothelial cells as well as aid the sequestration of neutrophils thereby leading to further injury after IR. Treatment with xanthine oxidase inhibitors, such as allopurinol or iodoxamide, has been shown to attenuate superoxide generation and lung IR injury in rabbit and mouse models of lung IR injury (Adkins & Taylor, 1990; Kennedy, et al., 1989; Lynch, et al., 1988). These investigations suggest an important role for xanthine oxidase in the production of ROS during lung IR.

4. Cytokines and transcription factors

A multitude of experimental studies have shown that IR injury entails a rapid release of pro-inflammatory cytokines and chemokines. Additionally, measurable amounts of pro- and anti-inflammatory cytokines have been reported in lung tissue after lung transplantation in humans (de Perrot, et al., 2002). Important roles for TNF-α, IL-8 (KC in mice), IL-10 and IL-17 in the initiation and progression of lung IR injury have now been demonstrated. Gene modulation of transcription factors like NF-κB and AP-1 has also been correlated to the sequential events involved in lung IR injury.

4.1 Cytokines and chemokines

Cytokines and chemokines are immunomodulating protein molecules secreted by bone marrow derived cells as well as resident lung cells after IR injury. Pro-inflammatory cytokines and chemokines are known to play roles in IR injury of the heart, kidney, small bowel, skin, and liver; however, until recently less was known about their role in lung IR. The C-C family of cytokines and chemokines includes many putative mediators of macrophages, lymphocytes, and granulocyte-derived responses in IR injury (Oppenheim, et al., 1991; Strieter & Kunkel, 1993). This family includes MCP-1 (CCL2), MIP-1α (CCL3), MIP-1β (CCL4), RANTES (CCL5), MCP-3 (CCL7), MCP-2 (CCL8), as well as others. In addition to serving as chemotactic factors, C-C chemokines can modulate cytokine production, adhesion molecule expression, and mononuclear cell proliferation. Krishnadasan *et al.* demonstrated that TNF-α and IL-1β promote lung IR injury likely by altering the expression of other pro-inflammatory cytokines and by influencing neutrophil recruitment (Krishnadasan, et al., 2003). Antibodies to TNF-α, IFN-γ, and MCP-1 have been utilized to demonstrate the importance of these mediators in lung IR injury (Eppinger, et al., 1997). A prominent role for TNF-α was demonstrated both in the acute (30 min) and delayed (4 hr) phases of IR injury, while IFN-γ and MCP-1 appear to have roles only in the acute phase (Eppinger, et al., 1997). Not only is TNF-α produced by stimulated alveolar macrophages, it can also have significant effects on the macrophage respiratory burst, which may lead to oxidative tissue injury (Phillips, et al., 1990). In human lung transplantation, cytokines such as TNF-α, IFN-γ, IL-8, IL-10, IL-12 and IL-18 have been detected in lung tissue (de Perrot, et al., 2002). Mal *et al.* showed that early failure of lung transplants is

associated with massive release of pro-inflammatory cytokines including TNF-α, IL-1β, IL-6 and IL-8 (Mal, et al., 1998).
Recent evidence has demonstrated a crucial role of IL-17 produced by iNKT cells in the initiation of lung IR injury via modulation of neutrophil infiltration and activation in an *in vivo* mouse model (Sharma, et al., 2011). On the other hand, a potent role for IL-10 as an anti-inflammatory molecule, promoting the abrogation of lung IR injury, has been shown in experimental lung IR models (Boehler, et al., 1998; de Perrot, et al., 2003; Fischer, et al., 2001; Martins, et al., 2004; McRae, et al., 2001). The cytotoxic and immunomodulatory effects of cytokines and chemokines are critical in the progression of lung IR injury. Taken together, the balance between pro- and anti-inflammatory cytokines is key to the outcome of lung injury after IR, and pharmacological modulation of these specific cytokine targets offers therapeutic potential for patients with primary graft dysfunction after lung transplantation.

4.2 Transcription factors

The activation of several aforementioned cytokines has been linked to the increased expression of key transcription factors like NF-κB and AP-1 after lung IR. A prominent role of gene regulation via these transcription factors in lung IR injury has been summarized by a number of previous studies.

4.2.1 NF-κB

In the cytoplasm, NF-κB is normally inhibited by IκB. Thus, a decrease in NF-κB activity, due to prevention of IκB degradation by pharmacological agents, leads to the attenuation of pro-inflammatory cytokine activation thereby leading to protection after lung IR. Inhibition of NF-κB via pharmacological agents like cyclosporine A or tacrolimus has been shown to offer protection from lung IR injury (Krishnadasan, et al., 2002). Treatment with pyrrolidine dithiocarbonate (another NF-κB inhibitor) has also been shown to improve lung function and attenuate lung IR injury in a porcine lung transplantation model (Ross, et al., 2000). Naidu *et al.* reported that simvastatin treatment attenuates lung IR injury via inhibition of NF-κB activity (Naidu, et al., 2003). Prevention of lung IR injury by pharmacological agents that inhibit NF-κB may offer a therapeutic strategy for patients with primary graft dysfunction after lung transplantation.

4.2.2 AP-1

The JNK/AP-1 pathway involves regulation of AP-1 by c-Jun kinase (JNK). Like NF-κB, AP-1 is also involved in the activation of several pro-inflammatory cytokines including TNF-α (Zhang, et al., 2002). For example, in a rat lung transplantation model, inhibition of AP-1 leads to decreased TNF-α expression in bronchoalveolar lavage fluid and a significant decrease in protein leakage resulting in decreased lung injury (Ishii, et al., 2004). Inhibition of the JNK/AP-1 pathway may also offer a potential therapeutic target to reduce lung IR injury.

5. Role of endogenous receptors in lung IR injury

Improving outcomes after lung transplantation and extending the donor pool and recipient criteria are predicated on the ability to minimize the deleterious inflammatory responses that occur with lung IR. Cellular receptor-mediated signaling is critical for the initiation and modulation of inflammation and injury after IR. Using pharmacological agents that regulate receptor activation or antagonism, several ubiquitous cellular receptors like adenosine receptors, toll like receptors (TLRs) and receptor for advanced glycation end products (RAGE) have been shown to orchestrate lung IR injury.

5.1 Adenosine receptors

Adenosine is an endogenous mediator that generally serves as a cytoprotective modulator in response to various stress stimuli, and the protective effects of adenosine in the setting of organ IR injury have been shown in various studies (Day, et al., 2005, 2006; Reece, et al., 2008; Rork, et al., 2008). Adenosine signals through 4 subtypes of the G protein-coupled receptors, A_1R, $A_{2A}R$, $A_{2B}R$, and A_3R, all of which are expressed in the lung. Protective effects of adenosine receptor signaling classically occur through second messenger pathways such as the cAMP/PKA or phospholipase C pathways. Most studies have provided evidence that A_1R, $A_{2A}R$ and A_3R may primarily be involved in anti-inflammatory actions whereas the $A_{2B}R$ may have more pro-inflammatory actions in the lung (Anvari, et al., 2010; Ellman, et al., 2008; Gazoni, et al., 2010; Reece, et al., 2005, 2008; Rivo, et al., 2004; Sharma, et al., 2009, 2010; Sun, et al., 2006). However, the role of the $A_{2B}R$ in IR injury remains less understood. $A_{2A}R$ activation has shown remarkable attenuation of lung inflammation, decreased neutrophil infiltration, decreased vascular permeability and improved lung function in rabbit, rat and murine models of lung IR injury (Ellman, et al., 2008; Gazoni, et al., 2008; Lau, et al., 2009; Sharma, et al., 2009) as well as in a pig lung transplant model (Reece, et al., 2005). The anti-inflammatory effects of $A_{2A}R$ activation on CD4+ T cells has been shown to attenuate lung IR injury (Sharma, et al., 2010). In recent literature involving lung IR injury, pharmacological compounds modulating adenosine receptor agonism or antagonism have shown tremendous potential as possible therapeutic strategies for clinical applications to prevent or treat primary graft dysfunction after lung transplantation.

5.2 Toll-like receptors (TLRs)

TLRs are transmembrane receptors that play a crucial role in the innate immune response to a variety of trigger factors including IR injury (Marshak-Rothstein & Rifkin, 2007). TLR-2 and TLR-4 have been implicated in various models of IR injury (Arslan, et al., 2010; Leemans, et al., 2005; Oyama, et al., 2004). Lung biopsies of patients after lung transplantation showed elevated expression of mRNA for multiple TLRs (Andrade, et al., 2006), and lungs from TLR-4 knockout mice showed marked protection from lung IR injury (Shimamoto, et al., 2006; Zanotti, et al., 2009). Shimamoto *et al.* reported that TLR-4-mediated injury appears to occur through activation of c-Jun NH_2-terminal kinase (JNK) and translocation of NF-κβ.

5.3 Receptor for advanced glycation end products (RAGE)

RAGE is a multi-ligand receptor of the immunoglobulin superfamily expressed in most tissues and present on a wide range of cells where it plays a key role in inflammatory processes, especially at sites where its ligands accumulate. High-mobility group box 1 (HMGB1) is an intracellular protein, readily released from necrotic or damaged cells, that can signal through RAGE, TLR-2 or TLR-4, initiating an inflammatory response to further damage viable cells (Scaffidi, et al., 2002). Prior studies suggest that HMGB1 can interact with both TLR-2 and TLR-4 to induce an inflammatory response during liver IR injury (Park, et al., 2006). Similarly, recent reports suggest a predominant role of RAGE and its ligand HMGB1 in the initiation of lung IR injury (Sternberg, et al., 2008). In a multi-center study, Christie *et al.* reported that an elevated plasma level of soluble RAGE (a truncated form of RAGE) was associated with primary graft dysfunction in patients undergoing lung transplantation (Christie, et al., 2009). An in depth characterization of the role of HMGB1, TLRs and RAGE remains to be elucidated in pulmonary injury after IR and transplantation.

5.4 Complement and fibrinolytic pathways

The complement system encompasses a collective term used for plasma and cell membrane proteins that play a role in cell defense processes. In lung IR injury, it has been shown that activation of the complement system leads to cellular injury through direct or indirect mechanisms (Bishop, et al., 1991; Naka, et al., 1997). In a swine single-lung transplantation model, the administration of soluble complement receptor 1, a potent inhibitor of complement activation, significantly reduces lung edema and improves lung function (Pierre, et al., 1998; Schmid, et al., 1998). In a clinical study, it was shown that complement inhibition by TP-10, a soluble complement receptor 1, significantly decreases the duration of mechanical ventilation in lung transplant recipients (Keshavjee, et al., 2005). This suggests that complement inhibition may offer additional therapeutic strategies for lung transplant patients. Further research is required to elucidate the specific pathways of the complement-mediated inflammation in lung IR pathophysiology.

The interplay between the fibrinolytic cascade and the inflammatory process in acute lung injury has been shown to be involved in lung IR injury. Tissue plasminogen activator (tPA), a member of the serine proteinase family, is expressed by vascular endothelial cells and functions to convert zymogen plasminogen to the active protease plasmin, thus initiating a potent fibrinolytic process. tPA knockout mice have attenuated lung inflammation by decreased neutrophil extravasation in a mouse model of lung IR (Zhao, et al., 2011). In the same study, it was shown that deletion of tPA leads to the concomitant downregulation of PECAM-1 expression via tPA/LRP/NF-κB signaling pathway and upregulation of P-selectin expression in small pulmonary vessels as well as to decreased MMP-9 expression. It has also been demonstrated that increased fibrinolysis through depletion of plasminogen activator inhibitor-1 (PAI-1), the endogenous tPA inhibitor, attenuated lung IR injury (Lau, et al., 2009). The complex molecular mechanisms involved in the fibrinolytic pathway and its potential role in clinical primary graft dysfunction remains to be further investigated.

6. Therapeutic strategies

Advancements in our understanding of molecular and pathophysiologic mechanisms for lung IR injury have supported significant research contributions aimed at improved allograft function. While no standardized treatment strategies specifically targeting IR injury exist, promising early results have demonstrated a potential role for *ex vivo* allograft treatment, nitric oxide therapy, and ischemic preconditioning in the prevention of IR injury.

6.1 Lung preservation strategies

A significant research commitment over the past decade has been invested in the creation of an ideal preservation and flush solution for lung transplantation. Intracellular solutions with high potassium and low sodium are the current standard for kidney and liver transplantation, while extracellular solutions such as Perfadex® (Vitrolife, Gothenburg, Sweden) with low potassium, high sodium and dextran have emerged as the superior method for lung preservation (de Perrot, et al., 2003; Fischer, et al., 2001). Dextran induces erythrocyte deformation and prevents aggregation, preserving the pulmonary microcirculation and endothelial-epithelial barrier (Keshavjee, et al., 1992). This inherent quality may limit ischemia in regions of microcirculation thrombosis while creating an osmotic gradient that reduces protein and water extravasation during the reperfusion period (de Perrot, et al., 2003). In a clinical study, the absence of dextrose in extracellular solutions has been associated with an increased incidence of primary graft dysfunction and mortality (Marasco, et al., 2011; Oto, et al., 2006). While long-term outcomes remain the focus of future investigation, these findings support the clinical adoption of low-potassium dextran solutions as the primary method for lung allograft preservation.

6.2 Ex vivo lung perfusion (EVLP)

EVLP is an emerging technique for normothermic donor lung perfusion during the preservation period. EVLP with warm acellular Steen Solution™ (Vitrolife, Gothenburg, Sweden) following a period of cold storage is a promising modality for lung preservation with a demonstrated efficacy in the maintenance of lung function (Cypel, et al., 2008). This novel treatment strategy prevents ongoing injury and accelerates lung recovery (Cypel, et al., 2009). Recent prospective clinical data has demonstrated the successful transplantation of high-risk donor lungs following EVLP with comparable physiology to lungs transplanted under conventional methods of selection and transplantation (Cypel, et al., 2011b). These studies promote EVLP as a potential strategy for donor pool expansion and pre-implantation pulmonary function testing. In addition, this promising treatment strategy for lung rehabilitation may serve as a vehicle for future therapeutic treatment of the donor allograft during the inherent ischemic period.

6.3 Nitric oxide (NO)

NO is a messenger gas molecule with potent vasoregulatory and immunomodulatory properties (de Perrot, et al., 2003; Meyer, et al., 1998). NO inhibits xanthine oxidase as well as neutrophil chemotaxis and activation (de Perrot, et al., 2003; Meyer, et al., 1998). This mechanism of action establishes therapeutic potential for inhaled NO in the prevention of lung IR injury. NO ventilation during ischemia and following graft implantation in experimental models with *ex vivo* perfusion has demonstrated a reduction in pulmonary edema, improvement in oxygenation capacity, reduction in pulmonary vascular resistance, and decreased TNF-α with treatment (Dong, et al., 2009). Treatment of experimental recipient lungs with inhalational NO during reperfusion improved the ventilation-perfusion mismatch and decreased pulmonary artery pressures associated with IR injury (Adatia, et al., 1994). Unfortunately, this promising experimental data for inhalational NO has had limited translation to the clinical prevention of human lung IR injury. In a randomized clinical trial to evaluate the use of inhaled NO treatment, no significant differences in immediate oxygenation, time to extubation, length of intensive care unit stay or 30-day mortality were demonstrated (Meade, et al., 2001). While experimental data supports improved gas exchange with inhaled NO treatment, clinical lung transplantation data has not yet demonstrated significant improvements in outcomes for lung transplantation recipients with inhaled NO treatment (de Perrot, et al., 2003) .

6.4 Preconditioning

Ischemic preconditioning enhances the ability of organs to withstand a sustained IR injury through repeated exposure to short periods of ischemia prior to the primary ischemic insult (Jun, et al., 2011). Ischemic preconditioning has demonstrated an ability to alter gene expression profiles within 6 hours of ischemia which is sustained until 24 hours following insult (Jun, et al., 2011). The proposed mechanism for ischemic preconditioning in the lung involves anti-inflammatory mediators, antioxidant stress, and the regulation of cellular energy metabolism (Jun, et al., 2011). Further experimental studies have suggested a role for adenosine A_1 receptor activation in the modulation of protective ischemic preconditioning (Yildiz, et al., 2007). Additional potential therapeutic preconditioning methods include hyperthermic and pharmacologic administration to improve the allograft response to the period of ischemia and subsequent reperfusion (Hiratsuka, et al., 1998; Schutte, et al., 2001). The role of preconditioning in clinical lung transplantation remains undefined (de Perrot, et al., 2003). Future application and study of preconditioning methods in the lung may demonstrate parallel beneficial effects to other organ systems, establishing this strategy for lung IR injury prevention.

7. Conclusions

Lung IR injury involves many cellular and molecular mechanisms making it a complex pathological process. Improvements in the technique of lung preservation and better understanding of the molecular mechanisms of IR injury are needed to prevent the occurrence of primary graft dysfunction after lung transplantation. The development of new strategies to improve the number of donor lungs available for transplantation could have a significant impact on the number of transplants performed and thus reduce the number of patients on the transplant waiting list. Additionally, improvements in lung preservation solution can help attenuate acute lung IR injury as well as chronic graft dysfunction. It is imperative that further experimental studies and multicenter clinical trials continue to be performed to reduce the morbidity and mortality associated with lung IR injury.
Research commitment to further define cellular responses to IR within the lung promises to support therapeutic advancement. Novel *ex vivo* treatment strategies may provide a therapeutic bridge for treatment of the donor allograft prior to recipient implantation. The combination of pharmacologic mechanistic inhibition and innovative approaches to sustained allograft perfusion support a promising future for lung transplantation. A dedicated and multidisciplinary approach to IR injury prevention is critical. Therapeutic advancement to ameliorate IR injury will increase the number of available donor grafts and improve lung transplantation outcomes for the increasing number of potential transplant recipients with end-stage pulmonary disease.

8. References

Adatia, I., Lillehei, C., Arnold, J. H., Thompson, J. E., Palazzo, R., Fackler, J. C. & Wessel, D. L. (1994). Inhaled nitric oxide in the treatment of postoperative graft dysfunction after lung transplantation. *Ann Thorac Surg*, Vol.57, No.5, (May), pp. 1311-1318, ISSN 0003-4975

Adkins, W. K. & Taylor, A. E. (1990). Role of xanthine oxidase and neutrophils in ischemia-reperfusion injury in rabbit lung. *J Appl Physiol*, Vol.69, No.6, (Dec), pp. 2012-2018, ISSN 8750-7587

Al-Mehdi, A., Shuman, H. & Fisher, A. B. (1994). Fluorescence microtopography of oxidative stress in lung ischemia-reperfusion. *Lab Invest*, Vol.70, No.4, (Apr), pp. 579-587, ISSN 0023-6837

Al-Mehdi, A. B., Shuman, H. & Fisher, A. B. (1997). Intracellular generation of reactive oxygen species during nonhypoxic lung ischemia. *Am J Physiol*, Vol.272, No.2 Pt 1, (Feb), pp. L294-300, ISSN 0002-9513

Al-Mehdi, A. B., Zhao, G., Dodia, C., Tozawa, K., Costa, K., Muzykantov, V., Ross, C., Blecha, F., Dinauer, M. & Fisher, A. B. (1998). Endothelial NADPH oxidase as the source of oxidants in lungs exposed to ischemia or high K+. *Circ Res*, Vol.83, No.7, (Oct 5), pp. 730-737, ISSN 0009-7330

Andrade, C. F., Kaneda, H., Der, S., Tsang, M., Lodyga, M., Chimisso Dos Santos, C., Keshavjee, S. & Liu, M. (2006). Toll-like receptor and cytokine gene expression in the early phase of human lung transplantation. *J Heart Lung Transplant*, Vol.25, No.11, (Nov), pp. 1317-1323, ISSN 1053-2498

Anvari, F., Sharma, A. K., Fernandez, L. G., Hranjec, T., Ravid, K., Kron, I. L. & Laubach, V. E. (2010). Tissue-derived proinflammatory effect of adenosine A2B receptor in lung ischemia-reperfusion injury. *J Thorac Cardiovasc Surg*, Vol.140, No.4, (Oct), pp. 871-877, ISSN 0022-5223

Arenzana-Seisdedos, F., Virelizier, J. L. & Fiers, W. (1985). Interferons as macrophage-activating factors. III. Preferential effects of interferon-gamma on the interleukin 1 secretory potential of fresh or aged human monocytes. *J Immunol*, Vol.134, No.4, (Apr), pp. 2444-2448, ISSN 0022-1767

Arslan, F., Keogh, B., McGuirk, P. & Parker, A. E. (2010). TLR2 and TLR4 in ischemia reperfusion injury. *Mediators Inflamm*, Vol.2010, pp. 704202, ISSN 0962-9351

Ayene, I. S., Dodia, C. & Fisher, A. B. (1992). Role of oxygen in oxidation of lipid and protein during ischemia/reperfusion in isolated perfused rat lung. *Arch Biochem Biophys*, Vol.296, No.1, (Jul), pp. 183-189, ISSN 0003-9861

Bacon, K. B., Premack, B. A., Gardner, P. & Schall, T. J. (1995). Activation of dual T cell signaling pathways by the chemokine RANTES. *Science*, Vol.269, No.5231, (Sep 22), pp. 1727-1730, ISSN 0036-8075

Balyasnikova, I. V., Visintine, D. J., Gunnerson, H. B., Paisansathan, C., Baughman, V. L., Minshall, R. D. & Danilov, S. M. (2005). Propofol attenuates lung endothelial injury induced by ischemia-reperfusion and oxidative stress. *Anesth Analg*, Vol.100, No.4, (Apr), pp. 929-936, ISSN 0003-2999

Bettelli, E., Korn, T. & Kuchroo, V. K. (2007). Th17: the third member of the effector T cell trilogy. *Curr Opin Immunol*, Vol.19, No.6, (Dec), pp. 652-657, ISSN 0952-7915

Bishop, M. J., Giclas, P. C., Guidotti, S. M., Su, M. L. & Chi, E. Y. (1991). Complement activation is a secondary rather than a causative factor in rabbit pulmonary artery ischemia/reperfusion injury. *Am Rev Respir Dis*, Vol.143, No.2, (Feb), pp. 386-390, ISSN 0003-0805

Boehler, A., Chamberlain, D., Xing, Z., Slutsky, A. S., Jordana, M., Gauldie, J., Liu, M. & Keshavjee, S. (1998). Adenovirus-mediated interleukin-10 gene transfer inhibits post-transplant fibrous airway obliteration in an animal model of bronchiolitis obliterans. *Hum Gene Ther*, Vol.9, No.4, (Mar 1), pp. 541-551, ISSN 1043-0342

Calfee, C. S., Budev, M. M., Matthay, M. A., Church, G., Brady, S., Uchida, T., Ishizaka, A., Lara, A., Ranes, J. L., deCamp, M. M. & Arroliga, A. C. (2007). Plasma receptor for advanced glycation end-products predicts duration of ICU stay and mechanical ventilation in patients after lung transplantation. *J Heart Lung Transplant*, Vol.26, No.7, (Jul), pp. 675-680, ISSN 1053-2498

Cho, H. Y., Reddy, S. P. & Kleeberger, S. R. (2006). Nrf2 defends the lung from oxidative stress. *Antioxid Redox Signal*, Vol.8, No.1-2, (Jan-Feb), pp. 76-87, ISSN 1523-0864

Christie, J. D., Shah, C. V., Kawut, S. M., Mangalmurti, N., Lederer, D. J., Sonett, J. R., Ahya, V. N., Palmer, S. M., Wille, K., Lama, V., Shah, P. D., Shah, A., Weinacker, A., Deutschman, C. S., Kohl, B. A., Demissie, E., Bellamy, S. & Ware, L. B. (2009). Plasma levels of receptor for advanced glycation end products, blood transfusion, and risk of primary graft dysfunction. *Am J Respir Crit Care Med*, Vol.180, No.10, (Nov 15), pp. 1010-1015, ISSN 1073-449X

Christie, J. D., Edwards, L. B., Kucheryavaya, A. Y., Aurora, P., Dobbels, F., Kirk, R., Rahmel, A. O., Stehlik, J. & Hertz, M. I. (2010). The Registry of the International Society for Heart and Lung Transplantation: twenty-seventh official adult lung and heart-lung transplant report--2010. *J Heart Lung Transplant*, Vol.29, No.10, (Oct), pp. 1104-1118, ISSN 1053-2498

Clavien, P. A., Harvey, P. R., Sanabria, J. R., Cywes, R., Levy, G. A. & Strasberg, S. M. (1993). Lymphocyte adherence in the reperfused rat liver: mechanisms and effects. *Hepatology*, Vol.17, No.1, (Jan), pp. 131-142, ISSN 0270-9139

Cottini, S. R., Lerch, N., de Perrot, M., Treggiari, M. M., Spiliopoulos, A., Nicod, L. & Ricou, B. (2006). Risk factors for reperfusion injury after lung transplantation. *Intensive Care Med*, Vol.32, No.4, (Apr), pp. 557-563, ISSN 0342-4642

Cypel, M., Yeung, J. C., Hirayama, S., Rubacha, M., Fischer, S., Anraku, M., Sato, M., Harwood, S., Pierre, A., Waddell, T. K., de Perrot, M., Liu, M. & Keshavjee, S. (2008). Technique for prolonged normothermic ex vivo lung perfusion. *J Heart Lung Transplant*, Vol.27, No.12, (Dec), pp. 1319-1325, ISSN 1053-2498

Cypel, M., Rubacha, M., Yeung, J., Hirayama, S., Torbicki, K., Madonik, M., Fischer, S., Hwang, D., Pierre, A., Waddell, T. K., de Perrot, M., Liu, M. & Keshavjee, S. (2009). Normothermic ex vivo perfusion prevents lung injury compared to extended cold preservation for transplantation. *Am J Transplant*, Vol.9, No.10, (Oct), pp. 2262-2269, ISSN 1600-6135

Cypel, M., Yeung, J. C. & Keshavjee, S. (2011a). Novel approaches to expanding the lung donor pool: donation after cardiac death and ex vivo conditioning. *Clin Chest Med*, Vol.32, No.2, (Jun), pp. 233-244, ISSN 0272-5231

Cypel, M., Yeung, J. C., Liu, M., Anraku, M., Chen, F., Karolak, W., Sato, M., Laratta, J., Azad, S., Madonik, M., Chow, C. W., Chaparro, C., Hutcheon, M., Singer, L. G.,

Slutsky, A. S., Yasufuku, K., de Perrot, M., Pierre, A. F., Waddell, T. K. & Keshavjee, S. (2011b). Normothermic ex vivo lung perfusion in clinical lung transplantation. *N Engl J Med*, Vol.364, No.15, (Apr 14), pp. 1431-1440, ISSN 0028-4793

Day, Y. J., Li, Y., Rieger, J. M., Ramos, S. I., Okusa, M. D. & Linden, J. (2005). A2A adenosine receptors on bone marrow-derived cells protect liver from ischemia-reperfusion injury. *J Immunol*, Vol.174, No.8, (Apr 15), pp. 5040-5046, ISSN 0022-1767

Day, Y. J., Huang, L., Ye, H., Li, L., Linden, J. & Okusa, M. D. (2006). Renal ischemia-reperfusion injury and adenosine 2A receptor-mediated tissue protection: the role of CD4+ T cells and IFN-gamma. *J Immunol*, Vol.176, No.5, (Mar 1), pp. 3108-3114, ISSN 0022-1767

de Perrot, M., Sekine, Y., Fischer, S., Waddell, T. K., McRae, K., Liu, M., Wigle, D. A. & Keshavjee, S. (2002). Interleukin-8 release during early reperfusion predicts graft function in human lung transplantation. *Am J Respir Crit Care Med*, Vol.165, No.2, (Jan 15), pp. 211-215, ISSN 1073-449X

de Perrot, M., Fischer, S., Liu, M., Imai, Y., Martins, S., Sakiyama, S., Tabata, T., Bai, X. H., Waddell, T. K., Davidson, B. L. & Keshavjee, S. (2003). Impact of human interleukin-10 on vector-induced inflammation and early graft function in rat lung transplantation. *Am J Respir Cell Mol Biol*, Vol.28, No.5, (May), pp. 616-625, ISSN 1044-1549

de Perrot, M., Liu, M., Waddell, T. K. & Keshavjee, S. (2003). Ischemia-reperfusion-induced lung injury. *Am J Respir Crit Care Med*, Vol.167, No.4, (Feb 15), pp. 490-511, ISSN 1073-449X

de Vleeschauwer, S. I., Wauters, S., Dupont, L. J., Verleden, S. E., Willems-Widyastuti, A., Vanaudenaerde, B. M., Verleden, G. M. & Van Raemdonck, D. E. (2011). Medium-term outcome after lung transplantation is comparable between brain-dead and cardiac-dead donors. *J Heart Lung Transplant*, (Jun 10), pp. ISSN 1053-2498

Deeb, G. M., Grum, C. M., Lynch, M. J., Guynn, T. P., Gallagher, K. P., Ljungman, A. G., Bolling, S. F. & Morganroth, M. L. (1990). Neutrophils are not necessary for induction of ischemia-reperfusion lung injury. *J Appl Physiol*, Vol.68, No.1, (Jan), pp. 374-381, ISSN 0161-7567

Diamond, J. M. & Christie, J. D. (2010). The contribution of airway and lung tissue ischemia to primary graft dysfunction. *Curr Opin Organ Transplant*, Vol.15, No.5, (Oct), pp. 552-557, ISSN 1087-2418

Dong, B. M., Abano, J. B. & Egan, T. M. (2009). Nitric oxide ventilation of rat lungs from non-heart-beating donors improves posttransplant function. *Am J Transplant*, Vol.9, No.12, (Dec), pp. 2707-2715, ISSN 1600-6135

Eckenhoff, R. G., Dodia, C., Tan, Z. & Fisher, A. B. (1992). Oxygen-dependent reperfusion injury in the isolated rat lung. *J Appl Physiol*, Vol.72, No.4, (Apr), pp. 1454-1460, ISSN 0161-7567

Eden, E. & Turino, G. M. (1986). Interleukin-1 secretion by human alveolar macrophages stimulated with endotoxin is augmented by recombinant immune (gamma) interferon. *Am Rev Respir Dis*, Vol.133, No.3, (Mar), pp. 455-460, ISSN 0003-0805

Edgerton, C., Crispin, J. C., Moratz, C. M., Bettelli, E., Oukka, M., Simovic, M., Zacharia, A., Egan, R., Chen, J., Dalle Lucca, J. J., Juang, Y. T. & Tsokos, G. C. (2008). IL-17 producing CD4(+) T cells mediate accelerated ischemia/reperfusion-induced injury in autoimmunity-prone mice. *Clin Immunol*, (Dec 3), pp. ISSN 1521-7035

Ellman, P. I., Reece, T. B., Law, M. G., Gazoni, L. M., Singh, R., Laubach, V. E., Linden, J., Tribble, C. G. & Kron, I. L. (2008). Adenosine A2A activation attenuates nontransplantation lung reperfusion injury. *J Surg Res*, Vol.149, No.1, (Sep), pp. 3-8, ISSN 0022-4804

Eppinger, M. J., Jones, M. L., Deeb, G. M., Bolling, S. F. & Ward, P. A. (1995). Pattern of injury and the role of neutrophils in reperfusion injury of rat lung. *J Surg Res*, Vol.58, No.6, (Jun), pp. 713-718, ISSN 0022-4804

Eppinger, M. J., Deeb, G. M., Bolling, S. F. & Ward, P. A. (1997). Mediators of ischemia-reperfusion injury of rat lung. *Am J Pathol*, Vol.150, No.5, (May), pp. 1773-1784, ISSN 0002-9440

Fischer, S., Liu, M., Maclean, A. A., De Perrot, M., Bai, X., Cardella, J., Imai, Y. & Keshavjee, S. (2001). In vivo donor adenoviral-mediated transtracheal transfection of human IL-10 (HIL-10) gene ameliorates ischemia-reperfusion (IR) injury and enhances transplanted lung function. *J Heart Lung Transplant*, Vol.20, No.2, (Feb), pp. 152-153, ISSN 1053-2498

Fischer, S., Matte-Martyn, A., De Perrot, M., Waddell, T. K., Sekine, Y., Hutcheon, M. & Keshavjee, S. (2001). Low-potassium dextran preservation solution improves lung function after human lung transplantation. *J Thorac Cardiovasc Surg*, Vol.121, No.3, (Mar), pp. 594-596, ISSN 0022-5223

Fiser, S. M., Tribble, C. G., Long, S. M., Kaza, A. K., Cope, J. T., Laubach, V. E., Kern, J. A. & Kron, I. L. (2001a). Lung transplant reperfusion injury involves pulmonary macrophages and circulating leukocytes in a biphasic response. *J Thorac Cardiovasc Surg*, Vol.121, No.6, (Jun), pp. 1069-1075, ISSN 0022-5223

Fiser, S. M., Tribble, C. G., Long, S. M., Kaza, A. K., Kern, J. A. & Kron, I. L. (2001b). Pulmonary macrophages are involved in reperfusion injury after lung transplantation. *Ann Thorac Surg*, Vol.71, No.4, (Apr), pp. 1134-1138, ISSN 0003-4975

Fiser, S. M., Tribble, C. G., Long, S. M., Kaza, A. K., Kern, J. A., Jones, D. R., Robbins, M. K. & Kron, I. L. (2002). Ischemia-reperfusion injury after lung transplantation increases risk of late bronchiolitis obliterans syndrome. *Ann Thorac Surg*, Vol.73, No.4, (Apr), pp. 1041-1047; discussion 1047-1048, ISSN 0003-4975

Fisher, A. B., Dodia, C., Tan, Z. T., Ayene, I. & Eckenhoff, R. G. (1991). Oxygen-dependent lipid peroxidation during lung ischemia. *J Clin Invest*, Vol.88, No.2, (Aug), pp. 674-679, ISSN 0021-9738

Fisher, A. J., Donnelly, S. C., Hirani, N., Haslett, C., Strieter, R. M., Dark, J. H. & Corris, P. A. (2001). Elevated levels of interleukin-8 in donor lungs is associated with early graft failure after lung transplantation. *Am J Respir Crit Care Med*, Vol.163, No.1, (Jan), pp. 259-265, ISSN 1073-449X

Gazoni, L. M., Laubach, V. E., Mulloy, D. P., Bellizzi, A., Unger, E. B., Linden, J., Ellman, P. I., Lisle, T. C. & Kron, I. L. (2008). Additive protection against lung ischemia-reperfusion injury by adenosine A2A receptor activation before procurement and during reperfusion. *J Thorac Cardiovasc Surg*, Vol.135, No.1, (Jan), pp. 156-165, ISSN 0022-5223

Gazoni, L. M., Walters, D. M., Unger, E. B., Linden, J., Kron, I. L. & Laubach, V. E. (2010). Activation of A1, A2A, or A3 adenosine receptors attenuates lung ischemia-reperfusion injury. *J Thorac Cardiovasc Surg*, Vol.140, No.2, (Aug), pp. 440-446, ISSN 0022-5223

Goyal, P., Weissmann, N., Grimminger, F., Hegel, C., Bader, L., Rose, F., Fink, L., Ghofrani, H. A., Schermuly, R. T., Schmidt, H. H., Seeger, W. & Hanze, J. (2004). Upregulation of NAD(P)H oxidase 1 in hypoxia activates hypoxia-inducible factor 1 via increase in reactive oxygen species. *Free Radic Biol Med*, Vol.36, No.10, (May 15), pp. 1279-1288, ISSN 0891-5849

Granton, J. (2006). Update of early respiratory failure in the lung transplant recipient. *Curr Opin Crit Care*, Vol.12, No.1, (Feb), pp. 19-24, ISSN 1070-5295

Hanschen, M., Zahler, S., Krombach, F. & Khandoga, A. (2008). Reciprocal activation between CD4+ T cells and Kupffer cells during hepatic ischemia-reperfusion. *Transplantation*, Vol.86, No.5, (Sep 15), pp. 710-718, ISSN 1534-6080

Hardy, J. D., Webb, W. R., Dalton, M. L. J. & Walker, G. R. J. (1963). Lung homotransplantation in man. *JAMA*, Vol.186, (Dec), pp. 1065-1074, ISSN 0098-7484

He, X., Han, B. & Liu, M. (2007). Long pentraxin 3 in pulmonary infection and acute lung injury. *Am J Physiol Lung Cell Mol Physiol*, Vol.292, No.5, (May), pp. L1039-1049, ISSN 1040-0605

Hidalgo, M. A., Shah, K. A., Fuller, B. J. & Green, C. J. (1996). Cold ischemia-induced damage to vascular endothelium results in permeability alterations in transplanted lungs. *J Thorac Cardiovasc Surg*, Vol.112, No.4, (Oct), pp. 1027-1035, ISSN 0022-5223

Hiratsuka, M., Yano, M., Mora, B. N., Nagahiro, I., Cooper, J. D. & Patterson, G. A. (1998). Heat shock pretreatment protects pulmonary isografts from subsequent ischemia-reperfusion injury. *J Heart Lung Transplant*, Vol.17, No.12, (Dec), pp. 1238-1246, ISSN 1053-2498

Ishii, M., Suzuki, Y., Takeshita, K., Miyao, N., Kudo, H., Hiraoka, R., Nishio, K., Sato, N., Naoki, K., Aoki, T. & Yamaguchi, K. (2004). Inhibition of c-Jun NH2-terminal kinase activity improves ischemia/reperfusion injury in rat lungs. *J Immunol*, Vol.172, No.4, (Feb 15), pp. 2569-2577, ISSN 0022-1767

Issekutz, A. C. & Issekutz, T. B. (1993). Quantitation and kinetics of blood monocyte migration to acute inflammatory reactions, and IL-1 alpha, tumor necrosis factor-alpha, and IFN-gamma. *J Immunol*, Vol.151, No.4, (Aug 15), pp. 2105-2115, ISSN 0022-1767

Jackson, S. H., Devadas, S., Kwon, J., Pinto, L. A. & Williams, M. S. (2004). T cells express a phagocyte-type NADPH oxidase that is activated after T cell receptor stimulation. *Nat Immunol*, Vol.5, No.8, (Aug), pp. 818-827, ISSN 1529-2908

Johnson, M. D., Bao, H. F., Helms, M. N., Chen, X. J., Tigue, Z., Jain, L., Dobbs, L. G. & Eaton, D. C. (2006). Functional ion channels in pulmonary alveolar type I cells support a role for type I cells in lung ion transport. *Proc Natl Acad Sci U S A*, Vol.103, No.13, (Mar 28), pp. 4964-4969, ISSN 0027-8424

Jun, N., Ke, J., Gang, C., Lin, C., Jinsong, L. & Jianjun, W. (2011). The protective effect of ischemic preconditioning associated with altered gene expression profiles in rat lung after reperfusion. *J Surg Res*, Vol.168, No.2, (Jun 15), pp. 281-293, ISSN 0022-4804

Kennedy, T. P., Rao, N. V., Hopkins, C., Pennington, L., Tolley, E. & Hoidal, J. R. (1989). Role of reactive oxygen species in reperfusion injury of the rabbit lung. *J Clin Invest*, Vol.83, No.4, (Apr), pp. 1326-1335, ISSN 0021-9738

Keshavjee, S., Davis, R. D., Zamora, M. R., de Perrot, M. & Patterson, G. A. (2005). A randomized, placebo-controlled trial of complement inhibition in ischemia-reperfusion injury after lung transplantation in human beings. *J Thorac Cardiovasc Surg*, Vol.129, No.2, (Feb), pp. 423-428, ISSN 0022-5223

Keshavjee, S. H., Yamazaki, F., Yokomise, H., Cardoso, P. F., Mullen, J. B., Slutsky, A. S. & Patterson, G. A. (1992). The role of dextran 40 and potassium in extended hypothermic lung preservation for transplantation. *J Thorac Cardiovasc Surg*, Vol.103, No.2, (Feb), pp. 314-325, ISSN 0022-5223

King, R. C., Binns, O. A., Rodriguez, F., Kanithanon, R. C., Daniel, T. M., Spotnitz, W. D., Tribble, C. G. & Kron, I. L. (2000). Reperfusion injury significantly impacts clinical outcome after pulmonary transplantation. *Ann Thorac Surg*, Vol.69, No.6, (Jun), pp. 1681-1685, ISSN 0003-4975

Kolls, J. K. & Linden, A. (2004). Interleukin-17 family members and inflammation. *Immunity*, Vol.21, No.4, (Oct), pp. 467-476, ISSN 1074-7613

Krishnadasan, B., Naidu, B., Rosengart, M., Farr, A. L., Barnes, A., Verrier, E. D. & Mulligan, M. S. (2002). Decreased lung ischemia-reperfusion injury in rats after preoperative administration of cyclosporine and tacrolimus. *J Thorac Cardiovasc Surg*, Vol.123, No.4, (Apr), pp. 756-767, ISSN 0022-5223

Krishnadasan, B., Naidu, B. V., Byrne, K., Fraga, C., Verrier, E. D. & Mulligan, M. S. (2003). The role of proinflammatory cytokines in lung ischemia-reperfusion injury. *J Thorac Cardiovasc Surg*, Vol.125, No.2, (Feb), pp. 261-272, ISSN 0022-5223

Larosa, D. F. & Orange, J. S. (2008). Lymphocytes. *J Allergy Clin Immunol*, Vol.121, No.2 Suppl, (Feb), pp. S364-369, ISSN 1097-6825

Lau, C. L., Zhao, Y., Kim, J., Kron, I. L., Sharma, A., Yang, Z., Laubach, V. E., Linden, J., Ailawadi, G. & Pinsky, D. J. (2009). Enhanced fibrinolysis protects against lung ischemia-reperfusion injury. *J Thorac Cardiovasc Surg*, Vol.137, No.5, (May), pp. 1241-1248, ISSN 0022-5223

Lau, C. L., Zhao, Y., Kron, I. L., Stoler, M. H., Laubach, V. E., Ailawadi, G. & Linden, J. (2009). The role of adenosine A2A receptor signaling in bronchiolitis obliterans. *Ann Thorac Surg*, Vol.88, No.4, (Oct), pp. 1071-1078, ISSN 1552-6259

Le Moine, O., Louis, H., Demols, A., Desalle, F., Demoor, F., Quertinmont, E., Goldman, M. & Deviere, J. (2000). Cold liver ischemia-reperfusion injury critically depends on liver T cells and is improved by donor pretreatment with interleukin 10 in mice. *Hepatology*, Vol.31, No.6, (Jun), pp. 1266-1274, ISSN 0270-9139

Leemans, J. C., Stokman, G., Claessen, N., Rouschop, K. M., Teske, G. J., Kirschning, C. J., Akira, S., van der Poll, T., Weening, J. J. & Florquin, S. (2005). Renal-associated

TLR2 mediates ischemia/reperfusion injury in the kidney. *J Clin Invest*, Vol.115, No.10, (Oct), pp. 2894-2903, ISSN 0021-9738
Li, L., Huang, L., Sung, S. S., Lobo, P. I., Brown, M. G., Gregg, R. K., Engelhard, V. H. & Okusa, M. D. (2007). NKT cell activation mediates neutrophil IFN-gamma production and renal ischemia-reperfusion injury. *J Immunol*, Vol.178, No.9, (May 1), pp. 5899-5911, ISSN 0022-1767
Lynch, M. J., Grum, C. M., Gallagher, K. P., Bolling, S. F., Deeb, G. M. & Morganroth, M. L. (1988). Xanthine oxidase inhibition attenuates ischemic-reperfusion lung injury. *J Surg Res*, Vol.44, No.5, (May), pp. 538-544, ISSN 0022-4804
Mal, H., Dehoux, M., Sleiman, C., Boczkowski, J., Leseche, G., Pariente, R. & Fournier, M. (1998). Early release of proinflammatory cytokines after lung transplantation. *Chest*, Vol.113, No.3, (Mar), pp. 645-651, ISSN 0012-3692
Marasco, S. F., Bailey, M., McGlade, D., Snell, G., Westall, G., Oto, T. & Pilcher, D. (2011). Effect of donor preservation solution and survival in lung transplantation. *J Heart Lung Transplant*, Vol.30, No.4, (Apr), pp. 414-419, ISSN 1557-3117
Marshak-Rothstein, A. & Rifkin, I. R. (2007). Immunologically active autoantigens: the role of toll-like receptors in the development of chronic inflammatory disease. *Annu Rev Immunol*, Vol.25, pp. 419-441, ISSN 0732-0582
Martins, S., de Perrot, M., Imai, Y., Yamane, M., Quadri, S. M., Segall, L., Dutly, A., Sakiyama, S., Chaparro, A., Davidson, B. L., Waddell, T. K., Liu, M. & Keshavjee, S. (2004). Transbronchial administration of adenoviral-mediated interleukin-10 gene to the donor improves function in a pig lung transplant model. *Gene Ther*, Vol.11, No.24, (Dec), pp. 1786-1796, ISSN 0969-7128
Maxey, T. S., Enelow, R. I., Gaston, B., Kron, I. L., Laubach, V. E. & Doctor, A. (2004). Tumor necrosis factor-alpha from resident lung cells is a key initiating factor in pulmonary ischemia-reperfusion injury. *J Thorac Cardiovasc Surg*, Vol.127, No.2, (Feb), pp. 541-547, ISSN 0022-5223
Mayer, A. M., Pittner, R. A., Lipscomb, G. E. & Spitzer, J. A. (1993). Effect of in vivo TNF administration on superoxide production and PKC activity of rat alveolar macrophages. *Am J Physiol*, Vol.264, No.1 Pt 1, (Jan), pp. L43-52, ISSN 0002-9513
McRae, K., De Perrot, M., Fischer, S., Waddell, T. K., Liu, M. & Keshavjee, S. (2001). Detection of IL-10 in the exhaled breath condensate, plasma and tissue during ischemia-reperfusion injury in experimental lung transplantation. *J Heart Lung Transplant*, Vol.20, No.2, (Feb), pp. 184, ISSN 1557-3117
Meade, M., Granton, J. T., Matte-Martyn, A., McRae, K., Cripps, P. M., Weaver, B. & Keshavjee, S. H. (2001). A randomized trial of inhaled nitric oxide to prevent reperfusion injury following lung transplantation. *J Heart Lung Transplant*, Vol.20, No.2, (Feb), pp. 254-255, ISSN 1557-3117
Meyer, K. C., Love, R. B. & Zimmerman, J. J. (1998). The therapeutic potential of nitric oxide in lung transplantation. *Chest*, Vol.113, No.5, (May), pp. 1360-1371, ISSN 0012-3692
Moore, T. M., Shirah, W. B., Khimenko, P. L., Paisley, P., Lausch, R. N. & Taylor, A. E. (2002). Involvement of CD40-CD40L signaling in postischemic lung injury. *Am J Physiol Lung Cell Mol Physiol*, Vol.283, No.6, (Dec), pp. L1255-1262, ISSN 1040-0605

Morimoto, R. I. (1993). Cells in stress: transcriptional activation of heat shock genes. *Science*, Vol.259, No.5100, (Mar 5), pp. 1409-1410, ISSN 0036-8075

Naidu, B. V., Woolley, S. M., Farivar, A. S., Thomas, R., Fraga, C. & Mulligan, M. S. (2003). Simvastatin ameliorates injury in an experimental model of lung ischemia-reperfusion. *J Thorac Cardiovasc Surg*, Vol.126, No.2, (Aug), pp. 482-489, ISSN 0022-5223

Naka, Y., Marsh, H. C., Scesney, S. M., Oz, M. C. & Pinsky, D. J. (1997). Complement activation as a cause for primary graft failure in an isogeneic rat model of hypothermic lung preservation and transplantation. *Transplantation*, Vol.64, No.9, (Nov 15), pp. 1248-1255, ISSN 0041-1337

Okazaki, M., Kreisel, F., Richardson, S. B., Kreisel, D., Krupnick, A. S., Patterson, G. A. & Gelman, A. E. (2007). Sphingosine 1-phosphate inhibits ischemia reperfusion injury following experimental lung transplantation. *Am J Transplant*, Vol.7, No.4, (Apr), pp. 751-758, ISSN 1600-6135

Oppenheim, J. J., Zachariae, C. O., Mukaida, N. & Matsushima, K. (1991). Properties of the novel proinflammatory supergene "intercrine" cytokine family. *Annu Rev Immunol*, Vol.9, pp. 617-648, ISSN 0732-0582

Oto, T., Griffiths, A. P., Rosenfeldt, F., Levvey, B. J., Williams, T. J. & Snell, G. I. (2006). Early outcomes comparing Perfadex, Euro-Collins, and Papworth solutions in lung transplantation. *Ann Thorac Surg*, Vol.82, No.5, (Nov), pp. 1842-1848, ISSN 1552-6259

Oyama, J., Blais, C., Jr., Liu, X., Pu, M., Kobzik, L., Kelly, R. A. & Bourcier, T. (2004). Reduced myocardial ischemia-reperfusion injury in toll-like receptor 4-deficient mice. *Circulation*, Vol.109, No.6, (Feb 17), pp. 784-789, ISSN 1524-4539

Park, J. S., Gamboni-Robertson, F., He, Q., Svetkauskaite, D., Kim, J. Y., Strassheim, D., Sohn, J. W., Yamada, S., Maruyama, I., Banerjee, A., Ishizaka, A. & Abraham, E. (2006). High mobility group box 1 protein interacts with multiple Toll-like receptors. *Am J Physiol Cell Physiol*, Vol.290, No.3, (Mar), pp. C917-924, ISSN 0363-6143

Pearse, D. B. & Dodd, J. M. (1999). Ischemia-reperfusion lung injury is prevented by apocynin, a novel inhibitor of leukocyte NADPH oxidase. *Chest*, Vol.116, No.1 Suppl, (Jul), pp. 55S-56S, ISSN 0012-3692

Phillips, W. A., Croatto, M. & Hamilton, J. A. (1990). Priming the macrophage respiratory burst with IL-4: enhancement with TNF-alpha but inhibition by IFN-gamma. *Immunology*, Vol.70, No.4, (Aug), pp. 498-503, ISSN 0019-2805

Pierre, A. F., Xavier, A. M., Liu, M., Cassivi, S. D., Lindsay, T. F., Marsh, H. C., Slutsky, A. S. & Keshavjee, S. H. (1998). Effect of complement inhibition with soluble complement receptor 1 on pig allotransplant lung function. *Transplantation*, Vol.66, No.6, (Sep 27), pp. 723-732, ISSN 0041-1337

Puri, V. & Patterson, G. A. (2008). Adult lung transplantation: technical considerations. *Semin Thorac Cardiovasc Surg*, Vol.20, No.2, (Summer), pp. 152-164, ISSN 1043-0679

Rabb, H., Daniels, F., O'Donnell, M., Haq, M., Saba, S. R., Keane, W. & Tang, W. W. (2000). Pathophysiological role of T lymphocytes in renal ischemia-reperfusion injury in mice. *Am J Physiol Renal Physiol*, Vol.279, No.3, (Sep), pp. F525-531, ISSN 1931-857X

Rachitskaya, A. V., Hansen, A. M., Horai, R., Li, Z., Villasmil, R., Luger, D., Nussenblatt, R. B. & Caspi, R. R. (2008). Cutting edge: NKT cells constitutively express IL-23 receptor and RORgammat and rapidly produce IL-17 upon receptor ligation in an IL-6-independent fashion. *J Immunol*, Vol.180, No.8, (Apr 15), pp. 5167-5171, ISSN 0022-1767

Reece, T. B., Laubach, V. E., Tribble, C. G., Maxey, T. S., Ellman, P. I., Warren, P. S., Schulman, A. M., Linden, J., Kern, J. A. & Kron, I. L. (2005). Adenosine A2A receptor agonist improves cardiac dysfunction from pulmonary ischemia-reperfusion injury. *Ann Thorac Surg*, Vol.79, No.4, (Apr), pp. 1189-1195, ISSN 1552-6259

Reece, T. B., Tribble, C. G., Okonkwo, D. O., Davis, J. D., Maxey, T. S., Gazoni, L. M., Linden, J., Kron, I. L. & Kern, J. A. (2008). Early adenosine receptor activation ameliorates spinal cord reperfusion injury. *J Cardiovasc Med (Hagerstown)*, Vol.9, No.4, (Apr), pp. 363-367, ISSN 1558-2027

Rivo, J., Zeira, E., Galun, E. & Matot, I. (2004). Activation of A3 adenosine receptor provides lung protection against ischemia-reperfusion injury associated with reduction in apoptosis. *Am J Transplant*, Vol.4, No.12, (Dec), pp. 1941-1948, ISSN 1600-6135

Rork, T. H., Wallace, K. L., Kennedy, D. P., Marshall, M. A., Lankford, A. R. & Linden, J. (2008). Adenosine A2A receptor activation reduces infarct size in the isolated, perfused mouse heart by inhibiting resident cardiac mast cell degranulation. *Am J Physiol Heart Circ Physiol*, Vol.295, No.5, (Nov), pp. H1825-1833, ISSN 0363-6135

Ross, S. D., Kron, I. L., Gangemi, J. J., Shockey, K. S., Stoler, M., Kern, J. A., Tribble, C. G. & Laubach, V. E. (2000). Attenuation of lung reperfusion injury after transplantation using an inhibitor of nuclear factor-kappaB. *Am J Physiol Lung Cell Mol Physiol*, Vol.279, No.3, (Sep), pp. L528-536, ISSN 1040-0605

Saemann, M. D., Haidinger, M., Hecking, M., Horl, W. H. & Weichhart, T. (2009). The multifunctional role of mTOR in innate immunity: implications for transplant immunity. *Am J Transplant*, Vol.9, No.12, (Dec), pp. 2655-2661, ISSN 1600-6143

Scaffidi, P., Misteli, T. & Bianchi, M. E. (2002). Release of chromatin protein HMGB1 by necrotic cells triggers inflammation. *Nature*, Vol.418, No.6894, (Jul 11), pp. 191-195, ISSN 0028-0836

Schmid, R. A., Zollinger, A., Singer, T., Hillinger, S., Leon-Wyss, J. R., Schob, O. M., Hogasen, K., Zund, G., Patterson, G. A. & Weder, W. (1998). Effect of soluble complement receptor type 1 on reperfusion edema and neutrophil migration after lung allotransplantation in swine. *J Thorac Cardiovasc Surg*, Vol.116, No.1, (Jul), pp. 90-97, ISSN 0022-5223

Schreck, R., Albermann, K. & Baeuerle, P. A. (1992). Nuclear factor kappa B: an oxidative stress-responsive transcription factor of eukaryotic cells (a review). *Free Radic Res Commun*, Vol.17, No.4, pp. 221-237, ISSN 8755-0199

Schutte, H., Witzenrath, M., Mayer, K., Rosseau, S., Seeger, W. & Grimminger, F. (2001). Short-term "preconditioning" with inhaled nitric oxide protects rabbit lungs against ischemia-reperfusion injury. *Transplantation*, Vol.72, No.8, (Oct 27), pp. 1363-1370, ISSN 0041-1337

Sharma, A. K., Fernandez, L. G., Awad, A. S., Kron, I. L. & Laubach, V. E. (2007). Proinflammatory response of alveolar epithelial cells is enhanced by alveolar macrophage-produced TNF-alpha during pulmonary ischemia-reperfusion injury. *Am J Physiol Lung Cell Mol Physiol*, Vol.293, No.1, (Jul), pp. L105-113, ISSN 1040-0605

Sharma, A. K., Yang, Z., Linden, J., Kron, I. L. & Laubach, V. E. (2008). Pulmonary ischemia-reperfusion injury is mediated by CD4+ T lymphocytes. *Am J Resp Crit Care Med*, Vol.177, No.Abstract Issue, pp. A38, ISSN

Sharma, A. K., Linden, J., Kron, I. L. & Laubach, V. E. (2009). Protection from pulmonary ischemia-reperfusion injury by adenosine A2A receptor activation. *Respir Res*, Vol.10, pp. 58, ISSN 1465-993X

Sharma, A. K., Laubach, V. E., Ramos, S. I., Zhao, Y., Stukenborg, G., Linden, J., Kron, I. L. & Yang, Z. (2010). Adenosine A2A receptor activation on CD4+ T lymphocytes and neutrophils attenuates lung ischemia-reperfusion injury. *J Thorac Cardiovasc Surg*, Vol.139, No.2, (Feb), pp. 474-482, ISSN 1097-685X

Sharma, A. K., Lapar, D. J., Zhao, Y., Li, L., Lau, C. L., Kron, I. L., Iwakura, Y., Okusa, M. D. & Laubach, V. E. (2011). Natural Killer T Cell-derived IL-17 Mediates Lung Ischemia-Reperfusion Injury. *Am J Respir Crit Care Med*, Vol.183, No.11, (Jun 1), pp. 1539-1549, ISSN 1535-4970

Shimamoto, A., Pohlman, T. H., Shomura, S., Tarukawa, T., Takao, M. & Shimpo, H. (2006). Toll-like receptor 4 mediates lung ischemia-reperfusion injury. *Ann Thorac Surg*, Vol.82, No.6, (Dec), pp. 2017-2023, ISSN 1552-6259

Shimoyama, T., Tabuchi, N., Kojima, K., Akamatsu, H., Arai, H., Tanaka, H. & Sunamori, M. (2005). Aprotinin attenuated ischemia-reperfusion injury in an isolated rat lung model after 18-hours preservation. *Eur J Cardiothorac Surg*, Vol.28, No.4, (Oct), pp. 581-587, ISSN 1010-7940

Shuvaev, V. V. & Muzykantov, V. R. (2011). Targeted modulation of reactive oxygen species in the vascular endothelium. *J Control Release*, (Mar 30), pp. ISSN 1873-4995

Sternberg, D. I., Gowda, R., Mehra, D., Qu, W., Weinberg, A., Twaddell, W., Sarkar, J., Wallace, A., Hudson, B., D'Ovidio, F., Arcasoy, S., Ramasamy, R., D'Armiento, J., Schmidt, A. M. & Sonett, J. R. (2008). Blockade of receptor for advanced glycation end product attenuates pulmonary reperfusion injury in mice. *J Thorac Cardiovasc Surg*, Vol.136, No.6, (Dec), pp. 1576-1585, ISSN 1097-685X

Strieter, R. M. & Kunkel, S. L. (1993). The immunopathology of chemotactic cytokines. *Adv Exp Med Biol*, Vol.351, pp. 19-28, ISSN 0065-2598

Sun, C. X., Zhong, H., Mohsenin, A., Morschl, E., Chunn, J. L., Molina, J. G., Belardinelli, L., Zeng, D. & Blackburn, M. R. (2006). Role of A2B adenosine receptor signaling in adenosine-dependent pulmonary inflammation and injury. *J Clin Invest*, Vol.116, No.8, (Aug), pp. 2173-2182, ISSN 0021-9738

Sundaresan, S., Semenkovich, J., Ochoa, L., Richardson, G., Trulock, E. P., Cooper, J. D. & Patterson, G. A. (1995). Successful outcome of lung transplantation is not compromised by the use of marginal donor lungs. *J Thorac Cardiovasc Surg*, Vol.109, No.6, (Jun), pp. 1075-1079, ISSN 0022-5223 van der Vliet, A. (2008). NADPH oxidases in lung biology and pathology: host defense enzymes, and more. *Free Radic Biol Med*, Vol.44, No.6, (Mar 15), pp. 938-955, ISSN 0891-5849

Wu, Q., Martin, R. J., Rino, J. G., Breed, R., Torres, R. M. & Chu, H. W. (2007). IL-23-dependent IL-17 production is essential in neutrophil recruitment and activity in mouse lung defense against respiratory Mycoplasma pneumoniae infection. *Microbes Infect*, Vol.9, No.1, (Jan), pp. 78-86, ISSN 1286-4579

Yang, Z., Sharma, A. K., Marshall, M., Kron, I. L. & Laubach, V. E. (2008). NADPH oxidase in bone marrow-derived cells mediates pulmonary ischemia-reperfusion injury. *Am J Respir Cell Mol Biol*, (Sep 11), pp. ISSN 1535-4989

Yang, Z., Sharma, A. K., Linden, J., Kron, I. L. & Laubach, V. E. (2009). CD4+ T lymphocytes mediate acute pulmonary ischemia-reperfusion injury. *J Thorac Cardiovasc Surg*, Vol.137, No.3, (Mar), pp. 695-702; discussion 702, ISSN 1097-685X

Yao, H., Yang, S. R., Kode, A., Rajendrasozhan, S., Caito, S., Adenuga, D., Henry, R., Edirisinghe, I. & Rahman, I. (2007). Redox regulation of lung inflammation: role of NADPH oxidase and NF-kappaB signalling. *Biochem Soc Trans*, Vol.35, No.Pt 5, (Nov), pp. 1151-1155, ISSN 0300-5127

Yen, D., Cheung, J., Scheerens, H., Poulet, F., McClanahan, T., McKenzie, B., Kleinschek, M. A., Owyang, A., Mattson, J., Blumenschein, W., Murphy, E., Sathe, M., Cua, D. J., Kastelein, R. A. & Rennick, D. (2006). IL-23 is essential for T cell-mediated colitis and promotes inflammation via IL-17 and IL-6. *J Clin Invest*, Vol.116, No.5, (May), pp. 1310-1316, ISSN 0021-9738

Yildiz, G., Demiryurek, A. T., Gumusel, B. & Lippton, H. (2007). Ischemic preconditioning modulates ischemia-reperfusion injury in the rat lung: role of adenosine receptors. *Eur J Pharmacol*, Vol.556, No.1-3, (Feb 5), pp. 144-150, ISSN 0014-2999

Zanotti, G., Casiraghi, M., Abano, J. B., Tatreau, J. R., Sevala, M., Berlin, H., Smyth, S., Funkhouser, W. K., Burridge, K., Randell, S. H. & Egan, T. M. (2009). Novel critical role of Toll-like receptor 4 in lung ischemia-reperfusion injury and edema. *Am J Physiol Lung Cell Mol Physiol*, Vol.297, No.1, (Jul), pp. L52-63, ISSN 1522-1504

Zhang, X., Bedard, E. L., Potter, R., Zhong, R., Alam, J., Choi, A. M. & Lee, P. J. (2002). Mitogen-activated protein kinases regulate HO-1 gene transcription after ischemia-reperfusion lung injury. *Am J Physiol Lung Cell Mol Physiol*, Vol.283, No.4, (Oct), pp. L815-829, ISSN 1040-0605

Zhao, G., al-Mehdi, A. B. & Fisher, A. B. (1997). Anoxia-reoxygenation versus ischemia in isolated rat lungs. *Am J Physiol*, Vol.273, No.6 Pt 1, (Dec), pp. L1112-1117, ISSN 0002-9513

Zhao, M., Fernandez, L. G., Doctor, A., Sharma, A. K., Zarbock, A., Tribble, C. G., Kron, I. L. & Laubach, V. E. (2006). Alveolar macrophage activation is a key initiation signal for acute lung ischemia-reperfusion injury. *Am J Physiol Lung Cell Mol Physiol*, Vol.291, No.5, (Nov), pp. L1018-1026, ISSN 1040-0605

Zhao, Y., Sharma, A. K., LaPar, D. J., Kron, I. L., Ailawadi, G., Liu, Y., Jones, D. R., Laubach, V. E. & Lau, C. L. (2011). Depletion of tissue plasminogen activator attenuates lung ischemia-reperfusion injury via inhibition of neutrophil extravasation. *Am J Physiol Lung Cell Mol Physiol*, Vol.300, No.5, (May), pp. L718-729, ISSN 1522-1504

Zhu, C., Bilali, A., Georgieva, G. S., Kurata, S., Mitaka, C. & Imai, T. (2008). Salvage of nonischemic control lung from injury by unilateral ischemic lung with apocynin, a nicotinamide adenine dinucleotide phosphate (NADPH) oxidase inhibitor, in isolated perfused rat lung. *Transl Res*, Vol.152, No.6, (Dec), pp. 273-282, ISSN 1878-1810

Zwacka, R. M., Zhang, Y., Halldorson, J., Schlossberg, H., Dudus, L. & Engelhardt, J. F. (1997). CD4(+) T-lymphocytes mediate ischemia/reperfusion-induced inflammatory responses in mouse liver. *J Clin Invest*, Vol.100, No.2, (Jul 15), pp. 279-289, ISSN 0021-9738

23

Superior Vena Cava Syndrome

Francesco Puma and Jacopo Vannucci
University of Perugia Medical School,
Thoracic Surgery Unit,
Italy

1. Introduction

1.1 Anatomy

The superior vena cava (SVC) originates in the chest, behind the first right sternocostal articulation, from the confluence of two main collector vessels: the right and left brachiocephalic veins which receive the ipsilateral internal jugular and subclavian veins. It is located in the anterior mediastinum, on the right side.

The internal jugular vein collects the blood from head and deep sections of the neck while the subclavian vein, from the superior limbs, superior chest and superficial head and neck.

Several other veins from the cervical region, chest wall and mediastinum are directly received by the brachiocephalic veins.

After the brachiocephalic convergence, the SVC follows the right lateral margin of the sternum in an inferoposterior direction. It displays a mild internal concavity due to the adjacent ascending aorta. Finally, it enters the pericardium superiorly and flows into the right atrium; no valve divides the SVC from right atrium.

The SVC's length ranges from 6 to 8 cm. Its diameter is usually 20-22 mm. The total diameters of both brachiocephalic veins are wider than the SVC's caliber. The blood pressure ranges from -5 to 5 mmHg and the flow is discontinuous depending on the heart pulse cycle.

The SVC can be classified anatomically in two sections: extrapericardial and intrapericardial. The extrapericardial segment is contiguous to the sternum, ribs, right lobe of the thymus, connective tissue, right mediastinal pleura, trachea, right bronchus, lymphnodes and ascending aorta. In the intrapericardial segment, the SVC enters the right atrium on the upper right face of the heart; in front it is close to the right main pulmonary artery. On the right side, the lung is in its proximity, separated only by mediastinal pleura. The right phrenic nerve runs next to the SVC for its entire course [1] (Figure 1).

The SVC receives a single affluent vein: the azygos vein. The azygos vein joins the SVC from the right side, at its mid length, above the right bronchus. The Azygos vein constantly receives the superior intercostal vein, a large vessel which drains blood from the upper two or three right intercostal spaces. In the case of SVC obstruction, the azygos vein is responsible for the most important collateral circulation. According to the expected collateral pathways, the SVC can be divided into two segments: the supra-azygos or preazygos and the infra-azygos or postazygos SVC. There are four possible collateral systems which were first described in 1949 by McIntire and Sykes. They are represented by the azygos venous system, the internal thoracic venous system, the vertebral venous system and the external thoracic venous system [2]. The azygos venous system is the only direct path into the SVC. The internal thoracic vein is the collector between SVC and inferior vena cava (IVC) via epigastric and iliac veins. The vertebral veins with intercostals, lumbar and sacral veins, represent the posterior network between SVC and IVC. The external thoracic vein system is the most superficial and it is represented by axillary, lateral thoracic and superficial epigastric veins.

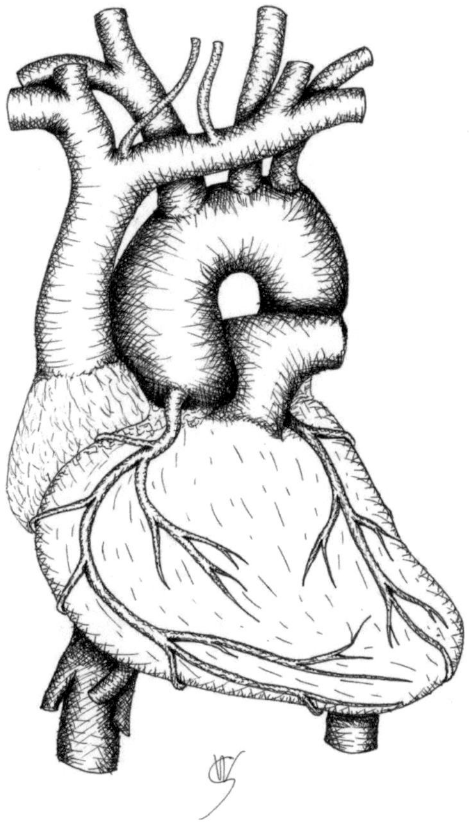

Fig. 1.

The SVC is a constituent part of the right paratracheal space (also called "*Barety's space*"), containing the main lymphatic route of the mediastinum, i.e. the right lateral tracheal chain. *Barety's space* is bounded laterally by the SVC, posteriorly by the tracheal wall, and medially by the ascending aorta. The nodes of the right paratracheal space are frequently involved in malignant growths: the SVC is undoubtedly the anatomical structure of this space which offers less resistance to compression, due to its thin wall and low internal pressure.

Anatomical anomalies are rare. The most frequent is the double SVC which has an embryologic etiology [1].

2. Etiology

SVC syndrome (SVCS) may be related to various etiological factors. Malignancies are predominant (95%) while, in the past, infectious diseases used to be common. During the last century, progression in anti-bacterial therapies and improvement in social conditions have led to a consistent decrease in the benign origin of this condition. The incidence of iatrogenic SVCS is currently increasing [3,4].
SVCS etiology is summarized as follows:

- Malignant
  - Lung cancer
  - Lymphomas
  - Thymoma
  - Mediastinal germ cell tumors
  - Mediastinal metastases
  - Mesothelioma
  - Leiomyosarcoma and angiosarcoma
  - Neoplastic thrombi
  - Anaplastic thyroid cancer
- Benign
  - Fibrosing mediastinitis (idiopathic or radiation-induced)
  - Infectious diseases (tubercolosis, histoplasmosis, echinococcosis, syphilis, aspergillosis, blastomycosis, filariasis, nocardiosis…)
  - Thrombosis (non-neoplastic)
  - Lymphadenopaties (sarcoidosis, Behçet's syndrome, Castelman's disease…)
  - Aortic aneurysm
  - Substernal goiter
  - Pericardial, thymic, bronchogenic cysts
- Iatrogenic
  - Pacemaker and defibrillator placement
  - Central venous catheters

3. Pathophysiology

The pathogenetic basis of SVCS is obstruction to the blood flow. It can result from intrinsic or extrinsic obstacles. The former are uncommon and are represented by thrombosis or invading tissue. Extrinsic factors develop from compression or stricture of the vein.
In physiologic conditions, blood return to the right atrium is facilitated by the pressure gradient between the right atrium and venae cavae. When obstruction of the SVC occurs, the vascular resistances rise and the venous return decreases. SVC pressure may increase consistently [4].
When SVC shows a significant stenosis (3/5 of the lumen or more), blood flow is redirected through the collateral circulation in order to bypass the obstruction and restore the venous

return [5]. The timing of the obstruction development is important for its clinical implications. In acute impairments, the blood flow is not rapidly distributed through the collateral network so symptoms arise markedly. In the case of slow-growing diseases, the collateral venous network has enough time to expand in order to receive the circulating volume. For this reason, long-lasting, severe SVC obstruction can sometimes be found without significant related signs and symptoms [3,6].

4. Clinical presentation

The SVC wall does not offer resistance to compression. When SVC lumen reduction is greater than 60%, hemodynamic changes occur: proximal dilatation, congestion and flow slowdown. The clinical signs of this condition are mainly represented by cyanosis (due to venous stasis with normal arterial oxygenation) and edema of the upper chest, arms, neck and face (periorbital initially). Swelling is usually more important on the right side, because of the better possibility of collateral circulation in the left brachiocephalic vein compared to the contralateral (Figure 2). Vein varicosities of the proximal tongue and dark purple ears are also typical. Other signs or symptoms are: coughing, epistaxis, hemoptysis, dysphagia, dysphonia and hoarseness (caused by vocal cord congestion), esophageal, retinal and conjuntival bleeding. In the case of significant cephalic venous stasis, headache, dizziness, buzzing, drowsiness, stupor, lethargy and even coma may be encountered. Headache is a common symptom and it is usually continuous and pressing, exacerbated by coughing. Epilepsy has been occasionally reported as well as psychosis, probably due to carbon dioxide accumulation [3,4,7-14]. Dyspnea can be directly related to the mediastinal mass or be caused by pleural effusion or cardiocirculatory impairment. Supine position may worsen the clinical scenarios.

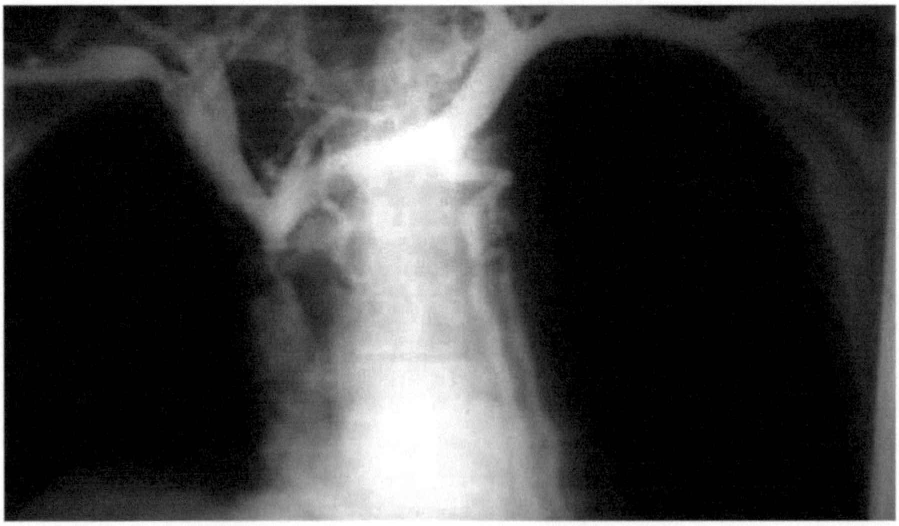

Fig. 2. Phlebogram showing obstruction of the SVC with azygos involvement. Blood return is distributed through a collateral circulation, mainly sustained by branches of the left brachiocephalic vein. Edema in this patient was more severe in the right arm than the left.

The clinical seriousness of the syndrome is related to several factors:

- Level of obstruction and rapidity of development, determining the effectiveness of collateral circulation
- Impairment of lymphatic drainage (pulmonary interstitial edema or pleural effusion)
- Involvement of other mediastinal structures (compression or invasion of heart, pulmonary artery and central airways, phrenic nerve paralysis…)

Intolerance of the supine position is always linked to a severe prognostic significance for patients with mediastinal syndromes [15]. The variation in decubitus may worsen the already existing signs and symptoms: in the supine position, an anterior mediastinal mass may compress the trachea or the heart by means of gravity, with possible cardiorespiratory problems. Direct compression of the common trunk of the pulmonary artery is also possible, although this is not as likely to happen, given that such structure is cranially protected by the aortic arch [16].

The presence of dyspnea at rest, especially in the sitting position, carries a severe prognostic significance in patients with mediastinal syndromes. Dyspnea at rest can be caused by either cardiovascular or respiratory problems:

- pulmonary congestion caused by lymphatic stasis
- combination with pulmonary atelectasis
- pleural effusion
- pericardial effusion
- direct compression of the mass on the airways, on the heart, or on the pulmonary artery
- laryngeal edema

Dyspnea at rest is not uncommon in the natural evolution of SVCS and it should always be considered as a high risk factor for invasive procedures under general anesthesia. If the shortness of breath is related to laryngeal edema, the patient should not be presented for general anesthesia and surgery.

Superficial dilated vascular routes are the main sign of collateral circulation and appear swollen and non-pulsating. In the case of marked obesity, superficial veins can be missing at inspection. The variety of collateral circulation and the differences in the venous re-arrangement are expression of the SVC obstruction site (Figure 3,4,5).

The anatomic classification includes three levels of obstruction:

1. Obstruction of the upper SVC, proximal to the azygos entry point.
2. Obstruction with azygos involvement.
3. Obstruction of the lower SVC, distal to the azygos entry point.

1. In this situation, there is no impediment to normal blood flow through the azygos vein which opens into the patent tract of the SVC. Venous drainage coming from the head neck, shoulders and arms cannot directly reach the right atrium. A longer but effective way is provided by several veins, the most important being the right superior intercostal vein. From the superior tract of the SVC, blood flow is reversed and directed to the azygos, mainly through the right superior intercostal vein. The azygos collateral system is eminently deep; therefore the presence of superficial vessels is usually lacking, even if possible in the area of the internal thoracic vein's superficial tributaries. The volumetric increase of the vessels can be consistent and capacity may increase up to eight times. The efficiency of this collateral route is reliable, thus the clinical compensation is unbalanced only in the case of a rapid development of the obstruction or if the stenosis is more than 90% (Figure 3).

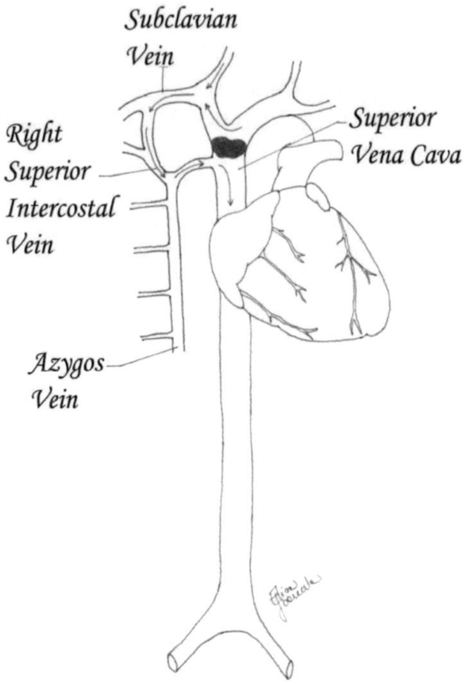

Fig. 3. Obstruction of the upper SVC, proximal to the azygos entry point. Collateral pathways.

2. In this case, the azygos vein cannot be available as collateral pathway and the only viable blood return is carried by minor vessels to IVC (cava-cava or anazygotic circulation). From the internal thoracic veins, blood is forced to the intercostal veins, then to azygos and emiazygos veins. The flow is thus reversed into the ascending lumbar veins to the iliac veins. Direct anastomosis between the azygos' origin and the IVC and between emiazygos and left renal vein are also active. In addition, the internal thoracic veins can flow into the superior epigastric veins. From the superior epigastric veins, blood is carried to the inferior epigastric veins across the superficial system of the cutaneous abdominal veins and finally to the iliac veins. Another course is between the thoraco-epigastric vein (collateral of the axillary vein) and the external iliac vein.

   In these conditions, the collateral circulation is partly deep and partly superficial. The physical examination often reveals SVC obstruction. The reversed circulation through the described pathways, remains less efficient than the azygos system and venous hypertension is usually more severe. For this reason, this kind of SVC obstruction is often related to important symptoms, dyspnea and pleural effusion. The ensuing slow blood flow may be responsible for superimposed thrombosis. In the disease progression, renal impairment can evolve as the SVC obstruction affects the lumbar plexus (mostly the ascending lumbar veins, left side) which congests the renal vein (Figure 4).

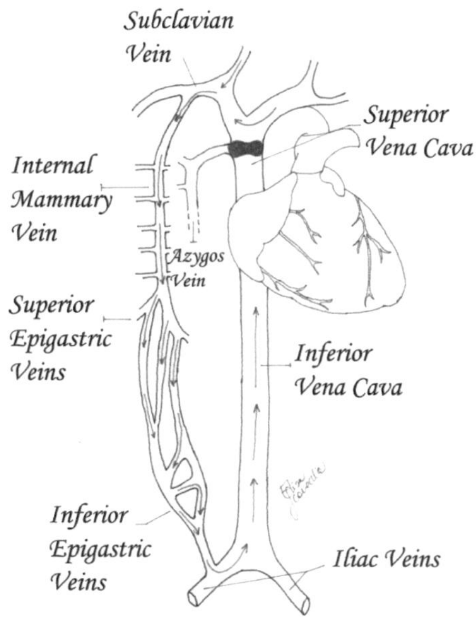

Fig. 4. Obstruction with azygos involvement. Collateral pathways.

3. In this condition, the obstruction is just below the azygos arch. The blood flow is distributed from the superior body into the azygos and emiazygos veins, in which the flow is inverted, to the IVC tributaries. In this type of case, the superficial collateral system is not always evident but the azygos and emiazygos congestion and dilatation are usually important. The hemodynamic changes lead to edema and cyanosis of the upper chest and pleural effusion. Pleural effusion is often slowly-growing and right-sided, probably due to anatomical reasons: there is a wider anastomosis between emiazygos and IVC than between azygos and IVC [17] (Figure 5).

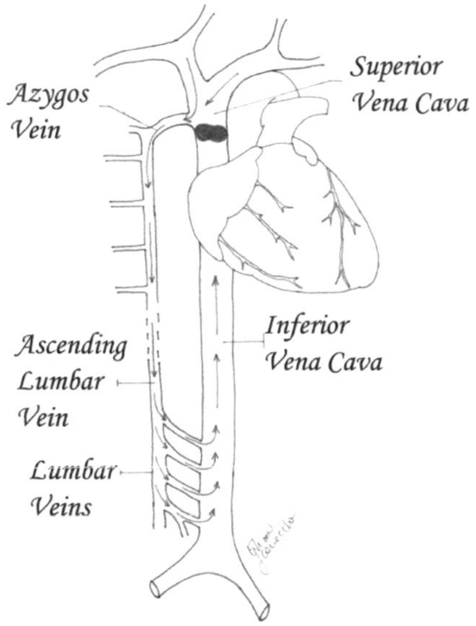

Fig. 5. Obstruction of the lower SVC, distal to the azygos entry point. Collateral pathways.

5. Classification of SVCS

Several classifications of SVCS have been proposed even though further investigations are required to achieve a definitive staging system. There are three main classification proposals which follow different methods of categorization [18-20].

1. Doty and Standford's classification (anatomical)
   - Type I: stenosis of up to 90% of the supra-azygos SVC
   - Type II: stenosis of more than 90% of the supra-azygos SVC
   - Type III: complete occlusion of SVC with azygos reverse blood flow
   - Type IV: complete occlusion of SVC with the involvement of the major tributaries and azygos vein
2. Yu's classification (clinical)
   - Grade 0: asymptomatic (imaging evidence of SVC obstruction)
   - Grade 1: mild (plethora, cyanosis, head and neck edema)
   - Grade 2: moderate (grade 1 evidence + functional impairment)
   - Grade 3: severe (mild/moderate cerebral or laryngeal edema, limited cardiac reserve)
   - Grade 4: life-threatening (significant cerebral or laryngeal edema, cardiac failure)
   - Grade 5: fatal
3. Bigsby's classification (operative risk)
   - Low risk
   - High risk

The authors proposed an algorithm for SVCS to assess the operative risk in order to submit the patient to invasive diagnostic procedures. The low risk patients present: no dyspnea at rest, no facial cyanosis in the upright position, no change of dyspnea and no worsening of facial edema and cyanosis, during the supine position. The high risk patients present facial cyanosis or dyspnea at rest in the sitting position.

6. Diagnosis

Physical examination is often crucial: the presence of edema and superficial venous network of the upper chest may support the clinical diagnosis. Imaging studies are however required. Most cases are suspected at the standard chest X-ray and the most common radiological findings are right mediastinal widening and pleural effusion [3].

Computed tomography (CT) with multislice detector is the most useful tool in the evaluation of the mediastinal syndromes. CT imaging is widely employed in SVCS assessment because of its large availability and short acquisition time. Intravenous contrast should be administered, in order to provide high-quality vascular imaging. Contrast enhanced multidetector CT may show the site of the obstruction, some aspects of the primary disease and eventual intraluminal thrombi. Multiplanar and 3D reconstructions may provide better image detection and definition. The contrast flow can also help to distinguish the extent of the collateral network (Figure 6) [21].

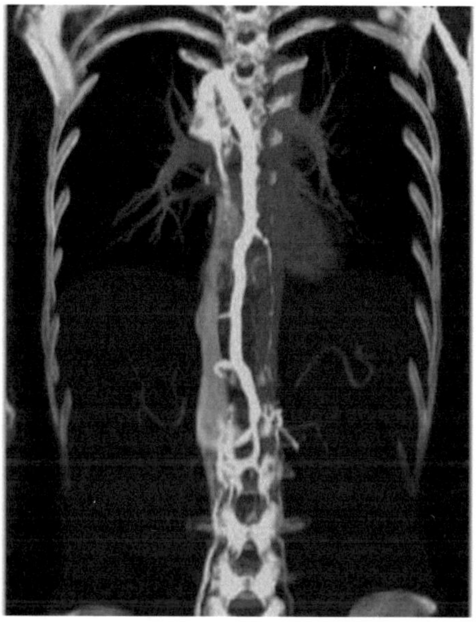

Fig. 6. Angio-CT scan: Obstruction of the lower SVC, distal to the azygos entry point. Collateral pathways: in the azygos vein system the blood flow is inverted and venous return occurs by means of IVC.

Magnetic resonance imaging (MRI) plays a side role; it is indicated when CT cannot be performed (e.g. pregnancy, endovenous contrast intollerance). The long acquisition times of MRI limit its use in critically ill patients.

Invasive venography is now rarely used due to the huge improvement in vascular CT imaging. It is currently performed only as a preliminary to operative procedures such as stent placement.

Once the thoracic imaging is obtained, the work-up should include brain, abdominal and bone studies in view of the probable malignant nature of the primary lesion. Recently Fluorodeoxyglucose-Positron Emission Tomography has gained an important role in oncology [22].

The histological definition remains the key factor for the causative treatment, in the case of neoplastic etiology. Superficial adenopathies have to be carefully investigated in order to find a possible source of tissue and the easiest target for biopsy. The invasive diagnostic procedure varies largely depending on the suspected malignancy and its site. The biopsy can be obtained through traditional bronchoscopy or echo-guided endoscopy, superficial node biopsy, mediastinoscopy, mediastinotomy, transthoracic needle biopsy, thoracoscopy, cervical or supraclavicular biopsies; thoracotomy and sternotomy are rarely indicated. Operative endoscopy has gained a new significance in the evaluation of SVCS since echography has been introduced but the best diagnostic result is still obtained by the mediastinoscopy. Venous hypertension may increase the procedure-related risk [23-27].

7. Treatment

Therapy should be causative. Syndrome management recognizes different levels of priority depending on the severity of symptoms, etiology and prognosis. SVCS needs a multidisciplinary approach and symptoms relief is often the first objective of complex care.

The therapeutic plan is usually targeted to clinical palliation. In fact, most cases are diagnosed as advanced-stage malignancies.

The patient must immediately assume an orthostatic position. Other supportive treatments are usually promptly established; oxygen, diuretics, and steroids are also suggested. The risk of an overlying thrombosis is particularly high and anticoagulant therapy should be introduced.

In case of malignancy, the treatment can have palliative or, rarely, curative intent. Chemotherapy is usually employed in lymphomas, small-cell lung cancer and germ cell tumors. Besides chemotherapy, radiotherapy is widely used in the treatment of non-small cell lung cancer. Radiation therapy can obtain good results but can also produce an initial inflammatory response with a possible temporary worsening [28,29]. Some cases must be approached as an emergency. In this type of situation, the treatment of choice is usually endovascular with the aim of restoring blood flow as soon as possible. The acute life-threatening presentation is the only situation in which radiotherapy before histological diagnosis can be considered. However, this approach should be avoided, whenever possible.

Endovascular stenting provides fast functional relief. It is the best option in an emergency and sometimes the clinical benefit is immediate. It is also advocated in the case of chemo-radiotherapy non-responders [3].

Surgery has a central role in the diagnosis but rarely in the therapy. A SVC resection and reconstruction is not often recommended and is a demanding procedure. The main proposal for SVC resection is direct infiltration in thymomas or in N0-N1 non-small cell lung cancer. In the case of infiltration of less than 30% of the SVC circumference, direct suture is favored (Figure 7). Larger involvements require a prosthetic repair. Different methods of SVC repair have been investigated using different materials (Figures 8, 9, 10a-b). Armoured PTFE grafts and biologic material are the preferred choices. Morbidity after SVC surgical procedures is high and the post-operative care must be intensive [4]. Long-term patency of a SVC by-pass graft is uncertain but, usually, the slow onset of the graft thrombosis favors the development of effective collateral circulation.

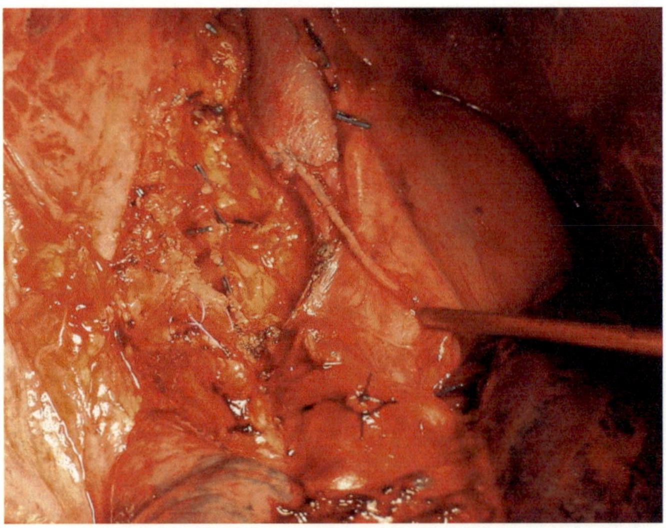

Fig. 7. SVC resection for limited infiltration by a right upper lobe NSCLC. The moderate stenosis following the direct SVC suture did not have hemodynamic consequences, in this patient.

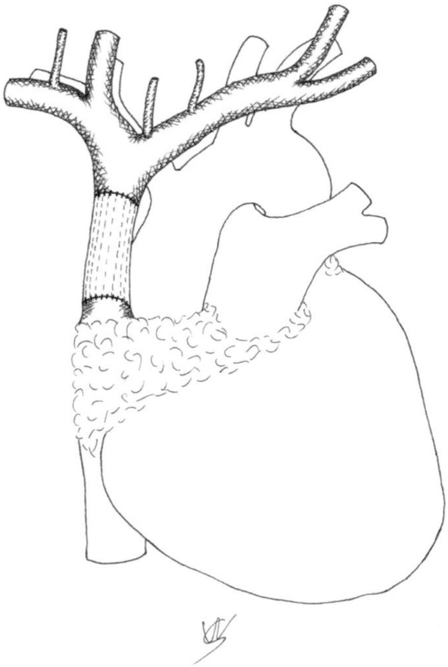

Fig. 8. Graft reconstruction by end-to-end anastomosis between proximal and distal SVC.

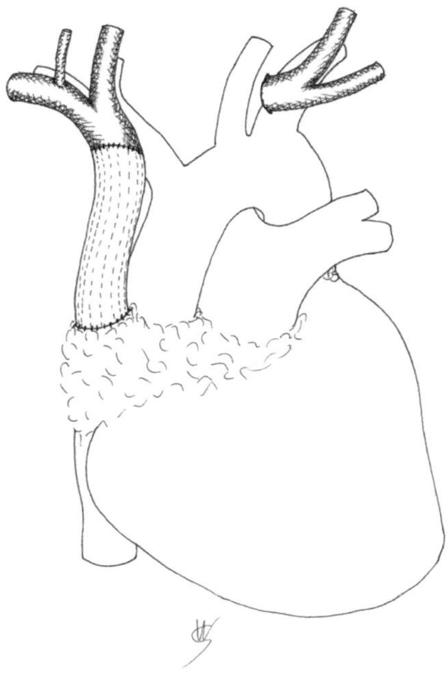

Fig. 9. Graft reconstruction of SVC by end-to-end anastomosis between the right brachiocephalic vein and the SVC.

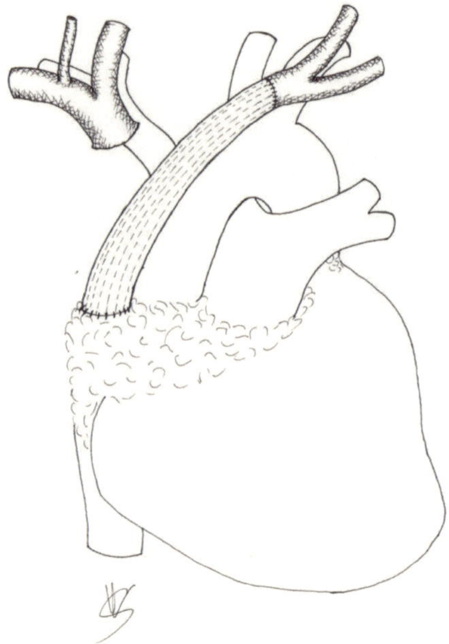

Fig. 10a. Graft reconstruction of SVC by end-to-end anastomosis between the left brachiocephalic vein and the SVC.

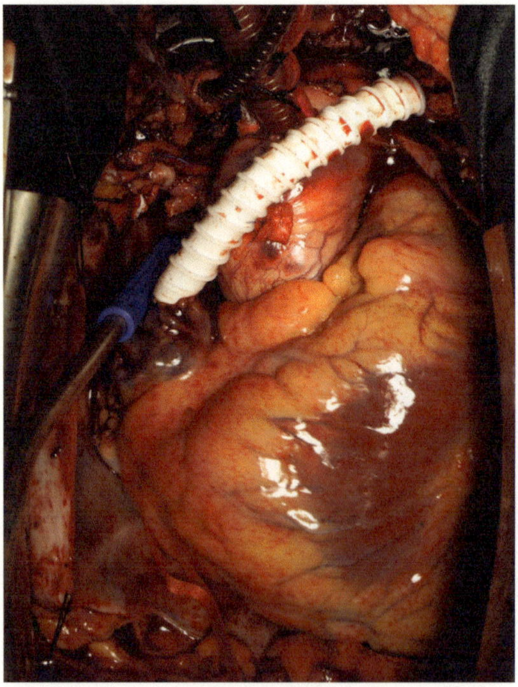

Fig. 10b. Armoured PTFE reconstruction of SVC by end-to-end anastomosis between the left brachiocephalic vein and the SVC.

Artworks by Walter Santilli R.N. and Elisa Scarnecchia M.D.

8. References

[1] Testut L, Latarjet A. Trattato di Anatomia Umana. 4th edition, Unione tipografica - Editrice Torinese. 1971. pp. 918-921

[2] McIntire FT, Sykes EM jr. Obstruction of the superior vena cava: A review of the literature and report of two personal cases. Ann Intern Med 1949; 30:925.

[3] Wan JF, Bezjak A. Superior vena cava syndrome. Hematol Oncol Clin North Am. 2010; 24:501-13

[4] Macchiarini P. Superior vena cava obstruction. In: Patterson GA, Cooper JD, Deslauriers J, Lerut AEM, Luketic JD, Rive TW, editors. Pearson's thoracic & esophageal surgery. 3rd edition, Philadelphia, PA: Churchill Livingstone, Elsevier; 2008. pp. 1684-96

[5] Sy WM, Lao RS. Collateral pathways in superior vena cava obstruction as seen on gamma images. Br J Radiol 1982; 55:294-300

[6] Rice TW, Rodriguez RM, Light RW. The superior vena cava syndrome: clinical characteristics and evolving etiology. Medicine (Baltimore) 2006; 85:37-42

[7] Ahmann FR. A reassessment of the clinical implications of the superior vena caval syndrome. J Clin Oncol 1984; 2:961-969

[8] Ganeshan A, Hon LQ, Warakaulle DR, Morgan R, Uberoi R. Superior vena caval stenting for SVC obstruction: current status. Eur J Radiol. 2009; 71:343-9

[9] Armstrong BA, Perez CA, Simpson JR, Hederman MA. Role of irradiation in the management of superior vena cava syndrome. Int J Radiat Oncol Biol Phys 1987; 13:531-539

[10] Yelling A, Rosen A, Reichert N, Lieberman Y. Superior vena cava syndrome: the Myth-the facts. Am Rev Respir Dis 1990; 141:1114-18

[11] Schraufnagel DE, Hill R, Leech JA, Pare JAP. Superior vena caval obstruction: is it a medical emergency? Am J Med 1981; 70:1169-74

[12] Chen JC, Bongard F, Klein SR. A contemporary perspective on superior vena cava syndrome. Am J Surg 1990; 160:207-11

[13] Rice TW, Rodriguez RM, Barnette R, Light RW. Prevalence and characteristics of pleural effusions in superior vena cava syndrome. Respirology 2006; 11:299-305

[14] Urruticoechea A, Mesía R, Domínguez J, Falo C, Escalante E, Montes A, Sancho C, Cardenal F, Majem M, Germà JR. Treatment of malignant superior vena cava syndrome by endovascular stent insertion. Experience on 52 patients with lung cancer. Lung Cancer 2004; 43:209-14

[15] Northrip DR, Bohman BK, Tsueda K. Total airway occlusion and superior vena cava syndrome in a child with an anterior mediastinal tumor. Anesth Analg 1986; 65:1079-82

[16] Levin H, Bursztein S, Haifetz M. Cardiac arrest in a child with an anterior mediastinal mass. Anesth Analg 1985; 64:1129-30

[17] Introzzi P. Trattato Italiano di Medicina Interna, parte quinta. 2nd edition, Industria grafica "l'impronta". 1974. pp.1514-25

[18] Stanford W, Doty DB. The role of venography and surgery in the management of patients with superior vena cava obstruction. Ann Thorac Surg 1986; 41:158

[19] Yu JB, Wilson LD, Detterbeck FC. Superior vena cava syndrome--a proposed classification system and algorithm for management. J Thorac Oncol 2008; 3:811-4

[20] Bigsby R, Greengrass R, Unruh H. Diagnostic algorithm for acute superior vena caval obstruction (SVCO). J Cardiovasc Surg 1993; 34:347-50

[21] Sheth S, Ebert MD, Fishman EK. Superior vena cava obstruction evaluation with MDCT. Am J Roentgenol 2010; 194:336-46

[22] Abner A: Approach to the patient who presents with superior vena cava obstruction. Chest 1993; 103:394-397

[23] Mineo TC, Ambrogi V, Nofroni I, Pistolese C. Mediastinoscopy in superior vena cava obstruction: analysis of 80 consecutive patients. Ann Thorac Surg 1999; 68:223-6

[24] Porte H, Metois D, Finzi L, Lebuffe G, Guidat A, Conti M, Wurtz A. Superior vena cava syndrome of malignant origin. Which surgical procedure for which diagnosis? Eur J Cardiothorac Surg 2000; 17:384-8

[25] Trinkle JK, Bryant LR, Malette WG, Playforth RH, Wood RC. Mediastinoscopy--diagnostic value compared to bronchoscopy: scalene biopsy and sputum cytology in 155 patients. Am Surg 1968; 34:740-3

[26] Jahangiri M, Taggart DP, Goldstraw P. Role of mediastinoscopy in superior vena cava obstruction. Cancer 1993; 71:3006-8

[27] Callejas MA, Rami R, Catalán M, Mainer A, Sánchez-Lloret J. Mediastinoscopy as an emergency diagnostic procedure in superior vena cava syndrome. Scand J Thorac Cardiovasc Surg 1991; 25:137-9

[28] Sculier JP, Evans WK, Feld R, DeBoer G, Payne DG, Shepherd FA, Pringle JF, Yeoh JL, Quirt IC, Curtis JE, et al. Superior vena caval obstruction syndrome in small cell lung cancer. Cancer 1986; 57:847-51

[29] Lonardi F, Gioga G, Agus G, Coeli M, Campostrini F. Double-flash, large-fraction radiation therapy as palliative treatment of malignant superior vena cava syndrome in the elderly. Support Care Cancer 2002; 10:156-60

24

Compensatory Lung Growth After Pneumonectomy

Lucas G. Fernández, James M. Isbell,
David R. Jones and Victor E. Laubach
University of Virginia Health System, Charlottesville, VA, USA

1. Introduction

Pneumonectomy, the surgical removal of a lung, elicits a number of anatomical changes within the thoracic cavity that augments the diffusion capacity of the remaining lung. Pneumonectomy directs the entire cardiac output into the remaining lung and creates an empty hemithorax that results in a shift of the mediastinum toward the vacated thoracic compartment. In a number of experimental animal models, pneumonectomy initiates compensatory, regenerative growth of the remaining lung tissue that restores normal mass, structure and function. This growth process, called compensatory lung growth (CLG), is qualitatively similar across species, but differs with gender, age and hormonal status. CLG involves unique structure-function interactions not seen in solid organs. Little is known about the regenerative potential of human lungs. Although CLG has been reported in children after major lung resection, CLG in adults rarely occurs and remains a significant challenge. Mechanical feedback between the lung and thorax constitutes a major signal that sustains both post-natal lung development as well as post-pneumonectomy CLG. After pneumonectomy, increased mechanical stress and strain on the remaining lung induce adaptive responses to augment oxygen transport, including 1) recruitment of alveolar-capillary reserves, 2) remodeling of existing tissue, and 3) regenerative growth of acinar tissue when strain exceeds a critical threshold. This chapter will discuss the clinical aspects of pneumonectomy and will primarily review cellular and molecular mechanisms of CLG via experimental pneumonectomy models, which offers powerful insights into regenerative organ growth.

2. Clinical pneumonectomy

2.1 Historical perspective

Before the 1930s, all pneumonectomies in humans were fatal due primarily to complications such as hemorrhage and sepsis. Another major challenge was to perform lung surgery with an open pneumothorax. A significant step to solve this problem was taken in 1903 by Ferdinand Sauerbruch, who designed a negative pressure chamber that allowed a team of surgeons to operate within the open chest without collapse of the lung (Sauerbruch, 1953). Sauerbruch brought his machine to New York in 1908, where Willy

Meyer modified it to work with positive and negative pressure. Meyer successfully performed pulmonary resections in dogs in 1909 using suture closure of the bronchus and individual vessel ligation (Meyer, 1909), but he did not attempt his technique in humans. Years later, Quinby and Morse used a modification of this technique in dogs and showed that after pneumonectomy, the hemithorax fills with fluid and the remaining lung will shift to this empty side (Quinby & Morse, 1911). After the experimental use of endotracheal delivery of oxygen and anesthetics (Meltzer & Auer, 1909), Howard Lilienthal performed the first thoracotomy under endotracheal anesthesia at Mount Sinai Hospital (Lilienthal, 1910). He also had the largest published series of lobectomies, which he considered dangerous, reaching a mortality rate of 70% if more than one lobe was removed (Lilienthal, 1922). The first successful case of total pneumonectomy was described in 1931 by Roudolph Nissen in Berlin. The patient was a 12 year-old girl with trauma injury of the left chest (Naef, 1987). She recovered completely after two months, and Nissen was quoted saying that the occlusion of the pulmonary artery did not cause cardiopulmonary collapse as predicted 20 years earlier by Quinby and Morse. A year later, Cameron Haight was the first surgeon to perform a successful pneumonectomy in the west at the University of Michigan, USA (Haight, 1934). This time, a 13 year-old girl developed pneumonia in the left lung and subsequent pyopneumothorax. After a small bronchial fistula, she recovered 3.5 months later. On April 1933, Evarts Graham performed the first successful pneumonectomy for cancer disease in a 48 year-old patient with a squamous cell cancer of the left upper lobe bronchus that survived almost 30 years after surgery (Graham & Berck, 1933). In his paper, Clarence Crawford standardized the pneumonectomy technique used for many years, including the use of periscapular incision, individual vessel ligation, suture closure of the bronchus and a new rhythmic ventilatory technique (O'Shaughnessy & Crawford, 1938). In 1950, the introduction of a new double lumen tube allowed the ventilatory exclusion of the operated side (Bjork & Carlens, 1950). By the 1970s, a new technique changed the surgical method with the design of surgical staplers for lung resection. The first successful thoracic surgery performed using video assisted thoracic surgery (VDATS) was for treatment of pneumothorax in 1990. Shortly thereafter the first descriptions of pulmonary lobectomies and pneumonectomies appeared (Davies & Panasuk, 1992). There has been steady progress in thoracic surgery and pneumonectomy in particular through the years, with advances in knowledge of respiratory physiology, anesthetics and ventilation techniques, as well as more sophisticated methods of lung resection. These advancements have transformed pneumonectomy surgery from a "dangerous procedure" to become a very useful treatment for both malignant and non malignant diseases of the lung and airways.

2.2 Indications and risk factors

Pneumonectomy is known to be associated with high morbidity and mortality. However, in certain instances, it offers the only chance for a cure. The indications for pneumonectomy are usually classified in two major groups: pneumonectomy for benign disease and pneumonectomy for malignant disease. Due to the improvement of antimicrobial therapies and better control of inflammatory diseases, pneumonectomy for benign diseases is not a routine procedure in our times. The conditions considered in this group belong to several categories including inflammatory, traumatic, congenital and other miscellaneous conditions (Conlan & Kopec, 1999). These conditions carry a high mortality rate in most cases, but some examples of non-malignant disease have an excellent cure rate. Indications for pneumonectomy in cases of bacterial or fungal infections include symptomatic patients with hemoptysis, productive cough or chronic empyema, as well as unilateral lung destruction documented by CT or bronchography (Blyth, 2000). In patients with pulmonary tuberculosis, pneumonectomy is indicated for either multidrug resistance disease or for complications or sequelae of tuberculosis infection. The most common fungal infection that requires pneumonectomy is produced by Aspergillum, which can produce severe infections with recurrent or massive hemoptysis in over 75% of patients (Conlan, et al., 1987). Pneumonectomy for trauma is uncommon, but is associated with high morbidity and mortality (66-75%). The most obvious indication of the procedure is the laceration of the lung and airways, which can produce massive hemorrhage and air leakage. Complications of congenital and other miscellaneous lung diseases, as well as completion pneumonectomy are rare indications for pneumonectomy, which can be associated with high mortality. Pneumonectomy for malignant disease has become the most common indication for lung resection today, which includes both primary lung tumors and metastatic lung disease. It is regarded as the only curative treatment for non small cell lung cancer (Shields, 1982) and also as an effective therapeutic option for pulmonary metastasis; however, these can be associated with high mortality (Spaggiari, et al., 1998).

2.3 Morbidity and mortality

Pneumonectomy is associated with a 38-59% rate of morbidity and a 30-day mortality ranging from 3-12%. Postoperative cardiac dysrhythmias (e.g., atrial fibrillation and supraventricular tachycardia) are relatively common complications occurring in approximately 20-40% of patients following pneumonectomy. Postpneumonectomy pulmonary edema (PPE) and acute respiratory distress syndrome (ARDS) occur in 4-7% of patients and are increasingly believed to be the same disease process. PPE/ARDS results in noncardiogenic pulmonary edema and is manifest by diffuse pulmonary infiltrates on chest radiograph combined with profound hypoxia and respiratory failure frequently requiring mechanical ventilation. One of the more devastating complications of pneumonectomy is an empyema involving the postpneumonectomy space. A postpneumonectomy empyema is usually associated with a bronchopleural fistula (BPF), which is a communication between the mainstem bronchial stump and the pleural cavity. The incidence of BPF and empyema ranges from 2-8%, but both complications are significantly more common in patients who undergo pneumonectomy for septic pulmonary disease (e.g., tuberculosis or fungal disease) (Deschamps, et al., 2001). Postpneumonectomy syndrome is a rare complication characterized by stridor, dyspnea and recurring pneumonia. Postpneumonectomy syndrome is more common following right pneumonectomy and results from severe shifting of the mediastinum and contralateral lung into the postpneumonectomy pleural space, which in turn leads to compression of the contralateral mainstem bronchus between the vertebral bodies and descending aorta (Kopec, et al., 1998).

2.4 Physiological changes

Pneumonectomy results in reduced lung function. Although residual volume (RV) declines after pneumonectomy, it decreases less than expected as a result of the hyperexpansion that occurs in the remaining lung. Forced expiratory volume in one second (FEV_1) and forced vital capacity (FVC) both typically decrease by 25-40%. Diffusion capacity usually decreases by less than 50% whereas PaO_2 and $PaCO_2$ typically remain unchanged from preoperative levels (Kopec, et al., 1998).

3. Experimental CLG following pneumonectomy

The removal of a lung entails profound mechanical, metabolic and vascular changes in response to the reduction in lung volume and the empty space in the hemithorax. These changes trigger a compensatory response in experimental models, known as CLG, which are directed toward reestablishing the normal rate of oxygen exchange capacity. This section describes a number of experimental animal models of CLG that are currently used to study this process, as well as a detailed evaluation of the CLG response in these models, including lung morphometry and imaging.

3.1 Animal models

In many animal models, pneumonectomy (or lobectomy) induces CLG of the remaining lung, resulting in rapid restoration of total lung volume, compliance, mass, DNA, protein, alveolar number, and normal lung cell populations. Pneumonectomy has proven to be a reliable model for characterizing the sources, mechanisms, and functional limits of the compensatory growth response after removal of lung tissue. Pulmonary resections in animals began in 1881 when it was documented that the remaining lung eventually expands to the same size as both lungs. Early animal studies established the basis for application of the procedure to humans, beginning in the 1900s. Cohn in 1939 first established mechanical forces as a major signal for the compensatory increase in lung mass following lobectomy. In the 1950s, Schilling detailed the well-preserved functional status in dogs that underwent removal in stages of up to nearly 70% of lung mass (Schilling, et al., 1958). The use of small animals (e.g. rabbit, rat, and mouse) from the 1960s to the current day has had a great impact in uncovering the hormonal, cellular, and molecular responses to pneumonectomy (Bennett, et al., 1985; Buhain & Brody, 1973; Rannels, et al., 1979; Romanova, et al., 1967). Significant progress in understanding the cellular and molecular pathways of tissue regeneration in vertebrates were achieved using both transgenic mice and molecular biology techniques (Leuwerke, et al., 2002; Sakamaki, et al., 2002; Sakuma, et al., 2002). Functional compensation to pneumonectomy has been described mainly in dogs to define the limits of such compensation (Ravikumar, et al., 2004; Takeda, et al., 1997).

3.2 Alveolar growth

Alveolar epithelial cells in pneumonectomized rats exhibit metabolic changes typical of accelerated cell growth. Studies in mice and rats indicate that type II epithelial cell hypertrophy, proliferation and differentiation into type I cells characterize CLG in a fashion similar to early postnatal lung growth and lung repair after injury (Kaza, et al., 2002).

The post-pneumonectomy CLG response is independent of the lobe or lobes removed in small animals; and all remaining lobes grow rapidly until normal total lung mass is restored. Increases in lung volume after pneumonectomy parallel accumulation of tissue growth. However, the increase of growth in the remaining lobes is not uniform (Fernandez, et al., 2007). Development of sophisticated morphometric methods has permitted accurate analysis of lung volume and alveolar number, and studies indicate that new alveoli are formed during post-pneumonectomy CLG (Kaza, et al., 2002; Sakamaki, et al., 2002). In dogs, however, it appears that the CLG response is initiated after a certain threshold is achieved (removal of >50% of total lung mass) (Hsia, et al., 1994). Bronchoalveolar stem cells (BASC) have also been implicated in CLG. Their proliferation and differentiation into alveolar epithelial cells type II and I, contribute between 0-25% to the regenerative lung growth process (Nolen-Walston, et al., 2008).

3.3 Vascular growth and angiogenesis

Vascular growth and angiogenesis during CLG has not been well characterized. Stimuli known to initiate angiogenesis include hypoxia, inflammation, and mechanical factors such as shear stress and stretch. Our laboratory has shown that angiogenesis is necessary for successful CLG by demonstrating that angiogenesis inhibitors such as fumagillin or thalidomide prevented increased lung weight and volume after pneumonectomy (Maxey, et al., 2003). We have also shown that pneumonectomy induces arterial growth including the increase in length and number of branches of pulmonary arteries and that these changes are proportional to the amount of tissue removed (Le Cras, et al., 2005). When a bilobectomy was performed in rats (24% of lung tissue removed), the arterial area of the remaining lung increased by 26% compared to sham animals. Furthermore, when lung resection was more extensive (trilobectomy, 52%) we found that the increase in arterial area increased by 47% (Le Cras, et al., 2005). Other researchers have shown the effects of exogenous angiogenic factors, such as vascular endothelial growth factor (VEGF) in the mouse model. Additional VEGF therapy accelerated the CLG response, which was completed in only 4 days compared to 10 days in the pneumonectomy control group (Sakurai, et al., 2007).

4. Initiation of CLG

Several general hypotheses have been advanced to account for events that initiate the cellular and molecular changes that lead to CLG. Mechanical signals, transient hypoxia associated with thoracotomy, and elevated blood flow have been considered; however, no single event has been proven to account for the growth response.

4.1 Mechanical forces

After resection of the lung, increased inflation of the remaining lung and increased blood flow will induce stretch in both alveolar and endothelial structures. The displacement of the lung to the empty hemithorax is also a feature of CLG. These mechanical forces have an important role in initiating and regulating CLG as it was demonstrated when lateral displacement of the lung was restricted by the use of an inflatable prosthesis. This prevention of the mediastinal shift significantly limited mechanical lung strain, and CLG was thus significantly impaired by 30-60% (Hsia, et al., 2001). Another factor, increased alveolar inflation, was also implicated when experiments using *in vitro* perfusion of lungs with or without constant positive pressure ventilation (CPAP) of 20 cmH_2O, demonstrated that lungs with increased inflation had cellular hyperplastic changes, such as elevated levels of cAMP and PKA activity, but perfusion alone did not account for these changes (Russo, et al., 1989). It is clear that CLG is very complex with multiple metabolic factors. Hyperinflation and stretch applied to the remaining lung after pneumonectomy are powerful signals to initiate CLG, and it is known that stretch of alveolar cells induces important changes associated with cell growth and septal formation, including signal transduction, protein turnover, growth factor production, proliferation, and apoptosis (Brody, 1975; Davies, et al., 1982; Fehrenbach, et al., 2008; Karl, et al., 1989). It appears that lung stress and strain generated after pneumonectomy, overlaid on a background of heightened developmental lung strain generated by the expanding thorax, intensifies the CLG responses. Importantly, minimizing post-pneumonectomy strain of the remaining lung with space-occupying, inert material blunts the CLG response.

4.2 Elevated blood flow

Post-pneumonectomy changes in pulmonary blood flow have been considered as possible signals for CLG. Increased perfusion, reflecting elevated cardiac output to the remaining lung, likely causes physical distention of the pulmonary vasculature, resulting in a mechanical signal for lung growth and a concurrent increase in the growth factor and/or nutrient availability to the lung. It has been described that, after banding of the left caudal pulmonary artery in ferrets that reduced blood flow to the lung by 25%, CLG still occurred after pneumonectomy. However, the caudal lobes in the banded animals were 17% smaller than those of non-banded animals and tended to have lower protein content (McBride, et al., 1992). In our laboratory, we have shown that after left pneumonectomy, increases in growth and proliferation were not uniform among the right lobes but were greater in the upper and cardiac lobes. These unequal changes coincided with a predominant vascular growth in the upper lobe, which received the highest fraction of relative blood flow (Fernandez, et al., 2007).

4.3 Hypoxia

Hypoxia has been shown to stimulate alveolar growth either directly or via interaction with other signals. The effects of hypoxia after pneumonectomy were initially described in the rat model, where pneumonectomized rats that recovered at hypoxic levels showed significant increases in lung weight and volume indices, increased alveolar surface area and total alveolar numbers compared to normoxic and hyperoxic rats (Sekhon, et al., 1993). Hypoxia-inducible factors (HIFs), which are activated in response to oxidative stress, hypoxia, injury, and physical forces, regulate transcription of genes involved in a wide array of functions including glycolysis, erythropoiesis, apoptosis, and angiogenesis. Most of these stressors are directly or indirectly associated with a change of intracellular oxygen tension, which leads to stabilization of the HIF-1α protein and increases the transcriptional activation of target genes. Elevated hypoxia-induced mitogenic factor (HIMF) and HIF-1α mRNA and protein expression has been documented during CLG, thus these pathways may play an important role in mediating CLG (Li, et al., 2005; Zhang, et al., 2006; Zhang, et al., 2007).

5. Molecular mediators of CLG

The molecular mediators of CLG remain poorly understood. CLG involves regulated pathways of cell cycle activity, cell differentiation, synthesis and organization of connective tissue components, tissue remodeling, and angiogenesis. Studies in animals have led to several hypotheses that various pathways play a role in the induction of CLG including post-operative release of hormones and growth factors, as well as changes in cellular behavior. This section describes several important aspects of post-pneumonectomy CLG regulatory mechanisms.

5.1 Hormones

The most substantial evidence for hormonal regulation of CLG stems from investigations that involved surgical ablation of the adrenal glands, or adrenalectomy, which alone does not stimulate lung growth. Adrenalectomy performed prior to pneumonectomy increases the rate and extent of CLG above that observed in rats after pneumonectomy alone. This stimulatory effect on lung growth was blocked by daily doses of hydrocortisone acetate, evidenced by parameters such as dry lung weigh and DNA content, which were similar to the pneumonectomy group (Bennett, et al., 1985). This blocking effect was found only if the therapy was used continuously for the entire period after surgery (Rannels, et al., 1987). A combination of dexamethasone, 8-bromo-3'-5'-cAMP and isobutylmethyl-xanthine (DCI) has been successfully used to accelerate CLG in mice, represented by an increase in lung dry weight index and an increased number of alveoli by morphometric analysis. The effect of a single airway dose was enough to maintain the effect for the entire 28-day period of study. This effect seems to be modulated by thyroid transcription factor 1 (TTF-1), since its transient inhibition attenuated CLG (Takahashi, et al., 2011). Adrenal glucocorticosteroids seem to have a role in the modulation of the accelerated CLG initiated by pneumonectomy. Several lines of evidence suggest a possible role of growth hormone in the regulation of CLG. Significantly higher serum levels of growth hormone were detected in pregnant rats 3 days after pneumonectomy when compared with sham and unoperated rats (Khadempour, et al., 1992). In diabetic rats, which normally have greater levels of growth hormone and adrenal corticosteroids, pneumonectomy was accompanied by an increased dry lung weight index as well as higher elastin and collagen content, when compared to control pneumonectomy and sham rats (Ofulue & Thurlbeck, 1995). Following pneumonectomy, rats implanted with a subcutaneous growth hormone-secreting tumor (MtTF4) underwent a CLG response similar to non-tumor-bearing controls; however, lung growth in MtTF4 rats was associated with a greater lung volume.

5.2 Growth factors

There is ample evidence that growth factors regulate CLG, and the production of many growth factors is known to be sensitive to mechanical strain. Each growth factor modulates different aspects of cellular growth, but any one growth factor cannot recapitulate the entire CLG response, and there is much functional overlap among growth factors. Our laboratory, among others, has demonstrated important roles for epidermal growth factor (EGF), hypoxia-induced mitogenic factor (HIMF), keratinocyte growth factor (KGF) and retinoic acid in CLG. Other growth factor signaling pathways have been found to be activated after PNX including insulin-like growth factor-1 (IGF-1), hepatocyte growth factor (HGF), erythropoietin receptor, and hypoxia-inducible factor-1α (HIF-1α). These growth factors will be discussed below.

5.2.1 Epidermal growth factor (EGF)

It is been shown that EGF via its receptor (EGFR) plays a role in prenatal and postnatal lung development. Its actions involve the synthesis of surfactant precursors and the differentiation of type 2 epithelial cells. Using a pig lobectomy model, our laboratory demonstrated an upregulation of EGFR expression two weeks after lobectomy, which coincided with an increased alveolar cell proliferation index of the remaining lung. At 3 months after surgery, there was an increase in the lung protein/DNA ratio in the lobectomy group compared to controls (Kaza, et al., 2001; Kaza, et al., 2002). We also have documented the effects of EGF in CLG using a rodent pneumonectomy model. When exogenous EGF was administered to rats after pneumonectomy, it caused significantly higher lung weight and volume indices when compared to pneumonectomy control animals. We also detected an upregulation of EGFR after exogenous EGF supplementation (Kaza, et al., 2000), suggesting that the upregulation of EGF signaling is a feature of this process and is capable of modulating post-pneumonectomy GLG.

5.2.2 Erythropoietin (EPO)

Erythropoietin (EPO) actions have been classically associated with the induction of erythropoiesis; however, organ specific EPO receptor (EPOR) signaling is also involved in development, angiogenesis and organ growth. Researchers have shown that EPOR is upregulated both during postnatal lung maturation and during CLG in adult dogs (Foster, et al., 2004). Furthermore, they demonstrated an upregulation of one of its upstream activators, HIF-1α, during the same processes. Using an *in vitro* system, the same group showed that upregulation of HIF-1α in cultured HEK-293 cells also caused the upregulation of endogenous EPOR expression (Zhang, et al., 2006). This also provided evidence of a possible role of EPOR in CLG after pneumonectomy.

5.2.3 Hepatocyte growth factor (HGF)

HGF is known to selectively stimulate epithelial and endothelial cells, and the major sources for HGF in the lung are macrophages, fibroblasts, and endothelial cells. The increase of serum HGF during the first week after major lung resections in humans has been documented (Dikmen, et al., 2006; Sugahara, et al., 1998). A more comprehensive study of the role of HGF in CLG was performed using a mouse pneumonectomy model (Sakamaki, et al., 2002). In this study, the authors demonstrated an increased level of both lung mRNA and protein expression of HGF after pneumonectomy, and serum HGF levels were also higher when compared to sham operated animals. These findings were accompanied by an increased proliferation index of alveolar and airway epithelial cells, which peaked at day 5 after surgery. They also detected an upregulation of the HGF receptor (c-Met) at day 3 post-pneumonectomy. In addition, injections of HGF twice daily enhanced the proliferative response of these cells as well as increased lung weight index at day 3 when compared to controls. Use of a neutralizing antibody against HGF resulted in the inhibition, although incomplete, of the increase in lung weight and DNA synthesis observed. Another interesting study evaluated the effects of CLG in a rat model of elastase-induced emphysema, with transfection of the human HGF cDNA into the lung (Shigemura, et al., 2005) or implantation of adipose tissue-derived stromal cells (ASCs), which produce a large amount of angiogenic factors including HGF (Shigemura, et al., 2006). Therapy with gene transfection was performed using the hemagglutinating virus of Japan (HVJ) envelope-plasmid complex. In the HGF- and ASC-treated animals, increased levels of both exogenous and endogenous HGF were detected; and furthermore, HGF enhanced the CLG response by increasing lung cell proliferation and improving functional parameters. Taken together, these studies provide strong evidence for a role of HGF in the proliferative responses during CLG.

5.2.4 Hypoxia-induced mitogenic factor (HIMF)

In a collaborative study, we demonstrated the role of HIMF in the context of CLG (Li, et al., 2005). The mRNA and protein expression of HIMF, which is known by its mitogenic and angiogenic properties, was upregulated after pneumonectomy (days 3-14) when compared to sham operated mice. The elevated HIMF expression also coincided with an increase in cell proliferation index in lungs of these animals. HIMF expression after pneumonectomy was mainly detected in airway epithelial, endothelial and type 2 epithelial cells. Intratracheal instillation of exogenous HIMF increased the proliferative activity in these cells, documenting its mitogenic properties and establishing its role in CLG.

5.2.5 Hypoxia-inducible factor-1α (HIF-1α)

Researchers have shown that HIF-1α expression is upregulated both during postnatal lung maturation and during adult CLG in dogs and that this coincides with the upregulation of one of its downstream targets, EPOR. *In vitro* experiments also provided evidence that upregulation of HIF-1α in cultured HEK-293 cells triggers the upregulation of endogenous EPOR expression (Zhang, et al., 2006). Another study found that lung expansion is a major contributor to the activation and stabilization of HIF-1α. Acute deflation of prosthesis in the chest cavity of pneumonectomized dogs triggered the increase of both HIF-1 and several HIF-1 targets including EPOR and VEGF compared to non-deflated animals. They concluded that these increases did not depend on hypoxia but instead were due to stretch-related signals after lung resection (Zhang, et al., 2007).

5.2.6 Insulin-like growth factor-I (IGF-I)

IGF-1, its receptor and binding proteins are naturally expressed in the lung during development, and IGF-1 is known to contribute to the regulation of postnatal lung cell proliferation. Researchers have shown that 2 and 6 days after pneumonectomy in rats, the bronchoalveolar lavage fluid from these animals demonstrated significantly increased mitogenic activity when applied *in vitro* to fibroblasts compared with controls. Importantly, such activity was partially inhibited by the use of neutralizing antibody against IGF-1, and the levels of IGF-1 were elevated by 100% at day 2 after pneumonectomy (McAnulty, et al., 1992). In a separate study, IGF-1 mRNA expression was again significantly increased after 21 days post-pneumonectomy in a model of neonatal CLG in lambs (Nobuhara, et al., 1998).

5.2.7 Keratinocyte growth factor-I (KGF)

KGF has been shown to play an important role in alveolar epithelial cell proliferation and lung development. In our laboratory, exogenous KGF administered to rats after pneumonectomy further enhanced several parameters of CLG compared to control animals. Changes in lung weight index, lung volume index as well as morphometric parameters were accompanied by a significant increase in pulmonary cell proliferation index, providing the first evidence for a role of KGF in CLG (Kaza, et al., 2002). A more recent study corroborated our findings where epithelial cell proliferation was further enhanced after *in vivo* transfection of a KGF cDNA vector in a model of CLG in rats, confirming KGF as an important lung mitogenic factor (Matsumoto, et al., 2009).

5.2.8 Retinoic acid

Retinoic acid, a metabolite of vitamin A, has been implicated in normal lung development and cell proliferation. Our laboratory described the effects of exogenous retinoic acid during CLG in a rat model (Kaza, et al., 2001). At 10 and 21 days after pneumonectomy, lung weight, lung volume and cellular proliferation indices were all significantly augmented in rats that received exogenous retinoic acid versus vehicle controls. Interestingly, we also found that pulmonary expression of EGFR was upregulated in lungs after retinoic acid treatment, uncovering a possible relationship between these two important growth factors in CLG. Another similarly designed study corroborated our results several years later (Karapolat, et al., 2008); however, these effects did not translate into functional recovery according to studies developed using the dog model (Dane, et al., 2004).

5.2.9 Vascular endothelial growth factor (VEGF)

Angiogenesis, the formation of new blood vessels, is a critical step in normal organ development and in abnormal processes such as tumor growth and metastasis. In the lung, alveolar growth and angiogenesis should occur concurrently in order to result in normal organ development or regeneration. One of the most important angiogenic growth factors, VEGF has been studied in CLG, revealing its importance in this regenerative process. Researchers described the effects of exogenous VEGF in the mouse model, showing that exogenous VEGF therapy accelerated the CLG response, which was completed in only 4 days compared to 10 days in control animals. However, these effects could not be blocked by the use of either VEGF receptor inhibitors or neutralizing antibodies (Sakurai, et al., 2007). Another study associated lung expansion and other signaling pathways to VEGF. The acute deflation of prosthesis in the chest cavity of pneumonectomized dogs triggered the increase of HIF-1α and its targets EPOR and VEGF compared to non-deflated animals, showing the interaction between these signals in the regulation of CLG (Zhang, et al., 2007). A recent paper studied the modulation of different VEGF isoforms along with its receptor during CLG, where VEGF 188 mRNA expression was decreased compared to sham animals and VEGF 164 and VEGF 120 mRNAs increased during days 1 and 3 respectively, describing what they believe is the recapitulation of the pattern of expression for these isoforms in the fetal lung (Jancelewicz, et al., 2010). A brief summary of evidence for the role of growth factors in CLG is shown in Table 1.

Growth Factor	Evidence	Species
EGF	• Pneumonectomy increased EGFR lung expression. • Exogenous EGF enhances CLG.	Rat, pig Rat
EPOR	• Pneumonectomy increased EPOR lung expression.	Dog
HGF	• Pneumonectomy increased serum HGF, along with expression of HGF and its receptor (c-Met) in lung. • Exogenous HGF enhances CLG. • Neutralizing antibody against HGF attenuate CLG.	Mouse Mouse, rat Mouse
HIMF	• Pneumonectomy increased lung HIMF mRNA and protein expression. • Exogenous HIMF enhances proliferation.	Mouse
HIF-1α	• Pneumonectomy increased lung HIF-1α mRNA and protein expression. • Lung expansion modulates HIF-1α expression.	Dog
IGF-1	• Pneumonectomy increased lung IGF-1 mRNA and protein expression. • Neutralizing antibody against IGF-1 attenuate mitogenic *in vitro* effects.	Lamb, rat Rat
KGF	• Pneumonectomy increased lung KGF mRNA. • Exogenous KGF enhances CLG.	Rat
Retinoic Acid	• Exogenous retinoic acid enhances CLG. • Exogenous retinoic acid induces EGFR.	Rat
VEGF	• Pneumonectomy increased lung VEGF 164 and 120 mRNA expressions. • Exogenous VEGF accelerates CLG.	Mouse

Table 1. Summary of potential roles of growth factors in CLG.

5.3 Transcription factors

Pneumonectomy induces shear stress in the lung, and several key transcription factors provide links between shear-mediated signaling and CLG. Mitogen-activated protein kinases (MAPKs), composed of extracellular signal-regulated kinases (ERKs), c-jun NH2-terminal kinases (JNKs), and p38 MAPKs, play a critical role in cell differentiation, growth and apoptosis and the regulation of various transcription factors and gene expression. One of the first reports about stretch-induced early gene expression demonstrated that in as early as 30 minutes post-pneumonectomy in rats, c-fos and JunB are significantly increased. These results were also reproduced when *in vitro* ventilation-perfusion was used (Gilbert & Rannels, 1998). Using array technology, researchers have also shown significant increases in six different transcription factors as early as 6 hours after pneumonectomy in mice including Erg-1 and Nur77, all of which have important roles in vascular biology, development and stress response (Landesberg, et al., 2001). In addition, a more recent paper found an important role for thyroid transcription factor 1 (TTF-1) in CLG (Takahashi, et al., 2010). These investigators detected a significant increase of TTF-1 expression 12 hours after pneumonectomy with TTF-1 expression primarily observed in cells of the alveolar ducts. When TTF-1 was repressed using small inhibitory RNAs (siRNAs), the CLG response was also temporally delayed.

5.4 Telomerase

Telomerase is an important enzyme for DNA repair and contributes to cell maintenance. Telomerase prevents the excess shortening of telomeres, and it has been demonstrated that telomerase is active in proliferating cells in a number of organs, including the lung. In humans, mutations of the telomerase gene results in a pathological condition known as idiopathic pulmonary fibrosis (IPF). Its role in preserving lung epithelial integrity was demonstrated in an experimental model in mice, where telomerase deficiency resulted in a reduction in the number and integrity of type 2 alveolar epithelial cells (AEC2) (Lee, et al., 2009). It is important to know that this defect may not be apparent in early generations, but after progressive inbreeding, it was possible to establish the deficiency in AEC2s as well as in bronchoalveolar stem cell (BASC) populations in the lung, due to shortening of the telomeres. In a recent study, the importance of telomerase was demonstrated for CLG after pneumonectomy using telomerase deficient mice from second (F2), third (F3) and fourth (F4) generation animals (Jackson, et al., 2011). In wild-type mice, the activity of telomerase was found to increase in isolated AEC2s up to 3.5-fold during post-pneumonectomy days 3 and 7. In addition, the total number of AEC2s and BASCs also increased at day 3 after pneumonectomy. However, pneumonectomy resulted in diminished CLG in F3 telomerase null animals, expressed as failure to induce an increase in lung mass by day 7 after pneumonectomy. In addition, the number of AEC2s and BASCs did not increase during the initial period after pneumonectomy when compared to wild-type mice. The normal CLG, both in lung mass and AEC2 numbers, in wild-type mice was also accompanied by an elevation in the proliferation marker Ki-67, early growth response gene (Egr-1) and repair transcription factors such as ERK 1/2, which were not observed in telomerase null mice. The authors concluded that telomerase deletion produces an attenuated CLG response after pneumonectomy by arresting cell growth and inducing DNA damage.

6. Conclusion

The extent of CLG in humans following pneumonectomy or lobectomy is incompletely investigated, but a number of long-term physiological studies suggest, however, that some degree of CLG may occur, especially in children (Nakajima, et al., 1998; Nonoyama, et al., 1986). The ability to manipulate the gain/loss of function for a particular gene in experimental animals has begun to provide a more detailed understanding of the molecular mediators and the pathologic consequences of CLG. Also, recent developments in cell therapy of diseased lungs with the use of adipose stem cells are indeed promising (Shigemura, et al., 2006). An important long-term goal of research into mechanisms of CLG is to generate knowledge that will allow the induction of alveolar regeneration or that rescues failed alveologenesis in humans. Such understanding will facilitate the development of therapies for the management of end-stage lung disease, lung volume reduction surgery, and transplantation. The potential clinical applications of this research are great. Specific examples of patients who would clearly benefit from lung regenerative therapies include chronic obstructive pulmonary disease (COPD), emphysema, pulmonary hypertension, bronchopulmonary dysplasia (BPD), as well as premature infants whose lungs are too underdeveloped to support life.

7. References

Bennett, R. A., Colony, P. C., Addison, J. L. & Rannels, D. E. (1985). Effects of prior adrenalectomy on postpneumonectomy lung growth in the rat. *Am J Physiol*, Vol.248, No.1 Pt 1, (Jan), pp. E70-74, ISSN 0002-9513

Bjork, V. O. & Carlens, E. (1950). The prevention of spread during pulmonary resection by the use of a double-lumen catheter. *J Thorac Surg*, Vol.20, No.1, (Jul), pp. 151-157, ISSN 0096-5588

Blyth, D. F. (2000). Pneumonectomy for inflammatory lung disease. *Eur J Cardiothorac Surg*, Vol.18, No.4, (Oct), pp. 429-434, ISSN 1010-7940

Brody, J. S. (1975). Time course of and stimuli to compensatory growth of the lung after pneumonectomy. *J Clin Invest*, Vol.56, No.4, (Oct), pp. 897-904, ISSN 0021-9738

Buhain, W. J. & Brody, J. S. (1973). Compensatory growth of the lung following pneumonectomy. *J Appl Physiol*, Vol.35, No.6, (Dec), pp. 898-902, ISSN 0021-8987

Conlan, A. A., Abramor, E. & Moyes, D. G. (1987). Pulmonary aspergilloma--indications for surgical intervention. An analysis of 22 cases. *S Afr Med J*, Vol.71, No.5, (Mar 7), pp. 285-288, ISSN 0256-9574

Conlan, A. A. & Kopec, S. E. (1999). Indications for pneumonectomy. Pneumonectomy for benign disease. *Chest Surg Clin N Am*, Vol.9, No.2, (May), pp. 311-326, ISSN 1052-3359

Dane, D. M., Yan, X., Tamhane, R. M., Johnson, R. L., Jr., Estrera, A. S., Hogg, D. C., Hogg, R. T. & Hsia, C. C. (2004). Retinoic acid-induced alveolar cellular growth does not improve function after right pneumonectomy. *J Appl Physiol*, Vol.96, No.3, (Mar), pp. 1090-1096, ISSN 8750-7587

Davies, A. L. & Panasuk, D. B. (1992). Video-assisted thoracic surgery: our first 20 cases. *Del Med J*, Vol.64, No.4, (Apr), pp. 267-272, ISSN 0011-7781

Davies, P., McBride, J., Murray, G. F., Wilcox, B. R., Shallal, J. A. & Reid, L. (1982). Structural changes in the canine lung and pulmonary arteries after pneumonectomy. *J Appl Physiol*, Vol.53, No.4, (Oct), pp. 859-864, ISSN 0161-7567

Deschamps, C., Bernard, A., Nichols, F. C., 3rd, Allen, M. S., Miller, D. L., Trastek, V. F., Jenkins, G. D. & Pairolero, P. C. (2001). Empyema and bronchopleural fistula after pneumonectomy: factors affecting incidence. *Ann Thorac Surg*, Vol.72, No.1, (Jul), pp. 243-247; ISSN 0003-4975

Dikmen, E., Kara, M., Kisa, U., Atinkaya, C., Han, S. & Sakinci, U. (2006). Human hepatocyte growth factor levels in patients undergoing thoracic operations. *Eur Respir J*, Vol.27, No.1, (Jan), pp. 73-76, ISSN 0903-1936

Fehrenbach, H., Voswinckel, R., Michl, V., Mehling, T., Fehrenbach, A., Seeger, W. & Nyengaard, J. R. (2008). Neoalveolarisation contributes to compensatory lung growth following pneumonectomy in mice. *Eur Respir J*, Vol.31, No.3, (Mar), pp. 515-522, ISSN 1399-3003

Fernandez, L. G., Le Cras, T. D., Ruiz, M., Glover, D. K., Kron, I. L. & Laubach, V. E. (2007). Differential vascular growth in postpneumonectomy compensatory lung growth. *J Thorac Cardiovasc Surg*, Vol.133, No.2, (Feb), pp. 309-316, ISSN 1097-685X

Foster, D. J., Moe, O. W. & Hsia, C. C. (2004). Upregulation of erythropoietin receptor during postnatal and postpneumonectomy lung growth. *Am J Physiol Lung Cell Mol Physiol*, Vol.287, No.6, (Dec), pp. L1107-1115, ISSN 1040-0605

Gilbert, K. A. & Rannels, D. E. (1998). Increased lung inflation induces gene expression after pneumonectomy. *Am J Physiol*, Vol.275, No.1 Pt 1, (Jul), pp. L21-29, ISSN 0002-9513

Graham, E. A. & Berck, M. (1933). Principle versus details in the treatment of acute empyema. *Ann Surg*, Vol.98, No.4, (Oct), pp. 520-527, ISSN 0003-4932

Haight, C. (1934). Total removal of the lung for bronchiectasis. *Surgery, Gynecology and Obstetrics*, Vol.58, pp. ISSN

Hsia, C. C., Herazo, L. F., Fryder-Doffey, F. & Weibel, E. R. (1994). Compensatory lung growth occurs in adult dogs after right pneumonectomy. *J Clin Invest*, Vol.94, No.1, (Jul), pp. 405-412, ISSN 0021-9738

Hsia, C. C., Wu, E. Y., Wagner, E. & Weibel, E. R. (2001). Preventing mediastinal shift after pneumonectomy impairs regenerative alveolar tissue growth. *Am J Physiol Lung Cell Mol Physiol*, Vol.281, No.5, (Nov), pp. L1279-1287, ISSN 1040-0605

Jackson, S. R., Lee, J., Reddy, R., Williams, G. N., Kikuchi, A., Freiberg, Y., Warburton, D. & Driscoll, B. (2011). Partial pneumonectomy of telomerase null mice carrying shortened telomeres initiates cell growth arrest resulting in a limited compensatory growth response. *Am J Physiol Lung Cell Mol Physiol*, Vol.300, No.6, (Jun), pp. L898-909, ISSN 1522-1504

Jancelewicz, T., Grethel, E. J., Chapin, C. J., Clifton, M. S. & Nobuhara, K. K. (2010). Vascular endothelial growth factor isoform and receptor expression during compensatory lung growth. *J Surg Res*, Vol.160, No.1, (May 1), pp. 107-113, ISSN 1095-8673

Karapolat, S., Sanli, A., Onen, A., Acikel, U. & Sivrikoz, O. (2008). Effects of retinoic acid on compensatory lung growth. *J Cardiothorac Surg*, Vol.3, pp. 37, ISSN 1749-8090

Karl, H. W., Russo, L. A. & Rannels, D. E. (1989). Inflation-associated increases in lung polyamine uptake: role of altered pulmonary vascular flow. *Am J Physiol*, Vol.257, No.5 Pt 1, (Nov), pp. E729-735, ISSN 0002-9513

Kaza, A. K., Laubach, V. E., Kern, J. A., Long, S. M., Fiser, S. M., Tepper, J. A., Nguyen, R. P., Shockey, K. S., Tribble, C. G. & Kron, I. L. (2000). Epidermal growth factor augments postpneumonectomy lung growth. *J Thorac Cardiovasc Surg*, Vol.120, No.5, (Nov), pp. 916-921, ISSN 0022-5223

Kaza, A. K., Kron, I. L., Kern, J. A., Long, S. M., Fiser, S. M., Nguyen, R. P., Tribble, C. G. & Laubach, V. E. (2001). Retinoic acid enhances lung growth after pneumonectomy. *Ann Thorac Surg*, Vol.71, No.5, (May), pp. 1645-1650, ISSN 0003-4975

Kaza, A. K., Kron, I. L., Long, S. M., Fiser, S. M., Stevens, P. M., Kern, J. A., Tribble, C. G. & Laubach, V. E. (2001). Epidermal growth factor receptor up-regulation is associated with lung growth after lobectomy. *Ann Thorac Surg*, Vol.72, No.2, (Aug), pp. 380-385, ISSN 0003-4975

Kaza, A. K., Cope, J. T., Fiser, S. M., Long, S. M., Kern, J. A., Tribble, C. G., Kron, I. L. & Laubach, V. E. (2002). Contrasting natures of lung growth after transplantation and lobectomy. *J Thorac Cardiovasc Surg*, Vol.123, No.2, (Feb), pp. 288-294, ISSN 0022-5223

Kaza, A. K., Kron, I. L., Leuwerke, S. M., Tribble, C. G. & Laubach, V. E. (2002). Keratinocyte growth factor enhances post-pneumonectomy lung growth by alveolar proliferation. *Circulation*, Vol.106, No.12 Suppl 1, (Sep 24), pp. I120-124, ISSN 1524-4539

Khadempour, M. H., Ofulue, A. F., Sekhon, H. S., Cherukupalli, K. M. & Thurlbeck, W. M. (1992). Changes of growth hormone, somatomedin C, and bombesin following pneumonectomy. *Exp Lung Res*, Vol.18, No.3, (May-Jun), pp. 421-432, ISSN 0190-2148

Kopec, S. E., Irwin, R. S., Umali-Torres, C. B., Balikian, J. P. & Conlan, A. A. (1998). The postpneumonectomy state. *Chest*, Vol.114, No.4, (Oct), pp. 1158-1184, ISSN 0012-3692

Landesberg, L. J., Ramalingam, R., Lee, K., Rosengart, T. K. & Crystal, R. G. (2001). Upregulation of transcription factors in lung in the early phase of postpneumonectomy lung growth. *Am J Physiol Lung Cell Mol Physiol*, Vol.281, No.5, (Nov), pp. L1138-1149, ISSN 1040-0605

Le Cras, T. D., Fernandez, L. G., Pastura, P. A. & Laubach, V. E. (2005). Vascular growth and remodeling in compensatory lung growth following right lobectomy. *J Appl Physiol*, Vol.98, No.3, (Mar), pp. 1140-1148, ISSN 8750-7587

Lee, J., Reddy, R., Barsky, L., Scholes, J., Chen, H., Shi, W. & Driscoll, B. (2009). Lung alveolar integrity is compromised by telomere shortening in telomerase-null mice. *Am J Physiol Lung Cell Mol Physiol*, Vol.296, No.1, (Jan), pp. L57-70, ISSN 1040-0605

Leuwerke, S. M., Kaza, A. K., Tribble, C. G., Kron, I. L. & Laubach, V. E. (2002). Inhibition of compensatory lung growth in endothelial nitric oxide synthase-deficient mice. *Am J Physiol Lung Cell Mol Physiol*, Vol.282, No.6, (Jun), pp. L1272-1278, ISSN 1040-0605

Li, D., Fernandez, L. G., Dodd-o, J., Langer, J., Wang, D. & Laubach, V. E. (2005). Upregulation of hypoxia-induced mitogenic factor in compensatory lung growth after pneumonectomy. *Am J Respir Cell Mol Biol*, Vol.32, No.3, (Mar), pp. 185-191, ISSN 1044-1549

Lilienthal, H. (1910). IV. The First Case of Thoracotomy in a Human Being under Anaesthesia by Intratracheal Insufflation. *Ann Surg*, Vol.52, No.1, (Jul), pp. 30-33, ISSN 0003-4932

Lilienthal, H. (1922). Resection of the Lung for Suppurative Infections with a Report Based on 31 Operative Cases in Which Resection Was Done or Intended. *Ann Surg*, Vol.75, No.3, (Mar), pp. 257-320, ISSN 0003-4932

Matsumoto, K., Nagayasu, T., Hishikawa, Y., Tagawa, T., Yamayoshi, T., Abo, T., Tobinaga, S., Furukawa, K. & Koji, T. (2009). Keratinocyte growth factor accelerates compensatory growth in the remaining lung after trilobectomy in rats. *J Thorac Cardiovasc Surg*, Vol.137, No.6, (Jun), pp. 1499-1507, ISSN 1097-685X

Maxey, T. S., Reece, T. B., Dimling, G. M., Tribble, C. G., Kron, I. L. & Laubach, V. E. (2003). Inhibition of angiogenesis prevents post-pneumonectomy compensatory lung growth. *Am J Respir Crit Care Med*, Vol.167, No.7, (April), pp. A575, ISSN 1073-449X

McAnulty, R. J., Guerreiro, D., Cambrey, A. D. & Laurent, G. J. (1992). Growth factor activity in the lung during compensatory growth after pneumonectomy: evidence of a role for IGF-1. *Eur Respir J*, Vol.5, No.6, (Jun), pp. 739-747, ISSN 0903-1936

McBride, J. T., Kirchner, K. K., Russ, G. & Finkelstein, J. (1992). Role of pulmonary blood flow in postpneumonectomy lung growth. *J Appl Physiol*, Vol.73, No.6, (Dec), pp. 2448-2451, ISSN 8750-7587

Meltzer, S. J. & Auer, J. (1909). Continuous Respiration without Respiratory Movements. *J Exp Med*, Vol.11, No.4, (Jul 17), pp. 622-625, ISSN 0022-1007

Meyer, W. (1909). Pneumonectomy with the aid of differential air pressure: an experimental study. *J Amer Acad Med*, Vol.53, pp. ISSN

Naef, A. P. (1987). [Development of thoracic surgery from 1880 to the present]. *Rev Med Suisse Romande*, Vol.107, No.11, (Nov), pp. 949-957, ISSN 0035-3655

Nakajima, C., Kijimoto, C., Yokoyama, Y., Miyakawa, T., Tsuchiya, Y., Kuroda, T., Nakano, M. & Saeki, M. (1998). Longitudinal follow-up of pulmonary function after lobectomy in childhood - factors affecting lung growth. *Pediatr Surg Int*, Vol.13, No.5-6, (Jul), pp. 341-345, ISSN 0179-0358

Nobuhara, K. K., DiFiore, J. W., Ibla, J. C., Siddiqui, A. M., Ferretti, M. L., Fauza, D. O., Schnitzer, J. J. & Wilson, J. M. (1998). Insulin-like growth factor-I gene expression in three models of accelerated lung growth. *J Pediatr Surg*, Vol.33, No.7, (Jul), pp. 1057-1060; discussion 1061, ISSN 0022-3468

Nolen-Walston, R. D., Kim, C. F., Mazan, M. R., Ingenito, E. P., Gruntman, A. M., Tsai, L., Boston, R., Woolfenden, A. E., Jacks, T. & Hoffman, A. M. (2008). Cellular kinetics and modeling of bronchioalveolar stem cell response during lung regeneration. *Am J Physiol Lung Cell Mol Physiol*, Vol.294, No.6, (Jun), pp. L1158-1165, ISSN 1040-0605

Nonoyama, A., Tanaka, K., Osako, T., Saito, Y., Umemoto, M., Masuda, A. & Kagawa, T. (1986). Pulmonary function after lobectomy in children under ten years of age. *Jpn J Surg*, Vol.16, No.6, (Nov), pp. 425-434, ISSN 0047-1909

O'Shaughnessy, L. & Crawford, J. H. (1938). The Surgical Treatment of Pulmonary Tuberculosis. *Postgrad Med J*, Vol.14, No.148, (Feb), pp. 38-48, ISSN 0032-5473

Ofulue, A. F. & Thurlbeck, W. M. (1995). Effects of streptozotocin-induced diabetes on postpneumonectomy lung growth and connective tissue levels. *Pediatr Pulmonol*, Vol.19, No.6, (Jun), pp. 365-370, ISSN 8755-6863

Quinby, W. & Morse, J. (1911). Experimental pneumonectomy, the implication of data obtained to surgery of the thorax. *Boston Medical and Surgical Journal*, Vol.165, pp. 121, ISSN

Rannels, D. E., White, D. M. & Watkins, C. A. (1979). Rapidity of compensatory lung growth following pneumonectomy in adult rats. *J Appl Physiol*, Vol.46, No.2, (Feb), pp. 326-333, ISSN 0161-7567

Rannels, D. E., Karl, H. W. & Bennett, R. A. (1987). Control of compensatory lung growth by adrenal hormones. *Am J Physiol*, Vol.253, No.4 Pt 1, (Oct), pp. E343-348, ISSN 0002-9513

Ravikumar, P., Yilmaz, C., Dane, D. M., Johnson, R. L., Jr., Estrera, A. S. & Hsia, C. C. (2004). Regional lung growth following pneumonectomy assessed by computed tomography. *J Appl Physiol*, Vol.97, No.4, (Oct), pp. 1567-1574; discussion 1549, ISSN 8750-7587

Romanova, L. K., Leikina, E. M. & Antipova, K. K. (1967). [Nucleic acid synthesis and mitotic activity during the development of compensatory pulmonary hypertrophy in rats]. *Biull Eksp Biol Med*, Vol.63, No.3, (Mar), pp. 96-100, ISSN 0365-9615

Russo, L. A., Rannels, S. R., Laslow, K. S. & Rannels, D. E. (1989). Stretch-related changes in lung cAMP after partial pneumonectomy. *Am J Physiol*, Vol.257, No.2 Pt 1, (Aug), pp. E261-268, ISSN 0002-9513

Sakamaki, Y., Matsumoto, K., Mizuno, S., Miyoshi, S., Matsuda, H. & Nakamura, T. (2002). Hepatocyte growth factor stimulates proliferation of respiratory epithelial cells during postpneumonectomy compensatory lung growth in mice. *Am J Respir Cell Mol Biol*, Vol.26, No.5, (May), pp. 525-533, ISSN 1044-1549

Sakuma, T., Sagawa, M., Hida, M., Nambu, Y., Osanai, K., Toga, H., Takahashi, K., Ohya, N. & Matthay, M. A. (2002). Time-dependent effect of pneumonectomy on alveolar epithelial fluid clearance in rat lungs. *J Thorac Cardiovasc Surg*, Vol.124, No.4, (Oct), pp. 668-674, ISSN 0022-5223

Sakurai, M. K., Lee, S., Arsenault, D. A., Nose, V., Wilson, J. M., Heymach, J. V. & Puder, M. (2007). Vascular endothelial growth factor accelerates compensatory lung growth after unilateral pneumonectomy. *Am J Physiol Lung Cell Mol Physiol*, Vol.292, No.3, (Mar), pp. L742-747, ISSN 1040-0605

Schilling, J. A., Lategola, M. T. & Massion, W. H. (1958). Physiologic effects of lung resection in dogs; mechanics of breathing, gas exchange, pulmonary arterial pressure, compliance, and lung weights. *Bull Soc Int Chir*, Vol.17, No.5-6, (Dec), pp. 310-319, ISSN 0037-945X

Sekhon, H. S., Smith, C. & Thurlbeck, W. M. (1993). Effect of hypoxia and hyperoxia on postpneumonectomy compensatory lung growth. *Exp Lung Res*, Vol.19, No.5, (Sep-Oct), pp. 519-532, ISSN 0190-2148

Shields, T. W. (1982). Surgical therapy for carcinoma of the lung. *Clin Chest Med*, Vol.3, No.2, (May), pp. 369-387, ISSN 0272-5231

Shigemura, N., Sawa, Y., Mizuno, S., Ono, M., Minami, M., Okumura, M., Nakamura, T., Kaneda, Y. & Matsuda, H. (2005). Induction of compensatory lung growth in pulmonary emphysema improves surgical outcomes in rats. *Am J Respir Crit Care Med*, Vol.171, No.11, (Jun 1), pp. 1237-1245, ISSN 1073-449X

Shigemura, N., Okumura, M., Mizuno, S., Imanishi, Y., Matsuyama, A., Shiono, H., Nakamura, T. & Sawa, Y. (2006). Lung tissue engineering technique with adipose stromal cells improves surgical outcome for pulmonary emphysema. *Am J Respir Crit Care Med*, Vol.174, No.11, (Dec 1), pp. 1199-1205, ISSN 1073-449X

Spaggiari, L., Grunenwald, D. H., Girard, P., Solli, P. & Le Chevalier, T. (1998). Pneumonectomy for lung metastases: indications, risks, and outcome. *Ann Thorac Surg*, Vol.66, No.6, (Dec), pp. 1930-1933, ISSN 0003-4975

Sugahara, K., Matsumoto, M., Baba, T., Nakamura, T. & Kawamoto, T. (1998). Elevation of serum human hepatocyte growth factor (HGF) level in patients with pneumonectomy during a perioperative period. *Intensive Care Med*, Vol.24, No.5, (May), pp. 434-437, ISSN 0342-4642

Takahashi, Y., Izumi, Y., Kohno, M., Kimura, T., Kawamura, M., Okada, Y., Nomori, H. & Ikeda, E. (2010). Thyroid transcription factor-1 influences the early phase of compensatory lung growth in adult mice. *Am J Respir Crit Care Med*, Vol.181, No.12, (Jun 15), pp. 1397-1406, ISSN 1535-4970

Takahashi, Y., Izumi, Y., Kohno, M., Kawamura, M., Ikeda, E. & Nomori, H. (2011). Airway administration of dexamethasone, 3'-5'-cyclic adenosine monophosphate, and isobutylmethylxanthine facilitates compensatory lung growth in adult mice. *Am J Physiol Lung Cell Mol Physiol*, Vol.300, No.3, (Mar), pp. L453-461, ISSN 1522-1504

Takeda, S., Wu, E. Y., Epstein, R. H., Estrera, A. S. & Hsia, C. C. (1997). In vivo assessment of changes in air and tissue volumes after pneumonectomy. *J Appl Physiol*, Vol.82, No.4, (Apr), pp. 1340-1348, ISSN 8750-7587

Zhang, Q., Moe, O. W., Garcia, J. A. & Hsia, C. C. (2006). Regulated expression of hypoxia-inducible factors during postnatal and postpneumonectomy lung growth. *Am J Physiol Lung Cell Mol Physiol*, Vol.290, No.5, (May), pp. L880-889, ISSN 1040-0605

Zhang, Q., Bellotto, D. J., Ravikumar, P., Moe, O. W., Hogg, R. T., Hogg, D. C., Estrera, A. S., Johnson, R. L., Jr. & Hsia, C. C. (2007). Postpneumonectomy lung expansion elicits hypoxia-inducible factor-1alpha signaling. *Am J Physiol Lung Cell Mol Physiol*, Vol.293, No.2, (Aug), pp. L497-504, ISSN 1040-0605

25

Pathophysiology of Extravascular Water in the Pleural Cavity and in the Lung Interstitium After Lung Thoracic Surgery

Giuseppe Miserocchi and Egidio Beretta
University of Milano-Bicocca, Department of Experimental Medicine, Italy

1. Introduction

Thoracic surgery implies a considerable imbalance of fluid dynamics in the pleural space and in the lung interstitium, and this is of relevance when considering that the volume of water in these compartments is physiologically very low thanks to very powerful mechanisms of control able to offset potential causes leading to an increase in this volume. There are reasons to believe that severe complications of lung fluid balance may occur after lung resection surgery and that the critical period is 24-48 hours after intervention. This paper wishes to present an updated review of pathophysiology of fluid balance in the respiratory system to be discussed within the specific frame of lung resection surgery. Some concept were only marginally considered in a paper previously published that was mostly dedicated to alterations in respiratory mechanics following lung resection surgery (Miserocchi et al, 2010).

2. Control of pleural liquid volume

Pleural fluid turnover occurs at parietal pleural level in physiological conditions: a pressure gradient causes fluid to filter from the capillaries of the parietal pleura into the cavity and is drained through the lymphatics stomata that connect the pleural space to the submesothelial lymphatic network of the parietal pleura itself (Miserocchi & Negrini, 1997).
Fig.1 highlights schematically that fluid filtration mostly occurs in less dependent regions and pleural fluid is drained towards preferential absorption sites at the bottom and in the mediastinal region. The absorption pressure of lymphatics (Fig. 2) sets a subatmospheric pressure of the pleural fluid that averages ~ -10 cmH_2O at mid heart level (it is more negative in the less dependent regions of the cavity and less negative at the bottom, where it reaches ~ 0 cmH_2O). This pressure acts to keep the lung in close apposition of the chest wall. Note that the lung and the chest wall develop an elastic recoil that would tend to pull them apart (red arrows in the insert in Fig. 2), however, the pressure generated by such recoil (about 4 cmH_2O at the functional residual capacity) is less subatmospheric than that generated by the lymphatic pump, therefore, lung and chest wall are actually pushing one against the other. This mechanical condition does not impair the reciprocal movements of the parietal and visceral pleura (about 25000 km in a life span) due to a very efficient lubrication system (see insert in Fig.2) based on reciprocal repulsive forces of negative charges carried by polar phospholipids adsorbed on the opposing pleural surfaces and assures a friction coefficient as low as 0.02 (comparable to that of ice on ice) (Hills, 1992).

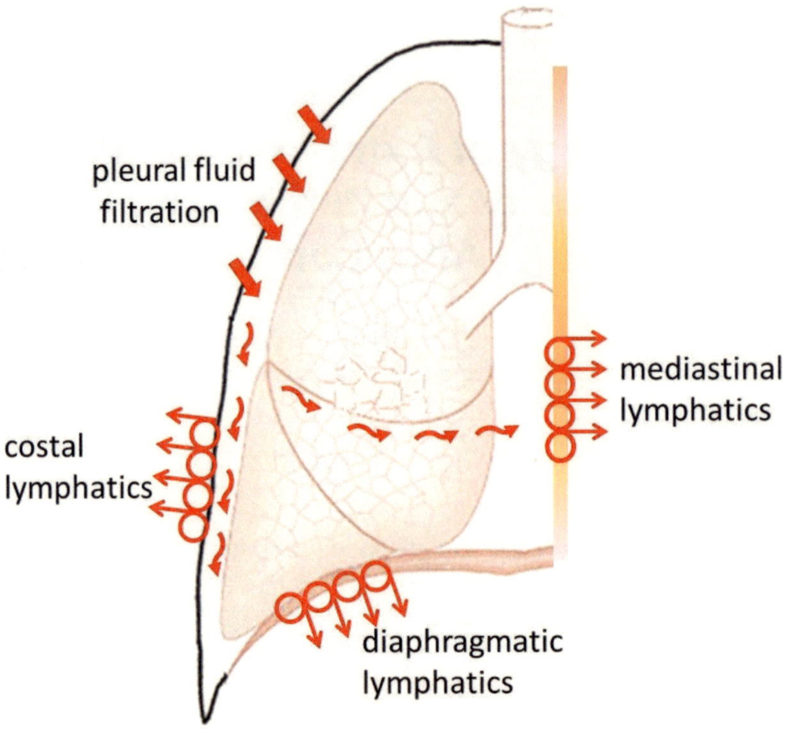

Fig. 1. Fluid turnover in the pleural cavity.

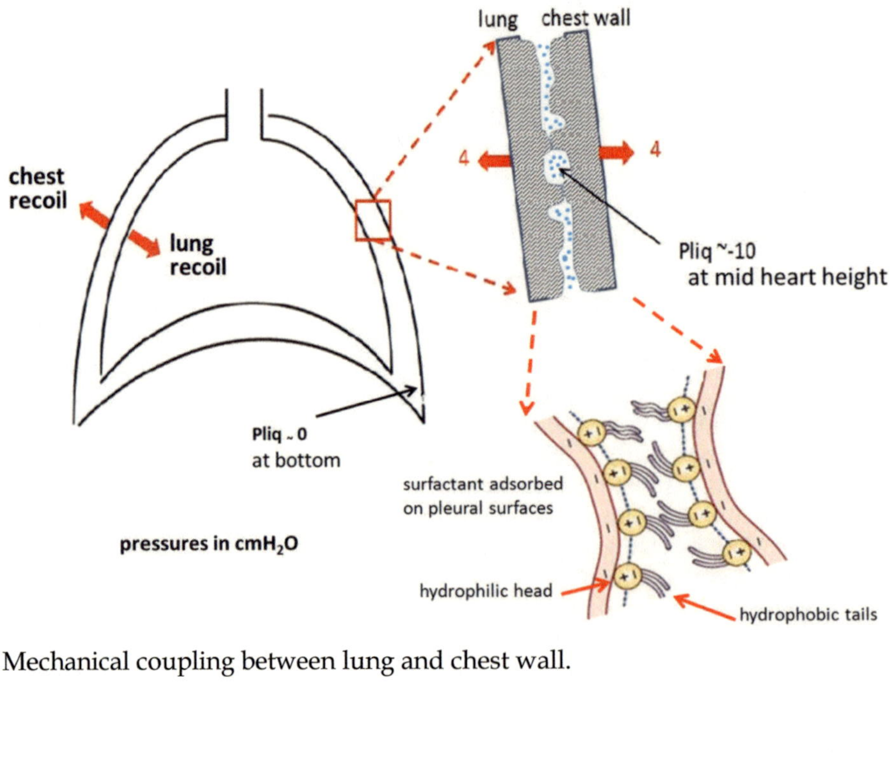

Fig. 2. Mechanical coupling between lung and chest wall.

2.1 Pathophysiology of pleural effusion

Pleural lymphatics act as efficient regulators of pleural liquid volume avoiding hydrothorax formation by increasing the draining flow (up to ~ 20 fold) in proportion to the increase in filtration rate (Miserocchi, 2009). As a matter of fact, for a tenfold increase in filtration rate, the volume of the pleural fluid would only be hardly doubled (Miserocchi, 2009). Any increase in pleural fluid filtration can in principle easily accumulate in the chest due to the opposite retraction of the lung and chest wall (Fig. 3).
When filtration exceeds the maximum lymphatic flow, pleural effusion results favoured by three conditions: an increase in systemic capillary pressure, an increase in permeability of the parietal/visceral pleura, a strong limitation to an increase in lymphatic flow. Pleural effusion are classified as exudates when the fluid/serum total protein ratio (indicated as TPR) exceeds 0.5 (Joseph et al, 2001; Joseph et al, 2002; Joseph et al, 2003). The degree of mesothelial lesion can be related to the concentration of lactic dehydrogenase (Joseph et al,2001) in the pleural fluid (indicated as FLDH); a cut off for FLDH at 163-200 U/L has been proposed for diagnostic.

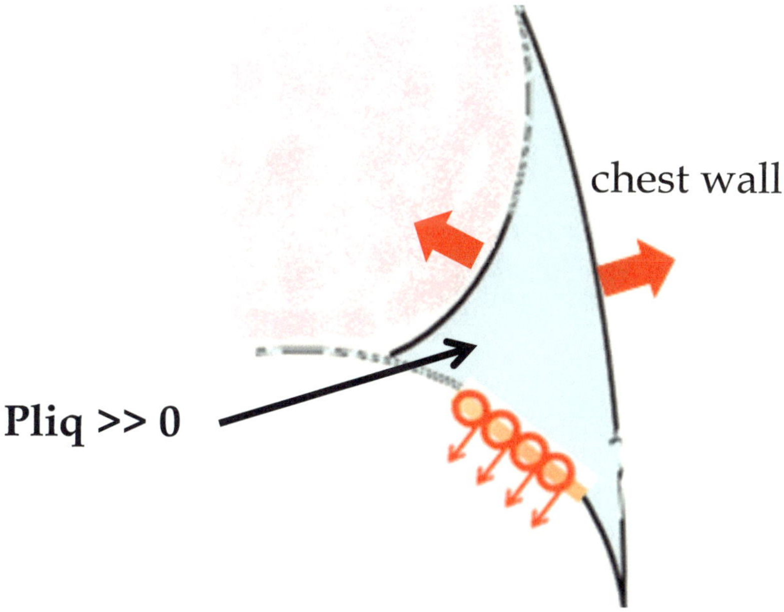

Fig. 3. Pleural lymphatics act as efficient regulators of pleural liquid volume.

3. Control of extravascular water volume

The thinness of the air-blood barrier (0.2-0.3 microns) reflects a functionally "dry" condition (Conforti et al, 2002), therefore, as much as for the pleural liquid, also for the extravascular space of the lung one can speak of a "minimum" volume of water. This ensures, in turn, a high efficiency of the gas diffusion. Similarly to the pleural fluid, also lung interstitial fluid is kept at a subatmospheric pressure (also ~ -10 cmH_2O, Fig.4) due to the powerful draining action of lymphatics in face of a very low microvascular permeability (Miserocchi, 2009). The latter feature allows to keep microvascular filtration as low as $1 \cdot 10^{-4}$ ml/cm^2 in 24h. Fig. 4 also presents important molecules, belonging to the proteoglycans (PGs) family, whose role appears crucial to control the extravascular water volume, as they act as highy hydroplhilic link proteins. Perlecan, an heparansulphate PG (MW 0.1-0.5 MDa) is placed in the basement membrane and controls the porosity to water and solutes; versican (MW 0.5 MDa), a large PG bound to hyaluronan (a random coiled molecule), provides rigidity to the tissue by establishing multiple non-covalent links with other molecules of the matrix and with cells (Roberts et al, 1997).

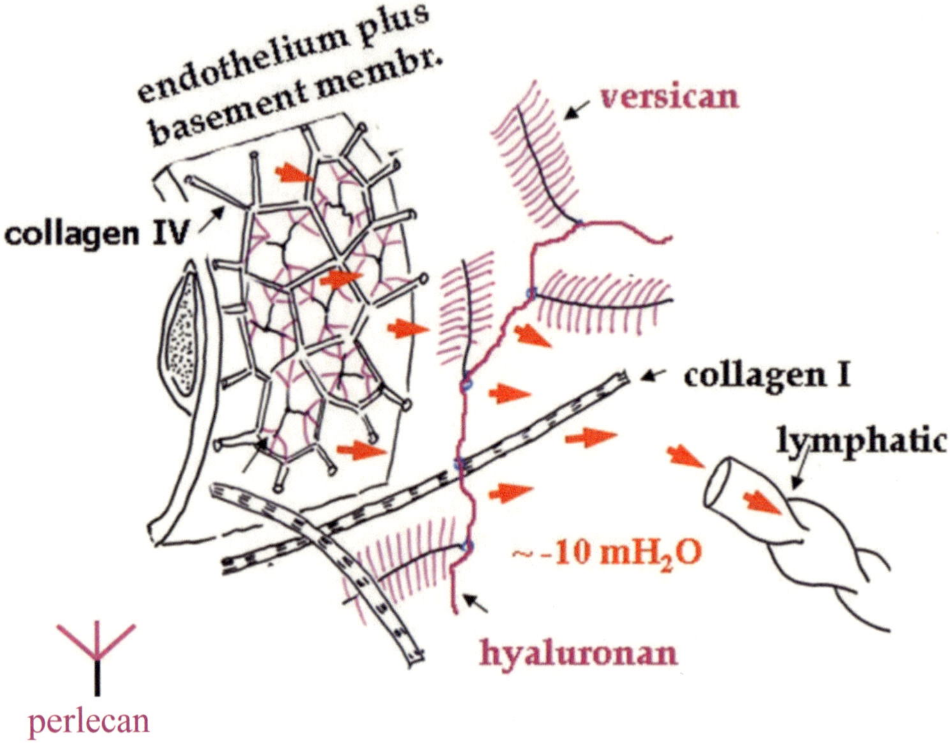

Fig. 4. Lung interstitial fluid dynamics and some macromolecular components of the interstitial matrix.

The volume of the extravascular water is strictly controlled so that the lung appears quite resistant to the development of edema. In fact, at least three mechanisms cooperate to allow only minimal variations in extravascular water volume relative to the steady state condition (Miserocchi, 2009). First, the glycosaminoglycan chains of PGs can bind excess water to form gel-like structures; this results in an increase in the steric hindrance of proteoglycans and corresponding decrease in the porosity of the basement membrane and thus also in microvascular permeability. Second, the assembly of large matrix PGs within the extracellular matrix provides low tissue compliance and this represents an important "tissue safety factor" against the development of edema. In fact, a minor increase in extravascular water in response to increased microvascular filtration, causes a marked increase in interstitial pressure (e.g., from ~ -10 to ~ 5 cmH_2O) (Miserocchi, 2009) that buffers further filtration. Third, arteriolar vasoconstriction represents an important reflex to avoid or actually decrease capillary pressure when filtration is increased due to an increase in microvascular permeability (Negrini, 1995, Rivolta et al, 2011).

4. Pathophysiology of lung edema

The development of severe edema is known as a tumultuous event taking place in minutes (Miserocchi et al, 2001a). Experimental models in animals allowed to attribute the sudden increase in extravascular lung water (Miserocchi et al, 2001a) to the loss of integrity of the proteoglycan components of the macromolecular structure of the lung interstitial space. Fragmentation/degradation of PGs of the basement membrane cause an increase in microvascular permeability of the paracellular pathway as pore size can reach 50-100 nm allowing easy leak of albumin. Finding of red blood cells in the alveolar fluid reflects major lesions of the air blood barrier. Fragmentation of matrix PGs removes the "tissue safety factor" by causing an increase in interstitial compliance. The loss of integrity of PGs reflects the sustained increase in parenchymal stresses, the weakening of the non-covalent bonds due to increased water binding, and the activation of tissue metalloproteases (Miserocchi et al, 2001a).

One shall consider interstitial edema as a sharp edge between tissue repair and severe disease: in fact, the transition from interstitial to severe lung edema occurs through an "accelerated" phase when the loss of integrity of the interstitial matrix proceeds beyond a critical threshold. Interestingly, the same pathophysiological mechanism can be extended to all forms of lung edema, the only difference being the time sequence of fragmentation of the families of PGs. The initial degradation process involves the large matrix PGs in cardiogenic edema, while in the lesional edema model, the initial process involves PGs of the basement membrane. In the hypoxia lung edema model, both PGs families are involved (Miserocchi et al, 2001a). Lung cellular activation for matrix remodelling and repair was documented as differential expression of signalling-transduction platforms on plasma membrane (Sabbadini et al, 2003; Palestini et al, 2002; Palestini et al, 2003; Daffara et al, 2004; Botto et al, 2006; Botto et al, 2008) and the hypothesis was put forward of differential activations of these platforms (lipid rafts or caveolae) to trigger redeposition of specific matrix components. A further peculiar feature of lung edema is that to develop in a patchy way, thus revealing regional differences in the efficiency of control of extravascular water volume. These differences have been recently documented in a hypoxic edema model (Rivolta et al, 2011) and the hypothesis was put forward that alterations in the geometry of the microvascular-alveolar design might favor an imbalance in interstitial fluid dynamics.

5. Specific conditions pertaining to thoracic surgery as potential causes of disturbance in extravascular water fluid dynamics

5.1 Pleural space

Evacuation of air from the cavity is the most immediate problem after thoracic surgery to allow re-expansion of the remaining lung. Air (and fluid) drainage are accomplished via a chest tube placement, and we address the reader to a recently published consensus definition (Brunelli et al, 2011). As a matter of fact, tube management is basically left to personal surgeon's evaluation despite the fact that such practice is a major factor affecting the length of recovery, the cost and the morbidity of patients undergoing lung resection surgery. Many surgeons use only a single drain, likely differently oriented, to drain both air and pleural fluid. The initial gas drainage is better performed by having the chest tube opening placed in the retrosternal region where air collects in the supine posture (see below). Conversely, pleural fluid is profitably drained by having the tube opening in the lowermost part of the pleural space (dorsal costodiaphragmatic sinus, both in supine and head up posture (Miserocchi et al, 1988; Haber et al, 2001) where fluid collects. Hydrothorax may develop due to surgical insult and/or to excessive subatmospehric pressure applied to the chest tube favouring fluid filtration. Note that pleural liquid pressure in the costodiaphragmatic sinus is close to 0 cmH_2O in physiological conditions and may become positive with increasing liquid pooling.

Thus, the recommended strategy is simply that of having the chest tube open to atmosphere (Fig. 5A): whenever pressure, in the hydrothorax will exceed atmospheric pressure fluid will drain into the tube. To avoid suction of liquid/air back into the pleural cavity when a subatmospheric pleural pressure is generated on inspiration, a one way valve should be placed on the tube outlet. In case fluid advances down the tube (by 10cm in Fig. 5B) a subatmospheric pressure (-10 cmH_2O) is generated at tip of chest tube in the pleural space, a condition speeding up the drainage.

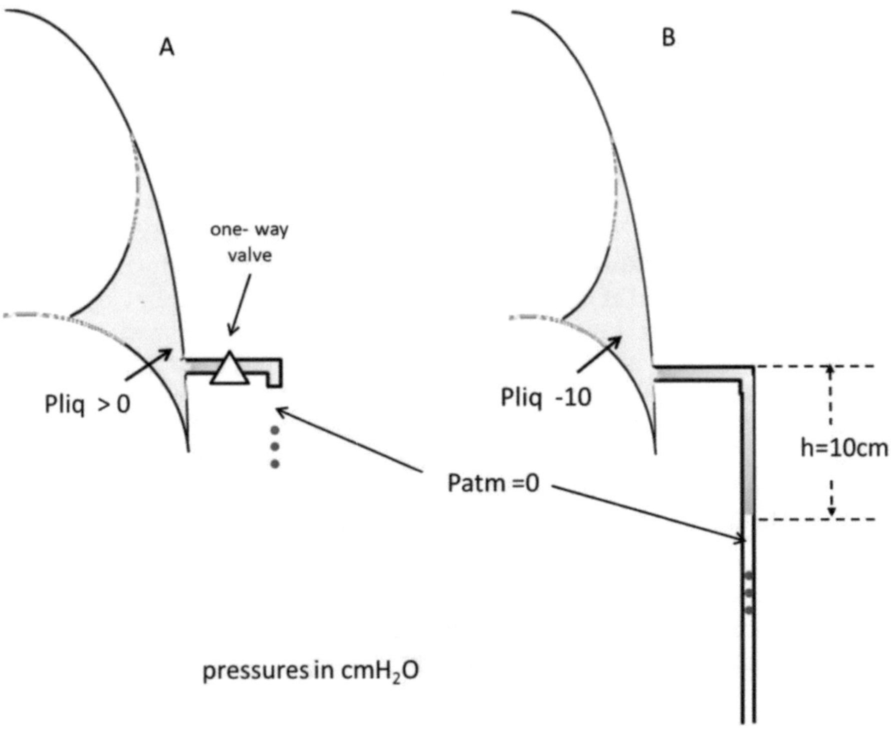

Fig. 5. Fluid mechanics of hydrothorax drainage from the costodiaphragmatic sinus.

For a pressure at tip of the order of about -60 cmH_2O (the case of a fluid column from patient bed down to the floor) the pressure gradient for fluid filtration into the cavity would be increased by about 10 times! No wonder that such pressure would contribute to increased fluid filtration and hydrothorax formation. Interestingly, the negative pressure generated at tip remains basically confined to the fluid pool and is not transmitted to the rest of the pleural space due to the extremely high flow resistance of the pleural space once the visceral pleura adheres to the parietal one (Miserocchi et al, 1992). Recovery from pleural effusion may be slow, ranging from weeks to months (Cohen & Sahn, 2001). Removal of chest tubes after fluid drainage of 400-450 cc /day or less appears reasonable (Cerfolio & Bryant, 2008; Cerfolio et al, 2010; Bertholet et al 2010) as it is in the range of physiological daily pleural fluid filtration (an estimated value of 350 ml/day (Miserocchi & Negrini, 1997).

5.2 Lung interstitium

The important point to be considered here is that the compliance ($\Delta V/\Delta P$) of the remaining lung is decreased in proportion to the amount of the resected portion: so, for example, a 50% reduction in lung volume, would entrain a similar reduction in lung compliance.

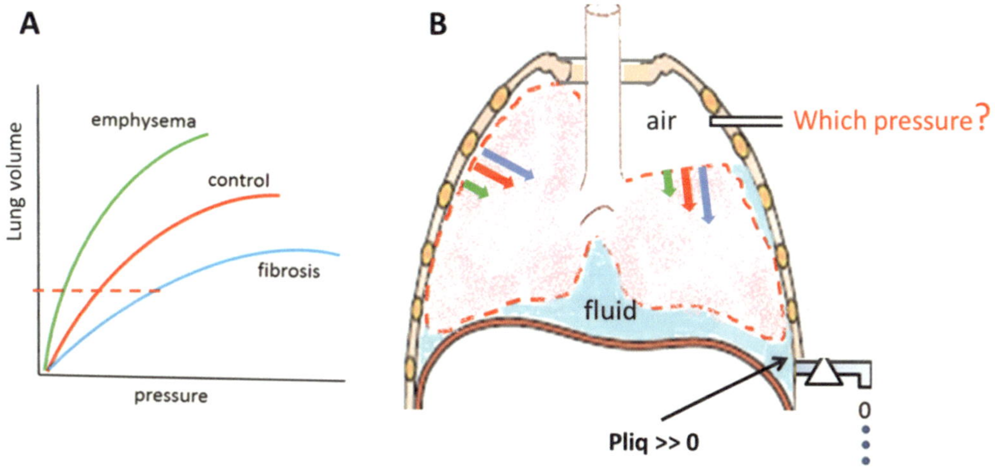

Fig. 6. Safe strategy to re-expand the lung after resection: gas pressure must generate the pre- operation lung distending pressure that depends upon the functional state of the lung.

Therefore re-expansion of the remaining lung to match the original chest volume would obviously require considerable greater distending pressure (over-distension) as well as a remarkable deformation of its natural shape. As thoroughly discussed in a previous paper (Miserocchi et al, 2010), to avoid lung over-distension re-expansion of the remaining lung should match the pre-operating distending pleural pressure that vary however as described by the volume-pressure relationship (Fig. 6A): fibrosis (blue) increases lung distending pressures on the abscissa and decreases compliance, while the opposite occurs in emphysema (green), relative to control (red). In practice, an air bubble ought to remain in the pleural cavity and the pressure generated by the suction line (Fig.6B) must be equal to that exerted by the lung before resection. The elastic properties of the lung can be described during a pneumological functional examination by relating lung volumes to the corresponding values of transpulmonary pressures as deduced from oesophageal pressure.

6. Lung over-distension: The risks of air leak and lung edema

6.1 Air leak

If no leaks are present, the gas bubble is reabsorbed (~1%/day), following the gradient in gas partial pressures in the blood and in the gas phase, until physical equilibration is reached. Reabsorption of the gas bubble is initially slow because the flow of O_2 to the blood is opposed by CO_2 flow to the bubble; furthermore, N_2 slows down the reabsorption process because of its low solubility in blood. Washing the cavity with oxygen would speed up the reabsorption process. The corresponding decrease in pleural pressure would increase fluid filtration so that, over time, liquid will replace gas.

Air leak after pulmonary resection may be due to bronchopleural or bronchoalveolar-pleural fistulas (Rice et al, 2002) due to failure to obtain a perfect surgical seal. An estimate of air leak would be useful to decide about chest drainage removal, however the methods of detecting air bubbles along the chest tube during forced expiratory maneuvers appears rather imprecise, while more refined methods are available (Varela et al, 2009). Measuring the change in pressure in the air bubble (ΔP) by a chest tube would allow an indirect estimate of the change in air volume (ΔV) considering that $\Delta V = Crs * \Delta P$, where *Crs* is the compliance of the respiratory system. Considering the mechanical arrangement of the lung and of the chest wall, one has:

$$\frac{1}{Crs} = \frac{1}{Cl} + \frac{1}{Cw}$$

where *Cl* and *Cw* are the compliance of lung and chest wall respectively. In physiological conditions, one has $Cl = Cw = 0.2$ L/cmH_2O, so that one has $Crs = 0.1Cl$. As mentioned above, *Cl* reflects the functional state of the lung and furthermore is decreased in proportion of the decrease in lung volume. No such measurements are considered so far in the clinical practice: yet, we believe that a pneumological functional evaluation would provide important information concerning the trend of an air leak.

6.2 Lung edema

Severe complications representing the major cause of morbidity after lung resection ("idiopathic edema", ALI, atelectasis, ARDS) share a similar patho-physiological basis essentially represented by an acute increase in microvascular filtration, thus, simply, edema formation (Miserocchi et al, 2010). In post lung resection surgery, this can be due to:

- lung overinflation on re-expansion and/or prolonged mechanical ventilation with excessive tidal volume (Miserocchi et al, 1991). Stretching of lung parenchyma results indeed in a marked subatmospheric interstitial pressure, that, in turn, favours microvascular filtration potentially evolving towards matrix fragmentation and an "accelerated phase" (Miserocchi et al, 2001a);
- lack of clearance of the fragments, neutrophil and macrophage activation (Adair-Kirk & Senior, 2008), production of reactive oxygen species, leading to diffuse alveolar damage and inhibition of the active alveolar fluid reabsorption (Khimenko et al, 1994);
- large amounts of intraoperative fluid administration (Zeltin et al, 1984; Slinger, 2006), particularly when coupled to increased microvascular permeability, as clearly shown by experimental models of lung edema (Miserocchi et al, 2001a);
- the remaining lung is hosting a greater blood flow and this is accomplished by capillary recruitment and increased blood flow velocity and shear rate that lead to an increase in microvascular permeability (Min-Ho et al, 2005);
- local hypoxia, a known factor favouring edema formation (Miserocchi et al, 2001b), may develop due to edema itself as well as to ventilation/perfusion mismatch;

- finally, due to the decrease in vascular bed, pulmonary vascular resistances are likely to increase leading to pulmonary hypertension that is potentially correlated to the risk of developing pulmonary edema (Grünig et al, 2000; Rivolta et al, 2011).

7. The "postoperative residual pleural space"

The "postoperative residual pleural space" refers to the fate of the volume left free by lung resection (Misthos et al, 2007). As much as in physiological conditions, **the main variable setting the volume of the postoperative residual pleural space is the absorption pressure of the pleural lymphatics**. If their capacity to drain flow and generate a subatmospheric pressure have remained unchanged, they will still tend to reduce pleural liquid volume to a minimum. However, the new "minimum" will reflect a state equilibrium resulting from the modified lung-chest wall coupling and the actual filtration/absorption balance of pleural fluid. In practice, the volume left free by lung resection will be occupied (Fig. 7) in part by pleural fluid, in part by an increase in volume of the remaining lung, and in part by the displacement of the diaphragm and of the mediastinum.

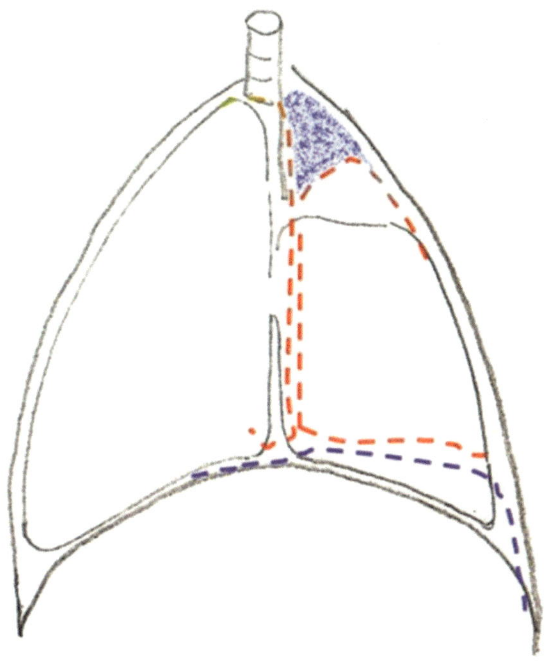

Fig. 7. The "postoperative residual pleural space"(blue area).

8. Cardiac output, lung fluid-balance and oxygen diffusion-transport

As delineated in section 2, control mechanisms are present in the lung to limit the increase in extravascular volume such as when lung capillary recruitment occurs in response to an increase in cardiac output. However the efficiency of these mechanisms, as from experimental models, varies among lung regions and among individuals, particularly when tissue hypoxia is also present (Rivolta et al, 2011).

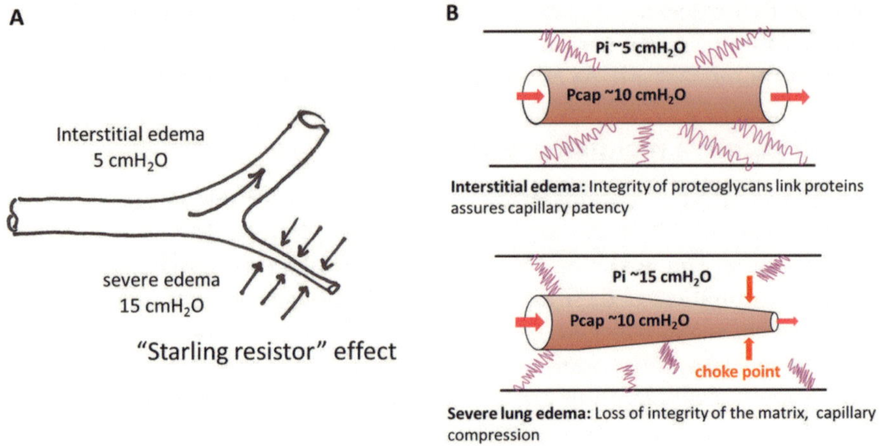

Fig. 8. A: lung capillary squeeze in relation to interstitial fluid pressure ("Starling resistor" effect). B: role of proteoglycans (in pink) fragmentation in favouring the squeeze of microvessels in severe edema.

Fig. 8A shows that in regions where severe edema develops, the increase in interstitial pressure is such as to squeeze the microcirculation ("Starling resistor" effect) thus impairing blood flow (Rivolta et al, 2011). In fact, the patency of microvessels is critically dependent upon the integrity of the proteoglycan molecules linking the matrix to the endothelial surface: as suggested in Fig. 8B, the integrity is preserved in interstitial edema, while massive fragmentation occurs when severe edema develops. The decrease in vascular bed causes a rise in pulmonary vascular resistances leading to an increase in pulmonary artery pressure, whose entity reflects the extension of severe edema (Rivolta et al, 2011). The variability concerning the proneness to develop lung edema and associated pulmonary hypertension in response to an increase in cardiac output, particularly when associated with alveolar hypoxia, is documented not only in animals but also in humans (Grünig et al, 2000). One can now remark that after resection surgery, the remaining lung, as described in section 4.2, is also exposed to increased blood flow and, owing to potential ventilation/perfusion mismatch, also to local hypoxia. Therefore, the risk of developing post-lung resection surgery pulmonary edema may depend upon the extension of the resection as well as on the individual proneness to develop lung edema. It appears therefore justified to assess the latter point by performing a pre-operation cardio-pulmonary exercise test and gather data on cardiac output, pulmonary artery pressure, pulmonary vascular resistance as well as indirect evidence of increase in lung water (see paragraph 7 below). These data may be compared to post-resection surgery condition.

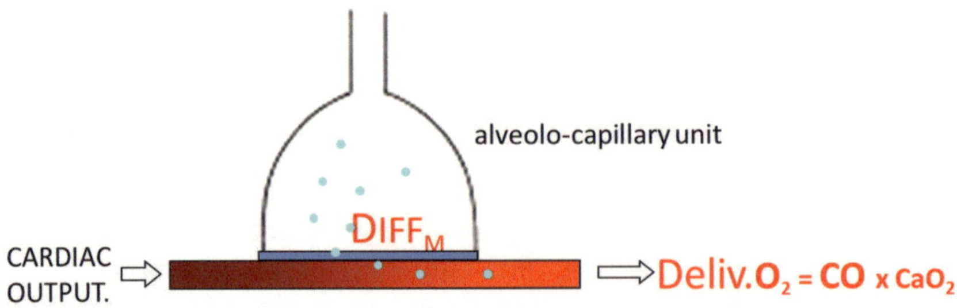

Fig. 9. Lung water balance related mechanisms limiting oxygen delivery

Fig. 9 summarizes the lung-water balance related mechanisms that may limit oxygen delivery defined as $DelivO_2$ = Cardiac Output x CaO_2, where CaO_2 is the oxygen concentration at the lung capillary outlet. A membrane "diffusion limitation" ($DIFF_M$) may result from the reduction in alveolar surface available for diffusion and/or from the presence of edema fluid. "Perfusion limitation" in oxygen transport has also to be envisaged because $DelivO_2$ is critically dependent upon regional lung blood flow and this, in turn, depends upon the local patency-compression condition of microvessels (see Fig. 8). Finally, the increase in blood flow velocity slows down the alveolo-capillary oxygen equilibration. All together, these alterations result in an alveolo-capillary oxygen pressure difference.

9. Indexes to assess alteration in pleural and lung interstitial fluid balance

Most of the complications of post-thoracic surgery relate to a severe disturbance in lung extravascular water and occur in the early postoperative period (Alvarez et al, 2007; Khan et al, 1999), similarly to what is observed after lung transplant (Khan et al, 1999).

Pre-operative:
- lung compliance: needs measurement of transpulmonary pressure by using an esophageal balloon (more easily performed once the patient is anesthetized)
- lung diffusion DLCO, Krogh factor (DLCO/alveolar volume). After lung resection DLCO will be reduced in proportion of resected volume, however, if the remaining lung works as an efficient diffusor, the Krogh factor will be normal.
- respiratory impedance (in particular reactance at low oscillation frequency , 1 Hz). A recent paper highlights that reactance significantly decreases for an increase in extravascular water of about 10% (Dellacà et al, 2008).
- lung comets determined by echocardiography, as a sign of interstitial lung edema (Picano et al, 2006).
- cardio-pulmonary exercise test to evaluate the efficiency of the oxygen diffusion-transport system and the proneness to develop pulmonary edema

Immediate Post-operative:
- measure lung compliance at the end of operation while the patient is still under anaesthesia
- sensitive methods to assess a disturbance in lung fluid (respiratory impedance, comets)
- time course of pressure in the pleural air bubble to monitor the trend of a potential air leak
- lung diffusion: DLCO, Krogh factor (DLCO/alveolar volume)

Later on:
- cardio-pulmonary exercise test to evaluate the efficiency of the oxygen diffusion-transport system

10. References

Adair-Kirk T.L. & Senior R.M. (2008). Fragments of extracellular matrix as mediators of inflammation. *Int J Bioch. Cell Biol*, Vol.40, pp. 1101–1110.

Alvarez JM, Tan J, Kejriwal N, Ghanim, K., Newman, M.A., Segal, A., Sterret, G. & Bulsara, M.K. (2007). Idiopathic postpneumonectomy pulmonary edema: Hyperinflation of the remaining lung is a potential etiologic factor, but the condition can be averted by balanced pleural drainage. *J Thorac Cardiovasc Surg*, Vol. 133, pp. 1439-4147.

Bertholet, J.W., Joosten J.J., Keemers-Gels M.E., van den Wildenberg F.J. & Barendregt W.B. (2010) Chest tube management following pulmonary lobectomy: change in protocol results in fewer air leaks. *Interact Cardiovasc Thorac Surg*, Vol. 12, No. 1, pp. 28-31.

Botto, L., Beretta, E., Bulbarelli, A., Rivolta I., Lettiero, B., Leone, B.E., Miserocchi, G. & Palestini, P. (2008). Hypoxia-induced modifications in plasma membranes and lipid microdomains in A549 cells and primary human alveolar cells. *J Cell Biochem*, Vol. 105, No 2, pp. 503-513.

Botto, L., Beretta, E., Daffara, R., Miserocchi, G. & Palestini P. (2006) Biochemical and morphological changes in endothelial cells in response to hypoxic interstitial edema. *Respir Res*, Vol. 7, No. 1, pp. 7.

Brunelli, A., Beretta, E., Cassivi, S.D., Cerfolio, R.J., Detterbeck, F., Kiefer, T., Miserocchi, G., Shrager, J., Singhal, S., Van Raemdonck, D. & Varela, G. (2011). Consensus definitions to promote an evidence-based approach to management of the pleural space. A collaborative proposal by ESTS, AATS, STS, and GTSC. *Eur J Cardiothorac Surg*. Vol. 40(2), pp.291-297.

Cerfolio, R.J. & Bryant, A.S. (2008). Results of a prospective algorithm to remove chest tubes after Pulmonary resection with high output. *J Thorac Cardiovasc Surg*, Vol. 135 pp. 269-273.

Cerfolio, R.J., Varela, G, & Brunelli, A. (2010). Digital and smart chest drainage systems to monitor air leaks: the birth of a new era? *Thorac Surg Clin*, Vol. 20, pp. 413-420.

Cohen, M. & Sahn, S.A. (2001). Resolution of Pleural Effusions. *Chest*, Vol. 119, pp. 1547–1562.

Conforti, E., Fenoglio, C., Bernocchi, G., Bruschi, O. & Miserocchi, G. (2002). Morpho-functional analysis of lung tissue in mild interstitial edema. *Am J Physiol* (*Lung Cell Mol Physiol*), Vol. 282, pp. L766-L774.

Daffara, R., Botto, L., Beretta, E., Conforti, E., Faini, A., Palestini, P. & Miserocchi, G. (2004). Endothelial cells as early sensors of pulmonary interstitial edema. *J Appl Physiol*, Vol. 97, No 4, pp. 1575-1583.

Dellacà, R.L., Zannin, E., Sancini, G., Rivolta, I., Leone, B,E,, Pedotti, A. & Miserocchi, G. (2008). Changes in the mechanical properties of the respiratory system during the development of interstitial lung edema. *Respir Res*, Vol. 12, No. 9, pp. 51-60.

Grünig E., Mereles D., Hildebrandt W., Swenson E.R., Kübler W., Kuecherer H. & Bärtsch P. (2000). Stress Doppler echocardiography for identification of susceptibility to high altitude pulmonary edema. *J Am Coll Cardiol*. Vol. 35, No. 4, pp. 980-987.

Haber, R., Grotberg, J.B., Glucksberg, M.R., Miserocchi, G., Venturoli, D., Del Fabbro, M. & Waters CM. (2001). Steady-state pleural fluid flow and pressure and the effects of lung buoyancy. *J Biomech Engineering*, Vol. 124, pp. 485-492T

Hills, B.A. (1992). Graphite-like lubrication of mesothelium by oligolamellar pleural surfactant. *J Appl Physiol*, Vol. 73, pp. 1034-1039.

Joseph, J., Badrinath, P., Basran, G.S. & Sahn, S.A. (2001). Is the pleural fluid transudate or exudate? A revisit of the diagnostic criteria. *Thorax*, Vol.56, pp. 867-870.

Joseph, J., Badrinath, P., Basran, G.S. & Sahn, S.A. (2003). Do we need all three criteria for the diagnostic separation of pleural fluid into transudates and exudates? An appraisal of the traditional criteria. *Med Sci Monit*, Vol. 9, No. 11, pp. CR474-476.

Joseph, J., Badrinath, P., Basran, G.S. & Sahn, S.A. (2002). Is albumin gradient or fluid to serum albumin ratio better than the pleural fluid lactate dehydroginase in the diagnostic of separation of pleural effusion? *BMC Pulmonary Medicine*, Vol. 22, No. 2, pp. 1.

Khan, S.U., Salloum, J., O'Donovan, P.B., Mascha, E.J., Mehta, A.C., Matthay, M.A. & Arroliga, A.C. (1999). Acute Pulmonary Edema After Lung transplantation. *Chest*, Vol.116, pp. 187-194.

Khimenko, P.L., Barnard, J.W., Moore, T.M., Wilson, P.S., Ballard, S.T. & Taylor, A.E. (1994). Vascular permeability and epithelial transport effects on lung edema formation in ischemia and reperfusion. *J Appl Physiol*, Vol. 77, No. 3, pp. 1116-1121.

Min-Ho, K., Harris, N.R. & Tarbell, J.M. (2005). Regulation of capillary hydraulic conductivity in response to an acute change in shear. *Am J Physiol Heart Circ Physiol*, Vol. 289, pp. H2126–H2135.

Miserocchi, G., Negrini, D., Pistolesi, M., Bellina, C.R., Gilardi, M.C., Bettinardi, V. & Rossitto F. Intrapleural liquid flow down a gravity dependent hydraulic pressure gradient. *J Appl Physiol*, Vol. 1988, No. 64, pp. 577-584.

Miserocchi, G., Negrini, D. & Gonano, C. (1991). Parenchymal stress affects interstitial and pleural pressures in in situ lung. *J Appl Physiol*, Vol. 71, No. 5, pp. 1967-1972.

Miserocchi, G., Venturoli, D., Negrini, D., Gilardi, M.C. & Bellina, R. (1992). Intrapleural fluid movements described by a porous flow model. *J Appl Physiol*, Vol. 73, pp. 2511-2516.

Miserocchi, G. & Negrini, D. (1997). Pleural space: pressure and fluid dynamics, In: *THE LUNG, Scientific Foundations,* Crystal, R.G. West, J.B., Weibel, E.R. & Barnes, P.J., pp. 1217-1225, Lippincott-Raven Pub, New York..

Miserocchi, G., Negrini, D., Passi, A. & De Luca, G. (2001a). Development of lung edema: interstitial fluid dynamics and molecular structure. *News Physiol Sci*, Vol. 16, pp. 66-71.

Miserocchi, G., Passi, A., Negrini, D., Del Fabbro, M. & De Luca. (2001b). Pulmonary interstitial pressure and tissue matrix structure in acute hypoxia. *Am J Physiol (Lung Cell Mol Physiol)*, Vol. 280, pp. L881-L887.

Miserocchi, G. (2009). Mechanisms controlling the volume of pleural liquid and extravascular lung water. *Eur Respir Rev*, Vol. 18, pp. 244–52.

Miserocchi, G., Beretta, E. & Rivolta, I. (2010). Respiratory mechanics and fluid dynamics after lung resection surgery. *Thorac Surg Clin*, Vol. 20, pp. 345-357.

Misthos, P., Kokotsakis, J., Konstantinou, M., Skottis, I. & Lioulias, A. (2007). Postoperative Residual Pleural Spaces: Characteristics and Natural History. *Asian Cardiovasc Thorac Ann*, Vol. 15, pp. 54–58.

Negrini, D. (1995). Pulmonary microvascular pressure profile during development of hydrostatic edema. *Microcirculation*, Vol. 2, pp. 173-180.

Palestini, P., Calvi, C., Conforti, E., Botto, L., Fenoglio, C. & Miserocchi, G. (2002). Composition, biophysical properties and morphometry of plasma membranes in pulmonary interstitial edema. *Am J Physiol Lung Cell Mol Physiol,* Vol. 282, pp. L1382-L1390.

Palestini, P., Calvi ,C., Conforti, E., Daffara, R., Botto, L. & Miserocchi, G. (2003). Compositional changes in lipid microdomains of air-blood barrier plasma membranes in pulmonary interstitial edema. *J Appl Physiol*, Vol. 95, pp. 1446-1452.

Picano, E., Frassi, F., Agricola, E., Gligorova, S., Gargani, L. & Mottola, G. (2006). Ultrasound lung comets: a clinically useful sign of extravascular lung water. *J Am Soc Echocardiogr*, Vol. 19, No. 3, pp. 356-363.

Rice, T.W., Okereke, I.C. & Blackstone, E.H. (2002). Persistent air-leak following pulmonary resection. *Chest Surg Clin N Am*, Vol. 12, pp. 529-539.

Rivolta, I., Lucchini, V., Rocchetti, M., Kolar, F., Palazzo, F., Zaza, A. & Miserocchi, G. (2011). Interstitial pressure and lung oedema in chronic hypoxia. *Eur Respir J*, Vol. 37, pp. 943–949.

Roberts, C.R., Wight, T.N. & Hascall, V.C. (1997). Proteoglycans. In: T*he LUNG scientific foundtaions.*, Crystal, R.G. West, J.B., Weibel, E.R. & Barnes, P.J. pp. 757-767, Lippincott-Raven Pub, New York.

Sabbadini, M., Barisani, D., Conforti, E., Marozzi, A., Ginelli, E., Miserocchi, G. & Meneveri, R. (2003). Gene expression analysis in interstitial lung edema induced by saline infusion. *Bioch Bioph Acta-Mol Basis of Dis,* Vol. 1638, pp. 149-156.

Slinger, P.D. (2006). Postpneumonectomy pulmonary edema. *Anesthesiology*, Vol. 105, pp. 2-5.

Varela, G., Jimenez, M.F., Novoa, N.M. & Aranda, J.L. (2009). Postoperative chest tube management: measuring air leak using an electronic device decreases variability in the clinical practice. *Eur J Cardiothorac Surg*, Vol. 35, pp. 28–31.

Zeldin, R.A., Normadin, D., Landwing, B.S. & Peters, R.M. (1984). Postpenumonectomy pulmonary edema. *J Thoracic Cardiovasc Surg*, Vol. 87, pp. 359-365.

26

The Role of PET-CT in the Clinical Management of Oesophageal Cancer

Reubendra Jeganathan, Jim McGuigan and Tom Lynch
Royal Victoria Hospital, Belfast,
United Kingdom

1. Introduction

Oesophageal cancer, once a relatively rare form of cancer, with a non-uniform geographical distribution, is the sixth most common cause of cancer related death in UK for 2005 (1-3). By the time of presentation, only 24-31% of patients are suitable for curative surgical resection and the overall 5-year survival is 20-30% (2, 4). PET-CT, a new staging modality is said to improve patient selection, by the detection of metastatic disease, which is not readily identifiable by other imaging modalities.

Recent published literature demonstrates an ever-evolving role for PET-CT in the management of various cancer types. PET-CT is not only used as a staging tool but can be used to assess early response to chemotherapy and radiotherapy (5). PET-CT can also be employed to identify disease recurrence, often detecting sites of relapse, before any other imaging modality (6). Additionally, metabolic parameters determined from the PET-CT study can provide prognostic information for individual patients (7).

The aim of this chapter is to provide the reader with an introduction to PET-CT, covering cellular metabolism, imaging of glucose metabolism, imaging protocols and the utility of standard uptake value. Following this, we will provide a pertinent review of the current published literature on the prognostic potential of standard uptake value of PET-CT in the management of oesophageal cancer and its ability to supplement the TNM classification. Finally, we will include future applications of PET-CT, including its role as a measure of tumour response following neo-adjuvant chemotherapy, and other de novo techniques currently being considered in the field of PET-CT.

2. Positron emission tomography and computed tomography

Positron Emission Tomography or PET involves an intravenous injection of a radioactive tracer, attached to a biological substance, which then distributes within the body in a recognised pattern. The radiation emitted from this injected substance can then be imaged to reveal the pattern of distribution within the body and abnormal areas of tracer accumulation, can therefore be identified. This creates a functional image. There are many radioactive tracers used, but in the context of this chapter, we will only consider fluourodeoxyglucose, FDG. FDG is a glucose analogue, which has a distribution, similar to simple glucose molecules within the body.

A CT scan uses X-rays to provide an anatomical image of the patient and a PET scan gives an image revealing the distribution of glucose like, metabolic function. Each on its own is a powerful tool but when combined they start to revolutionise cancer imaging. A PET-CT scanner is a single device that combines both modalities to produce an image that contains the metabolic functional information from the PET image and the anatomical information from the CT scan, displaying the resultant data as a fused PET-CT image.

2.1 Cellular metabolism

Cancer cells share similar traits to normal cells, in that they divide and multiply, but do so at a faster rate. Cancer cells also have an inherent tendency to metastasise, once they have overcome the body immunological defence. In order to achieve this objective the cancer cells must have an energy source capable of fuelling this division and growth. Otto Warburg, a German biochemist, noted over 80 years ago that many cancers use glucose as their primary energy substrate for this process (8). As the cancer cells grow, they often become starved of oxygen and therefore anaerobic metabolism of glucose becomes easier to sustain than aerobic metabolism, within the tricarboxylic acid cycle. The result of this is an increase in utilization of glucose within cancer cells, relative to most normal cells. Thus, a cancer cell will tend to have a much greater metabolic rate than the average normal cell.

Some cells within the body can use several different energy sources to fulfill their metabolic needs. Cardiac muscle, for example, preferentially uses free fatty acids as an energy source, but can also use glucose, lipids or amino acids if required. As a result the glucose uptake within the heart varies between people and can change considerably within an individual over a short period, in relation to the blood glucose at the time. Brain cells do not have the ability to use any fuel other than glucose and consequently the glucose activity within the normal brain is always high. In a fasting state, most body tissues, with the exception of the brain, actually use free fatty acids as their preferred energy source. After a glucose-rich meal, these cells may temporarily switch from free fatty acid to glucose metabolism, under the influence of rising insulin levels.

Transmembrane proteins, called glucose transporters, facilitate glucose uptake into the cell. At least 12 different glucose transporters have been identified and are known as GLUT 1, GLUT 2, and so forth.

When the glucose molecule enters the cell, it usually becomes phosphorylated by the enzyme hexokinase. The resultant compound is glucose-6-phosphate. Under normal circumstances the glucose-6-phosphate will undergo further enzymatic change to be converted into other smaller compounds thereby releasing energy, a process called 'glycolysis'. Alternatively the glucose-6-phosphate may be stored as a future energy reserve in the form of glycogen by the glyconeogenesis pathway, or it can be converted into either lipid or protein by other pathways.

The increased energy demands of a growing cancer cell necessitate a more rapid efficient delivery of glucose. As cellular division and growth proceed, a cancer cell uses some ingenious ways of meeting its energy requirements. First the cell can increase the number of transmembrane GLUT transporters to aid glucose delivery. If this is still not sufficient to meet demand, the cell can then increase the rate of phosphorylation, by up-regulating hexokinase activity. The resultant effect is that many cancer cells demonstrate a marked increase in glucose metabolism when compared to normal cells.

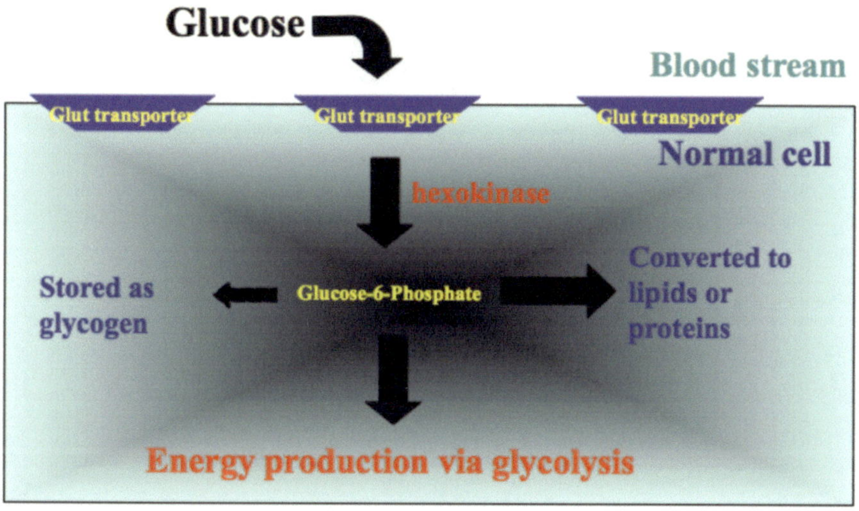

Fig. 1. Uptake and metabolism of glucose in a cell

2.2 Imaging glucose metabolism

FDG is produced in a device called a cyclotron. FDG is a radioactive positron emitter and decays with a half-life of approximately two hours. Due to the relatively long half-life of the FDG, a PET scanner can be located within a 2-hour drive from the cyclotron site. Other positron emitters such as Carbon-11 and Nitrogen-13 have much shorter half-lives and can only be used for PET scanners located in close proximity to a cyclotron.

FDG is injected intravenously and is taken up by normal and cancer cells alike. Cancer cells and normal cells compete with each other for cellular uptake using the GLUT transporters. Within a cell, FDG will be converted into FDG-6-phosphate by the action of hexokinase, just like normal glucose. Beyond this point, the fate of FDG and glucose are different. Due to the isomeric constitution of FDG, it cannot undergo further enzymatic change, unlike the glucose molecule. As a result, their pathways diverge; glucose is converted into either energy or stored as glycogen, whereas FDG undergoes no further metabolism and mostly remains trapped in the cell.

The distribution of radioactivity within the body can be imaged using a specialized camera called a PET scanner. An image gives a picture of the areas of the body that have FDG and therefore glucose uptake. The intense accumulation of FDG within many cancer cells allows those cells to be identified, compared to the less intense uptake in normal cells. Patients are imaged in the fasting state since most normal cells will more likely be using free fatty acids as their energy substrate. Figure 2 is a PET scan showing the normal distribution of glucose as identified by FDG uptake.

This image is called the maximum intensity projection image or MIP and is the two-dimensional representation of the accumulation of FDG uptake in the body as a whole. We can see that the brain has intense uptake, with less marked uptake in the heart, liver and spleen. We also see intense uptake in the renal system. Individuals, under normal circumstances, do not excrete glucose through the urinary system. Although FDG is an analogue of glucose, it behaves differently in this regard and is excreted in large amounts through the renal system. Whereas most normal glucose is freely filtered within the renal glomeruli and rapidly reabsorbed by the nephron, filtered FDG is poorly reabsorbed and a large proportion is excreted in the urine.

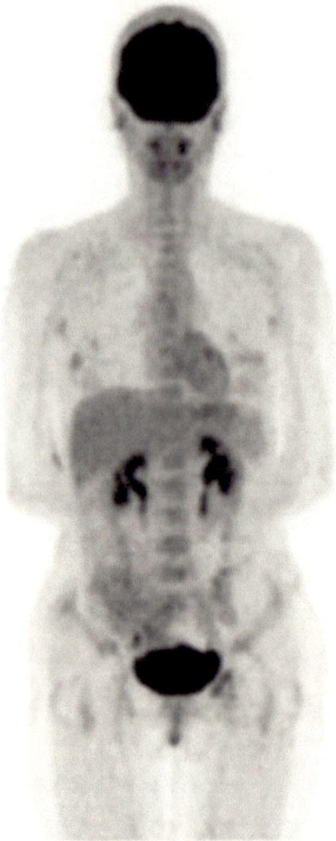

Fig. 2. The distribution of FDG within a normal individual

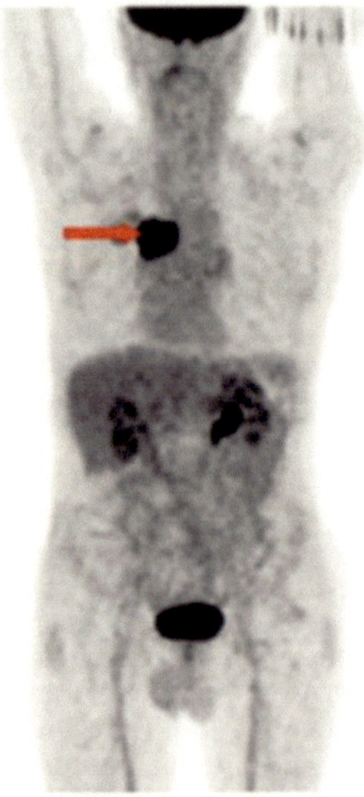

Fig. 3. A FDG +ve right hilar squamous cell carcinoma.

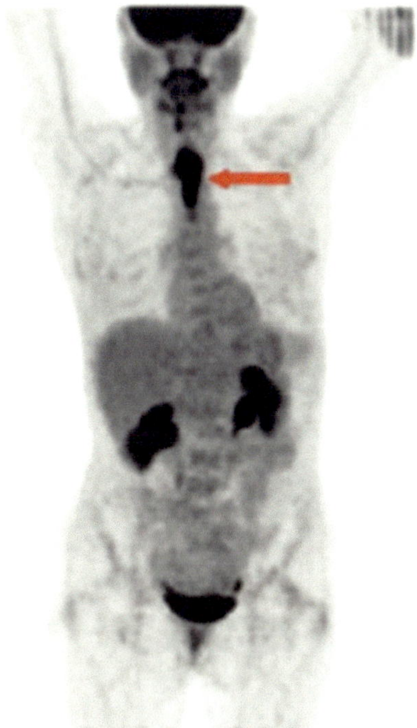

Fig. 4. An upper oesophageal squamous cell carcinoma.

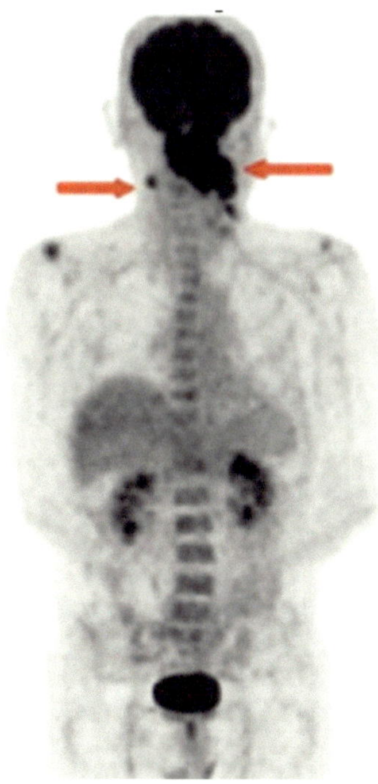

Fig. 5. A naso-pharyngeal lymphoma with bilateral neck node involvement.

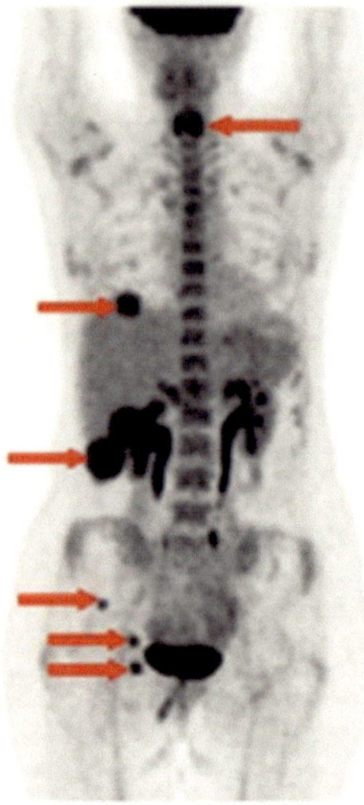

Fig. 6. Recurrent colorectal cancer with metabolically active deposits in the liver and right hemipelvis. The uptake in the neck is due to a coincidental thyroiditis.

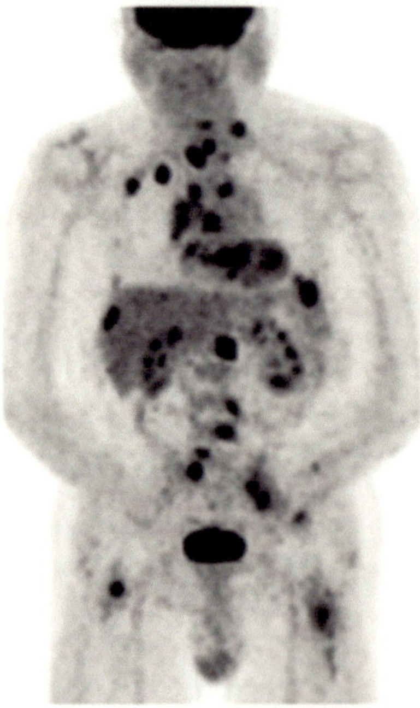

Fig. 7. Multiple bony metastatic deposits.

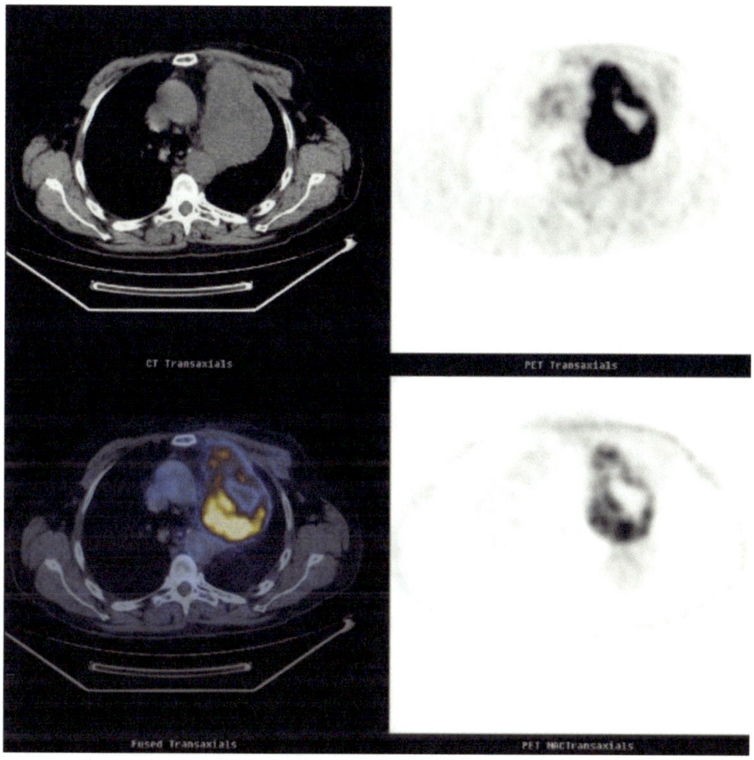

Fig. 8. Fused PET-CT image of a lung cancer.

Figure 3 to 7 is abnormal PET scans with the abnormality highlighted by arrows. Figure 8 is an example of a fused PET-CT image. The CT component is viewed in the top left hand corner and the attenuation-corrected PET in the top right hand corner. This image uses the CT data to correct for the effect of different positron absorption within different density tissues of the patient. The more intense the FDG (or glucose) uptake, the blacker it appears on the PET scan.

The fused PET-CT scan is seen in the bottom left hand corner of the image. This combines the anatomical data from the CT and the metabolic data from the PET, the colour scale chosen, shows the FDG uptake as increasingly orange to yellow, with increasing activity. The bottom right hand image is the non-attenuated PET image, which is effectively the raw PET data.

2.3 Scanning protocol and imaging sequence

Patients should arrive at the nuclear medicine department having fasted for at least four hours. This ensures most tissues are using free fatty acids as their energy source. Diabetic patients are advised to take their normal insulin or medication prior to arriving at the department.

After the staff has made all the necessary patient checks including correct patient identification and a check of blood glucose level, the injection of radioactive FDG can take place. The patient is advised to lie still for approximately 45 minutes to allow the FDG enough time to accumulate in metabolically active cells. Any unnecessary patient movement during this uptake period can result in muscular uptake than can cause confusion with later scan interpretation. Patients who are tense during this time often show physiological uptake within the muscles of the neck.

Following the uptake period, the patient is taken into the scanning room and lies supine on the table. A picture of a GE Discovery Lightspeed PET-CT scanner is shown in Figure 9.

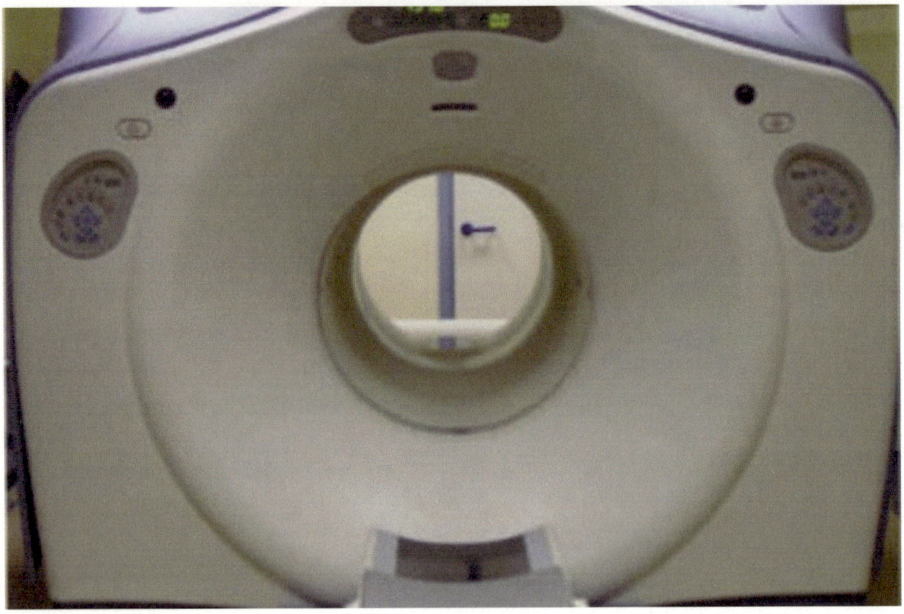

Fig. 9. GE Discovery Lightspeed PET-CT

Many centres now routinely use oral contrast enhancement to help visualise the bowel. Some centres also now recommend the use of intravenous contrast but this is presently not routine practice in the UK.

The CT scan is normally carried out from the base of skull to mid-thigh level. There are a number of reasons for performing this and not a whole body scan:

1. Brain metastases are difficult to detect using FDG as any brain lesion must have an intensity greater than or less than the surrounding brain tissue to be identified.
2. Only a few tumours have metastatic potential to disseminate to the distal lower limbs.
3. There is a decreased radiation burden to the patient from the CT.
4. There is a considerable amount of time saved which can be used to increase the patient throughput.

Whole body scans are carried out in some circumstances, for example patients with melanoma due to the widespread and unpredictable lymphatic dissemination that characterises this disease. A similar problem is encountered with the pattern of disease spread in non-Hodgkin's lymphoma, which often requires a larger scanning volume. Patients with head and neck disease often have scans that include the entire skull, and patients with soft tissue sarcomas may also require additional views.

After the CT images are acquired, which only takes a minute or so, when using a modern multislice scanner, the patient is then scanned again using the PET component of the machine. The detectors on the PET scanner can identify radioactive emissions from the FDG within the body. A ring of detectors surrounds the patient. This ring is approximately 15 cm long and images are therefore acquired in blocks of 15 cm from the base of the skull to mid thigh. In most individuals this area is covered in about five blocks (~75 cm), taller or shorter individuals will take more or less imaging time. The time required for each 15 cm image of the patient is between three and five minutes. This means that the PET component of the study can take at least 15-45 minutes to acquire. Any patient movement during this time will degrade the quality of the images obtained.

After the PET scan has been acquired the patient is free to go but is given warnings about exposure to individuals during the next few hours as the radioactivity decays and is excreted from the body.

2.4 Standard uptake value

A semi quantitative method is available to calculate the intensity of FDG uptake within a range of interest on the PET scan. This value is called the Standardised Uptake Value, SUV, and takes account of factors such as injected activity, patient weight and time from injection. Simply speaking, the SUV assumes that if there's an even distribution of radioactivity throughout the body the SUV would be measured as one. Obviously this is not the case but we can calculate the relative uptake within different parts of the body and relate them to each other. An area with an SUV of five means this area has five times the average uptake. Certain modifications can be made to the SUV calculation to take into account, for example, the patient's body fat, since FDG is not generally taken up into fatty tissue.

The SUV allows comparisons to be made between different parts of the body and between different scans on the same patient over a period of time. It must be emphasised that the SUV is only a semi-quantitative measurement and can vary considerably with changes in the patient's plasma glucose level and are dependent on the uptake time allowed prior to scanning. Therefore, is it important that PET facilities use a standard scanning and imaging protocol for all their patients.

It is the SUVmax that is usually quoted in PET reports and measured in research studies. However there is a growing interest in the measurement of SUVmean, as it is less susceptible to outliers. The maximum SUV represents only one single pixel (the pixel with the maximum SUV within the entire tumour), whereas, the mean SUV in a region of interest, represents the average SUV of the given number of pixels within the ROI. Some clinicians prefer to avoid numbers altogether, and simply use visual interpretation to compare the intensity of one area to another using the background blood pool as a guide to normality. There is evidence to suggest that both methods are equally accurate.

3. The prognostic potential of PET-CT in the clinical management of oesophageal cancer

3.1 Introduction

Oesophageal cancer is staged according to the current American Joint Committee on Cancer guidelines, which incorporate the T, N and M classification (9). The current staging modalities utilize an array of morphological imaging studies, and more recently, minimally invasive surgical techniques, to bridge the gap between clinical and pathological staging. The introduction of PET-CT has provided an incremental yield to the diagnostic accuracy in oesophageal cancer staging (10-11). PET-CT provides an increased sensitivity and specificity of metastatic disease compared to other morphological imaging techniques (PET-CT vs CT: sensitivity 71% vs 52% and specificity 93% vs 91%), changing the operability in up to 20% of patients (12-13).

PET-CT also provides a semi-quantitative value of biological aggressiveness of a malignancy by reporting the standard uptake value, which represents the amount of metabolic activity within the tumour. Like certain biochemical indices, this amount of metabolic activity has been shown to be related to the clinical behaviour for a specific type of tumour for a given patient (7, 14-19). Therefore, it has been suggested that the FDG SUV value, may have a role as a predictive tool for patient outcome in oesophageal cancer (7, 17-19). This has already been demonstrated in other types of malignancies such as lung cancer and head and neck cancer (20-21). However, to our knowledge, there are only limited data available with regards to oesophageal cancer (7, 17-19).

3.2 Methods and materials

3.2.1 Patient population

All patients diagnosed with oesophageal carcinoma that had undergone staging PET-CT imaging between the period of June 2002 and May 2008, were included in this study. The eligibility criteria included only patients diagnosed with adenocarcinoma or squamous carcinoma of the oesophagus, (specifically excluding lesions confined to the upper third of the oesophagus), including those who were suitable for curative surgery, either with or without neo-adjuvant chemotherapy.

Studies were performed at a single institution (Regional Thoracic Surgical Unit, Royal Victoria Hospital, Belfast) with a standardised procedure, a Total Thoracic Oesophagectomy with a cervical anastomosis and two field lymphadenectomy. All patients were discussed at a surgical cancer network multidisciplinary meeting that included a thoracic or upper gastrointestinal surgeon, a nuclear medicine radiologist, an oncologist and a pathologist.

The study protocol was approved by our local research ethics committee (08/NIR03/106). Only electronic patient files including cancer network meetings, pathology reports and nuclear medicine imaging were used to collect the clinical information.

3.2.2 Patient image acquisition of FGD PET-CT data

Patients were scanned after injection of 370MBq 18F-FDG and an uptake period of 45 minutes, on a GE Discovery Light Speed PET-CT scanner, using a standard diagnostic protocol.

3.2.3 Measurement of prognostic variables and clinical outcome

Standardised Uptake Value (SUVmean and SUVmax)

A region of interest (ROI) was created for every individual patient based on the diameter of the FDG avid oesophageal lesion, on the attenuated corrected PET image, with side by side comparison with the CT image. The ROI ranged from 1cm to 3cm in diameter accordingly. This was to prevent overestimation, if a large ROI was used from neighbouring structures especially the heart, or underestimation, if a small predetermined ROI was used. The SUVmean and SUVmax were calculated, with the SUVmean taken at the same corresponding level as the SUVmax for that particular patient.

Clinical Outcome

The outcome evaluated was overall survival, which was from the date of surgery to death, identified from the Hospital Episode Statistics Data. Follow-up was through March 2009, constituting our censoring date for survival.

3.2.4 Surgery and pathological staging

Only patients with middle, lower or OGJ tumours involved were included in this study, with a standard total thoracic oesophagectomy being performed in all patients. This consists of a left thorocolaparotomy incision, resection of all the thoracic and abdominal oesophagus with two field lymphadenectomy, mobilisation of the stomach on the right gastro-epiploic arcade, creating a neo-oesophagus that is then anastomosed in the neck via a left oblique cervical incison. The same experienced surgical team performed all procedures. A single pathologist reported all pathological specimens using the current TNM staging.

3.2.5 Statistical analysis

The associations between the SUVmax and SUVmean with clinical staging (T and N categories) were assessed using analysis of variance or t-test. Pearson's correlation was used to assess the association between the different prognostic variables. Log-Rank and Cox regression tests were performed for disease free survival analysis. A $p < 0.05$ was considered significant. All statistical analysis was performed using the SPSS Version 18 (SPSS, Chicago, IL).

3.3 Results

There were a total of 96 patients during this study period that underwent staging FDG PET-CT scans. Fifty-three patients proceeded to receive neo-adjuvant chemotherapy followed by surgery. A response scan was performed 3 weeks after completion of neo-adjuvant treatment. The remaining 43 patients proceeded directly to surgery following their staging PET-CT.

From the 96 patients, 68.7% had adenocarcinoma and 31.3% had squamous carcinoma. Tumours were located predominantly in the lower oesophagus, 59.4%, followed by OGJ and middle oesophageal lesions, with 25% and 15.6% respectively (Figure 10)

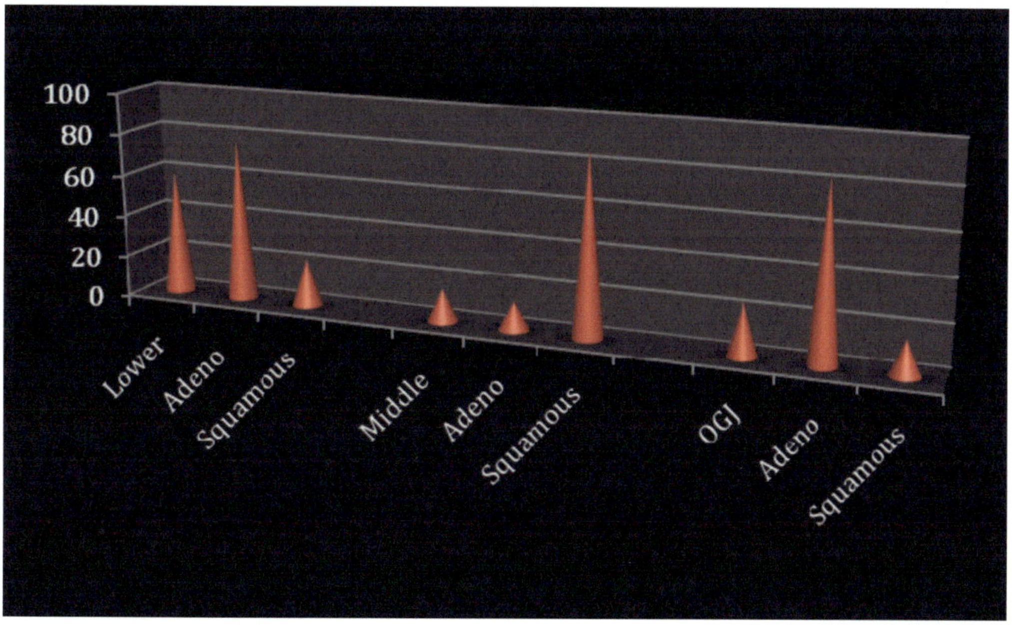

Fig. 10. Distribution of tissue type according to location.

The mean and median Staging SUV values were 10.3 and 9.3 for SUVmax, and, 6 and 5.8 for SUVmean, with a fairly normal distribution for SUVmean within the population studied (Figure 11 and 12).

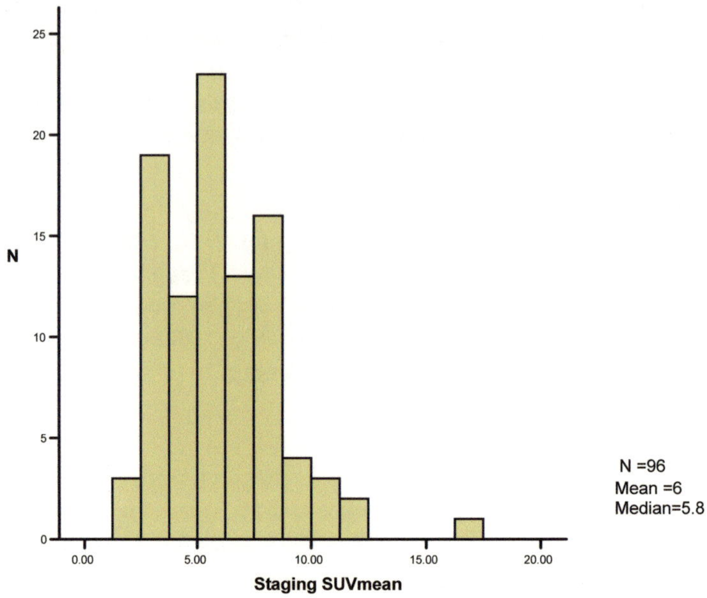

Fig. 11. Distribution of Staging SUVmean amongst study population.

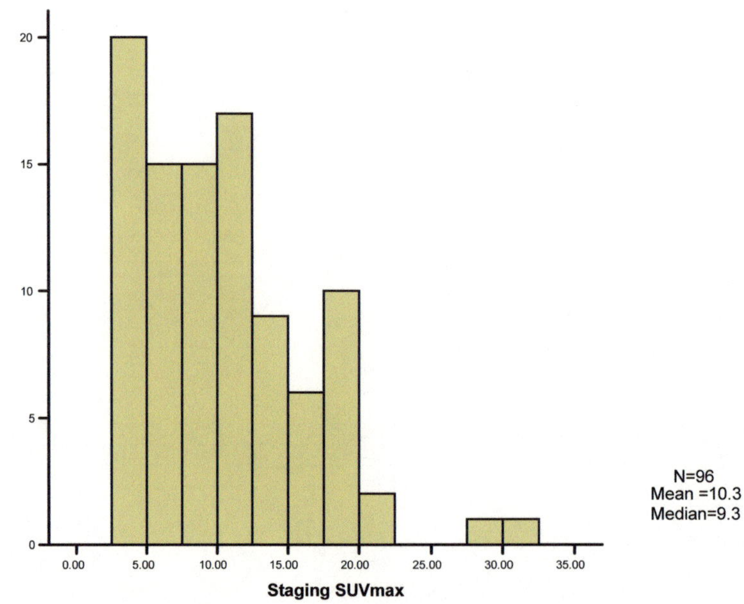

Fig. 12. Distribution of Staging SUVmax amongst the study population.

Both the Staging SUVmax and SUVmean correlated well, with a Pearson's correlation coefficient of 0.91 ($p<0.01$), Figure 13.

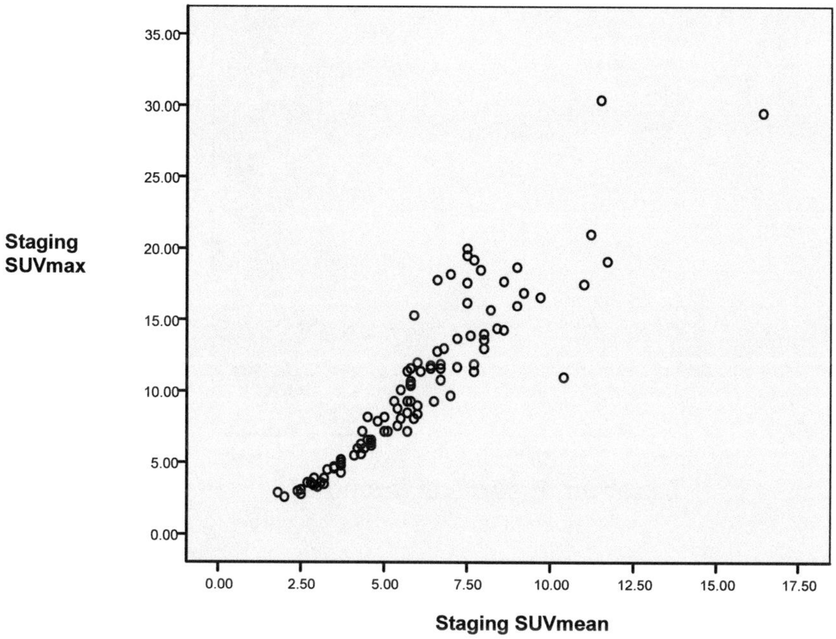

Fig. 13. Pearson's Correlation between SUVmax and SUVmean.

SUV_{max} and SUV_{mean} were both influenced by tissue type, with squamous carcinoma having a significantly higher uptake than adenocarcinoma, SUVmax 13.6 vs 8.8 ($p<0.01$) and SUVmean 7.3 vs 5.3 ($p<0.01$) respectively. SUVmax and SUVmean also varied according to locality, with tumours located in the middle oesophagus having the highest SUV uptake followed by the lower and then OGJ tumours. SUVmax varied from 13.4 to 10.5 to 8.0 ($p=0.02$) and for SUVmean from 6.7 to 6.1 to 5.2 ($p=0.14$) respectively. Logistic regression analysis demonstrated that the SUVmax dropped by 2.6 ($p<0.01$) and SUVmean by 0.8 ($p=0.05$) between tumour locations from proximal to distal oesophagus. However, the effect of tumour location on SUVmax ($p=0.23$) and SUVmean ($p=0.37$) lost its significance when corrected for tissue type.

Prognostically, staging SUVmean had a significant correlation with survival in patients with SUV values of less than 5 having a better survival than those above 5 ($p=0.02$), Figure 14. The risk of death was 2.4 times higher (95% CI 1.1, 5.0, $p=0.02$) in the latter group, after correcting for patients age, tumour type and tumour location. This survival advantage, however, wasn't demonstrated with a SUVmax of 10 and above ($p=0.14$), Figure 15. The effect of chemotherapy did not seem to influence survival in this cohort of patients ($p=0.20$).

Patients with advanced tumours, seemed to demonstrate an increase in metabolic activity, reflected by the increase in SUV uptake. The SUVmax for high-grade dysplasia, Stage I, II and III were 3.5, 5.1, 11.6 and 9.6 ($p=0.02$) and for SUVmean were 2.9, 3.9, 6.5 and 5.3 ($p=0.03$) respectively. Patients with nodal disease also demonstrated an increase in SUV uptake compared to N0 disease, with SUVmax of 11.4 versus 7.4 ($p=0.02$) and SUVmean of 6.1 versus 4.6 ($p=0.03$) respectively.

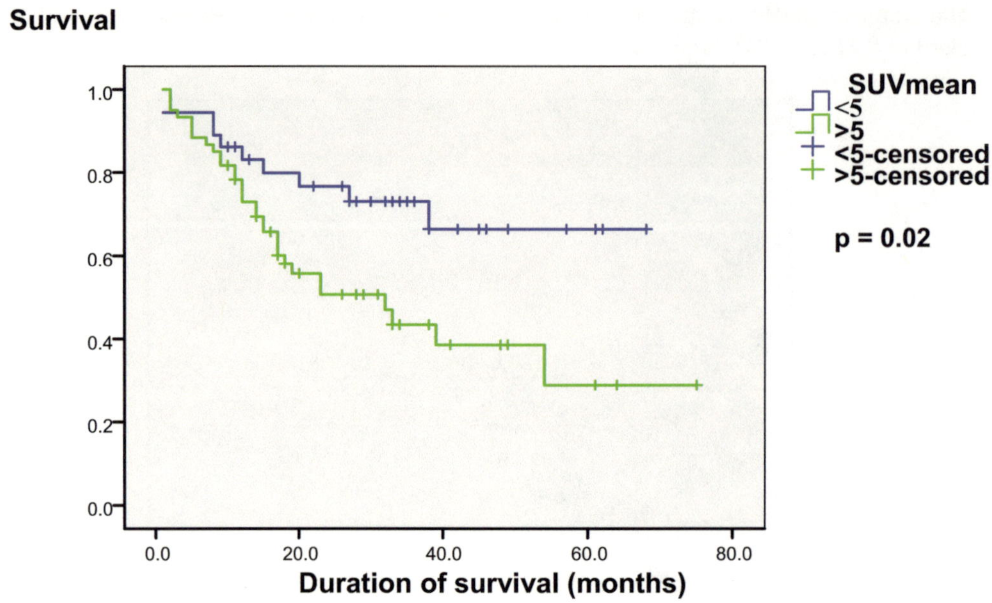

Fig. 14. Survival in operable oesophageal cancer patients around a SUVmean of 5.

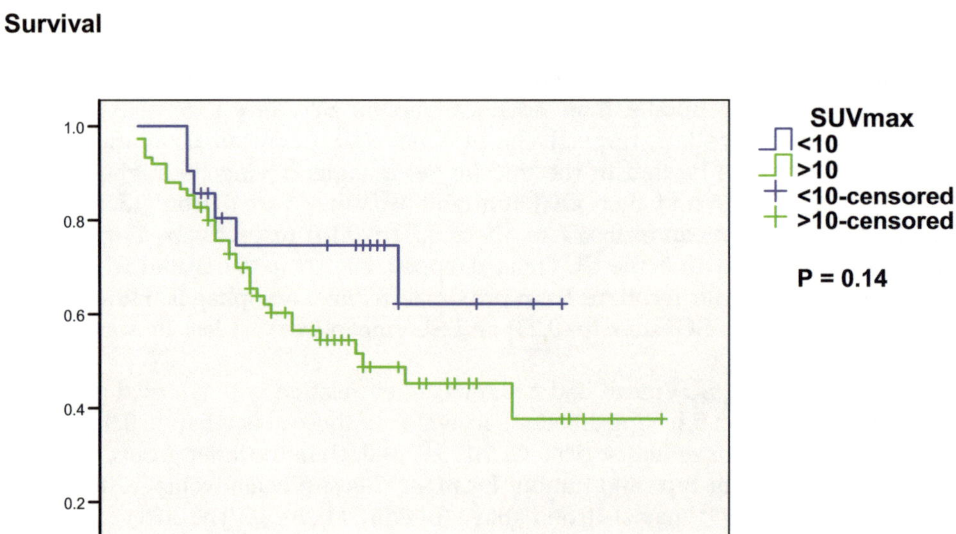

Fig. 15. Survival in operable oesophageal cancer patients around a SUVmax of 10.

3.4 Discussion

The treatment of oesophageal cancer, like any other solid organ tumour, is dependent of the stage of the cancer. However, the current TNM staging system is based only on anatomic and not on any biological factors. Interestingly, there is increasing evidence to suggest that biological factors influence prognosis just as much, if not more than, anatomical factors (22-24). FDG PET may aid in the detection of some of these biological factors that can't be identified with the current morphological imaging techniques. FDG PET has emerged as a useful metabolism-based whole body non-invasive imaging technique for the detection, characterization and staging of oesophageal cancer in recent years (25).

Van Westreenen et al. in a meta-analysis of the staging performance of FDG PET in oesophageal cancer, was able to demonstrate a moderate sensitivity and specificity for the detection of loco-regional metastases, but a reasonable sensitivity and specificity for the detection of distant metastases (26). The limited sensitivity and specificity for loco-regional metastases is due to the reduced spatial and contrast resolutions of PET-CT, and therefore limits visualization of the anatomic extent of the primary tumour as well as the ability to differentiate peri-oesophageal lymph nodes from the primary tumour (27). However, most morphological imaging scans as well as minimally invasive staging methods are able to compensate for this with a high accuracy for T and N staging. PET-CT, however, does have an excellent accuracy for the detection of M staging, accounting for up to 40% change in treatment strategies in patients as described by Chatterton et al. (28).

Recently, there is a growing body of evidence to suggest the prognostic potential of PET-CT in patients with oesophageal cancer, apart from its utility as a tool for radiotherapy planning or measuring tumour response in patients receiving neo-adjuvant treatment (7, 17-19). Its ability to identify metabolic activity within tumours reflects the biological aggressiveness of these cancers. This was first demonstrated by Fukunaga et al., who reported that patients with high SUV value within the primary tumour have a worse prognosis than those patients with a low SUV (29). A recent meta-analysis by Pan et al. demonstrated that patients with high SUV value not only have a worse survival prognosis, HR: 1.86, but also a reduced disease free survival with early recurrence, HR: 2.52 (30). The majority of these studies use SUVmax, to distinguish high from low SUV groups (30). Only one study utilized SUVmean (30).

From our data, we were able to demonstrate the independent predictor of survival using SUVmean and not SUVmax, both with univariate and multivariate analysis. SUVmean is less susceptible to outliers, but bear in mind, this study also showed both SUVmean and SUVmax to correlate well, with a correlation coefficient close to 1, and therefore it would be premature to disregard the prognostic potential of SUVmax. Hence, they should be used hand in hand to complement each other.

The metabolic activity is influenced by the biological properties of the tumour as we know. We demonstrated that squamous carcinomas have a higher SUVmax and SUVmean uptake compared to adenocarcinomas. Unfortunately, due to the small number in our series, we were unable to analyse the prognostic potential of the SUV values within the individual tumour types. Interestingly, both tumour types had a similar range distribution, with squamous carcinomas SUVmax and SUVmean ranging from 3.5 to 30.5 and 3.2 to 11.5 respectively, and, with adenocarcinomas SUVmax and SUVmean ranging from 2.6 to 29.5 and 2 to 16.4 respectively. Also, in the multivariate analysis, SUVmean was shown to be an independent predictor of survival after taking into account of tumour type.

The prognostic potential of SUV is strengthened by its relationship to the T and N staging. We found a linear increase in SUVmax and mean with the T staging apart for stage III, where there was a slight decrease. This could be attributed to the fact that there were more adenocarcinomas than squamous carcinomas (64% vs 36%). Also, the SUVmax and mean within the primary tumour also related significantly to nodal disease, with a higher incidence of nodal involvement when the SUVmean was greater than 5 (50% vs 23.5%). This relationship between metabolic activity and the current morphological staging has been correlated in only a handful number of papers (7, 17-18).

Finally, how do we translate the wealth of information we obtain from morphological, biological, biochemical and minimally invasive techniques to these patients diagnosed with oesophageal cancer? As we already now, the incidence of oesophageal cancer varies according to geographic location, as well as the treatment practices (31). Apart from the TNM staging which provides prognostic information to the clinician, it allows treatment based algorithms to be compared, with the idea of producing a uniform framework, enabling multi-disciplinary teams to tailor their treatment appropriately according to the disease stage. However, there are subgroups of patients where, surgery alone, even in early cancers (T2N0) will not provide cure, or cases, where surgery itself is prohibitive due to the significant co-morbidities of the patient. Here, the additional biological information provided by PET-CT can better inform the multi-disciplinary team and treat the patient accordingly.

For example patients who are currently staged as T2N0 oesophageal cancers, have no agreed consensus with regards to their optimal therapy. The risk-benefit analysis of proceeding directly to surgery, or being treated initially with neo-adjuvant treatment followed by surgery, fails to reach a clear consensus. When we analysed our data pertaining to this subgroup, it was interesting to find out that patients with a SUVmean < 5 (n=6), only 1 patient died, due to peri-operative complications. However, in patients with a SUVmean > 5 (n=11), 2 patients died due to recurrent disease, both of which were not treated with neo-adjuvant treatment. The remaining patients were alive, taking into account that nearly 90% of these patients had received neo-adjuvant treatment. Though these numbers seem small, the fact that these early tumours with an SUV > 5 demonstrate a greater malignant potential should alert the multi-disciplinary team to adjust their treatment accordingly.

In conclusion, apart from PET-CT serving as a staging modality for oesophageal cancer, it provides important biological information that reflects the metabolic activity of the tumour. This pre-treatment or staging SUV, can provide important prognostic information that can supplement the current TNM staging to improve our decision making process, to ensure patients with oesophageal cancer receive the appropriate treatment care.

4. Future developments of PET-CT

As technology improvements parallel the increase utility of PET-CT, we anticipate further development prospects within the field of metabolic imaging. One such area is the development of new novel tracers that mimic cellular mechanisms, other than glucose uptake. Already tracers exist which can identify regions of hypoxia, examples include, Flourine and Copper labelled compounds, such as, (18F-fluoromisonidazole, 18F-fluoroazomycinarabinofuranoside, 64Cu-ATSM, and 18F-EF5). These tracers can modify chemotherapy and radiotherapy by highlighting areas of hypoxia. These regions can be particularly difficult to treat, and resistant clonal elements can survive, due to the delivery of sub toxic therapies. With this knowledge, dose modification can be carried out, for example using Intensity Modulated Radiotherapy (IMRT). Other potential areas for research include the development of tracers to assess the rate of tumour proliferation and the prospective clinical application of the integrated MRI-PET.

Another growing utility of PET-CT is the ability to predict tumour response to neo-adjuvant treatment by PET-CT (6, 32-35). Metabolic response is suggested when there was a certain relative decrease of the SUV between staging and response PET-CT scans, Figure 16.

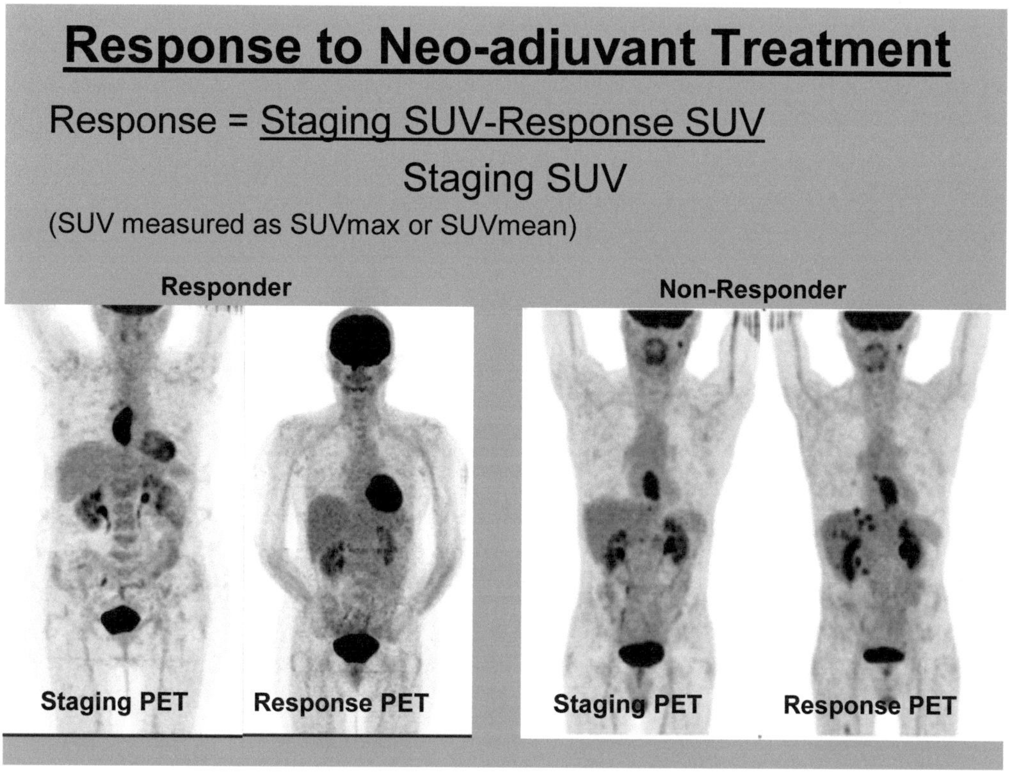

Fig. 16. Response measurement.

Several studies have concluded that FDG-PET is an effective modality for the non-invasive assessment of pathologic tumour response to neo-adjuvant treatment, but other investigations have seen no association between metabolic and histopathologic response (6, 32-35). The reason for these discrepancies between studies could be explained, at least in part, by various confounding factors that have an effect on SUV measurements; such as tissue activity factors, tissue state factors or normalisation factor; but also in part, by the definition of response in these respective studies (36). Simply using a specific cut-off value of SUV, to determine metabolic response from the response PET-CT scan, would be inappropriate, as we have demonstrated a wide distribution of SUV uptake amongst patients with oesophageal cancer, Figures 11 & 12 (34, 37). Additionally, the inflammatory response post neo-adjuvant treatment can complicate the interpretation of metabolic response, increasing the false positive rate of non-responders, as most of these patients have a background diffuse low FDG uptake, with an SUV value as high as 2.6 as demonstrated by Wieder et al (38). More importantly, as we have demonstrated, the biology tissue type influences the SUV uptake, both max and mean, and therefore using a percentage drop of the SUV from the staging to response PET-CT scan would be more judicious.

Recent evidence would suggest an interval PET-CT at 14 days after commencing neo-adjuvant treatment, to judge treatment response and therefore determine further treatment course. Wieder et al was able to demonstrate this, predicting histopathologic response with a sensitivity and specificity of 93% and 88%, respectively, with treatment induced oesophagitis observed in less than 15% of the scans (38). Furthermore, the decrease in metabolic activity at 14 days was significantly associated with overall survival (38). This was also confirmed in the

MUNICON trial, confirming the usefulness of early response evaluation by PET, and therefore tailoring multimodal treatment in accordance with individual tumour biology (39). We anticipate that PET-CT will have a significant impact on patient management by allowing a new means to individualize neo-adjuvant treatment in patients with oesophageal cancer.

5. References

[1] Office of National Statistics, 2010 Mortality Statistics: Deaths Registered in England & Wales, 2008.

[2] Northern Ireland Statistics & Research Agency: Registrar General Annual Report 2010

[3] General Register Office for Scotland, 2010 Deaths Time Series Data, 1997-2008

[4] Jeganathan R, Kinnear H, Campbell J, Jordan S, Graham A, Gavin A, et al. A surgeon's case volume of oesophagectomy for cancer does not influence patient outcome in a high volume hospital. Interact.Cardiovasc.Thorac.Surg. 2009 Jul;9(1):66-69.

[5] Bruzzi JF, Munden RF, Truong MT, Marom EM, Sabloff BS, Gladish GW, et al. PET/CT of esophageal cancer: its role in clinical management. Radiographics 2007 Nov-Dec;27(6):1635-1652.

[6] Ott K, Weber WA, Lordick F, Becker K, Busch R, Herrmann K, et al. Metabolic imaging predicts response, survival, and recurrence in adenocarcinomas of the esophagogastric junction. J.Clin.Oncol. 2006 Oct 10;24(29):4692-4698.

[7] Cerfolio RJ, Bryant AS. Maximum standardized uptake values on positron emission tomography of esophageal cancer predicts stage, tumor biology, and survival. Ann.Thorac.Surg. 2006 Aug;82(2):391-4; discussion 394-5.

[8] Warburg O, Wind F, Negelein E. The Metabolism of Tumors in the Body. J.Gen.Physiol. 1927 Mar 7;8(6):519-530.

[9] Greene F, Fritz A, Balch C, et al. Esophagus. In: Greene F, Fritz A, Balch C, et al, eds. AJCC cancer staging handbook part III: digestive system-9 esophagus. 6th ed. New York, NY: Springer- Verlag, 2002.

[10] Kato H, Miyazaki T, Nakajima M, Takita J, Kimura H, Faried A, et al. The incremental effect of positron emission tomography on diagnostic accuracy in the initial staging of esophageal carcinoma. Cancer 2005 Jan 1;103(1):148-156.

[11] Kato H, Fukuchi M, Miyazaki T, et al. Positron emission tomography in esophageal cancer. Esophagus. 2005;2:111-121.

[12] van Vliet EP, Heijenbrok-Kal MH, Hunink MG, Kuipers EJ, Siersema PD. Staging investigations for oesophageal cancer: a meta-analysis. Br.J.Cancer 2008 Feb 12;98(3):547-557.

[13] Weber WA, Ott K. Imaging of esophageal and gastric cancer. Semin.Oncol. 2004 Aug;31(4):530-541.

[14] Wayman J, O'Hanlon D, Hayes N, Shaw I, Griffin SM. Fibrinogen levels correlate with stage of disease in patients with oesophageal cancer. Br.J.Surg. 1997 Feb;84(2):185-188.

[15] Shimada H, Oohira G, Okazumi S, Matsubara H, Nabeya Y, Hayashi H, et al. Thrombocytosis associated with poor prognosis in patients with esophageal carcinoma. J.Am.Coll.Surg. 2004 May;198(5):737-741.

[16] Guillem P, Triboulet JP. Elevated serum levels of C-reactive protein are indicative of a poor prognosis in patients with esophageal cancer. Dis.Esophagus 2005;18(3):146-150.

[17] Kato H, Nakajima M, Sohda M, Tanaka N, Inose T, Miyazaki T, et al. The clinical application of (18)F-fluorodeoxyglucose positron emission tomography to predict

survival in patients with operable esophageal cancer. Cancer 2009 Jul 15;115(14):3196-3203.
[18] Rizk N, Downey RJ, Akhurst T, Gonen M, Bains MS, Larson S, et al. Preoperative 18[F]-fluorodeoxyglucose positron emission tomography standardized uptake values predict survival after esophageal adenocarcinoma resection. Ann.Thorac.Surg. 2006 Mar;81(3):1076-1081.
[19] Choi JY, Jang HJ, Shim YM, Kim K, Lee KS, Lee KH, et al. 18F-FDG PET in patients with esophageal squamous cell carcinoma undergoing curative surgery: prognostic implications. J.Nucl.Med. 2004 Nov;45(11):1843-1850.
[20] Downey RJ, Akhurst T, Gonen M, Vincent A, Bains MS, Larson S, et al. Preoperative F-18 fluorodeoxyglucose-positron emission tomography maximal standardized uptake value predicts survival after lung cancer resection. J.Clin.Oncol. 2004 Aug 15;22(16):3255-3260.
[21] Sanghera B, Wong WL, Lodge MA, Hain S, Stott D, Lowe J, et al. Potential novel application of dual time point SUV measurements as a predictor of survival in head and neck cancer. Nucl.Med.Commun. 2005 Oct;26(10):861-867.
[22] Wijnhoven BP, Pignatelli M, Dinjens WN, Tilanus HW. Reduced p120ctn expression correlates with poor survival in patients with adenocarcinoma of the gastroesophageal junction. J.Surg.Oncol. 2005 Nov 1;92(2):116-123.
[23] Yamazaki K, Hasegawa M, Ohoka I, Hanami K, Asoh A, Nagao T, et al. Increased E2F-1 expression via tumour cell proliferation and decreased apoptosis are correlated with adverse prognosis in patients with squamous cell carcinoma of the oesophagus. J.Clin.Pathol. 2005 Sep;58(9):904-910.
[24] Kato H, Takita J, Miyazaki T, Nakajima M, Fukai Y, Masuda N, et al. Correlation of 18-F-fluorodeoxyglucose (FDG) accumulation with glucose transporter (Glut-1) expression in esophageal squamous cell carcinoma. Anticancer Res. 2003 Jul-Aug;23(4):3263-3272.
[25] Kuipers EJ, Haringsma J. Diagnostic and therapeutic endoscopy. J.Surg.Oncol. 2005 Dec 1;92(3):203-209.
[26] van Westreenen HL, Westerterp M, Bossuyt PM, Pruim J, Sloof GW, van Lanschot JJ, et al. Systematic review of the staging performance of 18F-fluorodeoxyglucose positron emission tomography in esophageal cancer. J.Clin.Oncol. 2004 Sep 15;22(18):3805-3812.
[27] Rice TW. Clinical staging of esophageal carcinoma. CT, EUS, and PET. Chest Surg.Clin.N.Am. 2000 Aug;10(3):471-485.
[28] Chatterton BE, Ho Shon I, Baldey A, Lenzo N, Patrikeos A, Kelley B, et al. Positron emission tomography changes management and prognostic stratification in patients with oesophageal cancer: results of a multicentre prospective study. Eur.J.Nucl.Med.Mol.Imaging 2009 Mar;36(3):354-361.
[29] Fukunaga T, Okazumi S, Koide Y, Isono K, Imazeki K. Evaluation of esophageal cancers using fluorine-18-fluorodeoxyglucose PET. J.Nucl.Med. 1998 Jun;39(6):1002-1007.
[30] Pan L, Gu P, Huang G, Xue H, Wu S. Prognostic significance of SUV on PET/CT in patients with esophageal cancer: a systematic review and meta-analysis. Eur.J.Gastroenterol.Hepatol. 2009 Sep;21(9):1008-1015.
[31] Parkin DM, Bray F, Ferlay J, Pisani P. Global cancer statistics, 2002. CA Cancer.J.Clin. 2005 Mar-Apr;55(2):74-108.

[32] Downey RJ, Akhurst T, Ilson D, Ginsberg R, Bains MS, Gonen M, et al. Whole body 18FDG-PET and the response of esophageal cancer to induction therapy: results of a prospective trial. J.Clin.Oncol. 2003 Feb 1;21(3):428-432.

[33] Kato H, Kuwano H, Nakajima M, Miyazaki T, Yoshikawa M, Masuda N, et al. Usefulness of positron emission tomography for assessing the response of neoadjuvant chemoradiotherapy in patients with esophageal cancer. Am.J.Surg. 2002 Sep;184(3):279-283.

[34] Song SY, Kim JH, Ryu JS, Lee GH, Kim SB, Park SI, et al. FDG-PET in the prediction of pathologic response after neoadjuvant chemoradiotherapy in locally advanced, resectable esophageal cancer. Int.J.Radiat.Oncol.Biol.Phys. 2005 Nov 15;63(4):1053-1059.

[35] Brink I, Hentschel M, Bley TA, Walch A, Mix M, Kleimaier M, et al. Effects of neoadjuvant radio-chemotherapy on 18F-FDG-PET in esophageal carcinoma. Eur.J.Surg.Oncol. 2004 Jun;30(5):544-550.

[36] van Baardwijk A, Baumert BG, Bosmans G, van Kroonenburgh M, Stroobants S, Gregoire V, et al. The current status of FDG-PET in tumour volume definition in radiotherapy treatment planning. Cancer Treat.Rev. 2006 Jun;32(4):245-260.

[37] Swisher SG, Maish M, Erasmus JJ, Correa AM, Ajani JA, Bresalier R, et al. Utility of PET, CT, and EUS to identify pathologic responders in esophageal cancer. Ann.Thorac.Surg. 2004 Oct;78(4):1152-60; discussion 1152-60.

[38] Wieder HA, Brucher BL, Zimmermann F, Becker K, Lordick F, Beer A, et al. Time course of tumor metabolic activity during chemoradiotherapy of esophageal squamous cell carcinoma and response to treatment. J.Clin.Oncol. 2004 Mar 1;22(5):900-908.

[39] Lordick F, Ott k, Krause BJ, Weber WA, Becker K, Stein HJ, et al. PET to assess early metabolic response and to guide treatment of adenocarcinoma of the oesophagogastric junction: the MUNICON phase II trial. Lancet Oncol. 2007 Sep;8(9):797-805.

27

Extracorporeal Membrane Oxygenation in the Transition of Emergent Thoracic Surgery

Shao-Jung Hsu and Kuang-Yao Yang
Department of Chest Medicine, Taipei Veterans General Hospital, School of Medicine, National Yang-Ming University, Taiwan, Republic of China

1. Introduction

Extracorporeal membrane oxygenation (ECMO) has been used more extensively since it became known as a potential bridge therapy, in patients with severe respiratory failure even under optimum conventional mechanical ventilator support, for further definite therapy. In the area of thoracic surgery, ECMO may have already become a useful life-saving tool but studies on this treatment method remain scarce. Currently available reports and case series reveal that patients with massive hemoptysis or critical tracheal stenosis may be benefit from temporary ECMO therapy during the transition of emergent thoracic surgery.

2. ECMO

ECMO, also called extracorporeal life support, is a type of cardiopulmonary bypass. In May 1953, Gibbon (Gibbon, 1954) used artificial oxygenation and perfusion support for the first successful open heart surgery. Then it was first also effectively used in an adult patient with acute post-traumatic respiratory failure in 1972 (Hill et al., 1972). The following preliminary studies in 1970s suggested that ECMO could support oxygenation in patients with profound respiratory failure. Recently, the CESAR trial demonstrated that ECMO-based management can improve survival in patients with severe acute respiratory failure (Peek et al., 2009). As technological continues to advance, increasing indications and reports suggest that ECMO has a role to play in the transition of emergent thoracic surgery (Hsu et al., 2011).

There are two types of ECMO: venous-arterial (VA) and venous-venous (VV) ECMO. VV ECMO supports isolated oxygenation failure, whereas VA ECMO provides hemodynamic and respiratory support. Although VA ECMO applies cardiopulmonary bypass, it has more complications due to the alteration of hemodynamic system. As a result, VV ECMO is typically used for respiratory failure while VA ECMO is used for cardiac failure.

2.1 Initiation of ECMO

ECMO is composed of a pump, an oxygenator and a heat exchanger. Once cannulation established, a large volume of blood is extracted from vessels by the mechanical pump. It passes through the oxygenator and heat exchanger. The oxygenated blood is then finally re-infused into the vessels. A complete circuit can be established in 40 minutes by an experience team. In VV ECMO, blood is drawn distally into the right atrium and returned into right atrium in an attempt to minimize recirculation. To achieve this, a drainage cannula is inserted in the right common femoral vein and the other infusion cannula is inserted in the right internal jugular vein. The tip of each cannula should be placed near the junction of the vena cava and the right atrium (fig. 1A). Alternatively, a double lumen cannula can be placed in one major vein (fig. 1B).

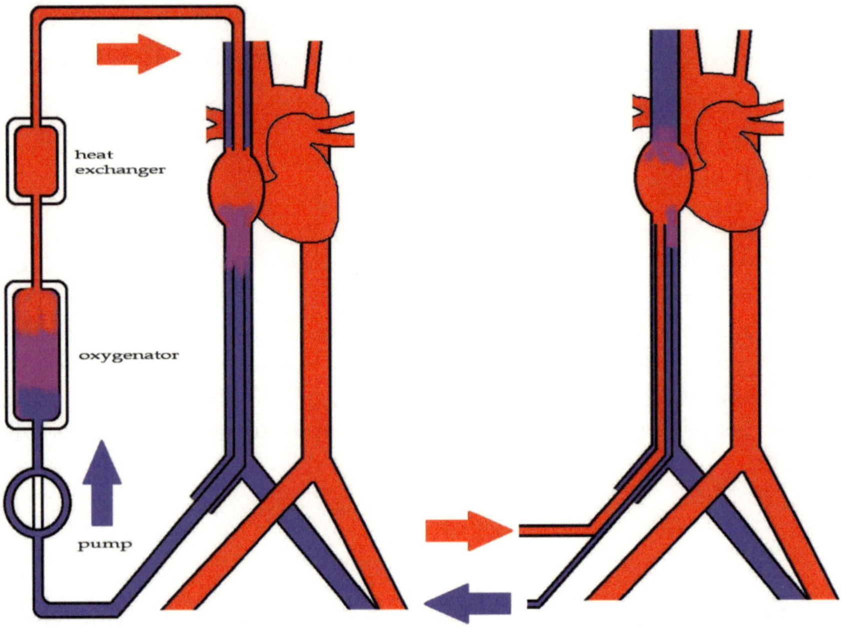

Fig. 1. A: Cannulation of VV ECMO through the femoral vein and jugular vein.
B: Alternative cannulation with a double lumen cannula through one major vein.

In VA ECMO, blood is drawn from the common femoral vein and returned into the femoral artery (fig. 2A). Venous blood is oxygenated and pumped back into arterial circulation. As a result, both the heart and lungs are bypassed. The main concern in femoral artery cannulation is hypoxia of the ipsilateral leg. On the other hand, if native heart function was presence, the oxygenated blood may not reach the proximal aorta and this would result in hypoxia of the heart and upper body. Alternatively, carotid artery cannulation could be performed (fig. 2B). But the risk of watershed cerebral infarction increases when utilizing this method. Because ECMO draw a large volume of blood from vessels, the circuit should be primed with fluid. In most cases, the circuit is re-circulated with normal saline, heparin and crystalloid first. A typical regimen is normal saline 2000ml with heparin 2000units/liter. Once ECMO activated, packed red blood cells are transfused to compensate for the diluting effects of the priming fluid. There is no consensus about the total amount of units that should be transfused. This depends on the volume of the circuit, the perfusion status of patients and the underlying disease. Typically, the goal is to make the hematocrit more than 30% and the mean arterial pressure more than 65mmHg.

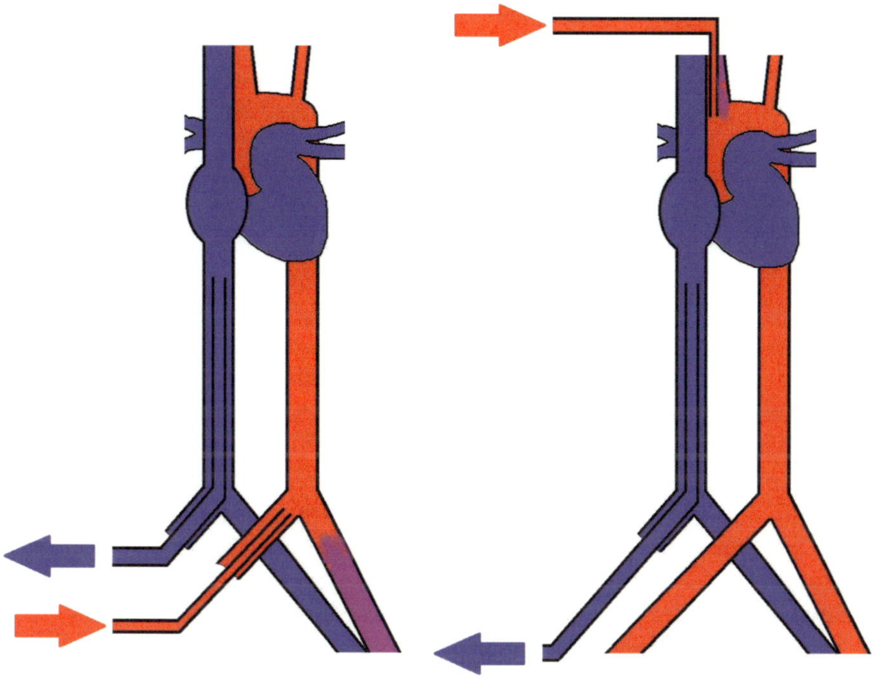

Fig. 2. A: Cannulation of VA ECMO through the femoral vein and artery. B: Cannulation through the femoral vein and carotid artery. Each path has its own unique risks with regards to complications.

2.2 Maintenance of ECMO

During the extracorporeal circulation, thrombosis may occur in the circuit and induce an embolism because of blood surface interaction. As a result, anticoagulation with a continuous infusion of unfractionated heparin is mandatory. The anticoagulant is monitored by activated clotting time (ACT). In general, ACT should be titrated to 210 to 230 seconds. The target should be decreased if the patients have a tendency towards bleeding. Platelets are continuously consumed because of the exposure to the foreign surface and the sheer force. As a result, platelet counts should also be monitored frequently. Sedation is definitely needed during ECMO. Adequate sedation can decrease the anxiety and suffering of patients and put the cardiopulmonary system at rest. The common agents for sedation in ICU are a continuous infusion of midazolam or propofol. Muscle relaxants could be added as well if the patients cannot tolerate use of mechanical ventilators well. Regardless, ECMO should only be utilized when patients are adequately sedated.

2.3 Complications

ECMO alters hemodynamic stability and induces a large amount of blood run in a device out of body. As a result, complications including localized tissues ischemia and hemostastic instability may occur. The VA ECMO also changes the direction of blood flow which may cause more complications than VV ECMO.

2.3.1 Complications in VV and VA ECMO

Bleeding tendency is usually increased and profound bleeding may even become life-threatening. The occurrence rate of bleeding ranges from 7-34%. The contributing factors are due to the mandatory continuous infusion of unfractionated heparin, platelet consumption and sometimes the underline diseases such as massive hemoptysis and sepsis-related DIC. Effective management depends upon the sites and the causes of bleeding. For example, if the bleeding source is mucosa or gastrointestinal tract, medical management including correcting thrombocytopenia and transfusing with fresh frozen plasma may be necessary. If the bleeding persists or develops into profound bleeding, unfractionated heparin infusion must be withheld temporarily. After the bleeding stops, heparin should be added once again but the target ACT could be adjusted. On the other hand, bleeding from the surgical or device-insertion wounds, including ECMO cannulation site, often requires surgical intervention. This ranges from bedside electrocautery to surgical exploration to achieve bleeding stoppage.

Thrombosis occurs at a rate of 8-17% and heparinization may help to reduce the incidence rate, but could also increase the potential for bleeding events. The balance between homeostasis and thrombosis require frequent clinical and laboratory monitoring. The pressure gradient across the oxygenator is a useful tool to be monitored, and a sudden change in the gradient may suggest a thrombus formation.

Bleeding from a cannulated site is not uncommon. Vascular perforation and arterial dissection may occur during the placement of the cannula. Thus, the utilization of an experienced surgeon is quite important to avoid such complications.

2.3.2 Complications only in VA ECMO

In VA ECMO, oxygenated blood is infused into carotid artery or femoral artery, which forms a countercurrent to native blood flow from the left ventricle. As a result, the increased afterload may worsen the cardiac output of the left ventricle. This results in left ventricle distension, acute pulmonary hypertension and then even pulmonary hemorrhage.

If the infusion cannula is placed in the femoral artery, not only the direction of blood flow of left ventricle, but also the blood flow of aorta is changed. Blood stasis in the aorta is induced if we are not able to maintain left ventricle output. Consequently, aorta thrombosis may develop.

In this type of situation, blood flow from ECMO supplies lower extremities and visceral organs, where as the brain, heart and upper extremities are supplied by the heart itself. It is obvious that the oxygen saturation from the blood vessels supplied by ECMO is much higher than that by heart. Under this type of condition, cerebral and cardiac hypoxia may occur without being recognized if saturation is only monitored by blood sampling from the lower extremities. As a result, monitoring blood saturation during VA ECMO only by digital oxymetry or single arterial line should be avoided.

2.4 Pumpless extracorporeal lung-assisted (pECLA) device

Pumpless extracorporeal lung-assisted device, a novel type of ECMO, had been developed in recent 10 years. In 1967, Rashkind and colleagues first proposed the concept of pECLA (Rashkind et al. 1967). In recent years, the commercialized devices are available and become more and more popular in intensive care unit (Walles, 2007).

During setting up, the blood was drawn from the common femoral artery and sent back to the femoral vein. The pressure gradient driving blood flow in the device was supplied by heart pumping. As a result, pECLA dose not need a centrifugal or roller pump. In this way, it could be set more easily with lower cost and lower dose of heparin than conventional ECMO. However, the device was built to remove carbon dioxide in patient with acute respiratory distress syndrome under lung protective ventilation strategy. Since the blood was drawn from the artery, the oxygenated ability of pECLA was not superior to conventional ECMO. In the management of massive hemoptysis or critical tracheal stenosis, the main problem encountered was hypoxemic respiratory failure, but not hypercapnia. As a result, the application of pECLA in these patients may need more strictly selection.

in summary, ECMO is a powerful therapeutic tool since it can replace the function of the heart and lungs. However, it has several potential complications and their risks increase as the duration of ECMO is prolonged. As a result, it can only serve as a salvage tool in life-threatening conditions and as a bridge to the definite therapy. There are two types of ECMO, the VA type and the VV type. Although VA type can supply perfusion pressure, it obviously has more complications than the VV type. In the field of emergent thoracic surgery, which we will introduce in the following sections, the cardiac function is usually preservative. As a result, VV type ECMO is the first choice in emergent thoracic surgery.

In thoracic surgery, there are 2 conditions, massive hemoptysis and major airway obstruction, where oxygenation is difficult to maintain. Under these conditions, if oxygenation could not be maintained by optimized mechanical ventilation or if the risk of life-threatening hypoxemia is very high, ECMO should be considered.

3. Massive hemoptysis

Massive hemoptysis is an important and potentially fatal event. It has been variably defined as an expectoration of blood amount ranging from 100-1000 ml in 24 hours (Dweik & Stoller, 1999). Since 200 ml of blood could fulfill the anatomical dead space of a major airway and 400 ml of blood might impede the oxygen exchange of alveolar space, massive hemoptysis can be defined as the expectorated blood volume that induces a life-threatening condition by virtue of airway obstruction or severe blood loss (Garzon et al., 1982).

3.1 Conventional management of massive hemoptysis

In the management of massive hemoptysis, protection of the non-bleeding lung and maintenance of adequate oxygen saturation are the major priorities. Then, the second step is to identify the source of the bleeding. The final step is the definite and specific treatment to prevent recurrent bleeding. Among the 3 steps, lung protection and maintenance of oxygenation are the most critical and could determine the outcome of patients. There are five methods for lung protection if the patient has continuous bleeding: decubitus position, selective intubation, double lumen intubation, Fogarty catheter placement and bronchoscope balloon tamponade (Lordan et al., 2003).

At first, an attempt should be made to identify the bleeding side of the lung. After that, the patient should be laid with the bleeding side down to isolate the bleeding lung and ventilate the normal lung. Single lung intubation could be performed if the amount of blood is too great (Gourin & Garzon, 1975). For right side bleeding, the bronchoscope could be placed in the left main bronchus and the endotracheal tube could be inserted in the left lung under the guidance of bronchoscope. For left side bleeding, the endotracheal tube could be placed in the right main bronchus simply by "pushing deeper"; however, this procedure has the risk of occluding the right upper lobe bronchus.

Double lumen endotracheal tube is an alternative method for lung isolation. However, it has four major disadvantages and is not routinely performed in ICU. First, it is difficult for a physician to decide whether double lumen tube should be inserted if the patient only has mild hemoptysis at presentation. Second, it is difficult for an operator to insert a double lumen catheter if the patient was under a hypoxemic status with large amount of blood in the trachea and pharynx. Third, an experienced operator is mandated to avoid the serious result of mal positioning, especially during the transference of patients from ICU to an angiography room. The last disadvantage is that there are still not enough trials to definitively demonstrate whether the double lumen catheter procedure is effective.

Fogarty catheter and bronchoscope balloon tamponade can be applied for lung isolation. A Fogarty catheter (14Fr/100cm length) can be placed over the bleeding bronchus under the guidance of bronchoscope. After inflated, the blood could be restricted in the bleeding side. Bronchoscope balloon tamponade may be more selective in restricting the blood. A 4-7 Fr balloon catheter is passed through the working channel of the bronchoscope and inflated to isolate the lung. However, both interventions need the guidance of bronchoscope. If the patient has massive bleeding, the large amount of blood in the trachea will impede the placement of a balloon catheter.

3.2 ECMO in massive hemoptysis

Several methods for lung isolation have been developed. Their aim is basically the same: to ventilate the good lung and to maintain adequate oxygenation. As a result, if a physician is able to establish a route for oxygenation without depending on inadequate ventilation support, the definite therapy could be applied more safely, even if we fail to protect the good lung. ECMO has such characteristics and might be useful in certain circumstances.

If the patient had "abrupt desaturation", ECMO can be implemented in 40 minutes by an experienced team. VV ECMO is the first choice, since most patients with massive hemoptysis are threatened by desaturation, rather than hypotension and shock. ECMO can be used as a bridge therapy for the definite treatment, such as angiography embolization and surgery.

Comprehensive review for ECMO use in life-threatening hemoptysis is lacking, and there are still no studies in the related literature on this topic. Since no original study has been published, the experience in application of ECMO in certain patients is largely based on case reports and case series. As early as in 1974, Hanson and colleague reported the first case with pulmonary hemorrhage rescued by ECMO (Hanson et al., 1974). However, not until the 1990s was there was a study or report about the use of ECMO in certain situations. There may be two reasons for this lack of reporting. The first, there is still the argument about the benefit of ECMO in an adult population at that era. And the second, heparinization during

Author, year (list in reference)	Underlie disease	Duration (days)	ACT (seconds)	Note
Hernandez et al., 2002	Wegener's granuloma	9	150	Pediatric
Kolovos et al., 2002	Autoimmune disease or sepsis	4.9	160-180	Pediatric, Case No. 8
Ahmed et al., 2004	ANCA vasculitis	12	Full anticoagulation since day 3	
Fujita et al., 2005	Fulminant hepatitis s/p liver transplant	4	N/A	
Agarwal et al., 2005	Microscopic polyangitis	7	160-180	
Arokianathana et al., 2005	Leptospirosis	7	N/A	
Sun et al., 2006	Idiopathic Pulmonary Hemosiderosis	5	170-200	
Zhong et al., 2008	Microscopic polyangitis	12	120-200	

Table 1. The application of ECMO in the 8 reported cases of diffuse alveolar hemorrhage.

ECMO may precipitate further lung hemorrhage. In 2002, Kolovos and colleague reported the largest series and again raised the profile of reconsidering the role of ECMO in severe hemoptysis and pulmonary hemorrhage (Kolovos et al., 2002). They reported 8 children, aged 2 months to 18 years, with pulmonary hemorrhage due to sepsis or autoimmune disease received ECMO as the final therapeutic method because of severe respiratory failure. The eight children exhibited varying degrees of coagulopathy but still received heparinization. The ACT was controlled between 160 to 180 seconds. There was no profound hemorrhage after they received ECMO and all of them were weaned from ECMO successfully after pulmonary hemorrhage was controlled. After that report, although bleeding tendency was still thought to be a relative contraindication for ECMO, it seems that some patients with severe pulmonary hemorrhage could be rescued by ECMO use.

As mentioned above, studies and reports in the related literature in this field are still scarce. To the best of our knowledge, there are only 13 reports about the application of ECMO in massive hemoptysis; 8 of them had diffused alveolar hemorrhage (DAH) (Table 1). In DAH, the use of ECMO has a stronger indication because there is no effective lung protective strategy. The patients in these reports were on ECMO support for 4 to 12 days. Heparin was used at a lower dosage to keep ACT around 120 to 200 seconds, instead of 210 to 230 seconds. Alternatively, delaying the application of heparin seems to be a safe method. All of the patients in these case reports were successfully weaned from ECMO after the underlying causes of severe hemoptysis were under control.

There are 5 reports about the use of ECMO in localized lung hemorrhage (Table 2). In 2 of them, the patients encountered abrupt desaturation during the procedure (bronchial artery embolization and operation), and lung protective therapy was difficult under that condition. Yuan et al. reported a patient with massive hemoptysis due to trauma and a double lumen endotracheal tube was intubated at the ER. However, the patient's clinical condition deteriorated and ECMO was used as a rescue method. In our experience, we have reported a case with bronchiectasis and massive hemoptysis (Hsu et al. 2011). The patient presented with acute respiratory failure due to a rapid progression of severe hemoptysis. A total of 4000 ml of packed red blood cells was transfused within 24 h to keep the hemoglobin level at around 10 mg/dl. The ventilator setting was in the volume control mode, at a positive end-expiratory pressure of 15 cm H2O, and a FiO2 of 100%; however, these setting only could maintain the arterial blood gas at a PaO2 of 62 mmHg. ECMO was applied due to high risk of transferring the patient from the intensive care unit to the angiography room and in-procedure mortality. After bronchial artery embolization successfully, ECMO was weaned 1 day later. No heparinization was performed because of the short term application of ECMO. The patient received left lower lobe lobectomy 2 weeks later due to intermittent small amount of hemoptysis. After the surgery, hemoptysis did not recur. He was discharged in ambulatory condition without any oxygen therapy.

Author, year (list in reference)	Underlie disease	Duration (days)	ACT (seconds)	Note
Fukui et al., 2006	Pulmonary hypertension	12	40-50 since day 3	
Bianchini et al., 2007	Swan-Ganz related trauma	2.5	N/A	During operation
Bedard et al., 2008	Aorto-pulmonary fistula	N/A	N/A	During bronchial arterial embolization
Yuan et al., 2008	Double lumen related trauma	10	60-80	
Hsu et al., 2011	Bronchiectasis	1	No heparin	

Table 2. The application of ECMO in the 4 reported cases of localized lung hemorrhage.

The use of ECMO in massive hemoptysis may be beneficial for certain populations. However, there are still a number of debates about the use of ECMO, since available data is not sufficient in this field. First, setting up ECMO is an invasive procedure, and physicians may not maximize the "conventional therapy" before initiating ECMO. Second, heparinization is usually necessary in ECMO, but it may produce a more severe hemorrhage. Third, ECMO itself may bring about some complications, such as platelet consumption, bleeding and/or thromboembolism.

In summary, maintenance of oxygenation is the most important object in the management of massive hemoptysis. ECMO should be used if all other methods fail or cannot be performed to maintain adequate oxygenation. However, there is still some uncertainty that needs to be addressed, such as the selection criteria of patients and the method of heparinization. Based on currently available evidence, the use of ECMO as a bridge tool for life-threatening hemoptysis can allow a patient to undergo definite therapy more safely.

4. Critical tracheal stenosis

Critical tracheal stenosis can be caused by either malignant or benign lesion. The symptoms may develop abruptly or slowly. In a chronic disease, such as malignancy, chronic inflammatory disease or collagen vascular disease, patients present with progressive dyspnea and stridor. While in acute conditions, such as blunt or penetrating neck trauma, patients may suffer from life-threatening asphyxia. The nature and severity of symptoms depends on the location and the magnitude of the lesion.

4.1 Conventional management of critical tracheal stenosis

Most patients with tracheal stenosis present with chronic symptoms. However, a 50% reduction in the cross-sectional area of the trachea usually results in dyspnea on exertion, whereas a 75% reduction in the cross-sectional area produces dyspnea and stridor at rest. This means that when these symptoms develop, the airway has been severely compromised with impending life-threatening obstruction (Wood, 2002). The patient may be compensated for airway obstruction, but even a small amount of secretion can be lethal. As a result, the strategies of management are different according to the time point of diagnosis.

If the tracheal stenosis is diagnosed early, physicians have enough time to make a complete study. The treatment options include surgical resection, reconstruction, therapeutic bronchoscopy with ablation and airway-stent placement. Before the management takes place, a secure airway could be performed utilizing an efficient method. The fiberoptic bronchoscope (FOB) provides a safe and effective way for airway control (Ovassapian, 2001). With FOB, the lesion could be evaluated vividly and the residual lumen of airway could be estimated. After that, the largest endotracheal tube (ETT) that can pass the lumen should be chosen, since the airway pressure is inversely proportional to the inner diameter of the ETT. To avoid trauma to the airway or the trachea lesion, the ideal size of FOB is 1mm smaller than the internal diameter of ETT. The ideal-sized FOB should be used if available. After determining the size of ETT and FOB, intubation could be performed by experienced anaesthesiologist.

If critical airway stenosis has developed, management will then become more difficult. The position of stenosis is important in this circumstance. For upper airway stenosis, FOB - assisted intubation or emergent tracheotomy can stabilize the airway. For severe mid-level tracheal stenosis, intubation above the stenotic portion can be performed first. After positive pressure ventilation, the residual lumen will be mildly dilated. Then a smaller tracheal tube is placed under the assistance of FOB through trachea or directly placed into main bronchus by the surgeon during surgery.

However, sometimes endotracheal intubation may be impossible, and even dangerous, possibly leading to complete airway obstruction. For most patients, emergent tracheotomy is ineffective because it cannot bypass the obstructive lesion. FOB may precipitate cough, bleeding or further mucosal edema and worsen the obstruction. There are only few choices for patients with this type of life-threatening major airway obstruction. One way is place the patient in a quiet room with very mild sedation and cool humidified oxygen. Nebulized epinephrine and dexamethasone help decrease the contraction and edema of the airway. It may temporary attenuate the symptoms and facilitate subsequent procedure, and FOB - assisted intubation.

4.2 ECMO in critical tracheal stenosis

In patients with critical tracheal stenosis, the key to saving their lives is to maintain safe and efficient gas exchange. However, conventional anesthetic technique has a high risk of causing airway total occlusion, and the risk is inversely proportional to the residual lumen of the airway. As a result, if intubation is performed under a "back up" system, that can maintain adequate oxygenation even under total airway occlusion, it becomes safer for patients and less challenging to anaesthesiologists. Thus, ECMO serves as an ideal tool in this situation.

In paediatric surgery, an increasing number of reports and small-scale patient studies have pointed out that ECMO, either elective or emergent, serves as a good-bridge tool for trachea reconstruction. In neonates with congenital trachea anomalies, ECMO reduces the risk of surgery to allow more precise and unrushed airway reconstruction (Huang et al., 2007)(Kunisaki et al., 2008). Elective ECMO uses in postoperative period also contribute to improve patients' outcome (Connonlly & McGuirt, 2001).
However, in the field of adults with critical trachea stenosis, we remain in the "case report era." In 1999, Onozawa and colleagues first reported a case with critical airway obstruction due to thyroid cancer. The diameter of residual lumen of trachea was only 5mm. VA ECMO was applied before induction and the surgery was performed smoothly. After the partial resection of the thyroid tumor and the insertion of tracheostomy, ECMO was decannulated successfully. Following that, there are total 7 case reports with 9 adult patients involving the application of ECMO during critical tracheal stenosis surgery (table 3). These physicians attempted to intubate the patients reported but failed in two of them. One of them even experienced hypoxia cardiac arrest. Emergent ECMO was activated and this saved the patient's life. Among them, the variable etiologies ranged from benign to malignant origin. The residual lumens of trachea are between 1mm to 5mm. The locations of trachea lesion distribute from 1.5cm above carina to upper level of trachea. VA ECMO was first used and more recently VV ECMO has been applied in cases of critical tracheal stenosis. Both types of ECMO can supply adequate oxygenation for performing the definite therapy.

Author, year (list in reference)	Underlie disease	Diameter & position of residual lumen	Ecmo type	Note
Onozawa et al., 1999	thyroid tumor	5mm	VA ECMO	
Kurokawa et al., 2000	tracheolysis	3mm	VV ECMO	
Chen et al., 2004	neurofibroma	more than 5.5mm, 5cm above carina	N/A	ETT, ECMO stand by only
Zhou et al., 2007	Post intubation trachea stenosis	2-3mm, 1.5cm above carina	VA ECMO	ETT but failure, emergent ECMO
	Leiomyoma	1mm, 6cm below vocal cords	VA ECMO	
Jeon et al., 2009	Thyroid tumor	N/A (3x4 cm)	VV ECMO	
Smith et al., 2009	Papilloma	N/A (2.5x2.8 cm), 2.5cm above carina	VV ECMO	
	Papilloma	N/A, extend 2 cm below vocal cords to just above carina	VV ECMO	Bronchoscope ETT related hypoxic cardiac arrest
Shao et al., 2009	Bilateral nodular goiter	5mm,	VA ECMO	

Table 3. The application of ECMO in critical airway stenosis during surgery

In summary, although there is still no original study published in this field, the related case reports have provided useful information. If the residual lumen of trachea is less than 5mm or the ETT cannot pass the lesion, a "stand by" ECMO should be considered before anaesthesia induction. VV ECMO is preferred since it can maintain adequate oxygenation with fewer complications.

And finally, it is worth noting that the criteria for patient selection still needs further investigation to demonstrate the benefits of ECMO as a bridge therapy in critical trachea stenosis. The cost-effectiveness of this method is also worthy of further investigation. Before a definitive conclusion can be made, ECMO should be kept in mind as one option for clinical physicians when handling a patient with critical tracheal stenosis.

5. Conclusion

During the transition of emergent thoracic surgery, the most important objective is to maintain vital signs, ensuring that they are stable. However, in cases of massive hemoptysis and critical airway stenosis, it remains difficult for physicians to achieve adequate oxygenation since these conditions share the same challenge: difficult airway maintenance. In this field, ECMO serves as the rationale option if conventional therapy cannot achieve adequate oxygenation. Due to the lack of an original study, the role of ECMO in the transition of emergent thoracic surgery still deserves further investigation regarding its utilization and cost-effectiveness. Based on the current evidence available, ECMO could make the transition of emergent thoracic surgery safer.

6. References

Ahmed, SH. et al. (2004). Use of extracorporeal membrane oxygenation in a patient with diffuse alveolar hemorrhage. *CHEST,* No.126, Vol.1, (July 2004), pp. 305–309, ISSN 0012-3692.

Arokianathana, D. et al. (2005). Leptospirosis: a case report of a patient with pulmonary haemorrhage successfully managed with extra corporeal membrane oxygenation. *The Journal of Infection,* Vol.50, No.2, (February 2005), pp. 158-162, ISSN 0163-4453.

Agarwal, HS. et al. (2005). Extra corporeal membrane oxygenation and plasmapheresis for pulmonary hemorrhage in microscopic polyangiitis. *Pediatric Nephrology,* Vol. 20, No.4, (April 2005), pp. 526-528, ISSN 0931-041X.

Bedard, E. et al. (2008). Life-threatening hemoptysis following the Fontan procedure. *The Canadian Journal of Cardiology,* Vol.24, No.2, (February 2008), pp. 145-147, ISSN 0828-282X.

Bianchini, R. et al. (2007). Extracorporeal membrane oxygenation for Swan-Ganz induced intraoperative hemorrhage. *Ann Annals of Thorac Surgery,* Vol.83, No.6, (Jun 2007), pp. 2213– 2214, ISSN 0003-4975.

Chen, PT. et al. (2004). Anesthetic management of a patient undergoing segmental resection of trachea with an endotracheal neurofibroma and nearly total occlusion of trachea. *Acta Anaesthesiology Taiwanica,* Vol.42, No.4, (December 2004), pp. 233-236, ISSN 1875-4597.

Connonlly, KM. & McGuirt, WF Jr. (2001). Elective extracorporeal membrane oxygenation: an improved perioperative technique in the treatment of tracheal obstruction. *The Annals of Otology, Rhinology and Laryngology*, Vol.110, No.3, (March 2001), pp. 205-209, ISSN 0003-4894.

Dweik, RA. & Stoller, JK. (1999). Role of bronchoscopy in massive hemoptysis. *Clinics in Chest Medicine,* Vol.20, No.1, (March 1999), pp. 89–105, ISSN 0272-5231

Fujita, S. et al. (2005). Expanded efficacy and indication of extracorporeal membrane oxygenation for preoperative pulmonary bleeding on pediatric cadaveric orthotopic liver transplantation. *Transplantation,* Vol.79, No.11, (June 2005), pp. 1637, ISSN 0041-1337.

Fukui, S. et al. (2006). Recovery from hemorrhagic pulmonary damage by combined use of a left ventricular assist system and right ventricular assist system and extracorporeal membrane oxygenation. *The Journal of Heart and Lung Transplantation*, Vol.25, No.2, (February 2006), pp. 248–250, ISSN 1053-2498.

Garzon AA.; Cerruti MM. & Golding ME. (1982). Exsanguinating hemoptysis. *The journal of Thoracic and Cardiovascular Surgery,* Vol.84, No.6, (December 1982), pp. 829–833, ISSN 0022-5223.

Gibbon, JH. Jr. (1954). Application of a mechanical heart and lung apparatus to cardiac surgery. *Minnesota Medicine,* Vol.37, No.3, (March 1954), pp. 171-178, ISSN 0026-556X.

Gourin, A. & Garzon, AA. (1975). Control of hemorrhage in emergency pulmonaryresection for massive hemoptysis. *Chest*, Vol.68, No.1, (July 1975), pp. 120–121, ISSN 0012-3692.

Hanson, EL. et al. (1974). Venoarterial bypass with a membrane oxygenator: Successful respiratory support in a woman following pulmonary hemorrhage secondary to renal failure. *Surgery,* Vol.75, No.4 (April 1974), pp. 557–565, ISSN 0039-6060.

Hernandez, ME. et al. (2002). Acute onset of Wegener's granulomatosis and diffuse alveolar hemorrhage treated successfully by extracorporeal membrane oxygenation. *Pediatric Critical Care Medicine,* Vol.3, No.1, (January 2002), pp. 63–66, ISSN 1529-7535.

Hill, JD. et al. (1972). Prolonged extracorporeal oxygenation for acute post-traumatic respiratory failure (shock-lung syndrome). Use of the Bramson membrane lung. *The New England Journal of Medicine,* Vol.286, No.12, (March 1972), pp. 629-634, ISSN 0028-4793.

Hsu, SJ. et al. (2011). Life-threatening hemoptysis due to left inferior phrenic artery to pulmonary artery fistula rescued by extracorporeal membrane oxygenation therapy. *Interactive Cardiovascular and Thoracic Surgery,* Vol.12, No.2, (February 2011), pp. 337-338, ISSN 1569-9293.

Huang, SC. et al. (2007). Perioperative extracorporeal membrane oxygenation support for critical pediatric airway surgery. *European Journals of Pediatrics,* Vol.166, No.11, (November 2007), pp. 1129-1133, ISSN 0340-6199.

Jeon, HK. et al. (2009). Extracorporeal oxygenation support for curative surgery in a patient with papillary thyroid carcinoma invading the trachea. *The Journal of Laryngology and Otology*, Vol.123, No.7, (July 2009), pp. 807-810, ISSN 0022-2151.

Kolovos, NS. et al. (2002). Extracorporal life support for pulmonary hemorrhage in children: A case series. *Critical Care Medicine*, Vol.30, No.3, (March 2002), pp. 577–580, ISSN 0090-3493.

Kunisaki, SM. et al. (2008). Extracorporeal membrane oxygenation as a bridge to definitive tracheal reconstruction in neonates. *Journal of Pediatric Surgery*, Vol.43, No. 5, (May 2008), pp. 800-804, ISSN 0022-3468.

Kurokawa, S. et al. (2000). Anesthetic management using extracorporeal circulation of a patient with severe tracheal stenosis by thyroid cancer. *The Japenese journal of anesthesiology*, Vol.49, No.11, (November 2000), pp. 1242-1246, ISSN 0021-4892.

Lordan, JL.; Gascoigne, A. & Corris, PA. (2003). The pulmonary physician in critical care * Illustrative case 7: Assessment and management of massive haemoptysis. *Thorax*, Vol. 58, No.9, (September 2003), pp. 814-819, ISSN 0040-6376.

Onozawa, H. et al. (1999). Anesthetic management using extracorporeal circulation of a patient with severe tracheal stenosis by thyroid cancer. *The Japenese journal of anesthesiology*, Vol.48, No.6, (June 1999), pp. 658-661, ISSN 0021-4892

Ovassapian, A. (2001). The flexible bronchoscope. A tool for anesthesiologists. Clinics in Chest Medicine, Vol.22, No.2, (June 2001), pp. 281-299, ISSN 0272-5231.

Peek, GJ. et al. (2009). Efficacy and economic assessment of conventional ventilatory support versus extracorporeal membrane oxygenation for severe adult respiratory failure (CESAR): a multicentre randomised controlled trial. *Lancet*, Vol.374, No.9698, (October 2009), pp. 1351–1363, ISSN 0140-6736.

Rashkind, WJ. et al. (1967). Hemodynamic effects of arteriovenous oxygenation with a small-volume artificial extracorporeal lung. *The Journal of Pediatrics*, Vol.70, No.2, (March 1967), pp. 425-429, ISSN 0022-3476

Shao, Y. et al. (2009). Extracorporeal membrane oxygenation-assisted resection of goiter causing severe extrinsic airway compression. *The Annals of Thoracic Surgery*, Vol.88, No.2, (August 2009), pp. 659-661, ISSN 0003-4975.

Smith, IJ. et al. (2009). Use of extracorporeal membrane oxygenation during resection of tracheal papillomatosis. *Anesthesiology*, Vol.110, No.2, (February 2009), pp.427-429, ISSN 0003-3022.

Sun, LC. et al. (2006). Extracorporeal membrane oxygenation to rescue profound pulmonary hemorrhage due to idiopathic pulmonary hemosiderosis in a child. *Pediatric Pulmonology*, Vol.41, No.9, (September 2006), pp.900–903, ISSN 8755-6863.

Walles, T. (2007). Clinical experience with the iLA Membrane Ventilator pumpless extracorporeal lung-assist device. *Expert Review of Medical Device*, Vol.4, No.3, (May 2007), pp. 297-305, ISSN 1743-4440

Wood, DE. (2002). Management of malignant tracheobronchial obstruction. *The Surgical Clinics of North America*, Vol.82, No.3, (June 2002), pp. 621–642, ISSN 0039-6109.

Yuan, KC. et al. (2008). Treatment of endobronchial hemorrhage after blunt chest trauma with extracorporeal membrane oxygenation. *The Journal of Trauma*, Vol.65, No.5, (November 2008), pp. 1151–1154, ISSN 0022-5282.

Zhong, H. et al. (2008). Extracorporeal membrane oxygenation for pulmonary hemorrhage in microscopic polyangiitis. *Chinese Medical Journal*, Vol.121, No.24, (December 2008) ,pp. 2622-2623, ISSN 0366-6999.

Zhou, YF. Et al. (2007). Anesthetic management of emergent critical tracheal stenosis. *Journal of Zhejiang University. Science. B.*, Vol.8, No.7, (July 2007), pp. 522-525, ISSN 1673-1581.